Medical Group Management Association

Physician Compensation and Production Survey

2008 REPORT BASED ON 2007 DATA

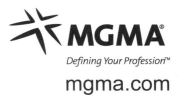

Defining Your Profession™

mgma.com

MGMA Survey Advisory Committee Members

The Medical Group Management Association® (MGMA®) Survey Advisory Committee provided guidance on the format and content of this report as well as the related questionnaire and guide to ensure that the survey addresses current and relevant practice management areas.

Chair
David P. Taylor, FACMPE, FACHE
Vice President
CoxHealth
Springfield, MO

Susan Gardner
Project Manager
Northwest Permanente, PC
500 NE Multnomah, Suite 100
Portland, OR

Robert Walker, MD
President/Director
Walker Medical Consulting, LLC
Medical Sciences MedImmune, Inc.
Columbia, SC

Terri McSorley
Office Manager
Women's Health Asociates
Voorhees, NJ

David Schlactus, MBA, CMPE
CEO
Willamette Surgery Center
Salem, OR

Jeff Milburn, CMPE
Senior Vice President
Colorado Springs Health Partners PC
Colorado Springs, CO

Daniel Caldwell, CMPE
Executive Director
Little Rock Cardiology Clinic PA
Little Rock, AR

Jason A. Whitmer, CPA
Senior Manager
Crowe Chizek & Company
South Bend, IN

Sherry C. Elliott, FACMPE
Vice Chair of Operations
Dept. of Radiology
Virginia Commonwealth University Health System
Richmond, VA

Academic Practice Committee Liason
Shirley Zwinggi, MBA, FACMPE
Administrator
Medical Center
University of Texas Southwestern
Dallas, TX

Staff Liaison
Bruce A. Johnson, JD, MPA
Principal
MGMA Health Care Consulting Group
Special Counsel, Faegre & Benson, LLP
Erie, CO

Desktop Publishing by: Glacier Publishing Services, Inc.
Cover Design by: Jeff Beene

For further information or questions, contact MGMA Survey Operations, toll-free 877.ASK.MGMA (275.6462), ext. 895.

Item # 7032
ISSN 1064-4563
ISBN 978-1-56829-250-2

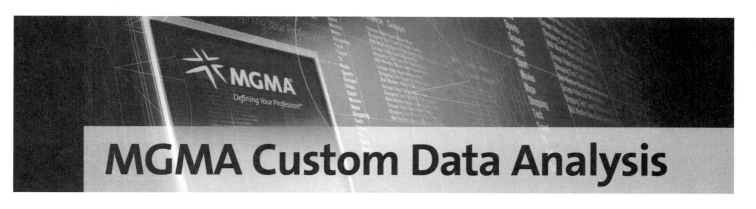

MGMA Custom Data Analysis

Looking for the right data for your board reports?
Searching for data you can't find anywhere else?

MGMA analysts can help you with your benchmarking needs.

Our survey analysts are experts in the medical field and have years of experience analyzing data and developing specialized benchmarking reports. They are available for special projects, such as tables that are not available in the reports, compensation by specialty and state, trending data and more. We can provide you with a professional, bound report with color tables and the MGMA logo, which will enhance the integrity of your presentation. This report will improve the quality of your presentations to your superiors or clients.

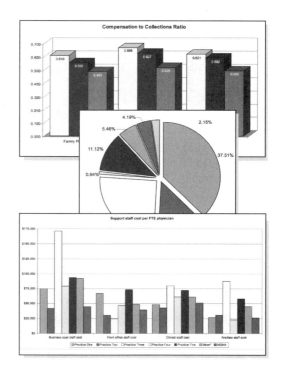

We can use your specific practice data and the raw data from our annual reports, including:

- Physician Compensation and Production

- Management Compensation

- Cost and Revenue

- Academic Faculty and Management Compensation and Production

Some examples of the custom work we've done:

- Analysis of costs, revenue and staffing levels comparing all of the practices within a large multispecialty network

- Report of compensation data for a large integrated delivery system compared to a major hospital

- Report determining the value of a practice for an attorney preparing for a court case

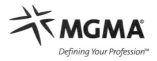
Defining Your Profession™

Call toll-free 877.ASK.MGMA, ext. 895 for pricing and availability.

Or visit mgma.com/surveys for more information.

MGMA Survey Operations

The *Physician Compensation and Production Survey: 2008 Report Based on 2007 Data* was compiled by MGMA Survey Operations. The MGMA Survey Operations staff members responsible for this and other MGMA reports are

Devon Broderick, Data Specialist
Donna Culmer, Project Assistant
Jennifer Dysert, Marketing Manager
Todd B. Evenson, MBA, Survey Analyst II
Meaghan Flynn, Systems Analyst
M. Michelle Hughes, Administrative Assistant
Michael J. Kasher, MPA, CMPE, Director

David Litzau, Survey Analyst I
Meghan McMahon, MS, Survey Analyst I
Aaron Nesbitt, Survey Analyst I
Erica Nikolaidis, MA, Production Manager
Eric Speer, Survey Analyst I
Crystal D. Taylor, MHA, Assistant Director
Jay Y. Whitten, Data Specialist

Important Notice and Disclaimer

The information contained in the *Physician Compensation and Production Survey: 2008 Report Based on 2007 Data* is presented solely for the purpose of informing readers of ranges of compensation and productivity measures reported by MGMA member and nonmember organizations. These data may not be used for the purpose of limiting competition, restraining trade or reducing or stabilizing salary or benefit levels. Such improper use is prohibited by federal and state antitrust laws and will violate the antitrust compliance program established and enforced by the MGMA Board of Directors.

MGMA publications are intended to provide current and accurate information, and are designed to assist readers in becoming more familiar with the subject matter covered. MGMA published the *Physician Compensation and Production Survey: 2008 Report Based on 2007 Data* for a general audience as well as for MGMA members. Such publications are distributed with the understanding that MGMA does not render any legal, accounting or professional advice that may be construed as specifically applicable to individual situations. No representations or warranties are made concerning the application of legal or other principles discussed in MGMA publications to any specific factual situation, nor is any prediction made concerning how any particular judge, government official or other person will interpret or apply such principles. Specific factual situations should be discussed with professional advisors. In addition, some specialties were not included in this report due to insufficient responses.

Confidentiality

The MGMA and MGMA Center for Research Policy on Data Confidentiality states: "All data submitted to MGMA and the MGMA Center for Research will be kept confidential. All submitted data and related materials that identify a specific organization or individual will be safeguarded and will not be published or voluntarily released within the public domain without written permission."

Only summary statistics will be published. A summary statistic will be reported only if there are sufficient responses to be statistically reliable and if the anonymity of those submitting data is protected. In compliance with the MGMA policy, an asterisk (*) denotes data that have been suppressed to ensure confidentiality.

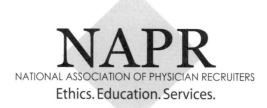

NAPR
NATIONAL ASSOCIATION OF PHYSICIAN RECRUITERS
Ethics. Education. Services.

What is the NAPR?

The National Association of Physician Recruiters (NAPR) is the premier professional organization for physician recruiters across the country, representing physician recruiting firms, in-house staff physician recruiters and contract staffing and management professionals. Since its inception in 1984, the NAPR has provided comprehensive healthcare recruiting and consulting services to the growing healthcare industry. Membership includes over 1000 recruiters who adhere to the highest professional standards in the physician recruiting industry. The NAPR promotes a positive industry image through the establishment of a practical, but strict, code of ethics. No other organization in the recruiting industry ensures that its members adhere to the most principled business practices. The NAPR's Code of Ethics can be viewed at www.napr.org/codeofethics.asp

Why work only with an NAPR member?

When you work with an NAPR member, you work with the best. Our members include the best physician recruiters in the country who understand the complexities within the physician recruiting and healthcare industries.

- Membership made up of the most experienced recruiters in the industry
- NAPR offers members continuing education in industry legislature and trends
- Members adhere to NAPR's Code of Ethics

Recruiters, why Join NAPR?

Members and member firms of the NAPR enjoy many great benefits.

- Participate in cost-effective cooperative recruitment mailing programs
- Post available positions on the NAPR's World Job Bank
- Gain access to the NAPR's database of over 10,000 physicians who are actively seeking positions
- Stay abreast of current legislative and industry news through quarterly newsletters and monthly electronic updates
- Attend two annual meetings that encourage roundtable discussions on industry trends and offer invaluable networking opportunities

For a complete listing of NAPR members and member firms, visit www.napr.org

Ethics. Education. Services.

To find out more about becoming an NAPR member, please contact Bill Kautter at NAPR Headquarters at 800-726-5613 or by e-mail at bkautter@kmgnet.com.

National Association of Physician Recruiters

222 S. Westmonte Dr. • Suite 101 • Altamonte Springs, FL 32714 • 800-726-5613

Dear Colleague:

We are proud to announce that in our second year of offering an online version of the survey, participation via the Web portal reached 78 percent. What's more is that another 21 percent of surveys were submitted via Excel format, which means we received just 1 percent of this year's response on paper. Not only are we making strides to provide you with a more efficient way to participate, you are opting for eco-friendly participation methods on your own. MGMA Survey Operations is moving closer to our goal of going green, and we have you to thank.

This year also marked a dramatic change in the timeline for the survey. Through the cooperation and hard work of our participants, we were able to complete the data collection period nearly two months earlier than years prior. The payoff is our ability to publish the reports much earlier, which translates to more opportunity for you to use relevant benchmarks in your practice.

This year's MGMA *Physician Compensation and Production Survey: 2008 Report Based on 2007 Data* spotlights the critical pay-performance relationship for physicians and nonphysician providers. It is a popular and powerful tool that has become the gold standard compensation benchmark reference of the medical group management profession. You can use this report, as I do, to manage, evaluate and compare strategic measures of your medical practice with your peers.

Take a look at the key findings tables and graphs to see the factors that affect compensation trends and the extensive table of contents that will guide you to the specific data table you need. If you are new to the report, review the statistical interpretation user's guide that explains the approach we use to present the summary statistics.

If you have this report because your practice participated in the survey, we appreciate your contribution. A major benefit of survey participation is a complimentary copy of the report. If you are involved in the management of a practice that did not submit data, I strongly encourage you to take part in next year's survey. Greater participation makes the survey report even more credible and valuable to you, your practice and your colleagues.

If you want an easier way to benchmark your physician compensation and productivity, you can purchase the interactive CD, which offers even more benchmarking tools and will generate reports for you. The CD also features additional data than that provided in the printed report, and includes each percentile from the 10th to 90th. Participants in the survey receive a $200 discount on the CD.

Again, thanks for helping to make MGMA survey reports the gold standard in our profession.

Sincerely,

David P. Taylor, FACMPE, FACHE
Chair, 2008 MGMA Survey Advisory Committee

Table of Contents

Overview

Introduction
Purpose 12
Description 12
What's New? 12
Data Collection 12
Response Rate 12

How to Use This Report
Report Organization 13
Appendices 13
Additional Information 13

Statistical Interpretation — A User's Guide
Introduction 14
Interpreting the Data 14
Using the Survey Report 14

Key Findings and Demographics — Section One

Key Findings
Factors Affecting Compensation 16
Compensation by Hospital Ownership 17
Compensation by Practice Total Medical Revenue 18
Table A: Median Compensation for Selected Specialties, 2003–2007 19
Table B: Median Gross Charges (TC/NPP Excluded) for Selected Specialties, 2003–2007 20
Table C: Median Collections for Professional Charges (TC/NPP Excluded) for Selected Specialties, 2003–2007 21
Graph 1: Changes in Compensation and Production for Primary Care Physicians, 1997–2007 22
Graph 2: Changes in Compensation and Production for Specialty Care Physicians, 1997–2007 22
Primary Care 23
Specialty Care 23
Nonphysician Provider Analyses 24

Medical Practice
1: Responses Received 25
2: Geographic Section 25
3: Demographic Classification 25
4: State 26
5: Legal Organization 27
6: Organization Ownership 27
7: Group Type 27
8: Single-Specialty Group Type 28
9: Integration Options 29
10: 2007 Total Medical Revenue 29
11: 2007 Percent of Capitation Revenue 29
12: Practice Plans to Change Compensation Methodology 29
13: Productivity Measures Used in Compensation Methodology 30
14: Basis for Incentive/Bonus Used in Compensation Methodology 30
15: Health Records Storage 31

Providers
16: Physician Specialty 32
17: Physician Years in Specialty 33
18: FTE Physicians 33
19: FTE Physicians per Group 33

20: Clinical FTE 33
21: On-call Duties 33
22: Gender 33
23: Compensation to Gross Charges (TC/NPP Excluded) Ratio Category 34
24: Reporting Technical Component in Collections and Professional Gross Charges 34
25: Reporting Nonphysician Providers in Production 34
26: Nonphysician Provider Specialty 35
27: FTE Nonphysician Providers 35
28: Nonphysician Provider Clinical FTE 36
29: Nonphysician Provider Gender 36
30: Nonphysician Provider per FTE Physician 36
31: FTE Nonphysician Providers per Group 36

Physician Compensation and Benefits — Section Two

Compensation
   Table 1: Physician Compensation 38
   Table 2: Physician Compensation by Group Type 40
   Table 3A: Physician Compensation by Size of Multispecialty Practice (50 or fewer FTE Physicians) 42
   Table 3B: Physician Compensation by Size of Multispecialty Practice (51 or more FTE Physicians) 44
   Table 4: Physician Compensation by Hospital Ownership 46
   Table 5A: Physician Compensation by Geographic Section for All Practices 48
   Table 5B: Physician Compensation by Geographic Section for Single-Specialty Practices 50
   Table 5C: Physician Compensation by Geographic Section for Multispecialty Practices 52
   Table 6: Physician Compensation by Demographic Classification 54
   Table 7A: Physician Compensation by Practice Total Medical Revenue 56
   Table 7B: Physician Compensation by Practice Total Medical Revenue 58
   Table 8A: Physician Compensation by Method of Compensation (more than Two Years in Specialty) ... 60
   Table 8B: Physician Compensation by Method of Compensation (more than Two Years in Specialty) ... 62
   Table 9A: Physician Compensation by Years in Specialty 64
   Table 9B: Physician Compensation by 1–2 Years in Specialty 66
   Table 10: Physician Compensation by Gender 68
   Table 11: Physician Compensation by Clinical Service Hours Worked per Week 70
   Table 12: Physician Compensation by Weeks Worked per Year 72
   Table 13: Physician Compensation by Partner/Shareholder in Practice 74

Benefits
   Table 14: Physician Retirement Benefits 76
   Table 15: Physician Retirement Benefits by Group Type 78

Physician Productivity — Section Three

Collections for Professional Charges
   Table 16: Collections for Professional Charges (TC/NPP Excluded) 82
   Table 17: Collections for Professional Charges (TC/NPP Excluded) by Group Type 84
   Table 18: Collections for Professional Charges (TC/NPP Excluded) by Hospital Ownership 86
   Table 19: Collections for Professional Charges (TC/NPP Excluded) by Geographic Section for All Practices 88
   Table 20: Collections for Professional Charges (TC/NPP Excluded) by Years in Specialty 90
   Table 21: Collections for Professional Charges (TC/NPP Excluded) by Gender 92
   Table 22: Collections for Professional Charges (TC/NPP Excluded) by Clinical Service Hours Worked per Week 94
   Table 23: Collections for Professional Charges (TC/NPP Excluded) by Weeks Worked per Year 96
   Table 24: Collections for Professional Charges (NPP Excluded) with 1–10% Technical Component 98
   Table 25: Collections for Professional Charges (NPP Excluded) with more than 10% Technical Component 100

Compensation to Collections Ratio
   Table 26: Physician Compensation to Collections Ratio (TC/NPP Excluded) 102
   Table 27: Physician Compensation to Collections Ratio (TC/NPP Excluded) by Group Type 104
   Table 28A: Physician Compensation to Collections Ratio (TC/NPP Excluded) by Geographic Section for
      All Practices 106

Table 28B: Physician Compensation to Collections Ratio (TC/NPP Excluded) by Geographic Section for Single-Specialty Practices 108

Table 28C: Physician Compensation to Collections Ratio (TC/NPP Excluded) by Geographic Section for Multispecialty Practices 110

Table 29: Physician Compensation to Collections Ratio (TC/NPP Excluded) by Clinical Service Hours Worked per Week 112

Table 30: Physician Compensation to Collections Ratio (TC/NPP Excluded) by Years in Specialty 114

Table 31: Physician Compensation to Collections Ratio (TC/NPP Excluded) by Hospital Ownership 116

Table 32: Physician Compensation to Collections Ratio (TC/NPP Excluded) by On-call Duties 118

Gross Charges

Table 33: Physician Gross Charges (TC/NPP Excluded) 120

Table 34: Physician Gross Charges (TC/NPP Excluded) by Group Type 122

Table 35A: Physician Gross Charges (TC/NPP Excluded) by Size of Multispecialty Practice (50 or fewer FTE Physicians) 124

Table 35B: Physician Gross Charges (TC/NPP Excluded) by Size of Multispecialty Practice (51 or more FTE Physicians) 126

Table 36: Physician Gross Charges (TC/NPP Excluded) by Hospital Ownership 128

Table 37: Physician Gross Charges (TC/NPP Excluded) by Geographic Section for All Practices 130

Table 38A: Physician Gross Charges (TC/NPP Excluded) by Method of Compensation (more than Two Years in Specialty) 132

Table 38B: Physician Gross Charges (TC/NPP Excluded) by Method of Compensation (more than Two Years in Specialty) 134

Table 39: Physician Gross Charges (TC/NPP Excluded) by Years in Specialty 136

Table 40: Physician Professional Gross Charges (TC/NPP Excluded) by Clinical Service Hours Worked per Week 138

Table 41: Physician Gross Charges (NPP Excluded) with 1–10% Technical Component 140

Table 42: Physician Gross Charges (NPP Excluded) with 1–10% Technical Component by Group Type 142

Table 43: Physician Gross Charges (NPP Excluded) with more than 10% Technical Component 144

Table 44: Physician Gross Charges (NPP Excluded) with more than 10% Technical Component by Group Type 146

Ambulatory Encounters

Table 45: Physician Ambulatory Encounters (NPP Excluded) 148

Table 46: Physician Ambulatory Encounters (NPP Excluded) by Group Type 150

Table 47: Physician Ambulatory Encounters (NPP Excluded) by Hospital Ownership 152

Table 48: Physician Ambulatory Encounters (NPP Excluded) by Geographic Section for All Practices 154

Table 49: Physician Ambulatory Encounters (NPP Excluded) by Years in Specialty 156

Table 50: Physician Ambulatory Encounters (NPP Excluded) by Gender 158

Hospital Encounters

Table 51: Physician Hospital Encounters (NPP Excluded) 160

Table 52: Physician Hospital Encounters (NPP Excluded) by Group Type 162

Surgery/Anesthesia Cases

Table 53: Physician Surgery/Anesthesia Cases (NPP Excluded) 164

Table 54: Physician Surgery/Anesthesia Cases (NPP Excluded) by Group Type 166

RVUs (CMS RBRVS Method)

Table 55: Total RVUs (CMS RBRVS Method) (TC/NPP Excluded) 168

Table 56: Total RVUs (CMS RBRVS Method) (TC/NPP Excluded) by Group Type 170

Table 57: Total RVUs (CMS RBRVS Method) (TC/NPP Excluded) by Hospital Ownership 172

Table 58: Physician Compensation to Total RVUs Ratio (CMS RBRVS Method) (TC/NPP Excluded) 174

Table 59: Physician Compensation to Total RVUs Ratio (CMS RBRVS Method) (TC/NPP Excluded) by Group Type 176

Table 60: Collections to Total RVUs Ratio (CMS RBRVS Method) (TC/NPP Excluded) 178

Table 61: Total RVUs to Total Encounters Ratio (TC/NPP Excluded) 180

Table 62: Physician Work RVUs (CMS RBRVS Method) (NPP Excluded) 182

Table 63: Physician Work RVUs (CMS RBRVS Method) (NPP Excluded) by Group Type 184

Table 64: Physician Work RVUs (CMS RBRVS Method) (NPP Excluded) by Hospital Ownership 186

Table 65: Physician Work RVUs (CMS RBRVS Method) (NPP Excluded) by Method of Compensation 188

Table 66: Physician Compensation to Physician Work RVUs Ratio (CMS RBRVS Method) (NPP Excluded) 190
Table 67: Physician Compensation to Physician Work RVUs Ratio (CMS RBRVS Method) (NPP Excluded)
    by Group Type 192
Table 68: Collections to Physician Work RVUs Ratio (CMS RBRVS Method) (NPP Excluded) 194
Table 69: Work RVUs to Total Encounters Ratio (CMS RBRVS Method) (NPP Excluded) 196

Physician Time Worked — Section Four

Table 70: Physician Weeks Worked per Year 200
Table 71: Physician Weeks Worked per Year by Years in Specialty 202
Table 72: Physician Clinical Service Hours Worked per Week 204
Table 73: Physician Clinical Service Hours Worked per Week by Years in Specialty 206

Summary Tables — Section Five

List of Summary Tables 209
Table 74: Allergy/Immunology 210
Table 75: Anesthesiology 211
Table 76: Anesthesiology: Pain Management 212
Table 77: Cardiology: Electrophysiology 213
Table 78: Cardiology: Invasive 214
Table 79: Cardiology: Invasive/Interventional 215
Table 80: Cardiology: Noninvasive 216
Table 81: Dermatology 217
Table 82: Emergency Medicine 218
Table 83: Endocrinology/Metabolism 219
Table 84: Family Practice (with OB) 220
Table 85: Family Practice (without OB) 221
Table 86: Family Practice: Ambulatory Only (no inpatient work) 222
Table 87: Gastroenterology 223
Table 88: Hematology/Oncology 224
Table 89: Hospitalist: Family Practice 225
Table 90: Hospitalist: Internal Medicine 226
Table 91: Hospitalist: Internal Medicine (fewer than 250 Ambulatory Encounters) 227
Table 92: Hospitalist: Pediatrics 228
Table 93: Infectious Disease 229
Table 94: Internal Medicine: General 230
Table 95: Internal Medicine: Ambulatory Only (no inpatient work) 231
Table 96: Nephrology 232
Table 97: Neurology 233
Table 98: Obstetrics/Gynecology 234
Table 99: Obstetrics/Gynecology: Gynecology (only) 235
Table 100: Ophthalmology 236
Table 101: Orthopedic Surgery: General 237
Table 102: Orthopedic Surgery: Sports Medicine 238
Table 103: Otorhinolaryngology 239
Table 104: Pathology: Anatomic and Clinical 240
Table 105: Pediatrics: General 241
Table 106: Physiatry (Physical Medicine and Rehabilitation) 242
Table 107: Podiatry: General 243
Table 108: Psychiatry: General 244
Table 109: Pulmonary Medicine: General 245
Table 110: Pulmonary Medicine: Critical Care 246
Table 111: Radiation Oncology 247
Table 112: Radiology: Diagnostic-Inv 248
Table 113: Radiology: Diagnostic-Non 249
Table 114: Rheumatology 250
Table 115: Surgery: General 251

Table 116: Surgery: Cardiovascular 252
Table 117: Surgery: Neurological 253
Table 118: Surgery: Vascular 254
Table 119: Urgent Care 255
Table 120: Urology 256

Nonphysician Providers — Section Six

Compensation
Table 121: Nonphysician Provider Compensation 258
Table 122: Nonphysician Provider Compensation by Group Type 259
Table 123: Nonphysician Provider Compensation by Hospital Ownership 260
Table 124: Nonphysician Provider Compensation by Geographic Section 261
Table 125A: Nonphysician Provider Compensation by Size of Practice (50 or fewer FTE Physicians) 262
Table 125B: Nonphysician Provider Compensation by Size of Practice (51 or more FTE Physicians) 263
Table 126: Nonphysician Provider Compensation by Years in Specialty 264
Table 127: Nonphysician Provider Compensation by Gender 265

Retirement Benefits
Table 128: Nonphysician Provider Retirement Benefits 266
Table 129: Nonphysician Provider Retirement Benefits by Group Type 267

Collections
Table 130: Nonphysician Provider Collections for Professional Charges (TC Excluded) 268
Table 131: Nonphysician Provider Collections for Professional Charges (TC Excluded) by Group Type 269
Table 132: Nonphysician Provider Compensation to Collections Ratio (TC Excluded) 270

Gross Charges
Table 133: Nonphysician Provider Gross Charges (TC Excluded) 271
Table 134: Nonphysician Provider Gross Charges (TC Excluded) by Group Type 272
Table 135: Nonphysician Provider Gross Charges (TC Excluded) by Geographic Section 273
Table 136: Nonphysician Provider Compensation to Gross Charges Ratio (TC Excluded) 274
Table 137: Nonphysician Provider Compensation to Gross Charges Ratio (TC Excluded) by Group Type 275

Ambulatory Encounters
Table 138: Nonphysician Provider Ambulatory Encounters 276
Table 139: Nonphysician Provider Ambulatory Encounters by Group Type 277

Hospital Encounters
Table 140: Nonphysician Provider Hospital Encounters 278
Table 141: Nonphysician Provider Hospital Encounters by Group Type 279
Table 142: Nonphysician Provider Surgery/Anesthesia Cases 280
Table 143: Nonphysician Provider Surgery/Anesthesia Cases by Group Type 281

RVUs (CMS RBRVS Method)
Table 144: Nonphysician Provider Total RVUs (TC Excluded) 282
Table 145: Nonphysician Provider Compensation to Total RVUs Ratio (CMS RBRVS Method) (TC Excluded) 283
Table 146: Nonphysician Provider Work RVUs (CMS RBRVS Method) 284
Table 147: Nonphysician Provider Work RVUs (CMS RBRVS Method) by Group Type 285
Table 148: Nonphysician Provider Compensation to Work RVUs Ratio (CMS RBRVS Method) 286

Appendices

Appendix A: Abbreviations, Acronyms and Geographic Sections 288
Appendix B: Terms Used in the Report 289
Appendix C: Formulas and Methodology 295
Appendix D: MGMA Survey Products 297
Appendix E: Compensation and Production Survey: 2008 Questionnaire Based on 2007 Data 299
Appendix F: Compensation and Production Survey: 2008 Guide to the Questionnaire Based on 2007 Data 307

Overview

Introduction

Purpose
Each year, MGMA surveys its membership to obtain the most recent physician compensation and production data. This year MGMA's *Physician Compensation and Production Survey: 2008 Report Based on 2007 Data* continues to be a significant benchmarking tool for medical group practices and will assist medical practice executives in evaluating the ranges of compensation and productivity for both full-time equivalent (FTE) physicians and nonphysician providers. The report also allows users to compare and learn more about the factors affecting compensation and production.

Description
In this report you will find
- Complete data on more than 50,000 physicians and nonphysician providers categorized by specialty;
- Complete data on more than 1,900 group practices categorized by their specialty or multispecialty;
- Data reported for more than 100 physician specialties and more than 25 nonphysician provider specialties;
- More than 10 performance ratios to illustrate the relationship between compensation and productivity; and
- Productivity measures of collections for professional charges, gross charges, ambulatory encounters, hospital encounters, surgical/anesthesia cases as well as total and physician work relative value units (RVUs).

What's New?
This year the report contains four new tables, including physician compensation by practice total medical revenue, physician compensation to collections ratio by on-call duties, physician work RVUs by method of compensation and nonphysician provider compensation by number of FTE physicians in practice. There are two new subspecialties included in the summary tables for primary care: family practice: ambulatory only and internal medicine: ambulatory only, both of which specify less than 250 hospital encounters a year. There are also four new hospitalist specialties, as well as hospice/palliative care.

Summary tables are now made available for the new hospitalist specialties. Productivity is also represented by work RVUs instead of total RVUs this year.

Data Collection
Invitations were mailed in January 2008 to MGMA member organizations that include both medical group practices and other types of organizations involved in physician practice management. Printed invitations were mailed with reminder magnets to selected organizations that were or were presumed to be affiliated with medical practices. Invitations to participate were also e-mailed to medical practices. The method of participation this year was almost completely electronic, at 99 percent via the Web portal and Excel survey.

Response Rate
The table illustrates the response rate for the *2008 Physician Compensation and Production Survey Report*.

Response Rate	Medical Practices	
	Count	Percent
Invitations mailed	9,975	100.00%
Undeliverable	202	2.03%
Invitations reaching recipients	9,773	97.97%
Responses	1,991	20.37%
Excel surveys	430	21.60%
Web surveys	1,548	77.75%
Paper surveys	13	0.65%
*Ineligible or incomplete surveys	48	2.41%
Completed surveys included in the report	1,943	
**Gross response rate		20.37%
***Net response rate		19.88%

*Missing required answers; not a full year of data; academic practices or ambulatory surgery centers.
**(Number of responses divided by the number of invitations reaching recipients) × 100.
***((Responses minus ineligible or incomplete surveys) divided by invitations reaching recipients) × 100.

How to Use This Report

Report Organization
Six sections appear in the report:

1. **Key findings and demographics** – provides changes in compensation and production over the years as well as tables broken down by various demographic categories such as state, group type and ownership.
2. **Physician compensation and benefits** – tables presented by specialty that include physician compensation data by group type, size of multispecialty practice, ownership, geographic section, method of compensation, years in specialty, gender, clinical service hours worked, weeks worked and shareholder in the practice.
3. **Physician productivity** – tables presented by specialty that include collections for professional charges, physician compensation to collections ratio, gross charges, compensation to gross charges ratio, ambulatory encounters, hospital encounters, surgery/anesthesia cases, RVUs and compensation per RVU ratios.
4. **Physician time worked** – tables presented by specialty that include physician weeks worked per year and physician clinical service hours worked per week.
5. **Summary tables** – tables presented by specialty, which include compensation, collections for professional charges, compensation to collections ratio and total RVUs by group type and geographic section.
6. **Nonphysician providers** – tables presented for select specialties that include compensation, retirement benefits, collections for professional charges, gross charges, compensation to gross charges ratio, ambulatory encounters, hospital encounters and surgical/anesthesia cases.

Appendices
More information can be found in the appendices that will explain how the information is collected and defined in the survey and report.

Appendix A contains a list of abbreviations and acronyms used in the report as well as the states included in the geographic sections.

Appendix B contains the terms used in the report and the term definitions.

Appendix C contains formulas and methodology used in the report.

Appendix D contains a list of MGMA survey products.

Appendices E and F feature the 2008 Compensation and Production Survey Questionnaire and Guide to the Questionnaire as references for the user.

Additional Information
Visit mgma.com for more information about the surveys and reports, and to find future educational Web casts. Any updates to this report can also be found on mgma.com.

To order MGMA products, visit the *Store* on mgma.com or call toll-free 877.ASK.MGMA (275.6462), ext. 888.

Statistical Interpretation — A User's Guide

Introduction

The MGMA *Physician Compensation and Production Survey: 2008 Report Based on 2007 Data* uses descriptive statistics to summarize the compensation and productivity of physicians and nonphysician providers from medical groups that participated in the survey. The statistics displayed in each table are

- **Physician count** – the number of physicians represented by the practices who reported the data used to create the variable
- **Medical practices count** – the number of practices that reported the data used to create the variable
- **Mean** – the arithmetic average calculated by summing the data and dividing by the count
- **Standard deviation** – an index of the variability of the data values for any given variable
- **25th percentile** – the value where one quarter (25%) of the responses are lower and the remainder greater
- **Median** – the midpoint of all responses when arrayed from lowest to highest
- **75th percentile** – the value where three quarters (75%) of the responses are lower and the remainder greater
- **90th percentile** – the value where nine tenths (90%) of the responses are lower and the remainder greater

Data tables for physician compensation and productivity measures are reported by physician subspecialty, while nonphysician providers are reported by type of nonphysician provider. Summary tables provide compensation, collections for professional charges, compensation to collections ratio and total RVU data by select physician specialties.

Interpreting the Data

Normally, the median should be used for comparisons. Since the median is the midpoint of all data, it is not subject to the distortion that often occurs in the mean when extremely high or low values are present. The extent of variability within the data set is measured by the standard deviation, another statistic presented in the report. A standard deviation that is similar in value to the mean indicates that the data are dispersed and there is weak central tendency. A standard deviation less than a third of the mean indicates that the data clustered tightly around the mean and there is strong central tendency.

Using the Survey Report

In examining the data presented in the report, practice administrators and other report users should consider the following:

1. What is the difference between your facility's data and the report median (or mean, if appropriate)?
2. Does the difference, if any, indicate that your medical group's performance is significantly out of line with the survey statistics? A substantial difference identifies an area that might require managerial attention.
3. Are the differences explainable? For example, the method of data collection, survey definitions, special circumstances or organization objectives can all affect the outcome of comparison analysis.
4. By what methods can the compensation or productivity indicator be internally and/or externally changed or controlled?
5. How should your medical group measure performance for this indicator? Do your systems and processes allow for the appropriate assessment of the compensation or productivity indicator?

Key Findings and Demographics

Key Findings

The following results and conclusions were reached by historical and current year trend analyses performed by the MGMA Survey Operations staff. These analyses provide more information on how compensation may change over time as well as factors that influence current compensation and productivity levels. The median was used in the analysis.

This report reflects data submitted for fiscal year 2007 or the medical practice's most recently completed 12-month period. A majority of practices, 78.7%, provided data for calendar year 2007; 11.0% of the respondents reported data for the fiscal year ending June 2007; another 7.4% of the respondents reported data for the fiscal year ending September 2007; and the remainder reported data for other fiscal periods.

Factors Affecting Compensation

The characteristics of the medical practice and individual provider may influence compensation levels. Examples include group type, geographic section and hospital ownership. The influence of these contributors may differ for primary care and specialty care physicians. The following sections discuss the association between direct compensation and various practice characteristics. Overall median compensation levels for primary care and specialty care physicians are below.

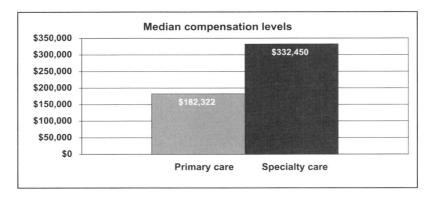

Group Type: Group type indicates whether physicians practiced in a single-specialty or multispecialty practice. Median compensation levels for primary care and specialty care physicians in both types of practices are below.

Compensation levels increased for physicians working in both single-specialty and multispecialty practices from 2006 to 2007. Primary care physicians in both types of practices had similar increases in compensation. This increase was 5.4% in a single-specialty practice and 6.2% in a multispecialty practice. For specialty care physicians, the gap between compensation at single-specialty practices and multispecialty practices grew significantly. Compensation for specialty care physicians in multispecialty practices increased 8.2% while their counterparts at single-specialty practices only saw a 1.7% increase.

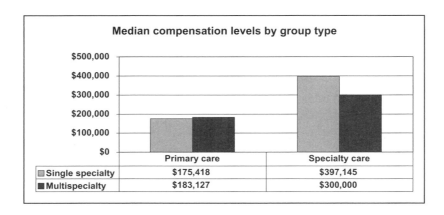

Geographic Section: Differences in compensation may also be reported by geographic section. The figures below present median compensation levels for primary care and specialty care physicians.

This year the western section had a large increase in compensation for primary care physicians, yielding the highest compensation levels of any section. This increase was 8.9% compared to 4.73% for the southern, 6.7% for the midwest and 3.2% for the eastern sections. Specialty care physician compensation also had the largest increase in the western section, increasing by 6.2%. The other sections had more modest increases, with the midwest section only increasing 0.6%. The increases for the eastern and southern sections were 2.2% and 2.3%, respectively.

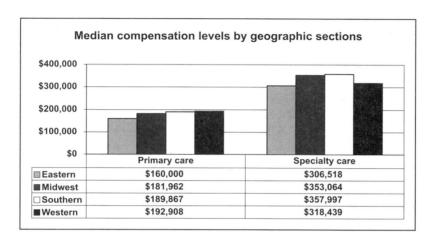

	Primary care	Specialty care
▨ Eastern	$160,000	$306,518
■ Midwest	$181,962	$353,064
☐ Southern	$189,867	$357,997
■ Western	$192,908	$318,439

Compensation by Hospital Ownership

The ownership of a practice can also effect compensation. Median compensation is reported for practices owned by a hospital and practices that are not owned by a hospital.

The figure below displays lower compensation for physicians who are employed by hospital-owned medical practices, which has been the trend over the past couple years.

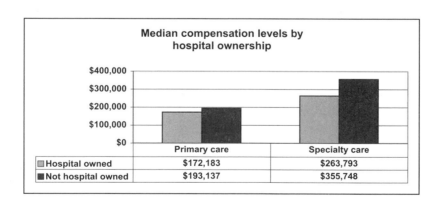

	Primary care	Specialty care
▨ Hospital owned	$172,183	$263,793
■ Not hospital owned	$193,137	$355,748

Compensation by Practice Total Medical Revenue

Primary Care Compensation by Practice Total Medical Revenue: For both family practice (without OB) and internal medicine: general, compensation tended to be greater in practices with greater total medical revenue. The exception to this for both groups was in practices with revenues of $2,000,001 to $5,000,000, where compensation was $164,327 and $175,400, respectively. This reflected greater compensation than practices with $5,000,001 to $10,000,000 in total medical revenue. In pediatric: general, the greatest compensation was in practices with $5,000,001 to $10,000,000 in total medical revenue ($199,732).

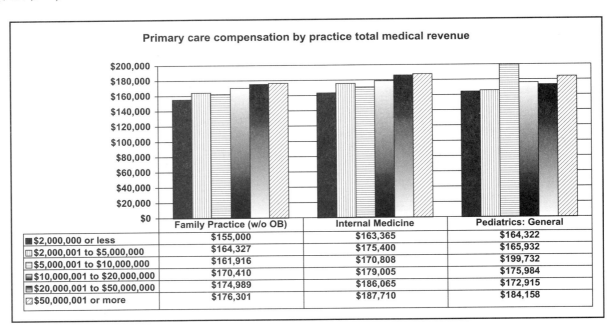

Primary care compensation by practice total medical revenue

	Family Practice (w/o OB)	Internal Medicine	Pediatrics: General
■ $2,000,000 or less	$155,000	$163,365	$164,322
▥ $2,000,001 to $5,000,000	$164,327	$175,400	$165,932
▤ $5,000,001 to $10,000,000	$161,916	$170,808	$199,732
▨ $10,000,001 to $20,000,000	$170,410	$179,005	$175,984
■ $20,000,001 to $50,000,000	$174,989	$186,065	$172,915
▨ $50,000,001 or more	$176,301	$187,710	$184,158

Specialty Care Compensation by Practice Total Medical Revenue: Compensation for specialty care physicians varied more across all total medical revenue categories. Anesthesiology showed the most consistent trend, as practices with $2,000,000 or less in total medical revenue reported $358,255 in compensation, while practices with total medical revenue of $50,000,001 or more reported $403,600 in compensation. OB/GYN physicians received a median of $318,742 in compensation in practices where total medical revenue was between $5,000,001 and $10,000,000, which was greater than any other category. Orthopedic surgery: general physicians received the greatest compensation in any practice with $20,000,001 to $50,000,000 in total medical revenue, where the median compensation was $494,346.

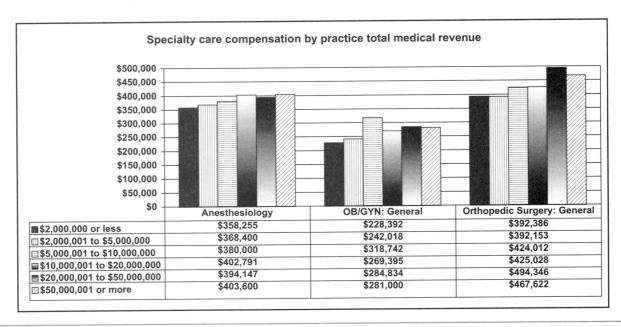

Specialty care compensation by practice total medical revenue

	Anesthesiology	OB/GYN: General	Orthopedic Surgery: General
■ $2,000,000 or less	$358,255	$228,392	$392,386
▥ $2,000,001 to $5,000,000	$368,400	$242,018	$392,153
▤ $5,000,001 to $10,000,000	$380,000	$318,742	$424,012
▨ $10,000,001 to $20,000,000	$402,791	$269,395	$425,028
■ $20,000,001 to $50,000,000	$394,147	$284,834	$494,346
▨ $50,000,001 or more	$403,600	$281,000	$467,622

Table A: Median Compensation for Selected Specialties, 2003–2007

	2003	03–04 change	2004	04–05 change	2005	05–06 change	2006	06–07 change	2007	03–07 change
All Primary Care:	$156,902	3.13%	$161,816	3.89%	$168,111	2.03%	$171,519	6.30%	$182,322	16.20%
Family Practice (without OB)	$152,478	2.32%	$156,011	3.02%	$160,729	2.05%	$164,021	5.97%	$173,812	13.99%
Internal Medicine*	$159,978	5.36%	$168,551	4.49%	$176,124	2.87%	$181,187	5.17%	$190,547	19.11%
Pediatric/Adolescent Medicine*	$158,853	1.47%	$161,188	3.72%	$167,178	4.21%	$174,209	4.89%	$182,727	15.03%
All Specialists:	$296,464	0.18%	$297,000	6.61%	$316,620	1.78%	$322,259	3.16%	$332,450	12.14%
Anesthesiology*	$323,491	0.78%	$325,999	10.34%	$359,699	1.59%	$365,409	9.47%	$400,000	23.65%
Cardiology: Invasive*	$410,272	4.28%	$427,815	8.41%	$463,801	-1.34%	$457,563	-0.18%	$456,747	11.33%
Cardiology: Noninvasive	$349,416	0.64%	$351,637	5.45%	$370,807	-0.84%	$367,704	11.72%	$410,784	17.56%
Dermatology*	$285,692	8.11%	$308,855	8.23%	$334,277	4.32%	$348,706	4.82%	$365,524	27.94%
Emergency Medicine	$215,859	2.70%	$221,679	9.82%	$243,449	2.70%	$250,030	2.71%	$256,800	18.97%
Gastroenterology	$351,614	4.87%	$368,733	4.14%	$384,015	5.81%	$406,345	2.90%	$418,139	18.92%
Hematology/Oncology*	$315,603	10.99%	$350,290	2.46%	$358,892	0.07%	$359,140	-16.83%	$298,689	-5.36%
Neurology	$190,973	10.54%	$211,094	2.42%	$216,199	1.76%	$220,000	3.49%	$227,670	19.22%
Obstetrics/Gynecology	$237,191	4.28%	$247,348	3.69%	$256,485	5.82%	$271,425	3.39%	$280,629	18.31%
Ophthalmology	$300,020	-6.56%	$280,353	7.84%	$302,321	-1.60%	$297,486	6.22%	$315,982	5.32%
Orthopedic Surgery*	$397,059	-0.10%	$396,650	7.93%	$428,119	4.30%	$446,517	3.02%	$459,992	15.85%
Otorhinolaryngology	$296,338	0.10%	$296,623	6.32%	$315,376	2.90%	$324,529	6.37%	$345,210	16.49%
Psychiatry*	$162,572	12.44%	$182,799	3.62%	$189,409	1.69%	$192,609	3.14%	$198,653	22.19%
Pulmonary Medicine	$229,173	0.66%	$230,688	1.58%	$234,336	9.16%	$255,807	7.25%	$274,358	19.72%
Radiology: Diagnostic*	$403,779	0.76%	$406,852	4.79%	$426,346	4.73%	$446,517	4.01%	$464,420	15.02%
Surgery: General	$264,375	6.86%	$282,504	6.48%	$300,800	1.77%	$306,115	3.53%	$316,909	19.87%
Urology	$344,038	-2.41%	$335,731	0.19%	$336,364	6.31%	$357,605	8.53%	$388,125	12.81%
All Nonphysician Providers:	$72,539	3.49%	$75,068	2.27%	$76,772	9.91%	$84,378	9.00%	$91,970	26.79%
Cert. Reg. Nurse Anes.	$123,166	3.16%	$127,054	3.42%	$131,400	5.02%	$138,000	1.45%	$140,000	13.67%
Nurse Practitioner*	$67,177	3.99%	$69,858	0.64%	$70,307	4.51%	$73,480	5.20%	$77,300	15.07%
Optometrist	$100,242	7.15%	$107,413	1.57%	$109,096	7.76%	$117,566	8.77%	$127,875	27.57%
Physician Asst. (surgical)*	$75,087	6.34%	$79,851	5.60%	$84,320	4.00%	$87,693	8.02%	$94,729	26.16%
Physician Asst. (primary care)*	$70,550	4.33%	$73,604	2.64%	$75,549	4.71%	$79,104	2.46%	$81,052	14.89%
Psychologist	$70,000	13.30%	$79,308	0.87%	$80,000	-1.48%	$78,816	5.85%	$83,423	19.18%

* Represents specialties that are combined.

Table B: Median Gross Charges (TC/NPP Excluded) for Selected Specialties, 2003–2007

	2003	03–04 change	2004	04–05 change	2005	05–06 change	2006	06–07 change	2007	03–06 change
All Primary Care:	**$466,283**	**0.99%**	**$470,901**	**6.76%**	**$502,746**	**3.78%**	**$521,733**	**7.59%**	**$561,354**	**20.39%**
Family Practice (without OB)	$453,062	-0.11%	$452,560	7.14%	$484,863	5.66%	$512,296	7.04%	$548,351	21.03%
Internal Medicine*	$437,462	4.55%	$457,384	2.38%	$468,270	3.27%	$483,601	10.04%	$532,161	21.65%
Pediatric/Adolescent Medicine*	$495,594	-0.19%	$494,647	10.48%	$546,469	3.58%	$566,057	11.06%	$628,635	26.84%
All Specialists:	**$954,239**	**-0.20%**	**$952,284**	**6.54%**	**$1,014,517**	**2.35%**	**$1,038,395**	**0.60%**	**$1,044,668**	**9.48%**
Anesthesiology*	$849,753	-2.92%	$824,967	18.78%	$979,880	4.38%	$1,022,754	16.36%	$1,190,117	40.05%
Cardiology: Invasive*	$1,751,214	-4.70%	$1,668,919	4.47%	$1,743,485	-2.50%	$1,699,984	3.53%	$1,759,983	0.50%
Cardiology: Noninvasive	$1,129,398	10.63%	$1,249,403	2.18%	$1,276,630	4.68%	$1,336,363	-2.25%	$1,306,322	15.67%
Dermatology*	$1,005,372	13.75%	$1,143,567	0.98%	$1,154,723	4.53%	$1,207,018	3.99%	$1,255,133	24.84%
Emergency Medicine	$669,736	2.08%	$683,680	17.46%	$803,035	-0.33%	$800,416	6.70%	$854,009	27.51%
Gastroenterology	$1,493,829	1.93%	$1,522,604	-1.37%	$1,501,752	9.71%	$1,647,541	-3.05%	$1,597,219	6.92%
Hematology/Oncology*	$632,329	8.06%	$683,317	18.90%	$812,488	-6.36%	$760,839	11.18%	$845,927	33.78%
Neurology	$627,336	2.90%	$645,548	8.82%	$702,513	-1.97%	$688,664	0.17%	$689,827	9.96%
Obstetrics/Gynecology	$872,045	2.66%	$895,253	2.28%	$915,622	7.35%	$982,918	0.62%	$989,024	13.41%
Ophthalmology	$1,251,441	-2.86%	$1,215,706	2.42%	$1,245,069	6.19%	$1,322,125	-0.38%	$1,317,143	5.25%
Orthopedic Surgery*	$1,490,484	5.57%	$1,573,488	4.99%	$1,652,014	4.13%	$1,720,293	-0.06%	$1,719,319	15.35%
Otorhinolaryngology	$1,196,694	3.51%	$1,238,732	7.65%	$1,333,505	1.38%	$1,351,858	3.47%	$1,398,708	16.88%
Psychiatry*	$343,057	8.28%	$371,460	-8.63%	$339,418	22.82%	$416,859	-16.23%	$349,216	1.80%
Pulmonary Medicine	$696,639	2.68%	$715,328	2.36%	$732,212	12.44%	$823,284	-0.36%	$820,336	17.76%
Radiology: Diagnostic*	$1,491,384	7.18%	$1,598,457	3.77%	$1,658,748	3.71%	$1,720,293	-8.08%	$1,581,303	6.03%
Surgery: General	$1,058,226	6.49%	$1,126,887	-2.76%	$1,095,735	11.15%	$1,217,944	-5.14%	$1,155,305	9.17%
Urology	$1,185,122	10.57%	$1,310,447	-9.27%	$1,188,933	8.06%	$1,284,714	8.76%	$1,397,303	17.90%
All Nonphysician Providers:	**$254,117**	**1.17%**	**$257,102**	**7.64%**	**$276,734**	**4.95%**	**$290,440**	**0.02%**	**$290,491**	**14.31%**
Cert. Reg. Nurse Anes.	$203,075	1.22%	$205,551	73.21%	$356,032	-23.70%	$271,670	-8.99%	$247,260	21.76%
Nurse Practitioner*	$249,579	-4.90%	$237,358	4.59%	$248,252	8.68%	$269,808	5.07%	$283,494	13.59%
Optometrist	$346,540	14.07%	$395,315	4.28%	$412,249	7.89%	$444,782	12.91%	$502,197	44.92%
Physician Asst. (surgical)*	$276,577	21.11%	$334,961	15.30%	$386,225	5.10%	$405,911	-6.69%	$378,746	36.94%
Physician Asst. (primary care)*	$298,937	5.37%	$315,000	-3.88%	$302,765	16.11%	$351,550	2.67%	$360,927	20.74%
Psychologist	$180,785	7.02%	$193,468	10.34%	$213,479	2.96%	$219,789	2.21%	$224,638	24.26%

* Represents specialties that are combined.

Table C: Median Collections for Professional Charges (TC/NPP Excluded) for Selected Specialties, 2003–2007

	2003	2004	03–04 change	2005	04–05 change	2006	05–06 change	2007	06–07 change	03–07 change
All Primary Care:	$325,522	$327,718	0.67%	$349,285	6.58%	$358,281	2.58%	$370,359	3.37%	13.77%
Family Practice (without OB)	$318,420	$310,613	-2.45%	$345,294	11.17%	$367,744	6.50%	$363,214	-1.23%	14.07%
Internal Medicine*	$300,753	$305,992	1.74%	$310,082	1.34%	$312,980	0.93%	$345,265	10.32%	14.80%
Pediatric/Adolescent Medicine*	$344,066	$355,798	3.41%	$370,810	4.22%	$380,893	2.72%	$407,592	7.01%	18.46%
All Specialists:	$536,811	$511,388	-4.74%	$525,531	2.77%	$505,525	-3.81%	$523,635	3.58%	-2.45%
Anesthesiology*	$440,866	$411,288	-6.71%	$434,716	5.70%	$475,716	9.43%	$531,716	11.77%	20.61%
Cardiology: Invasive*	$721,505	$724,186	0.37%	$718,478	-0.79%	$723,852	0.75%	$720,856	-0.41%	-0.09%
Cardiology: Noninvasive	$557,349	$510,356	-8.43%	$542,532	6.30%	$544,364	0.34%	$568,695	4.47%	2.04%
Dermatology*	$682,997	$708,076	3.67%	$719,357	1.59%	$742,951	3.28%	$765,120	2.98%	12.02%
Emergency Medicine	$345,254	$299,521	-13.25%	$324,145	8.22%	$314,190	-3.07%	$302,599	-3.69%	-12.35%
Gastroenterology	$719,958	$692,761	-3.78%	$740,094	6.83%	$741,927	0.25%	$743,867	0.26%	3.32%
Hematology/Oncology*	$464,368	$444,421	-4.30%	$585,395	31.72%	$554,639	-5.25%	$521,234	-6.02%	12.25%
Neurology	$399,171	$398,849	-0.08%	$415,419	4.15%	$396,279	-4.61%	$405,408	2.30%	1.56%
Obstetrics/Gynecology	$521,418	$549,597	5.40%	$567,915	3.33%	$583,752	2.79%	$588,871	0.88%	12.94%
Ophthalmology	$709,190	$663,439	-6.45%	$673,261	1.48%	$660,962	-1.83%	$669,795	1.34%	-5.55%
Orthopedic Surgery*	$767,752	$783,074	2.00%	$804,805	2.78%	$831,766	3.35%	$814,596	-2.06%	6.10%
Otorhinolaryngology	$648,104	$638,832	-1.43%	$679,257	6.33%	$670,485	-1.29%	$717,891	7.07%	10.77%
Psychiatry*	$232,978	$230,059	-1.25%	$219,327	-4.66%	$202,791	-7.54%	$194,667	-4.01%	-16.44%
Pulmonary Medicine	$394,806	$380,165	-3.71%	$404,276	6.34%	$464,313	14.85%	$446,582	-3.82%	13.11%
Radiology: Diagnostic*	$662,129	$624,429	-5.69%	$648,782	3.90%	$659,051	1.58%	$658,859	-0.03%	-0.49%
Surgery: General	$528,878	$521,526	-1.39%	$546,870	4.86%	$562,016	2.77%	$535,803	-4.66%	1.31%
Urology	$693,036	$716,262	3.35%	$628,064	-12.31%	$691,006	10.02%	$662,204	-4.17%	-4.45%
All Nonphysician Providers:	$172,556	$176,249	2.14%	$184,289	4.56%	$183,024	-0.69%	$185,556	1.38%	7.53%
Cert. Reg. Nurse Anes.	$203,075	$205,551	1.22%	$356,032	73.21%	$128,126	-64.01%	$219,103	71.01%	7.89%
Nurse Practitioner*	$166,481	$165,924	-0.33%	$171,270	3.22%	$179,698	4.92%	$176,964	-1.52%	6.30%
Optometrist	$346,540	$395,315	14.07%	$412,249	4.28%	$288,253	-30.08%	$316,906	9.94%	-8.55%
Physician Asst. (surgical)*	$112,442	$155,307	38.12%	$145,830	-6.10%	$151,684	4.01%	$145,016	-4.40%	28.97%
Physician Asst. (primary care)*	$209,389	$213,308	1.87%	$231,522	8.54%	$241,824	4.45%	$215,750	-10.78%	3.04%
Psychologist	$180,785	$193,468	7.02%	$213,479	10.34%	$141,917	-33.52%	$121,049	-14.70%	-33.04%

* Represents specialties that are combined.

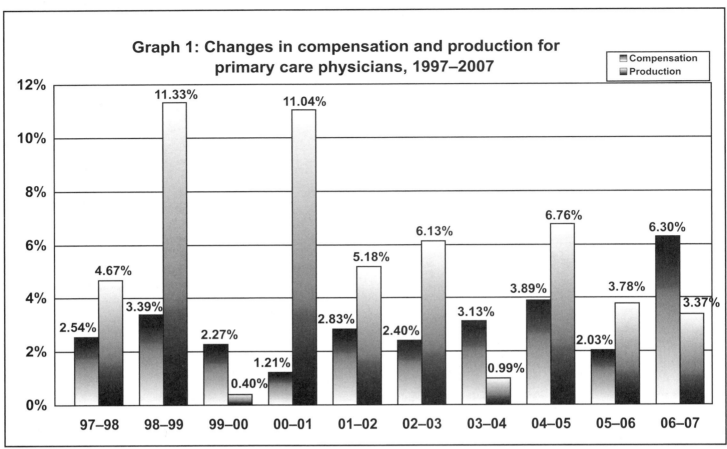

Graph 1: Changes in compensation and production for primary care physicians, 1997–2007

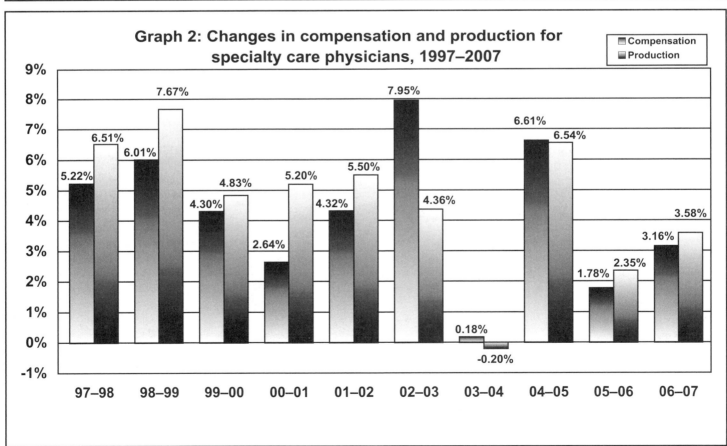

Graph 2: Changes in compensation and production for specialty care physicians, 1997–2007

Primary Care

Primary Care Multiyear Compensation, Gross Charges and Collections Analyses: The upper portions of Tables A, B and C focus on the primary care specialties of family practice, internal medicine and pediatrics.

Graph 1 on page 22 illustrates the year-to-year changes in both compensation and production (as measured by gross charges) for primary care physicians from 1997 to 2007.

Primary Care Compensation

Current Year: Compensation levels for all primary care physicians rose to $182,322 in 2007, a 6.30% increase. Each of the highlighted primary care specialties experienced increases from the previous year with family practice (without OB) experiencing the highest increase (5.97%).

Five-Year Trend: The last column in Table A on page 19 shows the change in compensation levels from 2003 to 2007. Compensation increased for all primary care specialties by 16.20%. Increases ranged from 13.99% for family practice (without OB) to 19.11% for internal medicine. The five-year increase of 16.20% for primary care physicians was greater than the 12.14% increase seen in specialty care physician compensation. The change in nonphysician provider compensation also increased during this five-year period by 26.79%.

Primary Care Gross Charges

Current Year: Gross charges for all primary care physicians increased by 7.59% in 2007 (Table B on page 20). Each of the highlighted primary care specialties experienced increases from the previous year, with pediatric/adolescent medicine experiencing the greatest increase at 11.06%.

Five-Year Trend: From 2003 to 2007, gross charges increased by 20.39%. Pediatric/adolescent medicine physicians' gross charges increased the most during this period at 26.84%, while family practitioners' and internists' gross charges rose 21.03% and 21.65%, respectively.

The year-to-year changes in compensation and gross charges for primary care physicians between 1997 and 2007 are shown in Graph 1 on page 22. Gross charges rose less than compensation for the first time in several years for primary care physicians.

Primary Care Collections for Professional Charges

Current Year: Collections for professional charges increased from 2006 to 2007 when all reporting primary care physicians were measured as a group. Individually, family practice (without OB) as a group reported a decrease in collections (-1.23%). The largest increase in collections was reported by internal medicine groups (10.23%).

Five-Year Trend: Primary care groups experienced a more than 10% increase in collections in the past five years (13.77%). The largest increase was reported by pediatric and adolescent medicine groups (18.46%). Collections for professional charges in primary groups as a whole have increased by a greater percentage than specialty care groups as a whole since 2003.

Specialty Care

Specialty Care Multiyear Compensation and Gross Charges Analyses: The middle portion of Tables A and B shows median compensation and gross charge levels for 17 selected specialties from 2003 to 2007. Graph 2 on page 22 illustrates the year-to-year changes for specialists since 1997.

Specialty Care Compensation

Current Year: All except two of the highlighted physician specialties experienced a compensation increase in 2007. The highest gains occurred in cardiology: noninvasive (11.72%), anesthesiology (9.47%) and urology (8.53%). The two specialties that did not see an increase were cardiology: invasive and hematology/oncology, which saw a very small decrease (-0.18%) and a much larger decrease (-16.83%), respectively.

Five-Year Trend: From 2003 to 2007, compensation levels for specialists increased by 12.14%. Of the selected specialties displayed in Table A, dermatology (27.94%), anesthesiology (23.65%) and psychiatry (22.19%) had the most significant gains. Hematology/oncology experienced the only decrease at -5.36%.

Specialty Care Gross Charges
Current Year: Gross charges for all specialty care physicians increased by 0.60% in 2007. Anesthesiology and hematology/oncology experienced the largest yearly increase in gross charges at 16.36% and 11.18%, respectively. Several specialties, including psychiatry (-16.23%), radiology: diagnostic (-8.08%) and surgery: general (-5.14%) exhibited declines in gross charges. Gross charges for all specialists who experienced a decrease in 2006 increased in 2007. They include cardiology: invasive, emergency medicine, hematology/oncology and neurology.

Five-Year Trend: In examining the change in gross charges since 2003, 4 of the 17 specialties experienced an increase of more than 20% in gross charges: anesthesiology (40.05%), hematology/oncology (33.78%), emergency medicine (27.51%) and dermatology (24.84%).

Specialty Care Collections for Professional Charges
Current Year: Specialty care groups as a whole reported an increase in collections from 2006 to 2007 (3.58%). The largest increase in collections was reported by anesthesiology groups (11.77%). Several specialty groups experienced decreases in collections including hematology/oncology (-6.02%), surgery: general (-4.66%) and urology (-4.17%).

Five-Year Trend: An overall decrease in collections was reported for the aggregate of specialty care groups from 2003 to 2007 (-2.45%). The group that experienced the largest increase in collections since 2003 is the same group that experienced the greatest increase since 2006: anesthesiology (20.61%). Five other groups reported an increase in collections greater than 10%: pulmonary medicine (13.11%), obstetrics/gynecology (12.94%), hematology/oncology (12.25%), dermatology (12.02%) and otorhinolaryngology (10.77%). Psychiatry reported the most significant decrease in collections at -16.44%.

Several caveats are necessary concerning multiyear analyses: year-to-year differences in response rate, measurement, editing and specialty mix exist that may distort results. Also, the respondent population was not held constant when analyzing the changes in compensation and gross charges over time.

Nonphysician Provider Analyses

The lower portion of Tables A and B show median compensation and gross charges for six select nonphysician providers. Compensation levels for all nonphysician providers increased by 9.00% while optometrists experienced the largest compensation increase for the highlighted providers at 8.77%. Gross charges for all nonphysician providers increased by 0.02% from 2006 to 2007. Optometrists experienced the greatest increase in gross charges at 12.91% this year, following an increase of 7.89% in the previous year.

Five-Year Trend: Optometrists experienced a 27.57% increase in compensation since 2003. Certified registered nurse anesthetists reported the lowest change in compensation over the five-year period at 13.67%. All the nonphysician providers listed in Table B reported an increase in gross charges since 2003.

Note: As of the 2006 questionnaire, anesthesia practices that recognize an equal-share compensation methodology were provided additional instructions allowing them to record compensation and productivity as an average by physician and nonphysician provider specialty. Therefore, some of the changes seen in anesthesia practices may be a result of these additional parameters for data submission.

Demographics — Medical Practice

1: Responses Received

	Medical Practices		All Providers	
	Count	Percent	Count	Percent
Questionnaires received	1,991	100.00%	51,884	100.00%
Ineligible/incomplete cases	48	2.41%	1,466	2.83%
Eligible/complete cases	1,943	97.59%	50,418	97.17%

2: Geographic Section

	Medical Practices		All Providers	
	Count	Percent	Count	Percent
Eastern	526	27.07%	9,979	19.79%
Midwest	466	23.98%	14,879	29.51%
Southern	642	33.04%	11,383	22.58%
Western	309	15.90%	14,177	28.12%
Total	1,943	100.00%	50,418	100.00%

3: Demographic Classification

	Medical Practices		All Providers	
	Count	Percent	Count	Percent
Nonmetropolitan (fewer than 50,000)	401	20.79%	5,469	10.94%
Metropolitan (50,000 to 250,000)	535	27.73%	13,483	26.96%
Metropolitan (250,001 to 1,000,000)	684	35.46%	15,476	30.94%
Metropolitan (more than 1,000,000)	309	16.02%	15,585	31.16%
Total	1,929	100.00%	50,013	100.00%

4: State

	Medical Practices		All Providers	
	Count	Percent	Count	Percent
Alabama	9	.46%	106	.21%
Alaska	6	.31%	24	.05%
Arizona	26	1.34%	405	.80%
Arkansas	30	1.54%	247	.49%
California	45	2.32%	5,792	11.49%
Colorado	52	2.68%	1,599	3.17%
Connecticut	15	.77%	281	.56%
Delaware	3	.15%	59	.12%
Florida	72	3.71%	1,403	2.78%
Georgia	58	2.99%	851	1.69%
Hawaii	4	.21%	156	.31%
Idaho	13	.67%	174	.35%
Illinois	72	3.71%	1,887	3.74%
Indiana	46	2.37%	1,188	2.36%
Iowa	40	2.06%	1,486	2.95%
Kansas	44	2.26%	830	1.65%
Kentucky	29	1.49%	541	1.07%
Louisiana	14	.72%	225	.45%
Maine	14	.72%	250	.50%
Maryland	19	.98%	248	.49%
Massachusetts	25	1.29%	1,946	3.86%
Michigan	112	5.76%	1,379	2.74%
Minnesota	43	2.21%	3,815	7.57%
Mississippi	14	.72%	394	.78%
Missouri	112	5.76%	1,300	2.58%
Montana	10	.51%	136	.27%
Nebraska	29	1.49%	491	.97%
Nevada	9	.46%	164	.33%
New Hampshire	11	.57%	182	.36%
New Jersey	18	.93%	269	.53%
New Mexico	2	.10%	31	.06%
New York	45	2.32%	922	1.83%
North Carolina	183	9.42%	1,953	3.87%
North Dakota	6	.31%	842	1.67%
Ohio	66	3.40%	1,183	2.35%
Oklahoma	19	.98%	418	.83%
Oregon	48	2.47%	1,784	3.54%
Pennsylvania	137	7.05%	2,942	5.84%
Rhode Island	2	.10%	60	.12%
South Carolina	14	.72%	350	.69%
South Dakota	11	.57%	135	.27%
Tennessee	70	3.60%	1,808	3.59%
Texas	157	8.08%	2,910	5.77%
Utah	15	.77%	990	1.96%
Vermont	4	.21%	68	.13%
Virginia	41	2.11%	684	1.36%
Washington	72	3.71%	2,875	5.70%
West Virginia	9	.46%	115	.23%
Wisconsin	41	2.11%	2,473	4.90%
Wyoming	7	.36%	47	.09%
Total	1,943	100.00%	50,418	100.00%

5: Legal Organization

	Medical Practices		All Providers	
	Count	Percent	Count	Percent
Business corporation	332	17.12%	5,191	10.42%
Limited liability company	189	9.75%	2,681	5.38%
Not-for-profit corporation/foundation	654	33.73%	19,845	39.82%
Partnership	69	3.56%	1,433	2.88%
Professional corporation/association	632	32.59%	19,768	39.66%
Sole proprietorship	9	.46%	19	.04%
Other	54	2.78%	904	1.81%
Total	1,939	100.00%	49,841	100.00%

6: Organization Ownership

	Medical Practices		All Providers	
	Count	Percent	Count	Percent
Government	11	.57%	378	.75%
Hospital/integrated delivery system	742	38.21%	17,358	34.45%
Insurance company or HMO	8	.41%	479	.95%
MSO or PPMC	35	1.80%	453	.90%
Physicians	1,080	55.61%	27,555	54.69%
University or medical school	3	.15%	116	.23%
Other	63	3.24%	4,046	8.03%
Total	1,942	100.00%	50,385	100.00%

7: Group Type

	Medical Practices		All Providers	
	Count	Percent	Count	Percent
Single Specialty	1,358	69.89%	13,874	27.52%
Multispecialty	585	30.11%	36,544	72.48%
Total	1,943	100.00%	50,418	100.00%

8: Single-Specialty Group Type

	Medical Practices		All Providers	
	Count	Percent	Count	Percent
Allergy/Immunology	9	.66%	38	.27%
Anesthesiology	112	8.25%	3,796	27.36%
Anesthesiology: Pain Management	21	1.55%	850	6.13%
Anesthesiology: Pain Management Only	5	.37%	34	.25%
Cardiology	94	6.92%	1,341	9.67%
Critical Care: Intensivist	1	.07%	3	.02%
Dermatology	11	.81%	40	.29%
Emergency Medicine	16	1.18%	475	3.42%
Endocrinology/Metabolism	11	.81%	27	.19%
Family Practice	298	21.94%	1,339	9.65%
Gastroenterology	41	3.02%	374	2.70%
Geriatrics	3	.22%	25	.18%
Hematology/Oncology	16	1.18%	90	.65%
Infectious Disease	6	.44%	22	.16%
Internal Medicine	79	5.82%	524	3.78%
Neonatal Medicine	5	.37%	31	.22%
Nephrology	10	.74%	65	.47%
Neurology	34	2.50%	152	1.10%
OB/GYN	87	6.41%	549	3.96%
OB/GYN: Gynecological Oncology	5	.37%	13	.09%
OB/GYN: Maternal/Fetal Med	6	.44%	16	.12%
OB/GYN: Reprod Endocrin	1	.07%	5	.04%
Occupational Medicine	1	.07%	4	.03%
Ophthalmology	42	3.09%	302	2.18%
Ophthalmology: Retina	2	.15%	13	.09%
Orthopedics (Nonsurgical)	1	.07%	1	.01%
Orthopedic Surgery	116	8.54%	1,229	8.86%
Otorhinolaryngology	21	1.55%	144	1.04%
Pathology	4	.29%	38	.27%
Pediatrics	80	5.89%	736	5.30%
Pediatrics: Cardiology	3	.22%	9	.06%
Pediatrics: Endocrinology	1	.07%	3	.02%
Pediatrics: Hematology/Oncology	2	.15%	8	.06%
Pediatrics: Hospitalist	1	.07%	10	.07%
Pediatrics: Neurology	3	.22%	5	.04%
Pediatrics: Pulmonology	2	.15%	5	.04%
Physiatry	6	.44%	34	.25%
Podiatry	1	.07%	1	.01%
Psychiatry	6	.44%	148	1.07%
Pulmonary Medicine	18	1.33%	95	.68%
Radiation Oncology	2	.15%	14	.10%
Radiology	22	1.62%	479	3.45%
Rheumatology	7	.52%	22	.16%
Surgery: Cardiovascular	14	1.03%	91	.66%
Surgery: General	36	2.65%	157	1.13%
Surgery: Neurological	15	1.10%	57	.41%
Surgery: Oral	3	.22%	9	.06%
Surgery: Pediatric	5	.37%	20	.14%
Surgery: Plastic/Recon	4	.29%	18	.13%
Surgery: Thoracic	3	.22%	10	.07%
Surgery: Transplant	1	.07%	8	.06%
Surgery: Trauma	3	.22%	11	.08%
Urology	28	2.06%	219	1.58%
Other Single Specialty	34	2.50%	165	1.19%
Total	1,358	100.00%	13,874	100.00%

9: Integration Options

	Medical Practices		All Providers	
	Count	Percent	Count	Percent
Hospital Owns Practice				
Yes	742	38.19%	17,358	34.43%
No	1,201	61.81%	33,060	65.57%
Total	1,943	100.00%	50,418	100.00%
Practice Receives Services from a PPMC/MSO				
Yes	361	18.83%	5,296	10.78%
No	1,556	81.17%	43,839	89.22%
Total	1,917	100.00%	49,135	100.00%

10: 2007 Total Medical Revenue

	Medical Practices		All Providers	
	Count	Percent	Count	Percent
$2,000,000 or less	527	27.32%	1,816	3.94%
$2,000,001 to $5,000,000	438	22.71%	2,507	5.43%
$5,000,001 to $10,000,000	367	19.03%	4,002	8.67%
$10,000,001 to $20,000,000	230	11.92%	4,837	10.48%
$20,000,001 to $50,000,000	210	10.89%	8,773	19.01%
$50,000,001 or more	157	8.14%	24,210	52.47%
Total	1,929	100.00%	46,145	100.00%

11: 2007 Percent of Capitation Revenue

	Medical Practices		All Providers	
	Count	Percent	Count	Percent
No capitation	1,601	90.91%	35,560	80.98%
5% or less	80	4.54%	3,501	7.97%
6% to 10%	17	.97%	801	1.82%
11% to 25%	30	1.70%	1,566	3.57%
26% to 50%	21	1.19%	1,082	2.46%
51% to 75%	8	.45%	715	1.63%
76% or more	4	.23%	687	1.56%
Total	1,761	100.00%	43,912	100.00%

12: Practice Plans to Change Compensation Methodology

	Medical Practices		All Providers	
	Count	Percent	Count	Percent
Yes	288	14.89%	8,365	16.81%
No	1,646	85.11%	41,396	83.19%
Total	1,934	100.00%	49,761	100.00%

13: Productivity Measures Used in Compensation Methodology

	Medical Practices		All Providers	
	Count	Percent	Count	Percent
Gross Charges				
Yes	221	11.37%	6,589	13.07%
No	1,722	88.63%	43,829	86.93%
Total	1,943	100.00%	50,418	100.00%
Adjusted Charges				
Yes	274	14.10%	6,531	12.95%
No	1,669	85.90%	43,887	87.05%
Total	1,943	100.00%	50,418	100.00%
Collections for Professional Charges				
Yes	776	39.94%	16,140	32.01%
No	1,167	60.06%	34,278	67.99%
Total	1,943	100.00%	50,418	100.00%
Number of Patient Encounters				
Yes	100	5.15%	3,097	6.14%
No	1,843	94.85%	47,321	93.86%
Total	1,943	100.00%	50,418	100.00%
Size of Physicians Patient Panel				
Yes	10	.51%	749	1.49%
No	1,933	99.49%	49,669	98.51%
Total	1,943	100.00%	50,418	100.00%
Number of RVUs				
Yes	330	16.98%	17,912	35.53%
No	1,613	83.02%	32,506	64.47%
Total	1,943	100.00%	50,418	100.00%

14: Basis for Incentive/Bonus Used in Compensation Methodology

	Medical Practices		All Providers	
	Count	Percent	Count	Percent
Patient Satisfaction				
Yes	139	7.15%	11,381	22.57%
No	1,804	92.85%	39,037	77.43%
Total	1,943	100.00%	50,418	100.00%
Peer Review				
Yes	145	7.46%	1,908	3.78%
No	1,798	92.54%	48,510	96.22%
Total	1,943	100.00%	50,418	100.00%
Administrative/Governance Responsibility				
Yes	215	11.07%	7,085	14.05%
No	1,728	88.93%	43,333	85.95%
Total	1,943	100.00%	50,418	100.00%
Service Quality				
Yes	122	6.28%	11,129	22.07%
No	1,821	93.72%	39,289	77.93%
Total	1,943	100.00%	50,418	100.00%
Seniority in the Medical Practice				
Yes	34	1.75%	1,104	2.19%
No	1,909	98.25%	49,314	97.81%
Total	1,943	100.00%	50,418	100.00%
Community Outreach				
Yes	65	3.35%	2,440	4.84%
No	1,878	96.65%	47,978	95.16%
Total	1,943	100.00%	50,418	100.00%

15: Health Records Storage

	Medical Practices		All Providers	
	Count	Percent	Count	Percent
Paper medical records	961	53.18%	14,416	30.57%
DIMS	105	5.81%	3,248	6.89%
EHR	559	30.94%	21,009	44.55%
Hybrid	133	7.36%	6,548	13.88%
Other	49	2.71%	1,942	4.12%
Total	1,807	100.00%	47,163	100.00%

page 31

Demographics — Providers

16: Physician Specialty

	Physicians	
	Count	Percent
Allergy/Immunology	186	0.43%
Anesthesiology	3,994	9.18%
Anesthesiology: Pain Management	207	0.48%
Anesthesiology: Pediatric	124	0.29%
Cardiology: Electrophysiology	210	0.48%
Cardiology: Invasive	583	1.34%
Cardiology: Inv-Intvl	690	1.59%
Cardiology: Noninvasive	563	1.29%
Critical Care: Intensivist	116	0.27%
Dentistry	67	0.15%
Dermatology	392	0.90%
Dermatology: Mohs Surgery	35	0.08%
Emergency Medicine	1,056	2.43%
Endocrinology/Metabolism	318	0.73%
Family Practice (w/ OB)	862	1.98%
Family Practice (w/o OB)	6,284	14.45%
Family Practice: Ambulatory Only (no inpatient work)	240	0.55%
Family Practice: Sports Med	47	0.11%
Gastroenterology	931	2.14%
Gastroenterology: Hepatology	22	0.05%
Genetics	12	0.03%
Geriatrics	119	0.27%
Hematology/Oncology	499	1.15%
Hematology/Oncology: Oncology (only)	306	0.70%
Hospice/Palliative Care	18	0.04%
Hospitalist: Family Practice	53	0.12%
Hospitalist: Pediatrics	1,255	2.89%
Hospitalist: Internal Medicine	9	0.02%
Hospitalist: Internal Medicine-Pediatrics	106	0.24%
Infectious Disease	240	0.55%
Internal Medicine: General	5,067	11.65%
Internal Medicine: Ambulatory Only (no inpatient work)	41	0.09%
Internal Med: Pediatrics	130	0.30%
Nephrology	301	0.69%
Neurology	681	1.57%
OB/GYN: General	2,086	4.80%
OB/GYN: Gynecology (only)	230	0.53%
OB/GYN: Gyn Oncology	61	0.14%
OB/GYN: Maternal & Fetal Med	131	0.30%
OB/GYN: Repro Endocrinology	27	0.06%
OB/GYN: Urogynecology	14	0.03%
Occupational Medicine	173	0.40%
Ophthalmology	646	1.49%
Ophthalmology: Pediatric	41	0.09%
Ophthalmology: Retina	71	0.16%
Orthopedic (nonsurgical)	51	0.12%
Orthopedic Surgery: General	1,082	2.49%
Orthopedic Surgery: Foot & Ankle	73	0.17%
Orthopedic Surgery: Hand	166	0.38%
Orthopedic Surgery: Hip & Joint	155	0.36%
Orthopedic Surgery: Pediatric	49	0.11%
Orthopedic Surgery: Spine	152	0.35%
Orthopedic Surgery: Trauma	46	0.11%
Orthopedic Surgery: Sports Med	216	0.50%

	Physicians	
	Count	Percent
Otorhinolaryngology	581	1.34%
Pathology: Anatomic & Clinical	247	0.57%
Pathology: Anatomic	40	0.09%
Pathology: Clinical	55	0.13%
Pediatrics: General	3,126	7.19%
Pediatrics: Adolescent Medicine	91	0.21%
Pediatrics: Allergy/Immunology	11	0.03%
Pediatrics: Cardiology	69	0.16%
Pediatrics: Child Development	20	0.05%
Pediatrics: Critical Care/Intensivist	101	0.23%
Pediatrics: Emergency Medicine	103	0.24%
Pediatrics: Endocrinology	47	0.11%
Pediatrics: Gastroenterology	48	0.11%
Pediatrics: Genetics	24	0.06%
Pediatrics: Hematology/Oncology	96	0.22%
Pediatrics: Infectious Disease	25	0.06%
Pediatrics: Neonatal Medicine	164	0.38%
Pediatrics: Nephrology	15	0.03%
Pediatrics: Neurology	69	0.16%
Pediatrics: Pulmonology	33	0.08%
Pediatrics: Rheumatology	11	0.03%
Physiatry (Phys Med & Rehab)	271	0.62%
Podiatry: General	154	0.35%
Podiatry: Surg-Foot & Ankle	139	0.32%
Podiatry: Surg-Forefoot Only	5	0.01%
Psychiatry: General	532	1.22%
Psychiatry: Child & Adolescent	106	0.24%
Psychiatry: Geriatric	8	0.02%
Pulmonary Medicine: General	272	0.63%
Pulmonary Med: Critical Care	101	0.23%
Pulmonary Med: Gen & Crit Care	188	0.43%
Radiation Oncology	147	0.34%
Radiology: Diagnostic-Inv	355	0.82%
Radiology: Diagnostic-Noninv	960	2.21%
Radiology: Nuclear Medicine	54	0.12%
Rheumatology	313	0.72%
Sleep Medicine	57	0.13%
Surgery: General	1,072	2.46%
Surgery: Bariatric	27	0.06%
Surgery: Cardiovascular	275	0.63%
Surgery: Colon and Rectal	51	0.12%
Surgery: Neurological	265	0.61%
Surgery: Oncology	27	0.06%
Surgery: Oral	29	0.07%
Surgery: Pediatric	62	0.14%
Surgery: Plastic & Reconstruction	150	0.34%
Surgery: Plastic & Recon-Hand	11	0.03%
Surgery: Thoracic (primary)	60	0.14%
Surgery: Transplant	34	0.08%
Surgery: Trauma	79	0.18%
Surgery: Trauma-Burn	4	0.01%
Surgery: Vascular (primary)	207	0.48%
Urgent Care	559	1.29%
Urology	592	1.36%
Urology: Pediatric	13	0.03%
Other physician specialty	105	0.24%
Total	43,494	100.00%

17: Physician Years in Specialty

	Physicians	
	Count	Percent
1 to 2 years	2,633	8.11%
3 to 7 years	6,816	20.99%
8 to 12 years	6,484	19.97%
13 to 17 years	5,267	16.22%
18 to 22 years	4,619	14.22%
23 years or more	6,653	20.49%
Total	32,472	100.00%

18: FTE Physicians

	Physicians	
	Count	Percent
4 or fewer	1,655	3.80%
5 to 10	3,802	8.73%
11 to 25	4,695	10.79%
26 to 50	5,946	13.66%
51 to 75	4,080	9.37%
76 to 100	2,943	6.76%
101 to 150	3,872	8.90%
151 or more	16,537	37.99%
Total	43,530	100.00%

19: FTE Physicians per Group

	Physicians	Mean	Std Deviation	25th %tile	Median	75th %tile	90th %tile
FTE Physicians	2,005	25.05	97.49	3.00	6.50	17.00	54.41

20: Clinical FTE

	Physicians	
	Count	Percent
.39 FTE or fewer	27	.06%
.40 to .60 FTE	1,330	3.07%
.61 to .69 FTE	375	.87%
.70 to .79 FTE	1,319	3.04%
.80 to .89 FTE	2,120	4.89%
.90 to .99 FTE	3,440	7.94%
1.00 FTE	34,737	80.14%
Total	43,348	100.00%

21: On-call Duties

	Physicians	
	Count	Percent
Physician had on-call duties	25,256	83.19%
Physician did not have on-call duties	5,105	16.81%
Total	30,361	100.00%

22: Gender

	Physicians	
	Count	Percent
Male	28,538	72.79%
Female	10,669	27.21%
Total	39,207	100.00%

page 33

23: Compensation to Gross Charges (TC/NPP Excluded) Ratio Category

	Physicians	
	Count	Percent
Less than .05	15	.08%
.10 to .14	458	2.35%
.15 to .19	1,171	6.01%
.20 to .24	2,889	14.82%
.25 to .29	3,350	17.18%
.30 to .34	3,213	16.48%
.35 to .39	2,598	13.32%
.40 to .44	1,912	9.81%
.45 to .49	1,408	7.22%
.50 to .54	803	4.12%
.55 to .59	518	2.66%
.60 to .64	358	1.84%
.65 to .69	237	1.22%
.70 to .74	157	.81%
.75 to .79	107	.55%
.80 to .84	103	.53%
.85 to .89	74	.38%
.90 to .94	68	.35%
.95 to 1.00	59	.30%
Total	19,498	100.00%

24: Reporting Technical Component in Collections and Professional Gross Charges

	Physicians	
	Count	Percent
0%	29,963	77.47%
1-10%	5,952	15.39%
> 10%	2,761	7.14%
Total	38,676	100.00%

25: Reporting Nonphysician Providers in Production

	Physicians	
	Count	Percent
Professional Gross Charges		
Yes	3,157	8.43%
No	34,307	91.57%
Total	37,464	100.00%
Ambulatory Encounters		
Yes	2,606	9.16%
No	25,849	90.84%
Total	28,455	100.00%
Total RVUs		
Yes	1,231	6.38%
No	18,066	93.62%
Total	19,297	100.00%
Work RVUs		
Yes	2,302	7.72%
No	27,514	92.28%
Total	29,816	100.00%

26: Nonphysician Provider Specialty

	Nonphysician Providers	
	Count	Percent
Audiologist	83	1.20%
Cert Reg Nurse Anesthetist	1,683	24.31%
Chiropractor	22	.32%
Dietician/Nutritionist	37	.53%
Midwife: Out-/In-patient	124	1.79%
Midwife: Outpatient (only)	11	.16%
Midwife: Inpatient (only)	15	.22%
Nurse Practitioner	1,435	20.73%
NP: Cardiology	26	.38%
NP: Family Practice (w/o OB)	40	.58%
NP: Gastroenterology	12	.17%
NP: Gerontology/Elder Health	17	.25%
NP: Hematology/Oncology	11	.16%
NP: Internal Medicine	58	.84%
NP: Pediatric/Child Health	60	.87%
NP: OB/GYN/Women's Health	69	1.00%
Occupational Therapist	45	.65%
Optometrist	271	3.91%
Perfusionist	13	.19%
Pharmacist	267	3.86%
Physical Therapist	432	6.24%
Physician Asst (surgical)	477	6.89%
PA: Orthopedic	58	.84%
PA: Surg: General	11	.16%
Physician Asst (primary care)	737	10.64%
PA: Family Practice (w/ OB)	54	.78%
PA: Family Practice (w/o OB)	43	.62%
PA: Internal Medicine	24	.35%
PA: Urgent Care	12	.17%
Phys Asst (nonsurgical/nonprimary care)	287	4.15%
PA: Cardiology	11	.16%
Psychologist	254	3.67%
Social Worker	168	2.43%
Speech Therapist	9	.13%
Surgeon Assistant	13	.19%
Other nonphysician provider	35	.51%
Total	6,924	100.00%

27: FTE Nonphysician Providers

	Nonphysician Providers	
	Count	Percent
No Nonphysician providers	12	.17%
3 or fewer	436	6.30%
4 to 9	915	13.21%
10 or more	5,561	80.31%
Total	6,924	100.00%

28: Nonphysician Provider Clinical FTE

	Nonphysician Providers	
	Count	Percent
.40 to .60 FTE	284	4.11%
.61 to .69 FTE	41	.59%
.70 to .79 FTE	238	3.44%
.80 to .89 FTE	457	6.61%
.90 to .99 FTE	605	8.75%
1.00 FTE	5,286	76.49%
Total	6,911	100.00%

29: Nonphysician Provider Gender

	Nonphysician Providers	
	Count	Percent
Male	1,542	29.98%
Female	3,601	70.02%
Total	5,143	100.00%

30: Nonphysician Provider per FTE Physician

	Nonphysician Providers	
	Count	Percent
0.01 to .49 FTE	3,592	51.92%
0.50 to .99 FTE	1,475	21.32%
1.00 to 1.49 FTE	646	9.34%
1.50 to 1.99 FTE	226	3.27%
2.00 to 2.49 FTE	374	5.41%
2.50 to 2.99 FTE	271	3.92%
3.00 to 3.49 FTE	34	.49%
3.50 to 3.99 FTE	88	1.27%
4.00 to 4.49 FTE	8	.12%
4.50 or more	205	2.96%
Total	6,919	100.00%

31: FTE Nonphysician Providers per Group

	NPPs	Mean	Std Deviation	25th %tile	Median	75th %tile	90th %tile
FTE Nonphysician Providers	1,943	13.81	147.82	.00	1.60	5.75	19.00

Physician Compensation and Benefits

Table 1: Physician Compensation

	Phys	Med Pracs	Mean	Std. Dev.	25th %tile	Median	75th %tile	90th %tile
Allergy/Immunology	175	85	$295,873	$136,255	$208,263	$267,688	$340,967	$539,160
Anesthesiology	3,903	184	$399,222	$127,132	$324,679	$398,925	$453,692	$558,712
Anesthesiology: Pain Management	191	62	$481,595	$166,135	$380,000	$457,604	$561,833	$660,002
Anesthesiology: Pediatric	105	10	$377,938	$87,948	$348,598	$399,437	$429,139	$478,300
Cardiology: Electrophysiology	203	96	$499,667	$183,539	$370,000	$491,231	$581,762	$760,093
Cardiology: Invasive	528	139	$452,970	$149,346	$352,211	$431,533	$541,442	$661,560
Cardiology: Inv-Intvl	627	161	$537,858	$221,905	$392,590	$485,006	$630,000	$880,473
Cardiology: Noninvasive	516	138	$418,451	$138,842	$330,514	$410,784	$509,374	$598,576
Critical Care: Intensivist	97	20	$288,499	$78,960	$242,200	$281,773	$316,301	$403,144
Dentistry	58	18	$146,839	$65,530	$104,854	$124,433	$162,479	$229,924
Dermatology	361	128	$400,834	$195,891	$271,484	$357,945	$467,764	$680,096
Dermatology: Mohs Surgery	32	22	$716,489	$359,612	$443,000	$610,483	$870,738	$1,304,604
Emergency Medicine	976	60	$260,790	$76,117	$217,827	$256,800	$302,397	$353,246
Endocrinology/Metabolism	291	137	$211,550	$67,221	$167,980	$199,006	$246,099	$302,168
Family Practice (w/ OB)	789	141	$199,650	$66,332	$150,725	$187,393	$233,616	$290,016
Family Practice (w/o OB)	5,959	630	$187,953	$72,042	$139,457	$173,812	$220,472	$283,010
FP: Amb Only (no inpatient work)	236	28	$170,721	$61,879	$134,784	$158,106	$190,067	$224,716
Family Practice: Sports Med	37	27	$215,809	$78,449	$164,714	$205,026	$226,157	$312,380
Family Practice: Urgent Care	110	25	$201,364	$83,104	$143,668	$183,947	$235,249	$324,477
Gastroenterology	887	198	$457,053	$184,066	$331,697	$418,139	$541,784	$715,593
Gastroenterology: Hepatology	10	7	$368,184	$120,376	$276,989	$351,228	$487,625	$534,783
Genetics	11	5	$205,968	$38,055	$181,742	$219,256	$234,659	$244,955
Geriatrics	104	33	$177,128	$50,619	$146,996	$171,010	$203,406	$225,699
Hematology/Oncology	460	111	$449,520	$261,932	$291,899	$363,428	$515,784	$777,783
Hematology/Oncology: Onc (only)	300	32	$277,654	$132,965	$211,930	$243,567	$266,705	$404,718
Hospice/Palliative Care	11	10	$178,375	$56,493	$135,000	$180,300	$220,000	$265,536
Hospitalist: Family Practice	53	16	$201,663	$57,148	$166,000	$194,259	$235,101	$283,988
Hospitalist: Internal Medicine	1,185	148	$206,768	$56,086	$172,999	$197,872	$227,878	$275,067
Hospitalist: IM-Pediatrics	8	4	*	*	*	*	*	*
Hospitalist: Pediatrics	97	19	$162,439	$47,341	$137,500	$161,000	$175,065	$202,491
Infectious Disease	213	68	$202,840	$58,949	$158,084	$192,454	$245,627	$268,837
Internal Medicine: General	4,745	461	$201,603	$76,495	$149,875	$190,547	$236,879	$295,394
IM: Amb Only (no inpatient work)	39	16	$174,735	$45,359	$132,038	$181,291	$205,800	$237,225
Internal Med: Pediatrics	128	45	$192,678	$57,710	$148,808	$185,052	$218,336	$268,537
Nephrology	277	80	$305,602	$109,873	$223,077	$299,121	$354,528	$446,793
Neurology	637	185	$260,536	$108,122	$191,154	$227,670	$294,586	$412,170
Obstetrics/Gynecology: General	2,012	307	$302,362	$115,661	$222,647	$280,629	$360,099	$450,289
OB/GYN: Gynecology (only)	211	94	$226,545	$98,195	$151,852	$209,867	$279,622	$376,261
OB/GYN: Gyn Oncology	59	31	$356,264	$117,850	$272,065	$368,756	$425,119	$495,227
OB/GYN: Maternal & Fetal Med	107	37	$411,679	$186,310	$285,085	$375,000	$500,000	$672,996
OB/GYN: Repro Endocrinology	21	11	$408,679	$142,522	$294,300	$428,160	$552,396	$587,259
OB/GYN: Urogynecology	14	7	$351,571	$90,309	$294,386	$350,899	$366,910	$504,014
Occupational Medicine	158	58	$220,088	$75,385	$171,358	$213,004	$249,966	$298,196
Ophthalmology	589	146	$349,766	$164,380	$245,415	$315,982	$407,705	$586,957
Ophthalmology: Pediatric	37	26	$281,561	$118,855	$191,326	$263,169	$361,880	$429,726
Ophthalmology: Retina	65	33	$613,331	$409,216	$412,817	$538,508	$636,919	$963,467
Orthopedic (Nonsurgical)	47	36	$212,532	$96,539	$139,778	$189,751	$280,000	$343,702
Orthopedic Surgery: General	1,029	240	$497,136	$233,403	$359,654	$446,303	$595,643	$799,883
Orthopedic Surgery: Foot & Ankle	68	46	$522,587	$278,156	$327,115	$461,092	$593,857	$998,282
Orthopedic Surgery: Hand	156	81	$523,050	$255,264	$363,663	$450,371	$599,307	$839,984
Orthopedic Surgery: Hip & Joint	136	66	$592,231	$275,694	$395,150	$548,863	$739,145	$1,016,567
Orthopedic Surgery: Pediatric	41	22	$451,015	$123,585	$365,740	$469,410	$515,000	$590,119
Orthopedic Surgery: Spine	139	78	$607,770	$295,173	$396,402	$586,116	$775,299	$933,959
Orthopedic Surgery: Trauma	41	24	$529,224	$265,391	$372,322	$488,627	$635,678	$991,292
Orthopedic Surgery: Sports Med	195	82	$610,641	$299,155	$404,515	$553,344	$773,722	$1,000,396

Table 1: Physician Compensation (continued)

	Phys	Med Pracs	Mean	Std. Dev.	25th %tile	Median	75th %tile	90th %tile
Otorhinolaryngology	541	159	$394,506	$186,754	$277,943	$345,210	$467,524	$641,344
Pathology: Anatomic and Clinical	210	26	$360,757	$165,267	$276,912	$319,405	$385,145	$538,460
Pathology: Anatomic	33	8	$331,326	$178,221	$239,863	$278,000	$345,350	$668,306
Pathology: Clinical	49	14	$301,270	$121,757	$235,562	$246,587	$376,510	$482,372
Pediatrics: General	2,862	354	$196,936	$78,868	$143,512	$183,265	$233,520	$301,010
Pediatrics: Adolescent Medicine	71	11	$167,607	$53,511	$135,000	$164,000	$199,086	$220,864
Pediatrics: Allergy/Immunology	8	5	*	*	*	*	*	*
Pediatrics: Cardiology	63	22	$303,416	$92,144	$236,187	$269,859	$345,234	$486,700
Pediatrics: Child Development	18	10	$155,094	$32,083	$137,561	$148,978	$170,639	$195,007
Pediatrics: Critical Care/Intensivist	91	23	$279,677	$92,282	$210,000	$255,162	$339,750	$432,314
Pediatrics: Emergency Medicine	92	10	$215,142	$56,772	$186,292	$213,061	$249,193	$294,212
Pediatrics: Endocrinology	40	24	$188,979	$64,643	$150,000	$174,700	$216,274	$254,797
Pediatrics: Gastroenterology	42	20	$274,582	$94,062	$227,359	$249,721	$276,182	$419,857
Pediatrics: Genetics	22	15	$166,988	$35,825	$138,862	$160,798	$185,788	$235,893
Pediatrics: Hematology/Oncology	86	25	$209,628	$56,682	$177,182	$202,444	$234,263	$293,840
Pediatrics: Infectious Disease	20	9	$179,629	$57,971	$129,685	$161,830	$237,089	$268,831
Pediatrics: Neonatal Medicine	150	27	$313,208	$105,498	$243,593	$276,810	$381,819	$486,199
Pediatrics: Nephrology	13	9	$232,577	$67,872	$176,917	$217,610	$288,155	$354,826
Pediatrics: Neurology	66	31	$232,720	$92,246	$169,959	$203,804	$276,448	$415,562
Pediatrics: Pulmonology	25	14	$278,161	$89,975	$207,919	$257,865	$328,580	$450,081
Pediatrics: Rheumatology	11	6	$282,712	$217,012	$160,014	$171,596	$404,337	$705,528
Physiatry (Phys Med & Rehab)	248	98	$261,555	$123,901	$199,538	$234,338	$290,044	$379,687
Podiatry: General	145	88	$207,587	$86,037	$146,708	$185,819	$256,182	$335,014
Podiatry: Surg-Foot & Ankle	135	32	$244,175	$67,115	$200,922	$243,575	$275,457	$321,339
Podiatry: Surg-Forefoot Only	5	3	*	*	*	*	*	*
Psychiatry: General	494	93	$200,518	$61,609	$159,364	$194,038	$230,486	$268,040
Psychiatry: Child & Adolescent	100	33	$236,998	$87,387	$184,422	$226,561	$266,069	$335,414
Psychiatry: Geriatric	8	4	*	*	*	*	*	*
Pulmonary Medicine	253	100	$297,555	$115,250	$207,497	$274,358	$367,649	$452,453
Pulmonary Medicine: Critical Care	91	21	$316,023	$97,063	$256,250	$315,779	$366,085	$464,440
Pulmonary Med: Gen & Crit Care	177	46	$318,977	$113,817	$239,028	$299,516	$382,329	$460,342
Radiation Oncology	140	37	$528,225	$197,178	$366,911	$463,293	$668,188	$866,655
Radiology: Diagnostic-Inv	341	52	$507,508	$179,652	$404,177	$494,801	$611,064	$715,534
Radiology: Diagnostic-Noninv	874	85	$470,939	$160,903	$376,974	$450,658	$522,789	$687,357
Radiology: Nuclear Medicine	52	23	$437,213	$164,283	$341,003	$412,553	$492,297	$658,845
Rheumatology	287	134	$238,574	$96,241	$176,497	$218,704	$273,966	$364,911
Sleep Medicine	55	31	$339,255	$177,856	$207,656	$289,223	$425,000	$647,633
Surgery: General	1,024	257	$339,362	$129,732	$251,361	$316,909	$396,004	$499,180
Surgery: Bariatric	25	15	$385,616	$211,276	$248,500	$325,812	$440,796	$595,357
Surgery: Cardiovascular	245	69	$479,624	$159,400	$382,950	$461,860	$560,180	$673,722
Surgery: Colon and Rectal	46	20	$412,560	$165,907	$302,204	$377,030	$457,028	$700,216
Surgery: Neurological	237	77	$721,458	$394,276	$483,067	$637,895	$841,047	$1,200,051
Surgery: Oncology	19	13	$369,772	$107,016	$300,573	$331,250	$444,790	$544,353
Surgery: Oral	27	12	$425,567	$175,473	$299,217	$366,482	$510,695	$739,038
Surgery: Pediatric	59	27	$461,357	$156,857	$365,830	$450,000	$581,487	$636,290
Surgery: Plastic & Reconstruction	139	57	$434,021	$204,439	$307,677	$370,471	$520,231	$656,642
Surgery: Plastic & Recon-Hand	11	7	$406,413	$113,269	$354,507	$411,015	$494,300	$552,878
Surgery: Thoracic (primary)	59	22	$417,823	$179,041	$295,721	$415,699	$496,611	$640,675
Surgery: Transplant	31	10	$441,381	$174,783	$332,509	$402,410	$502,945	$616,282
Surgery: Trauma	68	19	$380,190	$132,064	$276,028	$363,187	$445,940	$531,172
Surgery: Trauma-Burn	4	2	*	*	*	*	*	*
Surgery: Vascular (primary)	197	71	$390,563	$133,437	$306,680	$378,894	$468,333	$590,409
Urgent Care	407	78	$213,458	$75,869	$160,102	$204,528	$256,685	$306,563
Urology	557	150	$427,471	$192,729	$309,984	$388,125	$480,855	$644,304
Urology: Pediatric	13	7	$388,603	$91,111	$319,798	$391,500	$453,264	$533,912

Table 2: Physician Compensation by Group Type

	Single Specialty			Multispecialty		
	Phys	Med Pracs	Median	Phys	Med Pracs	Median
Allergy/Immunology	36	9	$263,548	139	76	$267,688
Anesthesiology	3,211	128	$403,600	692	56	$362,095
Anesthesiology: Pain Management	116	27	$461,140	75	35	$440,059
Anesthesiology: Pediatric	24	3	$416,565	81	7	$398,234
Cardiology: Electrophysiology	139	62	$488,554	64	34	$516,985
Cardiology: Invasive	243	61	$434,814	285	78	$430,253
Cardiology: Inv-Intvl	394	83	$469,778	233	78	$500,000
Cardiology: Noninvasive	260	63	$426,746	256	75	$393,375
Critical Care: Intensivist	9	3	*	88	17	$281,466
Dentistry	13	2	*	45	16	$137,873
Dermatology	27	11	$377,450	334	117	$356,462
Dermatology: Mohs Surgery	1	1	*	31	21	$620,671
Emergency Medicine	379	17	$264,116	597	43	$253,561
Endocrinology/Metabolism	18	11	$210,601	273	126	$197,186
Family Practice (w/ OB)	95	27	$187,396	694	114	$187,170
Family Practice (w/o OB)	947	272	$162,375	5,012	358	$176,233
FP: Amb Only (no inpatient work)	20	7	$178,500	216	21	$157,266
Family Practice: Sports Med	8	7	*	29	20	$205,026
Family Practice: Urgent Care	31	3	$146,315	79	22	$205,538
Gastroenterology	320	39	$431,228	567	159	$412,511
Gastroenterology: Hepatology	6	5	*	4	2	*
Genetics	*	*	*	11	5	$219,256
Geriatrics	28	5	$203,406	76	28	$167,949
Hematology/Oncology	77	16	$571,359	383	95	$348,780
Hematology/Oncology: Onc (only)	7	4	*	293	28	$241,300
Hospice/Palliative Care	5	5	*	6	5	*
Hospitalist: Family Practice	2	2	*	51	14	$194,259
Hospitalist: Internal Medicine	131	18	$228,088	1,054	130	$194,300
Hospitalist: IM-Pediatrics	*	*	*	8	4	*
Hospitalist: Pediatrics	9	1	*	88	18	$162,000
Infectious Disease	22	9	$227,666	191	59	$189,687
Internal Medicine: General	375	92	$182,121	4,370	369	$191,204
IM: Amb Only (no inpatient work)	1	1	*	38	15	$181,682
Internal Med: Pediatrics	0	*	*	128	45	$185,052
Nephrology	64	9	$308,943	213	71	$297,513
Neurology	126	34	$237,411	511	151	$225,000
Obstetrics/Gynecology: General	443	85	$296,138	1,569	222	$277,631
OB/GYN: Gynecology (only)	35	20	$205,104	176	74	$213,451
OB/GYN: Gyn Oncology	6	4	*	53	27	$368,756
OB/GYN: Maternal & Fetal Med	25	8	$432,083	82	29	$353,433
OB/GYN: Repro Endocrinology	4	1	*	17	10	$368,449
OB/GYN: Urogynecology	*	*	*	14	7	$350,899
Occupational Medicine	2	1	*	156	57	$213,004
Ophthalmology	180	38	$338,655	409	108	$307,192
Ophthalmology: Pediatric	16	13	$220,420	21	13	$297,984
Ophthalmology: Retina	32	16	$551,751	33	17	$473,088
Orthopedic (Nonsurgical)	28	20	$207,365	19	16	$184,274
Orthopedic Surgery: General	329	84	$472,606	700	156	$439,970
Orthopedic Surgery: Foot & Ankle	49	33	$468,022	19	13	$435,258
Orthopedic Surgery: Hand	99	49	$447,000	57	32	$455,153
Orthopedic Surgery: Hip & Joint	97	47	$495,877	39	19	$615,991
Orthopedic Surgery: Pediatric	18	9	$460,681	23	13	$469,410
Orthopedic Surgery: Spine	85	52	$542,049	54	26	$609,358
Orthopedic Surgery: Trauma	27	16	$482,619	14	8	$498,147
Orthopedic Surgery: Sports Med	122	54	$560,609	73	28	$537,388

Table 2: Physician Compensation by Group Type (continued)

	Single Specialty			Multispecialty		
	Phys	Med Pracs	Median	Phys	Med Pracs	Median
Otorhinolaryngology	110	18	$342,583	431	141	$345,951
Pathology: Anatomic and Clinical	63	5	$414,128	147	21	$313,723
Pathology: Anatomic	*	*	*	33	8	$278,000
Pathology: Clinical	2	2	*	47	12	$246,587
Pediatrics: General	622	81	$208,451	2,240	273	$179,766
Pediatrics: Adolescent Medicine	9	2	*	62	9	$167,286
Pediatrics: Allergy/Immunology	2	1	*	6	4	*
Pediatrics: Cardiology	7	3	*	56	19	$258,152
Pediatrics: Child Development	*	*	*	18	10	$148,978
Pediatrics: Critical Care/Intensivist	7	1	*	84	22	$261,834
Pediatrics: Emergency Medicine	10	1	*	82	9	$211,542
Pediatrics: Endocrinology	4	2	*	36	22	$172,913
Pediatrics: Gastroenterology	2	2	*	40	18	$251,000
Pediatrics: Genetics	9	5	*	13	10	$158,542
Pediatrics: Hematology/Oncology	6	2	*	80	23	$202,444
Pediatrics: Infectious Disease	*	*	*	20	9	$161,830
Pediatrics: Neonatal Medicine	25	6	$262,428	125	21	$280,000
Pediatrics: Nephrology	*	*	*	13	9	$217,610
Pediatrics: Neurology	4	2	*	62	29	$195,756
Pediatrics: Pulmonology	4	2	*	21	12	$257,865
Pediatrics: Rheumatology	*	*	*	11	6	$171,596
Physiatry (Phys Med & Rehab)	58	24	$252,051	190	74	$226,775
Podiatry: General	5	5	*	140	83	$186,065
Podiatry: Surg-Foot & Ankle	2	2	*	133	30	$244,052
Podiatry: Surg-Forefoot Only	1	1	*	4	2	*
Psychiatry: General	44	5	$149,722	450	88	$199,173
Psychiatry: Child & Adolescent	5	2	*	95	31	$228,526
Psychiatry: Geriatric	4	1	*	4	3	*
Pulmonary Medicine	27	7	$329,263	226	93	$273,180
Pulmonary Medicine: Critical Care	7	4	*	84	17	$314,252
Pulmonary Med: Gen & Crit Care	56	10	$275,492	121	36	$306,075
Radiation Oncology	20	5	$866,555	120	32	$452,946
Radiology: Diagnostic-Inv	189	19	$512,000	152	33	$476,762
Radiology: Diagnostic-Noninv	273	21	$475,249	601	64	$436,535
Radiology: Nuclear Medicine	15	8	$423,882	37	15	$386,421
Rheumatology	22	11	$183,478	265	123	$222,274
Sleep Medicine	4	1	*	51	30	$272,755
Surgery: General	129	34	$275,000	895	223	$322,707
Surgery: Bariatric	6	3	*	19	12	$385,041
Surgery: Cardiovascular	94	23	$447,841	151	46	$468,382
Surgery: Colon and Rectal	*	*	*	46	20	$377,030
Surgery: Neurological	46	13	$712,497	191	64	$626,712
Surgery: Oncology	1	1	*	18	12	$331,250
Surgery: Oral	8	3	*	19	9	$366,482
Surgery: Pediatric	18	5	$473,816	41	22	$438,573
Surgery: Plastic & Reconstruction	15	4	$380,305	124	53	$366,145
Surgery: Plastic & Recon-Hand	2	2	*	9	5	*
Surgery: Thoracic (primary)	12	5	$322,921	47	17	$419,179
Surgery: Transplant	6	1	*	25	9	$402,410
Surgery: Trauma	10	3	$357,005	58	16	$363,187
Surgery: Trauma-Burn	*	*	*	4	2	*
Surgery: Vascular (primary)	25	10	$374,776	172	61	$379,225
Urgent Care	17	5	$199,292	390	73	$204,704
Urology	186	23	$414,537	371	127	$378,606
Urology: Pediatric	5	3	*	8	4	*

Table 3A: Physician Compensation by Size of Multispecialty Practice (50 or fewer FTE Physicians)

	10 FTE or fewer		11 to 25 FTE		26 to 50 FTE	
	Phys	Median	Phys	Median	Phys	Median
Allergy/Immunology	7	*	3	*	13	$245,758
Anesthesiology	12	$254,196	30	$430,275	19	$359,800
Anesthesiology: Pain Management	8	*	8	*	7	*
Anesthesiology: Pediatric	*	*	*	*	11	*
Cardiology: Electrophysiology	*	*	6	*	15	$593,732
Cardiology: Invasive	5	*	16	$439,450	47	$320,917
Cardiology: Inv-Intvl	*	*	26	$554,866	34	$477,872
Cardiology: Noninvasive	2	*	7	*	66	$473,370
Critical Care: Intensivist	6	*	*	*	6	*
Dentistry	1	*	11	$106,500	*	*
Dermatology	5	*	2	*	34	$328,861
Dermatology: Mohs Surgery	*	*	1	*	5	*
Emergency Medicine	10	*	18	$273,465	57	$236,450
Endocrinology/Metabolism	5	*	9	*	39	$199,436
Family Practice (w/ OB)	46	$192,201	132	$184,333	120	$194,346
Family Practice (w/o OB)	224	$156,501	418	$165,744	816	$175,847
FP: Amb Only (no inpatient work)	9	*	24	$152,711	43	$142,608
Family Practice: Sports Med	1	*	2	*	7	*
Family Practice: Urgent Care	3	*	2	*	37	$200,243
Gastroenterology	6	*	22	$389,469	74	$429,430
Geriatrics	*	*	16	*	2	*
Hematology/Oncology	8	*	18	$380,495	56	$476,426
Hematology/Oncology: Onc (only)	1	*	5	*	12	$291,500
Hospice/Palliative Care	2	*	*	*	*	*
Hospitalist: Family Practice	1	*	1	*	9	*
Hospitalist: Internal Medicine	24	$220,847	71	$199,000	94	$192,077
Hospitalist: IM-Pediatrics	*	*	*	*	1	*
Hospitalist: Pediatrics	*	*	2	*	4	*
Infectious Disease	3	*	5	*	9	*
Internal Medicine: General	128	$162,076	326	$172,330	534	$192,470
IM: Amb Only (no inpatient work)	4	*	6	*	8	*
Internal Med: Pediatrics	24	$174,917	15	$215,126	25	$201,720
Nephrology	4	*	18	$346,437	21	$281,555
Neurology	19	$240,492	23	$222,200	64	$238,695
Obstetrics/Gynecology: General	30	$273,725	104	$278,423	237	$273,144
OB/GYN: Gynecology (only)	4	*	9	*	22	$179,008
OB/GYN: Gyn Oncology	2	*	2	*	1	*
OB/GYN: Maternal & Fetal Med	3	*	2	*	3	*
OB/GYN: Repro Endocrinology	1	*	*	*	*	*
Occupational Medicine	4	*	3	*	15	$215,000
Ophthalmology	14	$421,457	4	*	30	$304,594
Ophthalmology: Pediatric	0	*	*	*	2	*
Ophthalmology: Retina	3	*	*	*	1	*
Orthopedic (Nonsurgical)	*	*	*	*	3	*
Orthopedic Surgery: General	38	$387,118	47	$425,335	86	$452,811
Orthopedic Surgery: Foot & Ankle	2	*	5	*	0	*
Orthopedic Surgery: Hand	4	*	9	*	1	*
Orthopedic Surgery: Hip & Joint	4	*	9	*	0	*
Orthopedic Surgery: Pediatric	*	*	1	*	*	*
Orthopedic Surgery: Spine	3	*	7	*	2	*
Orthopedic Surgery: Trauma	*	*	3	*	*	*
Orthopedic Surgery: Sports Med	7	*	13	$668,666	2	*

Table 3A: Physician Compensation by Size of Multispecialty Practice (50 or fewer FTE Physicians) (continued)

	10 FTE or fewer		11 to 25 FTE		26 to 50 FTE	
	Phys	Median	Phys	Median	Phys	Median
Otorhinolaryngology	16	$585,718	6	*	53	$374,638
Pathology: Anatomic and Clinical	5	*	5	*	*	*
Pathology: Clinical	*	*	0	*	*	*
Pediatrics: General	70	$160,470	135	$168,262	262	$164,319
Pediatrics: Adolescent Medicine	3	*	1	*	4	*
Pediatrics: Cardiology	*	*	*	*	1	*
Pediatrics: Child Development	2	*	2	*	2	*
Pediatrics: Critical Care/Intensivist	*	*	5	*	15	$266,403
Pediatrics: Emergency Medicine	30	*	3	*	17	*
Pediatrics: Endocrinology	5	*	1	*	5	*
Pediatrics: Gastroenterology	*	*	1	*	3	*
Pediatrics: Genetics	2	*	*	*	1	*
Pediatrics: Hematology/Oncology	11	*	9	*	9	*
Pediatrics: Infectious Disease	3	*	*	*	*	*
Pediatrics: Neonatal Medicine	*	*	*	*	8	*
Pediatrics: Nephrology	*	*	*	*	2	*
Pediatrics: Neurology	1	*	*	*	7	*
Pediatrics: Pulmonology	*	*	2	*	5	*
Pediatrics: Rheumatology	2	*	*	*	*	*
Physiatry (Phys Med & Rehab)	6	*	12	$256,125	7	*
Podiatry: General	3	*	9	*	26	$156,962
Podiatry: Surg-Foot & Ankle	1	*	5	*	1	*
Podiatry: Surg-Forefoot Only	*	*	2	*	*	*
Psychiatry: General	9	*	8	*	40	$194,813
Psychiatry: Child & Adolescent	4	*	*	*	4	*
Pulmonary Medicine	1	*	13	$250,000	25	$264,438
Pulmonary Medicine: Critical Care	18	*	11	*	6	*
Pulmonary Med: Gen & Crit Care	12	$370,000	15	$440,783	18	$305,890
Radiation Oncology	5	*	7	*	13	$561,043
Radiology: Diagnostic-Inv	3	*	*	*	19	$453,032
Radiology: Diagnostic-Noninv	8	*	2	*	32	$395,381
Radiology: Nuclear Medicine	*	*	2	*	1	*
Rheumatology	8	*	8	*	26	$221,118
Sleep Medicine	2	*	3	*	5	*
Surgery: General	36	$265,873	61	$275,018	118	$294,371
Surgery: Bariatric	2	*	*	*	4	*
Surgery: Cardiovascular	4	*	10	$489,483	19	$453,333
Surgery: Colon and Rectal	4	*	4	*	1	*
Surgery: Neurological	14	$538,854	22	$776,032	9	*
Surgery: Oncology	2	*	4	*	*	*
Surgery: Oral	*	*	*	*	2	*
Surgery: Pediatric	*	*	5	*	6	*
Surgery: Plastic & Reconstruction	1	*	1	*	6	*
Surgery: Plastic & Recon-Hand	*	*	*	*	2	*
Surgery: Thoracic (primary)	*	*	5	*	3	*
Surgery: Trauma	2	*	9	*	*	*
Surgery: Vascular (primary)	5	*	8	*	23	$339,424
Urgent Care	6	*	11	$161,157	22	$171,912
Urology	10	$524,848	9	*	47	$325,523
Urology: Pediatric	*	*	*	*	4	*

Table 3B: Physician Compensation by Size of Multispecialty Practice (51 or more FTE Physicians)

	51 to 75 FTE		76 to 150 FTE		151 FTE or more	
	Phys	Median	Phys	Median	Phys	Median
Allergy/Immunology	15	$300,450	23	$272,298	78	$259,644
Anesthesiology	116	$352,867	94	$396,245	421	$360,677
Anesthesiology: Pain Management	13	*	19	$528,336	20	$385,414
Anesthesiology: Pediatric	25	*	20	*	25	*
Cardiology: Electrophysiology	3	*	14	$402,499	26	$465,614
Cardiology: Invasive	9	*	60	$465,363	148	$429,126
Cardiology: Inv-Intvl	20	$551,924	54	$508,355	99	$483,402
Cardiology: Noninvasive	5	*	40	$350,657	136	$390,226
Critical Care: Intensivist	1	*	7	*	68	$282,664
Dentistry	17	*	9	*	7	*
Dermatology	31	$425,402	81	$378,959	181	$353,898
Dermatology: Mohs Surgery	*	*	4	*	21	$519,000
Emergency Medicine	27	$195,655	98	$256,800	387	$255,878
Endocrinology/Metabolism	24	$195,163	69	$199,006	127	$195,375
Family Practice (w/ OB)	43	$186,948	95	$184,043	258	$184,935
Family Practice (w/o OB)	537	$181,116	899	$178,862	2,118	$178,422
FP: Amb Only (no inpatient work)	14	*	26	$166,850	100	$170,021
Family Practice: Sports Med	4	*	5	*	10	$198,216
Family Practice: Urgent Care	4	*	23	$235,000	10	*
Gastroenterology	51	$385,250	139	$443,656	275	$404,391
Gastroenterology: Hepatology	*	*	3	*	1	*
Genetics	*	*	1	*	10	$224,671
Geriatrics	6	*	12	$168,215	40	$166,765
Hematology/Oncology	21	$514,598	72	$407,670	208	$310,469
Hematology/Oncology: Onc (only)	10	$675,825	8	*	257	$237,979
Hospice/Palliative Care	*	*	*	*	4	*
Hospitalist: Family Practice	3	*	25	$200,154	12	*
Hospitalist: Internal Medicine	87	$189,288	186	$204,772	592	$189,452
Hospitalist: IM-Pediatrics	*	*	7	*	*	*
Hospitalist: Pediatrics	30	*	21	$148,913	31	$166,000
Infectious Disease	5	*	30	$218,388	139	$185,422
Internal Medicine: General	422	$187,298	847	$193,348	2,113	$194,285
IM: Amb Only (no inpatient work)	10	*	6	*	4	*
Internal Med: Pediatrics	2	*	26	$197,850	36	$175,316
Nephrology	16	$339,222	54	$292,223	100	$294,325
Neurology	33	$253,914	121	$239,928	251	$220,210
Obstetrics/Gynecology: General	117	$317,493	256	$290,872	825	$275,004
OB/GYN: Gynecology (only)	20	$215,433	41	$225,529	80	$216,181
OB/GYN: Gyn Oncology	*	*	7	*	41	$368,756
OB/GYN: Maternal & Fetal Med	1	*	33	$354,466	40	$356,539
OB/GYN: Repro Endocrinology	*	*	*	*	16	$376,234
OB/GYN: Urogynecology	*	*	1	*	13	$349,594
Occupational Medicine	4	*	23	$195,171	107	$221,009
Ophthalmology	40	$295,406	79	$355,000	242	$302,029
Ophthalmology: Pediatric	1	*	7	*	11	$297,984
Ophthalmology: Retina	0	*	4	*	25	$454,221
Orthopedic (Nonsurgical)	3	*	3	*	10	$194,876
Orthopedic Surgery: General	48	$440,928	130	$512,840	351	$438,580
Orthopedic Surgery: Foot & Ankle	*	*	6	*	6	*
Orthopedic Surgery: Hand	4	*	13	$652,841	26	$434,500
Orthopedic Surgery: Hip & Joint	1	*	6	*	19	$574,224
Orthopedic Surgery: Pediatric	1	*	8	*	13	$458,058
Orthopedic Surgery: Spine	4	*	18	$552,773	20	$670,251
Orthopedic Surgery: Trauma	0	*	6	*	5	*
Orthopedic Surgery: Sports Med	4	*	24	$763,846	23	$373,845

Table 3B: Physician Compensation by Size of Multispecialty Practice (51 or more FTE Physicians) (continued)

	51 to 75 FTE		76 to 150 FTE		151 FTE or more	
	Phys	Median	Phys	Median	Phys	Median
Otorhinolaryngology	31	$368,444	107	$324,670	218	$345,103
Pathology: Anatomic and Clinical	4	*	16	$281,783	117	$316,688
Pathology: Anatomic	*	*	4	*	29	$278,000
Pathology: Clinical	*	*	26	$261,350	21	$239,400
Pediatrics: General	250	$182,952	506	$179,642	1,017	$185,022
Pediatrics: Adolescent Medicine	1	*	*	*	53	$169,500
Pediatrics: Allergy/Immunology	*	*	1	*	5	*
Pediatrics: Cardiology	7	*	8	*	40	$267,891
Pediatrics: Child Development	*	*	1	*	11	$150,000
Pediatrics: Critical Care/Intensivist	24	*	13	$255,000	27	$269,145
Pediatrics: Emergency Medicine	7	*	*	*	25	$274,782
Pediatrics: Endocrinology	3	*	3	*	19	$197,222
Pediatrics: Gastroenterology	5	*	4	*	27	$260,000
Pediatrics: Genetics	3	*	2	*	5	*
Pediatrics: Hematology/Oncology	5		15	$180,271	31	$226,939
Pediatrics: Infectious Disease	*	*	4	*	13	$195,545
Pediatrics: Neonatal Medicine	11	*	34	$431,139	72	$266,099
Pediatrics: Nephrology	2	*	*	*	9	*
Pediatrics: Neurology	7	*	12	$156,543	35	$205,604
Pediatrics: Pulmonology	0	*	2	*	12	$252,872
Pediatrics: Rheumatology	2	*	5	*	2	*
Physiatry (Phys Med & Rehab)	5	*	34	$233,887	126	$225,822
Podiatry: General	16	$189,393	32	$192,781	54	$203,046
Podiatry: Surg-Foot & Ankle	8	*	17	$300,365	101	$242,433
Podiatry: Surg-Forefoot Only	*	*	*	*	2	*
Psychiatry: General	22	$208,917	88	$171,680	283	$207,804
Psychiatry: Child & Adolescent	3	*	7	*	77	$234,495
Psychiatry: Geriatric	*	*	2	*	2	*
Pulmonary Medicine	24	$280,720	70	$286,750	93	$274,731
Pulmonary Medicine: Critical Care	19	$327,431	10	$300,109	20	$318,546
Pulmonary Med: Gen & Crit Care	8	*	22	$323,191	46	$266,392
Radiation Oncology	16	*	13	$458,213	66	$412,694
Radiology: Diagnostic-Inv	17	$450,087	20	$535,292	93	$496,147
Radiology: Diagnostic-Noninv	100	$459,642	70	$474,823	389	$429,168
Radiology: Nuclear Medicine	7	*	2	*	25	$365,922
Rheumatology	26	$240,841	71	$241,540	126	$212,160
Sleep Medicine	3	*	16	$264,484	22	$293,345
Surgery: General	64	$320,827	190	$324,844	426	$333,537
Surgery: Bariatric	*	*	7	*	6	*
Surgery: Cardiovascular	1	*	25	$450,000	92	$496,225
Surgery: Colon and Rectal	2	*	16	$453,472	19	$353,814
Surgery: Neurological	7	*	32	$666,896	107	$600,000
Surgery: Oncology	*	*	5	*	7	*
Surgery: Oral	1	*	6	*	10	$350,779
Surgery: Pediatric	3	*	6	*	21	$435,752
Surgery: Plastic & Reconstruction	7		28	$431,415	81	$354,287
Surgery: Plastic & Recon-Hand	1	*	*	*	6	*
Surgery: Thoracic (primary)	1	*	3	*	35	$450,802
Surgery: Transplant	*	*	4	*	21	$400,000
Surgery: Trauma	0	*	10	$463,446	37	$351,957
Surgery: Trauma-Burn	*	*	*	*	4	*
Surgery: Vascular (primary)	12	$379,907	44	$396,588	80	$393,861
Urgent Care	21	$161,827	115	$209,637	215	$218,148
Urology	35	$376,746	78	$402,798	192	$384,777
Urology: Pediatric	1	*	2	*	1	*

Table 4: Physician Compensation by Hospital Ownership

	Hospital Owned			Not Hospital Owned		
	Phys	Med Pracs	Median	Phys	Med Pracs	Median
Allergy/Immunology	31	21	$246,380	144	64	$271,061
Anesthesiology	217	29	$385,673	3,653	154	$400,000
Anesthesiology: Pain Management	20	11	$400,967	171	51	$461,140
Anesthesiology: Pediatric	43	3	$423,155	62	7	$370,739
Cardiology: Electrophysiology	38	18	$546,823	165	78	$469,024
Cardiology: Invasive	105	28	$471,765	423	111	$422,641
Cardiology: Inv-Intvl	89	31	$502,499	538	130	$480,644
Cardiology: Noninvasive	118	33	$414,223	398	105	$409,204
Critical Care: Intensivist	23	8	$226,345	74	12	$291,940
Dentistry	9	6	*	49	12	$116,646
Dermatology	84	37	$320,385	277	91	$362,956
Dermatology: Mohs Surgery	7	5	*	25	17	$724,441
Emergency Medicine	343	28	$235,370	633	32	$272,844
Endocrinology/Metabolism	131	60	$189,824	160	77	$203,671
Family Practice (w/ OB)	347	66	$186,900	442	75	$187,421
Family Practice (w/o OB)	3,361	370	$167,231	2,598	260	$185,273
FP: Amb Only (no inpatient work)	134	15	$142,078	102	13	$178,321
Family Practice: Sports Med	16	11	$178,503	21	16	$212,366
Family Practice: Urgent Care	48	11	$210,109	62	14	$171,091
Gastroenterology	145	50	$404,300	742	148	$425,280
Gastroenterology: Hepatology	3	1	*	7	6	*
Genetics	3	2	*	8	3	*
Geriatrics	48	18	$167,949	56	15	$172,854
Hematology/Oncology	115	31	$309,361	345	80	$382,958
Hematology/Oncology: Onc (only)	14	11	$313,918	286	21	$241,094
Hospice/Palliative Care	8	7	*	3	3	*
Hospitalist: Family Practice	35	10	$180,000	18	6	$227,078
Hospitalist: Internal Medicine	755	81	$194,300	430	67	$206,601
Hospitalist: IM-Pediatrics	6	3	*	2	1	*
Hospitalist: Pediatrics	52	13	$167,114	45	6	$155,000
Infectious Disease	66	30	$189,349	147	38	$193,489
Internal Medicine: General	2,067	227	$173,359	2,678	234	$204,319
IM: Amb Only (no inpatient work)	33	11	$183,235	6	5	*
Internal Med: Pediatrics	69	21	$168,607	59	24	$203,343
Nephrology	44	22	$243,992	233	58	$306,914
Neurology	229	74	$213,271	408	111	$238,796
Obstetrics/Gynecology: General	688	122	$265,381	1,324	185	$290,001
OB/GYN: Gynecology (only)	96	34	$218,830	115	60	$196,594
OB/GYN: Gyn Oncology	31	20	$340,000	28	11	$388,167
OB/GYN: Maternal & Fetal Med	59	22	$361,375	48	15	$385,012
OB/GYN: Repro Endocrinology	6	5	*	15	6	$462,983
OB/GYN: Urogynecology	6	5	*	8	2	*
Occupational Medicine	46	26	$177,200	112	32	$223,475
Ophthalmology	93	29	$305,029	496	117	$318,139
Ophthalmology: Pediatric	4	3	*	33	23	$263,169
Ophthalmology: Retina	7	5	*	58	28	$538,714
Orthopedic (Nonsurgical)	5	4	*	42	32	$183,637
Orthopedic Surgery: General	212	61	$398,905	817	179	$455,619
Orthopedic Surgery: Foot & Ankle	3	2	*	65	44	$467,183
Orthopedic Surgery: Hand	6	6	*	150	75	$449,500
Orthopedic Surgery: Hip & Joint	7	4	*	129	62	$548,126
Orthopedic Surgery: Pediatric	11	5	$511,183	30	17	$463,734
Orthopedic Surgery: Spine	10	6	$646,398	129	72	$567,734
Orthopedic Surgery: Trauma	3	3	*	38	21	$489,387
Orthopedic Surgery: Sports Med	14	9	$399,213	181	73	$563,866

Table 4: Physician Compensation by Hospital Ownership (continued)

	Hospital Owned			Not Hospital Owned		
	Phys	Med Pracs	Median	Phys	Med Pracs	Median
Otorhinolaryngology	107	41	$315,900	434	118	$351,433
Pathology: Anatomic and Clinical	43	8	$314,415	167	18	$321,086
Pathology: Anatomic	9	3	*	24	5	$276,500
Pathology: Clinical	20	5	$239,400	29	9	$256,240
Pediatrics: General	1,347	162	$178,592	1,515	192	$188,606
Pediatrics: Adolescent Medicine	21	6	$172,543	50	5	$159,266
Pediatrics: Allergy/Immunology	1	1	*	7	4	*
Pediatrics: Cardiology	35	12	$270,000	28	10	$267,891
Pediatrics: Child Development	13	7	$154,570	5	3	*
Pediatrics: Critical Care/Intensivist	54	16	$263,548	37	7	$250,000
Pediatrics: Emergency Medicine	71	6	$212,060	21	4	$223,329
Pediatrics: Endocrinology	26	16	$174,700	14	8	$185,108
Pediatrics: Gastroenterology	20	10	$257,038	22	10	$246,793
Pediatrics: Genetics	14	10	$159,306	8	5	*
Pediatrics: Hematology/Oncology	52	15	$200,352	34	10	$209,252
Pediatrics: Infectious Disease	11	5	$149,895	9	4	*
Pediatrics: Neonatal Medicine	75	17	$252,000	75	10	$284,954
Pediatrics: Nephrology	4	4	*	9	5	*
Pediatrics: Neurology	36	17	$208,529	30	14	$192,131
Pediatrics: Pulmonology	17	10	$254,821	8	4	*
Pediatrics: Rheumatology	3	2	*	8	4	*
Physiatry (Phys Med & Rehab)	83	34	$220,165	165	64	$236,462
Podiatry: General	47	26	$173,782	98	62	$189,279
Podiatry: Surg-Foot & Ankle	19	6	$230,888	116	26	$244,867
Podiatry: Surg-Forefoot Only	*	*	*	5	3	*
Psychiatry: General	219	60	$183,000	275	33	$203,038
Psychiatry: Child & Adolescent	46	21	$205,762	54	12	$242,243
Psychiatry: Geriatric	3	2	*	5	2	*
Pulmonary Medicine	105	33	$251,265	148	67	$294,827
Pulmonary Medicine: Critical Care	18	5	$335,434	73	16	$289,670
Pulmonary Med: Gen & Crit Care	24	11	$299,657	153	35	$299,516
Radiation Oncology	43	15	$434,802	97	22	$538,089
Radiology: Diagnostic-Inv	43	12	$612,878	298	40	$491,049
Radiology: Diagnostic-Noninv	124	18	$428,000	750	67	$461,594
Radiology: Nuclear Medicine	11	6	$500,000	41	17	$379,808
Rheumatology	107	45	$205,245	180	89	$225,755
Sleep Medicine	12	10	$294,195	43	21	$289,223
Surgery: General	345	98	$307,206	679	159	$323,971
Surgery: Bariatric	10	7	$296,681	15	8	$395,543
Surgery: Cardiovascular	87	28	$501,950	158	41	$454,116
Surgery: Colon and Rectal	9	4	*	37	16	$374,509
Surgery: Neurological	93	35	$561,665	144	42	$700,323
Surgery: Oncology	10	6	$323,041	9	7	*
Surgery: Oral	3	2	*	24	10	$370,042
Surgery: Pediatric	26	14	$425,877	33	13	$466,875
Surgery: Plastic & Reconstruction	43	19	$350,000	96	38	$392,464
Surgery: Plastic & Recon-Hand	*	*	*	11	7	$411,015
Surgery: Thoracic (primary)	21	11	$467,500	38	11	$349,210
Surgery: Transplant	15	5	$421,644	16	5	$401,205
Surgery: Trauma	53	15	$354,870	15	4	$403,830
Surgery: Trauma-Burn	4	2	*	*	*	*
Surgery: Vascular (primary)	48	20	$441,390	149	51	$364,534
Urgent Care	145	29	$180,346	262	49	$221,797
Urology	90	40	$348,672	467	110	$396,349
Urology: Pediatric	5	2	*	8	5	*

Table 5A: Physician Compensation by Geographic Section for All Practices

	Eastern		Midwest		Southern		Western	
	Phys	Median	Phys	Median	Phys	Median	Phys	Median
Allergy/Immunology	21	$329,994	56	$273,542	37	$272,298	61	$237,857
Anesthesiology	912	$403,600	731	$412,694	857	$433,990	1,403	$358,252
Anesthesiology: Pain Management	46	$403,600	75	$472,496	50	$494,413	20	$459,372
Anesthesiology: Pediatric	4	*	28	$418,637	56	$397,551	17	*
Cardiology: Electrophysiology	41	$469,527	61	$526,543	72	$497,993	29	$368,802
Cardiology: Invasive	71	$439,489	122	$441,140	172	$466,700	163	$397,659
Cardiology: Inv-Intvl	88	$455,586	171	$511,141	206	$543,228	162	$440,000
Cardiology: Noninvasive	187	$400,000	158	$468,124	111	$400,281	60	$375,707
Critical Care: Intensivist	20	$223,960	11	$250,000	5	*	61	$295,361
Dentistry	16	$181,327	*	*	18	$113,609	24	$120,749
Dermatology	63	$290,570	94	$391,815	58	$362,628	146	$361,122
Dermatology: Mohs Surgery	6	*	12	$780,111	2	*	12	$457,341
Emergency Medicine	240	$239,778	220	$276,827	146	$256,800	370	$263,598
Endocrinology/Metabolism	69	$177,815	69	$209,364	81	$204,863	72	$210,746
Family Practice (w/ OB)	97	$159,330	386	$195,268	149	$190,012	157	$174,146
Family Practice (w/o OB)	1,087	$156,782	2,100	$173,782	1,451	$182,589	1,321	$182,322
FP: Amb Only (no inpatient work)	33	$130,474	34	$153,509	91	$167,360	78	$162,265
Family Practice: Sports Med	10	$206,612	12	$165,300	7	*	8	*
Family Practice: Urgent Care	18	$187,943	34	$220,200	47	$160,000	11	$168,434
Gastroenterology	146	$396,697	263	$466,130	195	$407,539	283	$404,300
Gastroenterology: Hepatology	1	*	1	*	3	*	5	*
Genetics	0	*	3	*	1	*	7	*
Geriatrics	14	$155,548	17	$181,924	14	$187,971	59	$170,844
Hematology/Oncology	102	$373,300	108	$413,974	113	$429,790	137	$324,000
Hematology/Oncology: Onc (only)	10	$404,509	11	$501,179	12	$446,584	267	$238,604
Hospice/Palliative Care	4	*	1	*	3	*	3	*
Hospitalist: Family Practice	6	*	16	$209,305	24	$197,498	7	*
Hospitalist: Internal Medicine	266	$181,443	330	$193,971	249	$219,170	340	$191,819
Hospitalist: IM-Pediatrics	5	*	*	*	3	*	*	*
Hospitalist: Pediatrics	6	*	10	$169,819	32	$170,392	49	$154,145
Infectious Disease	53	$189,010	91	$175,838	26	$206,800	43	$242,000
Internal Medicine: General	981	$163,365	1,189	$188,261	1,028	$197,307	1,547	$203,791
IM: Amb Only (no inpatient work)	18	$180,691	4	*	12	$205,800	5	*
Internal Med: Pediatrics	27	$179,837	63	$198,763	26	$163,251	12	$198,716
Nephrology	70	$245,364	69	$307,214	44	$317,926	94	$298,923
Neurology	183	$212,538	147	$242,985	135	$248,300	172	$227,795
Obstetrics/Gynecology: General	375	$237,053	569	$307,381	410	$300,100	658	$278,674
OB/GYN: Gynecology (only)	56	$200,000	82	$251,771	50	$187,206	23	$183,000
OB/GYN: Gyn Oncology	10	$324,556	13	$400,000	17	$300,870	19	$410,972
OB/GYN: Maternal & Fetal Med	24	$334,605	28	$355,014	26	$336,996	29	$436,441
OB/GYN: Repro Endocrinology	3	*	3	*	6	*	9	*
OB/GYN: Urogynecology	5	*	1	*	*	*	8	*
Occupational Medicine	8	*	42	$206,807	21	$177,840	87	$222,692
Ophthalmology	87	$275,000	179	$360,802	140	$343,038	183	$301,035
Ophthalmology: Pediatric	6	*	11	$337,167	12	$223,396	8	*
Ophthalmology: Retina	7	*	26	$556,958	14	$595,934	18	$436,737
Orthopedic (Nonsurgical)	6	*	22	$180,613	12	$226,015	7	*
Orthopedic Surgery: General	154	$414,389	312	$525,513	200	$405,394	363	$434,088
Orthopedic Surgery: Foot & Ankle	13	$435,258	23	$405,365	19	$497,844	13	$578,953
Orthopedic Surgery: Hand	29	$432,000	49	$448,099	28	$498,616	50	$440,602
Orthopedic Surgery: Hip & Joint	35	$519,927	50	$576,597	24	$533,661	27	$549,601
Orthopedic Surgery: Pediatric	2	*	6	*	23	$458,058	10	$495,026
Orthopedic Surgery: Spine	31	$472,687	40	$590,355	30	$523,305	38	$600,413
Orthopedic Surgery: Trauma	9	*	8	*	13	$539,873	11	$482,619
Orthopedic Surgery: Sports Med	50	$464,259	39	$621,384	51	$563,866	55	$551,171

Table 5A: Physician Compensation by Geographic Section for All Practices (continued)

	Eastern		Midwest		Southern		Western	
	Phys	Median	Phys	Median	Phys	Median	Phys	Median
Otorhinolaryngology	66	$335,650	137	$384,123	136	$357,000	202	$335,434
Pathology: Anatomic and Clinical	38	$258,920	59	$382,512	32	$416,359	81	$319,766
Pathology: Anatomic	8	*	17	$272,571	3	*	5	*
Pathology: Clinical	11	*	6	*	23	$258,543	9	*
Pediatrics: General	493	$160,000	848	$181,997	746	$203,247	775	$191,481
Pediatrics: Adolescent Medicine	8	*	3	*	48	$160,720	12	*
Pediatrics: Allergy/Immunology	*	*	3	*	3	*	2	*
Pediatrics: Cardiology	8	*	10	$293,168	22	$364,568	23	$255,104
Pediatrics: Child Development	5	*	5	*	7	*	1	*
Pediatrics: Critical Care/Intensivist	11	$222,900	29	$255,000	27	$339,750	24	$250,000
Pediatrics: Emergency Medicine	1	*	47	$203,216	32	*	12	$200,800
Pediatrics: Endocrinology	9	*	14	$174,700	11	$231,682	6	*
Pediatrics: Gastroenterology	10	$260,000	7	*	7	*	18	$246,793
Pediatrics: Genetics	11	$155,557	2	*	3	*	6	*
Pediatrics: Hematology/Oncology	8	*	22	$205,567	31	$200,704	25	$206,929
Pediatrics: Infectious Disease	1	*	4	*	8	*	7	*
Pediatrics: Neonatal Medicine	29	$243,965	36	$286,076	11	$376,106	74	$280,396
Pediatrics: Nephrology	1	*	4	*	3	*	5	*
Pediatrics: Neurology	9	*	20	$239,607	18	$241,620	19	$182,229
Pediatrics: Pulmonology	4	*	6	*	11	$267,599	4	*
Pediatrics: Rheumatology	1	*	2	*	3	*	5	*
Physiatry (Phys Med & Rehab)	41	$216,803	63	$226,825	54	$236,157	90	$239,833
Podiatry: General	12	$160,080	63	$180,003	32	$186,000	38	$199,493
Podiatry: Surg-Foot & Ankle	10	$238,639	38	$273,227	1	*	86	$234,886
Podiatry: Surg-Forefoot Only	*	*	2	*	2	*	1	*
Psychiatry: General	113	$171,912	153	$180,001	54	$183,349	174	$218,038
Psychiatry: Child & Adolescent	13	$339,465	26	$164,790	14	$212,484	47	$252,378
Psychiatry: Geriatric	5	*	1	*	*	*	2	*
Pulmonary Medicine	49	$270,133	70	$299,929	73	$269,043	61	$266,511
Pulmonary Medicine: Critical Care	1	*	39	$290,763	18	$312,603	33	$349,937
Pulmonary Med: Gen & Crit Care	34	$255,650	48	$306,648	53	$352,166	42	$265,507
Radiation Oncology	12	$348,000	27	$427,000	35	$631,669	66	$434,803
Radiology: Diagnostic-Inv	35	$483,760	58	$565,304	137	$517,000	111	$468,739
Radiology: Diagnostic-Noninv	164	$398,708	192	$498,862	132	$462,542	386	$428,722
Radiology: Nuclear Medicine	5	*	9	*	15	$461,000	23	$350,017
Rheumatology	49	$206,422	80	$222,056	68	$246,821	90	$212,455
Sleep Medicine	13	$188,966	6	*	25	$297,346	11	$307,860
Surgery: General	150	$264,415	317	$361,218	216	$298,517	341	$325,427
Surgery: Bariatric	12	$256,463	7	*	3	*	3	*
Surgery: Cardiovascular	51	$446,588	60	$460,633	81	$452,277	53	$488,099
Surgery: Colon and Rectal	18	$346,488	10	$424,546	9	*	9	*
Surgery: Neurological	48	$565,186	43	$807,650	66	$605,981	80	$634,548
Surgery: Oncology	8	*	*	*	8	*	3	*
Surgery: Oral	10	$433,621	7	*	3	*	7	*
Surgery: Pediatric	5	*	15	$458,604	25	$489,029	14	$455,265
Surgery: Plastic & Reconstruction	31	$336,305	28	$451,895	27	$406,610	53	$364,789
Surgery: Plastic & Recon-Hand	1	*	5	*	2	*	3	*
Surgery: Thoracic (primary)	11	$337,500	10	$369,983	6	*	32	$420,345
Surgery: Transplant	7	*	7	*	6	*	11	$458,614
Surgery: Trauma	24	$277,505	11	$403,830	31	$404,138	2	*
Surgery: Trauma-Burn	3	*	*	*	1	*	*	*
Surgery: Vascular (primary)	39	$362,921	47	$362,500	53	$430,316	58	$384,758
Urgent Care	26	$183,632	111	$207,976	69	$180,346	201	$212,125
Urology	86	$384,584	117	$388,125	189	$414,043	165	$380,000
Urology: Pediatric	1	*	5	*	3	*	4	*

Table 5B: Physician Compensation by Geographic Section for Single-Specialty Practices

	Eastern		Midwest		Southern		Western	
	Phys	Median	Phys	Median	Phys	Median	Phys	Median
Allergy/Immunology	9	*	3	*	17	$199,000	7	*
Anesthesiology	814	$403,600	609	$424,954	691	$438,404	1,097	$356,101
Anesthesiology: Pain Management	34	$403,600	48	$507,090	19	$448,204	15	$461,140
Anesthesiology: Pediatric	1	*	16	*	*	*	7	*
Cardiology: Electrophysiology	22	$490,810	42	$517,361	59	$482,052	16	$368,449
Cardiology: Invasive	30	$431,078	66	$440,140	104	$459,682	43	$373,715
Cardiology: Inv-Intvl	60	$458,239	111	$456,810	156	$500,849	67	$399,728
Cardiology: Noninvasive	83	$425,000	86	$494,096	79	$403,344	12	$273,903
Critical Care: Intensivist	3	*	1	*	5	*	*	*
Dentistry	*	*	*	*	1	*	12	*
Dermatology	15	$299,251	7	*	3	*	2	*
Dermatology: Mohs Surgery	1	*	0	*	*	*	*	*
Emergency Medicine	100	$262,500	83	$280,945	81	$273,629	115	$238,860
Endocrinology/Metabolism	9	*	3	*	6	*	*	*
Family Practice (w/ OB)	12	$155,665	37	$251,518	9	*	37	$149,285
Family Practice (w/o OB)	310	$160,797	165	$150,681	357	$172,268	115	$147,049
FP: Amb Only (no inpatient work)	1	*	2	*	10	*	7	*
Family Practice: Sports Med	2	*	2	*	2	*	2	*
Family Practice: Urgent Care	*	*	*	*	30	*	1	*
Gastroenterology	47	$450,000	123	$473,354	93	$412,882	57	$392,800
Gastroenterology: Hepatology	1	*	1	*	3	*	1	*
Geriatrics	2	*	0	*	5	*	21	*
Hematology/Oncology	24	$619,597	12	$683,420	31	$385,696	10	*
Hematology/Oncology: Onc (only)	4	*	1	*	*	*	2	*
Hospice/Palliative Care	1	*	*	*	3	*	1	*
Hospitalist: Family Practice	*	*	*	*	2	*	*	*
Hospitalist: Internal Medicine	31	$223,468	31	$212,124	59	$234,026	10	*
Hospitalist: Pediatrics	*	*	*	*	9	*	*	*
Infectious Disease	9	*	4	*	8	*	1	*
Internal Medicine: General	141	$179,195	69	$185,171	138	$185,988	27	$160,934
IM: Amb Only (no inpatient work)	1	*	*	*	*	*	*	*
Internal Med: Pediatrics	0	*	*	*	*	*	*	*
Nephrology	37	$327,912	11	$309,880	5	*	11	*
Neurology	63	$237,174	7	*	38	$245,936	18	$224,042
Obstetrics/Gynecology: General	103	$261,699	98	$300,701	146	$319,990	96	$285,528
OB/GYN: Gynecology (only)	11	$205,104	5	*	16	$225,225	3	*
OB/GYN: Gyn Oncology	*	*	4	*	2	*	*	*
OB/GYN: Maternal & Fetal Med	7	*	3	*	9	*	6	*
OB/GYN: Repro Endocrinology	*	*	*	*	4	*	*	*
Occupational Medicine	0	*	2	*	*	*	*	*
Ophthalmology	41	$285,000	64	$371,928	65	$323,482	10	$267,577
Ophthalmology: Pediatric	4	*	8	*	4	*	0	*
Ophthalmology: Retina	3	*	19	$548,467	10	$595,934	*	*
Orthopedic (Nonsurgical)	5	*	13	$179,547	8	*	2	*
Orthopedic Surgery: General	64	$406,109	131	$537,169	89	$471,611	45	$407,212
Orthopedic Surgery: Foot & Ankle	8	*	18	$417,922	15	$497,844	8	*
Orthopedic Surgery: Hand	18	$483,059	31	$436,322	20	$507,748	30	$430,914
Orthopedic Surgery: Hip & Joint	25	$475,047	44	$542,827	14	$496,400	14	$474,056
Orthopedic Surgery: Pediatric	1	*	3	*	14	$496,332	*	*
Orthopedic Surgery: Spine	19	$472,687	30	$590,355	21	$536,453	15	$494,509
Orthopedic Surgery: Trauma	6	*	6	*	6	*	9	*
Orthopedic Surgery: Sports Med	29	$459,639	28	$658,443	34	$571,712	31	$513,877

Table 5B: Physician Compensation by Geographic Section for Single-Specialty Practices (continued)

	Eastern		Midwest		Southern		Western	
	Phys	Median	Phys	Median	Phys	Median	Phys	Median
Otorhinolaryngology	14	$310,267	7	*	63	$395,115	26	$285,625
Pathology: Anatomic and Clinical	*	*	27	$306,693	27	*	9	*
Pathology: Clinical	*	*	*	*	1	*	1	*
Pediatrics: General	161	$173,265	121	$215,885	272	$232,108	68	$201,221
Pediatrics: Adolescent Medicine	2	*	*	*	7	*	*	*
Pediatrics: Allergy/Immunology	*	*	*	*	*	*	2	*
Pediatrics: Cardiology	2	*	2	*	3	*	*	*
Pediatrics: Critical Care/Intensivist	*	*	7	*	*	*	*	*
Pediatrics: Emergency Medicine	0	*	*	*	10	*	*	*
Pediatrics: Endocrinology	*	*	*	*	3	*	1	*
Pediatrics: Gastroenterology	1	*	1	*	*	*	*	*
Pediatrics: Genetics	9	*	*	*	*	*	*	*
Pediatrics: Hematology/Oncology	*	*	*	*	5	*	1	*
Pediatrics: Neonatal Medicine	4	*	*	*	10	$387,813	11	*
Pediatrics: Neurology	*	*	2	*	2	*	*	*
Pediatrics: Pulmonology	*	*	*	*	4	*	0	*
Physiatry (Phys Med & Rehab)	15	$238,913	8	*	24	$244,118	11	$304,874
Podiatry: General	2	*	2	*	*	*	1	*
Podiatry: Surg-Foot & Ankle	1	*	1	*	*	*	*	*
Podiatry: Surg-Forefoot Only	*	*	*	*	*	*	1	*
Psychiatry: General	17	$155,000	18	*	9	*	*	*
Psychiatry: Child & Adolescent	*	*	3	*	2	*	*	*
Psychiatry: Geriatric	4	*	*	*	*	*	*	*
Pulmonary Medicine	16	$367,649	1	*	10	$241,353	*	*
Pulmonary Medicine: Critical Care	1	*	3	*	1	*	2	*
Pulmonary Med: Gen & Crit Care	5	*	20	*	20	$329,847	11	*
Radiation Oncology	2	*	7	*	11	*	*	*
Radiology: Diagnostic-Inv	15	$508,784	24	$561,713	108	$514,608	42	$488,734
Radiology: Diagnostic-Noninv	65	$505,044	86	$499,621	72	$467,263	50	$426,143
Radiology: Nuclear Medicine	3	*	2	*	9	*	1	*
Rheumatology	*	*	11	$175,200	10	$306,947	1	*
Sleep Medicine	*	*	*	*	4	*	*	*
Surgery: General	37	$254,500	13	$320,049	62	$275,865	17	$305,949
Surgery: Bariatric	4	*	*	*	2	*	*	*
Surgery: Cardiovascular	27	$406,895	16	$449,755	41	$449,966	10	$625,000
Surgery: Neurological	*	*	6	*	22	$652,609	18	$700,323
Surgery: Oncology	1	*	*	*	*	*	*	*
Surgery: Oral	6	*	*	*	2	*	*	*
Surgery: Pediatric	*	*	7	*	11	*	*	*
Surgery: Plastic & Reconstruction	7	*	1	*	7	*	*	*
Surgery: Plastic & Recon-Hand	1	*	*	*	1	*	*	*
Surgery: Thoracic (primary)	6	*	1	*	1	*	4	*
Surgery: Transplant	*	*	*	*	6	*	*	*
Surgery: Trauma	*	*	3	*	7	*	*	*
Surgery: Vascular (primary)	5	*	7	*	13	$408,725	0	*
Urgent Care	3	*	9	*	3	*	2	*
Urology	16	$422,149	10	$373,254	135	$416,105	25	$449,266
Urology: Pediatric	1	*	*	*	3	*	1	*

Table 5C: Physician Compensation by Geographic Section for Multispecialty Practices

	Eastern		Midwest		Southern		Western	
	Phys	Median	Phys	Median	Phys	Median	Phys	Median
Allergy/Immunology	12	$273,672	53	$272,234	20	$299,712	54	$243,754
Anesthesiology	98	$327,000	122	$387,620	166	$380,981	306	$361,506
Anesthesiology: Pain Management	12	$429,098	27	$410,956	31	$520,268	5	*
Anesthesiology: Pediatric	3	*	12	*	56	$397,551	10	*
Cardiology: Electrophysiology	19	$457,978	19	$547,240	13	$598,184	13	$369,770
Cardiology: Invasive	41	$439,489	56	$445,497	68	$477,285	120	$403,443
Cardiology: Inv-Intvl	28	$452,097	60	$574,496	50	$651,987	95	$445,234
Cardiology: Noninvasive	104	$382,644	72	$447,551	32	$388,573	48	$390,226
Critical Care: Intensivist	17	$226,345	10	$250,000	0	*	61	$295,361
Dentistry	16	$181,327	*	*	17	$113,905	12	*
Dermatology	48	$288,169	87	$390,548	55	$358,049	144	$361,122
Dermatology: Mohs Surgery	5	*	12	$780,111	2	*	12	$457,341
Emergency Medicine	140	$223,567	137	$274,248	65	$226,824	255	$270,141
Endocrinology/Metabolism	60	$175,503	66	$204,690	75	$204,863	72	$210,746
Family Practice (w/ OB)	85	$160,805	349	$191,779	140	$187,340	120	$181,158
Family Practice (w/o OB)	777	$154,980	1,935	$175,333	1,094	$185,254	1,206	$186,374
FP: Amb Only (no inpatient work)	32	$130,459	32	$147,581	81	$167,360	71	$161,012
Family Practice: Sports Med	8	*	10	$165,014	5	*	6	*
Family Practice: Urgent Care	18	$187,943	34	$220,200	17	$235,000	10	$174,134
Gastroenterology	99	$382,836	140	$450,297	102	$406,586	226	$409,034
Gastroenterology: Hepatology	*	*	*	*	*	*	4	*
Genetics	0	*	3	*	1	*	7	*
Geriatrics	12	$145,056	17	$181,924	9	*	38	$165,200
Hematology/Oncology	78	$331,107	96	$402,962	82	$432,769	127	$320,561
Hematology/Oncology: Onc (only)	6	*	10	$459,946	12	$446,584	265	$238,504
Hospice/Palliative Care	3	*	1	*	0	*	2	*
Hospitalist: Family Practice	6	*	16	$209,305	22	$201,444	7	*
Hospitalist: Internal Medicine	235	$177,697	299	$192,071	190	$216,831	330	$191,298
Hospitalist: IM-Pediatrics	5	*	*	*	3	*	*	*
Hospitalist: Pediatrics	6	*	10	$169,819	23	$175,065	49	$154,145
Infectious Disease	44	$174,500	87	$175,894	18	$206,800	42	$242,164
Internal Medicine: General	840	$161,472	1,120	$188,676	890	$197,849	1,520	$204,319
IM: Amb Only (no inpatient work)	17	$182,073	4	*	12	$205,800	5	*
Internal Med: Pediatrics	27	$179,837	63	$198,763	26	$163,251	12	$198,716
Nephrology	33	$215,404	58	$301,238	39	$340,544	83	$298,401
Neurology	120	$206,472	140	$242,889	97	$248,300	154	$228,386
Obstetrics/Gynecology: General	272	$231,953	471	$308,804	264	$289,753	562	$277,708
OB/GYN: Gynecology (only)	45	$198,984	77	$253,524	34	$160,733	20	$171,989
OB/GYN: Gyn Oncology	10	$324,556	9	*	15	$309,918	19	$410,972
OB/GYN: Maternal & Fetal Med	17	$312,203	25	$341,091	17	$375,309	23	$436,441
OB/GYN: Repro Endocrinology	3	*	3	*	2	*	9	*
OB/GYN: Urogynecology	5	*	1	*	*	*	8	*
Occupational Medicine	8	*	40	$206,807	21	$177,840	87	$222,692
Ophthalmology	46	$259,684	115	$343,736	75	$365,950	173	$301,664
Ophthalmology: Pediatric	2	*	3	*	8	*	8	*
Ophthalmology: Retina	4	*	7	*	4	*	18	$436,737
Orthopedic (Nonsurgical)	1	*	9	*	4	*	5	*
Orthopedic Surgery: General	90	$420,317	181	$512,093	111	$375,000	318	$434,924
Orthopedic Surgery: Foot & Ankle	5	*	5	*	4	*	5	*
Orthopedic Surgery: Hand	11	$393,000	18	$484,726	8	*	20	$493,316
Orthopedic Surgery: Hip & Joint	10	$580,669	6	*	10	$631,086	13	$574,224
Orthopedic Surgery: Pediatric	1	*	3	*	9	*	10	$495,026
Orthopedic Surgery: Spine	12	$476,575	10	$566,303	9	*	23	$631,393
Orthopedic Surgery: Trauma	3	*	2	*	7	*	2	*
Orthopedic Surgery: Sports Med	21	$530,663	11	$486,133	17	$464,517	24	$763,846

Table 5C: Physician Compensation by Geographic Section for Multispecialty Practices (continued)

	Eastern		Midwest		Southern		Western	
	Phys	Median	Phys	Median	Phys	Median	Phys	Median
Otorhinolaryngology	52	$359,932	130	$384,712	73	$350,956	176	$337,407
Pathology: Anatomic and Clinical	38	$258,920	32	$382,512	5	*	72	$314,695
Pathology: Anatomic	8	*	17	$272,571	3	*	5	*
Pathology: Clinical	11	*	6	*	22	$258,505	8	*
Pediatrics: General	332	$159,044	727	$179,994	474	$186,832	707	$191,152
Pediatrics: Adolescent Medicine	6	*	3	*	41	$164,000	12	*
Pediatrics: Allergy/Immunology	*	*	3	*	3	*	0	*
Pediatrics: Cardiology	6	*	8	*	19	$384,135	23	$255,104
Pediatrics: Child Development	5	*	5	*	7	*	1	*
Pediatrics: Critical Care/Intensivist	11	$222,900	22	$261,834	27	$339,750	24	$250,000
Pediatrics: Emergency Medicine	1	*	47	$203,216	22	*	12	$200,800
Pediatrics: Endocrinology	9	*	14	$174,700	8	*	5	*
Pediatrics: Gastroenterology	9	*	6	*	7	*	18	$246,793
Pediatrics: Genetics	2	*	2	*	3	*	6	*
Pediatrics: Hematology/Oncology	8	*	22	$205,567	26	$214,555	24	$199,280
Pediatrics: Infectious Disease	1	*	4	*	8	*	7	*
Pediatrics: Neonatal Medicine	25	$250,859	36	$286,076	1	*	63	$282,483
Pediatrics: Nephrology	1	*	4	*	3	*	5	*
Pediatrics: Neurology	9	*	18	$226,136	16	$252,846	19	$182,229
Pediatrics: Pulmonology	4	*	6	*	7	*	4	*
Pediatrics: Rheumatology	1	*	2	*	3	*	5	*
Physiatry (Phys Med & Rehab)	26	$214,344	55	$221,321	30	$222,605	79	$234,819
Podiatry: General	10	$165,763	61	$180,003	32	$186,000	37	$199,925
Podiatry: Surg-Foot & Ankle	9	*	37	$273,533	1	*	86	$234,886
Podiatry: Surg-Forefoot Only	*	*	2	*	2	*	*	*
Psychiatry: General	96	$175,722	135	$189,939	45	$183,270	174	$218,038
Psychiatry: Child & Adolescent	13	$339,465	23	$165,720	12	$214,183	47	$252,378
Psychiatry: Geriatric	1	*	1	*	*	*	2	*
Pulmonary Medicine	33	$248,549	69	$299,077	63	$269,750	61	$266,511
Pulmonary Medicine: Critical Care	*	*	36	$304,690	17	$312,481	31	$327,431
Pulmonary Med: Gen & Crit Care	29	$244,435	28	$330,397	33	$353,631	31	$266,717
Radiation Oncology	10	$348,000	20	$411,735	24	$560,518	66	$434,803
Radiology: Diagnostic-Inv	20	$472,913	34	$591,877	29	$649,413	69	$458,385
Radiology: Diagnostic-Noninv	99	$384,211	106	$496,955	60	$444,767	336	$428,722
Radiology: Nuclear Medicine	2	*	7	*	6	*	22	$349,793
Rheumatology	49	$206,422	69	$231,437	58	$241,392	89	$213,620
Sleep Medicine	13	$188,966	6	*	21	$270,351	11	$307,860
Surgery: General	113	$270,321	304	$361,351	154	$300,819	324	$325,518
Surgery: Bariatric	8	*	7	*	1	*	3	*
Surgery: Cardiovascular	24	$461,138	44	$460,633	40	$467,468	43	$486,861
Surgery: Colon and Rectal	18	$346,488	10	$424,546	9	*	9	*
Surgery: Neurological	48	$565,186	37	$704,607	44	$567,391	62	$611,658
Surgery: Oncology	7	*	*	*	8	*	3	*
Surgery: Oral	4	*	7	*	1	*	7	*
Surgery: Pediatric	5	*	8	*	14	$478,957	14	$455,265
Surgery: Plastic & Reconstruction	24	$314,056	27	$464,859	20	$386,056	53	$364,789
Surgery: Plastic & Recon-Hand	*	*	5	*	1	*	3	*
Surgery: Thoracic (primary)	5	*	9	*	5	*	28	$418,082
Surgery: Transplant	7	*	7	*	*	*	11	$458,614
Surgery: Trauma	24	$277,505	8	*	24	$438,259	2	*
Surgery: Trauma-Burn	3	*	*	*	1	*	*	*
Surgery: Vascular (primary)	34	$386,961	40	$354,314	40	$433,213	58	$384,758
Urgent Care	23	$182,940	102	$220,817	66	$178,827	199	$212,125
Urology	70	$380,500	107	$394,308	54	$387,936	140	$373,922
Urology: Pediatric	*	*	5	*	*	*	3	*

Table 6: Physician Compensation by Demographic Classification

	Nonmetropolitan (fewer than 50,000)		Metropolitan (50,000 to 250,000)		Metropolitan (250,001 to 1,000,000)		Metropolitan (more than 1,000,000)	
	Phys	Median	Phys	Median	Phys	Median	Phys	Median
Allergy/Immunology	8	*	45	$268,128	53	$292,008	68	$242,064
Anesthesiology	189	$348,178	848	$397,886	1,431	$403,600	1,435	$370,086
Anesthesiology: Pain Management	12	$376,636	55	$500,000	92	$440,644	31	$461,140
Anesthesiology: Pediatric	*	*	1	*	31	$418,496	73	$388,423
Cardiology: Electrophysiology	6	*	59	$513,537	71	$469,024	67	$442,152
Cardiology: Invasive	32	$477,761	179	$457,828	118	$425,584	196	$412,778
Cardiology: Inv-Intvl	36	$554,077	202	$508,181	174	$469,411	211	$454,082
Cardiology: Noninvasive	38	$382,644	161	$389,600	159	$431,206	156	$400,437
Critical Care: Intensivist	8	*	17	$250,000	20	$253,484	52	$290,739
Dentistry	10	$153,577	4	*	21	$117,639	23	$125,008
Dermatology	33	$314,705	89	$390,548	97	$367,208	140	$343,909
Dermatology: Mohs Surgery	4	*	5	*	11	$765,938	12	$457,341
Emergency Medicine	64	$223,123	295	$256,800	191	$245,180	426	$263,737
Endocrinology/Metabolism	23	$199,436	87	$199,006	108	$184,672	69	$225,304
Family Practice (w/ OB)	263	$189,320	261	$195,394	167	$173,499	95	$175,860
Family Practice (w/o OB)	1,040	$170,643	1,793	$178,862	1,842	$172,465	1,204	$173,668
FP: Amb Only (no inpatient work)	26	$155,743	100	$163,487	62	$140,457	31	*
Family Practice: Sports Med	7	*	12	$211,354	12	$208,949	6	*
Family Practice: Urgent Care	2	*	44	$232,015	38	$179,918	26	$145,829
Gastroenterology	57	$425,216	259	$445,124	235	$399,780	333	$408,765
Gastroenterology: Hepatology	*	*	1	*	1	*	8	*
Genetics	*	*	1	*	2	*	8	*
Geriatrics	4	*	32	$164,755	36	$196,680	32	$169,273
Hematology/Oncology	43	$280,210	142	$457,929	119	$365,900	149	$335,053
Hematology/Oncology: Onc (only)	9	*	19	$653,046	8	*	264	$238,371
Hospice/Palliative Care	3	*	4	*	2	*	2	*
Hospitalist: Family Practice	4	*	44	$183,606	4	*	*	*
Hospitalist: Internal Medicine	80	$180,403	317	$218,312	446	$197,878	335	$189,811
Hospitalist: IM-Pediatrics	1	*	0	*	7	*	*	*
Hospitalist: Pediatrics	4	*	6	*	16	$166,986	71	$155,094
Infectious Disease	8	*	40	$204,407	65	$189,687	100	$189,008
Internal Medicine: General	478	$177,565	1,347	$184,387	1,329	$181,567	1,551	$203,791
IM: Amb Only (no inpatient work)	7	*	23	$199,416	6	*	*	*
Internal Med: Pediatrics	15	$209,598	43	$179,837	45	$209,777	23	$171,634
Nephrology	30	$274,428	89	$328,860	68	$285,108	85	$291,131
Neurology	61	$229,765	186	$239,443	211	$213,196	179	$237,426
Obstetrics/Gynecology: General	269	$277,122	525	$275,000	567	$294,786	633	$276,852
OB/GYN: Gynecology (only)	16	$192,998	78	$195,497	64	$199,492	52	$241,017
OB/GYN: Gyn Oncology	1	*	15	$404,435	25	$365,000	18	$372,027
OB/GYN: Maternal & Fetal Med	5	*	29	$307,262	48	$343,258	25	$437,260
OB/GYN: Repro Endocrinology	1	*	2	*	4	*	14	$470,445
OB/GYN: Urogynecology	2	*	*	*	4	*	8	*
Occupational Medicine	6	*	47	$193,763	33	$210,674	72	$221,258
Ophthalmology	55	$321,806	167	$353,064	158	$324,407	206	$302,029
Ophthalmology: Pediatric	3	*	7	*	10	$214,736	17	$337,546
Ophthalmology: Retina	2	*	17	$651,257	14	$595,934	32	$458,855
Orthopedic (Nonsurgical)	1	*	13	$184,274	17	$212,918	16	$182,340
Orthopedic Surgery: General	178	$469,898	265	$414,100	267	$464,708	317	$448,001
Orthopedic Surgery: Foot & Ankle	6	*	10	$307,468	28	$496,507	24	$504,376
Orthopedic Surgery: Hand	9	*	29	$538,819	63	$432,000	55	$450,742
Orthopedic Surgery: Hip & Joint	12	$572,634	22	$617,411	50	$454,927	52	$554,798
Orthopedic Surgery: Pediatric	1	*	4	*	7	*	29	$488,395
Orthopedic Surgery: Spine	17	$611,670	30	$492,636	45	$526,262	47	$631,393
Orthopedic Surgery: Trauma	4	*	11	$549,284	22	$480,051	4	*
Orthopedic Surgery: Sports Med	17	$405,000	38	$484,405	81	$564,562	59	$576,038

Table 6: Physician Compensation by Demographic Classification (continued)

	Nonmetropolitan (fewer than 50,000)		Metropolitan (50,000 to 250,000)		Metropolitan (250,001 to 1,000,000)		Metropolitan (more than 1,000,000)	
	Phys	Median	Phys	Median	Phys	Median	Phys	Median
Otorhinolaryngology	71	$320,792	139	$383,796	171	$369,752	158	$334,473
Pathology: Anatomic and Clinical	29	$287,199	47	$365,434	2	*	132	$321,670
Pathology: Anatomic	*	*	5	*	12	$271,786	16	$296,570
Pathology: Clinical	3	*	20	$393,681	13	$256,240	13	$239,400
Pediatrics: General	330	$168,670	780	$177,311	730	$182,499	1,007	$196,090
Pediatrics: Adolescent Medicine	4	*	5	*	1	*	61	$164,000
Pediatrics: Allergy/Immunology	*	*	3	*	3	*	2	*
Pediatrics: Cardiology	5	*	7	*	13	$257,369	38	$292,896
Pediatrics: Child Development	2	*	3	*	5	*	8	*
Pediatrics: Critical Care/Intensivist	3	*	24	$225,595	26	$266,404	38	$295,725
Pediatrics: Emergency Medicine	1	*	3	*	18	$195,000	70	$214,303
Pediatrics: Endocrinology	3	*	7	*	13	$174,700	17	$191,027
Pediatrics: Gastroenterology	5	*	6	*	10	$253,038	21	$247,479
Pediatrics: Genetics	1	*	1	*	11	$155,557	8	*
Pediatrics: Hematology/Oncology	3	*	9	*	18	$195,781	56	$205,567
Pediatrics: Infectious Disease	*	*	1	*	2	*	17	$173,765
Pediatrics: Neonatal Medicine	4	*	19	$250,000	50	$285,794	77	$282,483
Pediatrics: Nephrology	1	*	*	*	4	*	8	*
Pediatrics: Neurology	6	*	8	*	26	$192,274	26	$219,421
Pediatrics: Pulmonology	2	*	2	*	9	*	12	$256,343
Pediatrics: Rheumatology	1	*	*	*	3	*	7	*
Physiatry (Phys Med & Rehab)	14	$216,000	53	$246,305	83	$224,819	97	$234,662
Podiatry: General	28	$143,151	59	$203,358	36	$173,749	21	$199,060
Podiatry: Surg-Foot & Ankle	9	*	11	$245,844	23	$297,799	92	$238,664
Podiatry: Surg-Forefoot Only	*	*	2	*	3	*	*	*
Psychiatry: General	57	$189,025	104	$183,000	149	$173,705	165	$220,400
Psychiatry: Child & Adolescent	4	*	16	$186,727	22	$210,865	55	$237,617
Psychiatry: Geriatric	*	*	4	*	1	*	3	*
Pulmonary Medicine	31	$245,487	94	$294,685	82	$287,810	46	$263,834
Pulmonary Medicine: Critical Care	*	*	26	$267,778	57	$337,010	8	*
Pulmonary Med: Gen & Crit Care	18	$269,824	83	$352,166	40	$296,975	31	$260,907
Radiation Oncology	12	$410,035	16	$582,239	35	$398,440	75	$508,320
Radiology: Diagnostic-Inv	16	$611,064	92	$503,537	161	$520,993	72	$470,000
Radiology: Diagnostic-Noninv	52	$475,839	136	$476,716	333	$467,059	352	$434,350
Radiology: Nuclear Medicine	1	*	7	*	14	$420,695	30	$377,089
Rheumatology	26	$236,771	82	$213,292	88	$230,644	91	$208,640
Sleep Medicine	6	*	21	$272,755	13	$295,588	15	$340,450
Surgery: General	192	$309,897	292	$308,848	253	$324,660	284	$326,151
Surgery: Bariatric	1	*	7	*	15	$325,812	2	*
Surgery: Cardiovascular	14	$490,216	67	$467,468	84	$408,638	80	$474,447
Surgery: Colon and Rectal	2	*	13	$408,709	21	$395,086	10	$293,587
Surgery: Neurological	9	*	69	$653,963	81	$653,099	76	$636,128
Surgery: Oncology	2	*	4	*	7	*	6	*
Surgery: Oral	2	*	10	$481,845	1	*	14	$348,673
Surgery: Pediatric	2	*	9	*	20	$408,248	28	$478,032
Surgery: Plastic & Reconstruction	12	$277,692	42	$422,075	39	$374,913	46	$362,115
Surgery: Plastic & Recon-Hand	1	*	2	*	1	*	7	*
Surgery: Thoracic (primary)	2	*	14	$332,671	8	*	35	$416,986
Surgery: Transplant	2	*	1	*	11	$400,000	17	$434,804
Surgery: Trauma	4	*	22	$442,418	25	$335,535	17	$344,464
Surgery: Trauma-Burn	*	*	1	*	3	*	*	*
Surgery: Vascular (primary)	14	$372,629	46	$417,883	69	$392,291	68	$362,991
Urgent Care	24	$171,298	132	$206,356	146	$210,260	104	$205,135
Urology	59	$365,732	135	$418,047	142	$409,893	219	$385,383
Urology: Pediatric	*	*	*	*	6	*	7	*

Table 7A: Physician Compensation by Practice Total Medical Revenue

	$2,000,000 or less		$2,000,001 to $5,000,000		$5,000,001 to $10,000,000	
	Phys	Median	Phys	Median	Phys	Median
Allergy/Immunology	6	*	11	$225,000	8	*
Anesthesiology	67	$358,255	126	$368,400	486	$380,000
Anesthesiology: Pain Management	2	*	10	$427,796	22	$561,833
Cardiology: Electrophysiology	2	*	7	*	17	$438,900
Cardiology: Invasive	5	*	3	*	56	$398,023
Cardiology: Inv-Intvl	8	*	26	$363,662	65	$469,923
Cardiology: Noninvasive	4	*	7	*	34	$415,506
Critical Care: Intensivist	5	*	5	*	2	*
Dentistry	1	*	*	*	9	*
Dermatology	8	*	10	$405,769	13	$299,251
Dermatology: Mohs Surgery	*	*	1	*	*	*
Emergency Medicine	10	*	23	$266,128	128	$262,500
Endocrinology/Metabolism	16	$199,980	9	*	3	*
Family Practice (w/ OB)	50	$179,832	55	$204,124	91	$177,537
Family Practice (w/o OB)	425	$155,000	437	$164,327	409	$161,916
FP: Amb Only (no inpatient work)	23	$141,547	22	$163,932	26	$144,778
Family Practice: Sports Med	*	*	3	*	2	*
Family Practice: Urgent Care	7	*	2	*	2	*
Gastroenterology	8	*	27	$419,477	125	$359,084
Gastroenterology: Hepatology	1	*	*	*	2	*
Geriatrics	16	*	5	*	9	*
Hematology/Oncology	9	*	4	*	8	*
Hematology/Oncology: Onc (only)	1	*	2	*	1	*
Hospice/Palliative Care	6	*	*	*	1	*
Hospitalist: Family Practice	7	*	2	*	4	*
Hospitalist: Internal Medicine	61	$233,871	85	$215,026	75	$214,858
Hospitalist: Pediatrics	12	*	*	*	2	*
Infectious Disease	15	$219,934	12	$227,708	2	*
Internal Medicine: General	127	$163,365	217	$175,400	244	$170,808
IM: Amb Only (no inpatient work)	3	*	3	*	8	*
Internal Med: Pediatrics	11	$137,128	8	*	9	*
Nephrology	1	*	19	$293,559	25	$306,914
Neurology	39	$228,034	66	$225,535	44	$240,512
Obstetrics/Gynecology: General	42	$228,392	159	$242,018	276	$318,742
OB/GYN: Gynecology (only)	3	*	19	$183,000	16	$275,952
OB/GYN: Gyn Oncology	5	*	1	*	3	*
OB/GYN: Maternal & Fetal Med	3	*	12	$255,067	5	*
OB/GYN: Repro Endocrinology	*	*	*	*	5	*
Occupational Medicine	3	*	3	*	3	*
Ophthalmology	11	$250,000	19	$301,116	76	$361,581
Ophthalmology: Pediatric	*	*	2	*	3	*
Ophthalmology: Retina	1	*	0	*	5	*
Orthopedic (Nonsurgical)	3	*	*	*	4	*
Orthopedic Surgery: General	35	$392,386	40	$392,153	117	$424,012
Orthopedic Surgery: Foot & Ankle	*	*	1	*	13	$468,022
Orthopedic Surgery: Hand	7	*	4	*	35	$423,319
Orthopedic Surgery: Hip & Joint	1	*	6	*	18	$491,039
Orthopedic Surgery: Pediatric	*	*	9	*	2	*
Orthopedic Surgery: Spine	4	*	3	*	22	$421,901
Orthopedic Surgery: Trauma	*	*	*	*	4	*
Orthopedic Surgery: Sports Med	2	*	8	*	25	$459,707

Table 7A: Physician Compensation by Practice Total Medical Revenue (continued)

	$2,000,000 or less		$2,000,001 to $5,000,000		$5,000,001 to $10,000,000	
	Phys	Median	Phys	Median	Phys	Median
Otorhinolaryngology	5	*	25	$381,842	53	$395,085
Pathology: Anatomic and Clinical	5	*	7	*	23	*
Pediatrics: General	92	$164,322	201	$165,932	199	$199,732
Pediatrics: Adolescent Medicine	3	*	2	*	7	*
Pediatrics: Cardiology	5	*	2	*	*	*
Pediatrics: Child Development	2	*	2	*	2	*
Pediatrics: Critical Care/Intensivist	10	*	6	*	3	*
Pediatrics: Emergency Medicine	36	*	3	*	*	*
Pediatrics: Endocrinology	9	*	3	*	1	*
Pediatrics: Gastroenterology	3	*	*	*	1	*
Pediatrics: Genetics	5	*	*	*	6	*
Pediatrics: Hematology/Oncology	19	$205,567	3	*	7	*
Pediatrics: Infectious Disease	3	*	*	*	*	*
Pediatrics: Neonatal Medicine	14	$252,000	7	*	1	*
Pediatrics: Nephrology	0	*	2	*	*	*
Pediatrics: Neurology	6	*	2	*	*	*
Pediatrics: Pulmonology	5	*	3	*	2	*
Pediatrics: Rheumatology	2	*	*	*	*	*
Physiatry (Phys Med & Rehab)	15	$225,340	21	$224,362	12	$231,686
Podiatry: General	2	*	1	*	5	*
Podiatry: Surg-Foot & Ankle	*	*	*	*	2	*
Psychiatry: General	16	$155,983	20	$181,389	6	*
Psychiatry: Child & Adolescent	3	*	3	*	1	*
Psychiatry: Geriatric	4	*	*	*	*	*
Pulmonary Medicine	14	$241,353	2	*	8	*
Pulmonary Medicine: Critical Care	5	*	17	$282,288	11	*
Pulmonary Med: Gen & Crit Care	11	$304,483	41	$316,907	13	$507,796
Radiation Oncology	4	*	1	*	2	*
Radiology: Diagnostic-Inv	9	*	20	$470,500	12	$502,500
Radiology: Diagnostic-Noninv	17	$490,370	40	$420,900	22	$415,186
Radiology: Nuclear Medicine	*	*	3	*	3	*
Rheumatology	4	*	4	*	16	$187,148
Sleep Medicine	4	*	1	*	5	*
Surgery: General	37	$262,570	92	$293,387	58	$250,950
Surgery: Bariatric	1	*	4	*	3	*
Surgery: Cardiovascular	18	$440,678	10	$606,230	42	$400,000
Surgery: Colon and Rectal	*	*	4	*	1	*
Surgery: Neurological	18	$551,018	22	$712,497	11	$893,208
Surgery: Oncology	*	*	3	*	*	*
Surgery: Oral	*	*	2	*	6	*
Surgery: Pediatric	6	*	8	*	11	$489,029
Surgery: Plastic & Reconstruction	3	*	*	*	6	*
Surgery: Plastic & Recon-Hand	*	*	*	*	2	*
Surgery: Thoracic (primary)	6	*	*	*	1	*
Surgery: Transplant	*	*	*	*	6	*
Surgery: Trauma	12	$382,585	*	*	7	*
Surgery: Vascular (primary)	2	*	8	*	6	*
Urgent Care	12	$169,916	12	$162,798	5	*
Urology	12	$328,894	25	$342,358	43	$465,040
Urology: Pediatric	*	*	1	*	1	*

Table 7B: Physician Compensation by Practice Total Medical Revenue

	$10,000,001 to $20,000,000		$20,000,001 to $50,000,000		$50,000,001 or more	
	Phys	Median	Phys	Median	Phys	Median
Allergy/Immunology	24	$229,657	14	$281,869	97	$268,230
Anesthesiology	716	$402,791	1,148	$394,147	1,154	$403,600
Anesthesiology: Pain Management	36	$435,108	47	$489,064	72	$408,780
Anesthesiology: Pediatric	12	*	26	$387,459	57	$397,300
Cardiology: Electrophysiology	36	$486,777	78	$524,272	63	$437,686
Cardiology: Invasive	69	$431,583	158	$444,247	180	$461,398
Cardiology: Inv-Intvl	130	$478,451	192	$507,333	174	$506,840
Cardiology: Noninvasive	88	$431,757	158	$423,591	191	$420,000
Critical Care: Intensivist	*	*	9	*	28	$240,125
Dentistry	15	$103,272	11	*	22	$172,942
Dermatology	12	$263,634	40	$339,098	224	$359,596
Dermatology: Mohs Surgery	2	*	3	*	19	$724,441
Emergency Medicine	83	$261,274	238	$262,834	297	$236,912
Endocrinology/Metabolism	13	$162,005	45	$213,242	185	$194,723
Family Practice (w/ OB)	114	$186,325	139	$192,030	340	$185,952
Family Practice (w/o OB)	464	$170,410	1,096	$174,989	2,955	$176,301
FP: Amb Only (no inpatient work)	19	*	22	$167,452	93	$158,600
Family Practice: Sports Med	4	*	13	$207,692	15	$205,026
Family Practice: Urgent Care	32	$145,172	19	$229,029	48	$210,350
Gastroenterology	116	$552,042	115	$402,488	403	$439,040
Gastroenterology: Hepatology	3	*	*	*	4	*
Genetics	*	*	*	*	4	*
Geriatrics	14	*	11	$170,000	44	$165,200
Hematology/Oncology	4	*	82	$433,793	290	$381,699
Hematology/Oncology: Onc (only)	5	*	15	$421,184	21	$505,366
Hospice/Palliative Care	*	*	*	*	4	*
Hospitalist: Family Practice	*	*	*	*	37	$206,196
Hospitalist: Internal Medicine	62	$207,760	146	$172,451	726	$195,290
Hospitalist: IM-Pediatrics	1	*	*	*	7	*
Hospitalist: Pediatrics	31	$155,000	*	*	52	$165,958
Infectious Disease	4	*	10	$181,079	149	$183,254
Internal Medicine: General	318	$179,005	776	$186,065	2,362	$187,710
IM: Amb Only (no inpatient work)	5	*	10	*	10	$205,800
Internal Med: Pediatrics	9	*	31	$198,763	60	$180,721
Nephrology	39	$338,427	28	$300,418	114	$298,948
Neurology	30	$247,783	67	$224,744	337	$222,277
Obstetrics/Gynecology: General	69	$269,395	341	$284,834	839	$281,000
OB/GYN: Gynecology (only)	6	*	37	$194,350	127	$225,000
OB/GYN: Gyn Oncology	*	*	4	*	37	$335,094
OB/GYN: Maternal & Fetal Med	6	*	10	$400,723	59	$335,654
OB/GYN: Repro Endocrinology	*	*	*	*	10	$297,150
OB/GYN: Urogynecology	*	*	*	*	6	*
Occupational Medicine	10	$163,749	10	$176,420	86	$210,777
Ophthalmology	70	$336,825	64	$328,935	247	$307,500
Ophthalmology: Pediatric	10	$243,496	4	*	15	$297,984
Ophthalmology: Retina	14	$548,901	16	$564,060	15	$538,508
Orthopedic (Nonsurgical)	9	*	12	$200,079	19	$184,274
Orthopedic Surgery: General	103	$425,029	185	$494,346	417	$467,622
Orthopedic Surgery: Foot & Ankle	12	$388,268	21	$497,844	21	$435,258
Orthopedic Surgery: Hand	19	$549,950	42	$450,863	48	$501,721
Orthopedic Surgery: Hip & Joint	21	$618,884	55	$496,923	35	$607,086
Orthopedic Surgery: Pediatric	3	*	5	*	21	$469,410
Orthopedic Surgery: Spine	25	$542,049	35	$536,453	41	$611,670
Orthopedic Surgery: Trauma	5	*	20	$485,623	12	$498,147
Orthopedic Surgery: Sports Med	38	$517,766	63	$611,473	59	$555,300

Table 7B: Physician Compensation by Practice Total Medical Revenue (continued)

	$10,000,001 to $20,000,000		$20,000,001 to $50,000,000		$50,000,001 or more	
	Phys	Median	Phys	Median	Phys	Median
Otorhinolaryngology	45	$293,295	73	$393,641	257	$349,520
Pathology: Anatomic and Clinical	9	*	29	*	71	$313,723
Pathology: Anatomic	*	*	3	*	30	$280,000
Pathology: Clinical	1	*	4	*	44	$249,102
Pediatrics: General	180	$175,984	472	$172,915	1,452	$184,158
Pediatrics: Adolescent Medicine	1	*	5	*	53	$169,500
Pediatrics: Allergy/Immunology	2	*	*	*	6	*
Pediatrics: Cardiology	7	*	1	*	40	$252,274
Pediatrics: Child Development	*	*	*	*	12	$148,978
Pediatrics: Critical Care/Intensivist	25	*	*	*	44	$266,158
Pediatrics: Emergency Medicine	28	$226,665	*	*	25	$274,782
Pediatrics: Endocrinology	5	*	0	*	20	$174,907
Pediatrics: Gastroenterology	6	*	*	*	24	$264,743
Pediatrics: Genetics	3	*	1	*	7	*
Pediatrics: Hematology/Oncology	8	*	2	*	38	$183,217
Pediatrics: Infectious Disease	*	*	*	*	14	$149,450
Pediatrics: Neonatal Medicine	20	$240,000	2	*	80	$280,794
Pediatrics: Nephrology	2	*	0	*	7	*
Pediatrics: Neurology	6	*	4	*	44	$189,411
Pediatrics: Pulmonology	1	*	0	*	12	$249,346
Pediatrics: Rheumatology	2	*	*	*	6	*
Physiatry (Phys Med & Rehab)	10	$348,732	26	$294,647	110	$221,928
Podiatry: General	13	$151,564	27	$158,822	94	$198,713
Podiatry: Surg-Foot & Ankle	5	*	9	*	53	$273,533
Podiatry: Surg-Forefoot Only	*	*	3	*	2	*
Psychiatry: General	3	*	57	$170,000	253	$181,244
Psychiatry: Child & Adolescent	2	*	6	*	48	$197,917
Psychiatry: Geriatric	*	*	*	*	4	*
Pulmonary Medicine	29	$329,263	33	$273,611	165	$287,045
Pulmonary Medicine: Critical Care	15	*	6	*	37	$317,257
Pulmonary Med: Gen & Crit Care	20	$260,896	21	$325,344	63	$306,075
Radiation Oncology	15	$871,173	13	$496,321	91	$466,057
Radiology: Diagnostic-Inv	45	$508,784	59	$472,439	154	$567,100
Radiology: Diagnostic-Noninv	59	$438,648	140	$448,801	440	$475,226
Radiology: Nuclear Medicine	3	*	8	*	21	$462,501
Rheumatology	12	$159,687	35	$222,285	189	$220,245
Sleep Medicine	3	*	4	*	30	$302,194
Surgery: General	39	$316,849	148	$309,260	528	$328,029
Surgery: Bariatric	*	*	3	*	14	$392,521
Surgery: Cardiovascular	12	*	42	$453,138	109	$469,436
Surgery: Colon and Rectal	3	*	2	*	32	$404,453
Surgery: Neurological	4	*	42	$694,515	120	$580,815
Surgery: Oncology	1	*	4	*	11	$303,818
Surgery: Oral	*	*	2	*	11	$453,000
Surgery: Pediatric	7	*	*	*	24	$469,416
Surgery: Plastic & Reconstruction	10	$442,432	7	*	89	$374,913
Surgery: Plastic & Recon-Hand	1	*	2	*	6	*
Surgery: Thoracic (primary)	2	*	11	$295,721	20	$496,691
Surgery: Transplant	*	*	*	*	22	$401,205
Surgery: Trauma	2	*	0	*	47	$360,714
Surgery: Trauma-Burn	*	*	*	*	4	*
Surgery: Vascular (primary)	14	$367,979	36	$344,359	95	$411,000
Urgent Care	12	$195,655	24	$146,985	342	$214,618
Urology	40	$487,508	145	$376,725	218	$392,493
Urology: Pediatric	5	*	3	*	3	*

Table 8A: Physician Compensation by Method of Compensation (more than Two Years in Specialty)

	100% prod less allocated overhead		1–99% prod less allocated overhead		100% prod-based share of prac comp pool		1–99% prod-based share of prac comp pool	
	Phys	Median	Phys	Median	Phys	Median	Phys	Median
Allergy/Immunology	29	$308,199	6	*	18	$281,153	10	$217,165
Anesthesiology	386	$387,890	53	$438,083	486	$380,371	52	$402,373
Anesthesiology: Pain Management	28	$422,127	2	*	11	$419,289	2	*
Anesthesiology: Pediatric	1	*	*	*	8	*	*	*
Cardiology: Electrophysiology	28	$547,461	12	$674,894	8	*	38	$546,390
Cardiology: Invasive	86	$428,400	14	$409,123	28	$469,777	93	$515,606
Cardiology: Inv-Intvl	112	$506,454	39	$467,291	41	$500,393	114	$547,248
Cardiology: Noninvasive	41	$347,391	14	$398,887	41	$389,046	49	$495,009
Critical Care: Intensivist	5	*	*	*	5	*	2	*
Dentistry	6	*	*	*	*	*	*	*
Dermatology	56	$444,631	20	$410,527	41	$328,798	37	$341,278
Dermatology: Mohs Surgery	3	*	0	*	4	*	2	*
Emergency Medicine	36	$265,098	24	*	29	$317,037	15	*
Endocrinology/Metabolism	51	$214,781	14	$211,668	20	$247,482	25	$194,348
Family Practice (w/ OB)	100	$182,390	44	$220,714	120	$223,443	53	$191,303
Family Practice (w/o OB)	1,291	$185,509	408	$175,157	512	$198,926	370	$178,037
FP: Amb Only (no inpatient work)	12	$149,839	1	*	8	*	46	*
Family Practice: Sports Med	7	*	2	*	2	*	*	*
Family Practice: Urgent Care	10	$250,391	18	$208,384	1	*	2	*
Gastroenterology	219	$431,071	42	$436,524	66	$482,610	86	$497,739
Gastroenterology: Hepatology	2	*	1	*	*	*	2	*
Geriatrics	8	*	2	*	4	*	2	*
Hematology/Oncology	57	$454,665	7	*	40	$367,945	56	$406,429
Hematology/Oncology: Onc (only)	6	*	5	*	2	*	7	*
Hospitalist: Family Practice	*	*	7	*	3	*	*	*
Hospitalist: Internal Medicine	83	$206,742	7	*	53	$270,757	46	$204,575
Hospitalist: IM-Pediatrics	2	*	*	*	*	*	*	*
Hospitalist: Pediatrics	*	*	2	*	2	*	*	*
Infectious Disease	25	$237,909	8	*	8	*	64	$167,745
Internal Medicine: General	735	$200,280	197	$210,016	439	$211,444	285	$170,893
IM: Amb Only (no inpatient work)	3	*	*	*	2	*	3	*
Internal Med: Pediatrics	37	$204,866	1	*	12	$171,875	2	*
Nephrology	32	$296,340	14	$324,589	25	$316,769	12	$222,241
Neurology	103	$274,416	51	$255,132	49	$216,339	41	$219,590
Obstetrics/Gynecology: General	283	$281,122	110	$347,930	142	$334,436	176	$285,681
OB/GYN: Gynecology (only)	74	$216,270	4	*	21	$170,277	14	$194,169
OB/GYN: Gyn Oncology	7	*	1	*	3	*	3	*
OB/GYN: Maternal & Fetal Med	6	*	7	*	10	$268,411	*	*
OB/GYN: Repro Endocrinology	*	*	*	*	5	*	*	*
Occupational Medicine	14	$230,688	7	*	9	*	3	*
Ophthalmology	119	$347,482	34	$302,655	50	$302,553	50	$344,084
Ophthalmology: Pediatric	9	*	4	*	2	*	1	*
Ophthalmology: Retina	11	$601,465	4	*	1	*	9	*
Orthopedic (Nonsurgical)	19	$228,378	2	*	1	*	4	*
Orthopedic Surgery: General	340	$470,423	68	$437,854	66	$454,940	58	$504,173
Orthopedic Surgery: Foot & Ankle	28	$576,452	5	*	8	*	1	*
Orthopedic Surgery: Hand	54	$519,671	20	$479,205	10	$544,453	14	$408,000
Orthopedic Surgery: Hip & Joint	48	$608,285	19	$495,877	10	$533,661	4	*
Orthopedic Surgery: Pediatric	11	$412,469	7	*	6	*	*	*
Orthopedic Surgery: Spine	51	$620,959	18	$564,083	9	*	2	*
Orthopedic Surgery: Trauma	13	$754,913	3	*	6	*	1	*
Orthopedic Surgery: Sports Med	80	$656,112	23	$563,866	8	*	10	$534,026

Table 8A: Physician Compensation by Method of Compensation (more than Two Years in Specialty) (continued)

	100% prod less allocated overhead		1–99% prod less allocated overhead		100% prod-based share of prac comp pool		1–99% prod-based share of prac comp pool	
	Phys	Median	Phys	Median	Phys	Median	Phys	Median
Otorhinolaryngology	158	$417,739	44	$446,784	40	$318,004	26	$389,681
Pathology: Anatomic and Clinical	2	*	4	*	5	*	1	*
Pathology: Anatomic	*	*	*	*	3	*	10	*
Pathology: Clinical	10	$265,478	3	*	0	*	*	*
Pediatrics: General	470	$200,504	155	$199,223	261	$211,417	259	$173,785
Pediatrics: Adolescent Medicine	3	*	*	*	*	*	1	*
Pediatrics: Allergy/Immunology	1	*	2	*	2	*	*	*
Pediatrics: Cardiology	1	*	2	*	2	*	*	*
Pediatrics: Critical Care/Intensivist	3	*	*	*	0	*	*	*
Pediatrics: Endocrinology	4	*	1	*	0	*	*	*
Pediatrics: Gastroenterology	5	*	1	*	0	*	*	*
Pediatrics: Genetics	*	*	2	*	*	*	*	*
Pediatrics: Hematology/Oncology	3	*	3	*	7	*	*	*
Pediatrics: Infectious Disease	5	*	3	*	1	*	*	*
Pediatrics: Neonatal Medicine	5	*	20	*	18	$460,116	*	*
Pediatrics: Nephrology	1	*	*	*	1	*	*	*
Pediatrics: Neurology	9	*	5	*	2	*	*	*
Pediatrics: Pulmonology	1	*	2	*	0	*	5	*
Pediatrics: Rheumatology	3	*	2	*	*	*	*	*
Physiatry (Phys Med & Rehab)	27	$266,194	9	*	27	$220,165	13	$222,535
Podiatry: General	47	$172,264	10	$235,734	16	$178,577	7	*
Podiatry: Surg-Foot & Ankle	13	$247,996	0	*	4	*	13	$197,886
Psychiatry: General	27	$199,327	10	$307,035	58	$165,733	31	$170,980
Psychiatry: Child & Adolescent	5	*	7	*	7	*	1	*
Psychiatry: Geriatric	*	*	1	*	*	*	1	*
Pulmonary Medicine	55	$262,940	8	*	24	$310,066	25	$287,045
Pulmonary Medicine: Critical Care	6	*	13	$282,288	8	*	7	*
Pulmonary Med: Gen & Crit Care	40	$409,312	6	*	19	$352,166	8	*
Radiation Oncology	18	$462,965	*	*	8	*	4	*
Radiology: Diagnostic-Inv	31	$502,074	4		10	$586,131	16	$566,090
Radiology: Diagnostic-Noninv	38	$444,767	2	*	50	$478,988	77	$499,908
Radiology: Nuclear Medicine	2	*	*	*	5	*	*	*
Rheumatology	48	$265,886	16	$220,832	21	$236,781	24	$223,373
Sleep Medicine	14	$282,970	1	*	4	*	10	$247,834
Surgery: General	185	$319,316	52	$322,996	92	$340,898	80	$323,692
Surgery: Bariatric	*	*	2	*	*	*	2	*
Surgery: Cardiovascular	26	$452,277	*	*	12	$475,361	24	$464,728
Surgery: Colon and Rectal	10	$440,495	1	*	4	*	*	*
Surgery: Neurological	38	$851,374	23	$772,007	16	$545,631	3	*
Surgery: Oncology	1	*	1	*	1	*	3	*
Surgery: Oral	7	*	1	*	*	*	3	*
Surgery: Pediatric	6	*	2	*	3	*	*	*
Surgery: Plastic & Reconstruction	37	$406,610	5	*	8	*	10	$422,039
Surgery: Plastic & Recon-Hand	1	*	2	*	*	*	5	*
Surgery: Thoracic (primary)	2	*	5	*	1	*	*	*
Surgery: Transplant	*	*	*	*	6	*	*	*
Surgery: Trauma	4	*	*	*	*	*	6	*
Surgery: Vascular (primary)	15	$277,784	2	*	12	$387,601	19	$438,183
Urgent Care	24	$222,777	23	$236,983	43	$254,213	64	$205,777
Urology	92	$426,368	41	$444,088	36	$360,927	52	$406,998
Urology: Pediatric	1	*	1	*	1	*	*	*

Table 8B: Physician Compensation by Method of Compensation (more than Two Years in Specialty)

	100% straight/guaranteed salary		1–99% base salary plus incentive		100% equal share of prac comp pool	
	Phys	Median	Phys	Median	Phys	Median
Allergy/Immunology	5	*	21	$304,607	5	*
Anesthesiology	369	$403,600	276	$418,959	699	$428,479
Anesthesiology: Pain Management	25	$403,600	12	$395,324	21	$561,833
Anesthesiology: Pediatric	16	*	14	*	1	*
Cardiology: Electrophysiology	9	*	28	$449,061	25	$527,875
Cardiology: Invasive	24	$386,858	46	$425,742	45	$516,554
Cardiology: Inv-Intvl	27	$360,696	64	$455,930	76	$517,328
Cardiology: Noninvasive	47	$307,489	83	$409,630	96	$515,773
Critical Care: Intensivist	6	*	8	*	1	*
Dentistry	8	*	12	*	*	*
Dermatology	19	$241,217	24	$310,529	1	*
Dermatology: Mohs Surgery	*	*	4	*	*	*
Emergency Medicine	69	$220,644	114	$250,531	*	*
Endocrinology/Metabolism	18	$153,209	16	$190,644	*	*
Family Practice (w/ OB)	15	$154,876	79	$204,346	1	*
Family Practice (w/o OB)	205	$136,574	585	$162,188	6	*
FP: Amb Only (no inpatient work)	22	$137,500	36	$175,300	*	*
Family Practice: Sports Med	0	*	8	*	*	*
Family Practice: Urgent Care	10	$152,641	19	$194,629	*	*
Gastroenterology	32	$303,000	51	$393,937	37	$589,333
Gastroenterology: Hepatology	0	*	1	*	*	*
Genetics	*	*	1	*	*	*
Geriatrics	16	$176,338	10	$172,074	*	*
Hematology/Oncology	33	$250,000	56	$448,216	18	$686,230
Hematology/Oncology: Onc (only)	1	*	6	*	0	*
Hospice/Palliative Care	3	*	3	*	*	*
Hospitalist: Family Practice	1	*	2	*	9	*
Hospitalist: Internal Medicine	97	$191,070	230	$202,989	*	*
Hospitalist: IM-Pediatrics	*	*	1	*	*	*
Hospitalist: Pediatrics	21	$173,715	15	$164,561	*	*
Infectious Disease	10	$174,500	13	$169,370	*	*
Internal Medicine: General	235	$146,784	429	$186,814	11	$141,000
IM: Amb Only (no inpatient work)	2	*	5	*	*	*
Internal Med: Pediatrics	3	*	14	$179,256	*	*
Nephrology	19	$186,393	13	$257,895	28	$374,004
Neurology	43	$211,470	70	$212,904	*	*
Obstetrics/Gynecology: General	89	$220,351	161	$254,292	54	$296,319
OB/GYN: Gynecology (only)	11	$218,000	16	$216,583	*	*
OB/GYN: Gyn Oncology	7	*	4	*	*	*
OB/GYN: Maternal & Fetal Med	13	$292,644	10	$333,521	*	*
OB/GYN: Repro Endocrinology	*	*	1	*	*	*
OB/GYN: Urogynecology	*	*	4	*	*	*
Occupational Medicine	10	$155,427	19	$199,303	*	*
Ophthalmology	19	$236,500	27	$316,063	*	*
Ophthalmology: Pediatric	*	*	2	*	*	*
Ophthalmology: Retina	*	*	5	*	*	*
Orthopedic (Nonsurgical)	2	*	5	*	*	*
Orthopedic Surgery: General	40	$374,115	53	$441,722	19	$461,887
Orthopedic Surgery: Foot & Ankle	2	*	4	*	2	*
Orthopedic Surgery: Hand	4	*	12	$391,762	3	*
Orthopedic Surgery: Hip & Joint	1	*	7	*	7	*
Orthopedic Surgery: Pediatric	5	*	4	*	*	*
Orthopedic Surgery: Spine	1	*	9	*	4	*
Orthopedic Surgery: Trauma	1	*	3	*	1	*
Orthopedic Surgery: Sports Med	5	*	10	$384,860	6	*

Table 8B: Physician Compensation by Method of Compensation (more than Two Years in Specialty) (continued)

	100% straight/guaranteed salary		1–99% base salary plus incentive		100% equal share of prac comp pool	
	Phys	Median	Phys	Median	Phys	Median
Otorhinolaryngology	10	$283,853	40	$322,042	*	*
Pathology: Anatomic and Clinical	18	$344,693	25	$267,756	25	*
Pathology: Anatomic	13	*	1	*	*	*
Pathology: Clinical	14	$236,500	1	*	4	*
Pediatrics: General	137	$129,700	374	$189,591	6	*
Pediatrics: Adolescent Medicine	6	*	4	*	*	*
Pediatrics: Cardiology	4	*	6	*	8	*
Pediatrics: Child Development	5	*	2	*	*	*
Pediatrics: Critical Care/Intensivist	26	$254,529	11	$287,482	*	*
Pediatrics: Emergency Medicine	22	$200,800	19	*	*	*
Pediatrics: Endocrinology	5	*	5	*	*	*
Pediatrics: Gastroenterology	4	*	6	*	*	*
Pediatrics: Genetics	1	*	1	*	*	*
Pediatrics: Hematology/Oncology	10	$199,996	13	$210,403	*	*
Pediatrics: Infectious Disease	*	*	1	*	*	*
Pediatrics: Neonatal Medicine	21	$290,000	12	$241,621	*	*
Pediatrics: Nephrology	*	*	3	*	*	*
Pediatrics: Neurology	6	*	9	*	8	*
Pediatrics: Pulmonology	4	*	7	*	*	*
Pediatrics: Rheumatology	*	*	1	*	*	*
Physiatry (Phys Med & Rehab)	13	$211,875	28	$214,565	*	*
Podiatry: General	4	*	3	*	*	*
Podiatry: Surg-Foot & Ankle	2	*	11	$205,044	*	*
Psychiatry: General	24	$160,448	39	$175,876	*	*
Psychiatry: Child & Adolescent	5	*	13	$219,628	*	*
Psychiatry: Geriatric	*	*	4	*	*	*
Pulmonary Medicine	4	*	12	$201,520	*	*
Pulmonary Medicine: Critical Care	11	*	3	*	3	*
Pulmonary Med: Gen & Crit Care	22	$222,250	16	$244,248	20	$261,179
Radiation Oncology	40	$472,500	20	$503,075	11	*
Radiology: Diagnostic-Inv	40	$480,108	33	$458,850	39	$491,135
Radiology: Diagnostic-Noninv	157	$377,329	116	$444,330	92	$519,390
Radiology: Nuclear Medicine	9	*	4	*	7	*
Rheumatology	19	$158,484	23	$206,422	*	*
Sleep Medicine	3	*	3	*	1	*
Surgery: General	64	$260,552	110	$275,861	13	$345,000
Surgery: Bariatric	*	*	5	*	*	*
Surgery: Cardiovascular	46	$461,637	21	$461,860	26	$504,383
Surgery: Colon and Rectal	5	*	4	*	1	*
Surgery: Neurological	21	$550,000	30	$593,191	1	*
Surgery: Oncology	1	*	3	*	*	*
Surgery: Oral	1	*	4	*	*	*
Surgery: Pediatric	11	$405,000	11	$489,029	3	*
Surgery: Plastic & Reconstruction	5	*	12	$289,656	*	*
Surgery: Plastic & Recon-Hand	1	*	*	*	*	*
Surgery: Thoracic (primary)	7	*	7	*	1	*
Surgery: Transplant	10	$400,000	2	*	*	*
Surgery: Trauma	6	*	12	$295,575	5	*
Surgery: Vascular (primary)	15	$325,500	27	$364,534	19	$341,436
Urgent Care	40	$163,836	52	$178,941	*	*
Urology	32	$303,047	51	$419,981	10	$536,328
Urology: Pediatric	5	*	*	*	*	*

Table 9A: Physician Compensation by Years in Specialty

	1 to 2 years		3 to 7 years		8 to 17 years		18 years or more	
	Phys	Median	Phys	Median	Phys	Median	Phys	Median
Allergy/Immunology	9	*	22	$228,928	36	$275,622	66	$274,707
Anesthesiology	215	$327,525	372	$371,525	1,353	$403,600	953	$397,500
Anesthesiology: Pain Management	5	*	38	$403,600	47	$472,496	33	$428,574
Anesthesiology: Pediatric	15	$359,168	21	$397,802	31	$423,693	26	$399,791
Cardiology: Electrophysiology	16	$292,228	44	$466,928	72	$529,412	41	$522,000
Cardiology: Invasive	32	$342,438	94	$446,955	184	$453,338	131	$424,481
Cardiology: Inv-Intvl	27	$357,515	87	$464,583	205	$518,800	225	$489,450
Cardiology: Noninvasive	27	$343,769	71	$410,591	124	$466,682	214	$398,744
Critical Care: Intensivist	11	$237,854	23	$282,190	22	$292,805	24	$316,822
Dentistry	4	*	6	*	7	*	13	$142,011
Dermatology	19	$331,706	69	$350,035	97	$363,778	103	$378,711
Dermatology: Mohs Surgery	5	*	7	*	8	*	5	*
Emergency Medicine	67	$235,554	167	$261,707	179	$268,475	161	$263,115
Endocrinology/Metabolism	20	$189,118	49	$190,905	56	$198,096	83	$214,781
Family Practice (w/ OB)	35	$149,922	146	$171,838	232	$200,582	175	$196,577
Family Practice (w/o OB)	304	$147,456	933	$170,617	1,560	$178,126	1,554	$181,928
FP: Amb Only (no inpatient work)	14	$163,568	29	$155,632	43	$153,787	75	$160,320
Family Practice: Sports Med	8	*	8	*	8	*	6	*
Family Practice: Urgent Care	4	*	9	*	22	$183,000	31	$216,235
Gastroenterology	57	$347,120	134	$408,597	230	$437,734	277	$423,537
Gastroenterology: Hepatology	*	*	1	*	2	*	3	*
Genetics	*	*	2	*	4	*	3	*
Geriatrics	3	*	12	$160,040	23	$179,694	23	$203,406
Hematology/Oncology	35	$269,699	76	$309,815	112	$376,829	139	$432,975
Hematology/Oncology: Onc (only)	82	*	92	$238,554	73	$258,425	43	$277,920
Hospice/Palliative Care	1	*	3	*	3	*	1	*
Hospitalist: Family Practice	4	*	16	$219,947	5	*	4	*
Hospitalist: Internal Medicine	142	$189,185	306	$202,832	231	$210,000	67	$206,182
Hospitalist: IM-Pediatrics	1	*	2	*	1	*	*	*
Hospitalist: Pediatrics	3	*	16	$159,111	24	$165,446	11	$180,578
Infectious Disease	14	$154,209	38	$184,123	65	$194,991	55	$196,882
Internal Medicine: General	236	$179,406	728	$195,225	1,210	$207,890	1,263	$196,000
IM: Amb Only (no inpatient work)	*	*	*	*	3	*	12	$167,214
Internal Med: Pediatrics	9	*	25	$197,082	51	$192,889	2	*
Nephrology	25	$195,140	70	$294,325	64	$298,184	67	$319,382
Neurology	49	$219,210	117	$232,000	156	$242,105	180	$232,906
Obstetrics/Gynecology: General	159	$231,766	335	$269,381	571	$299,946	433	$297,538
OB/GYN: Gynecology (only)	1	*	22	$230,714	38	$240,126	98	$192,464
OB/GYN: Gyn Oncology	2	*	8	*	19	$368,756	11	$423,619
OB/GYN: Maternal & Fetal Med	3	*	14	$316,868	31	$397,513	22	$447,949
OB/GYN: Repro Endocrinology	4	*	*	*	5	*	6	*
OB/GYN: Urogynecology	1	*	7	*	*	*	4	*
Occupational Medicine	7	*	25	$208,054	35	$228,300	49	$241,081
Ophthalmology	34	$236,476	69	$303,568	175	$334,310	184	$322,292
Ophthalmology: Pediatric	2	*	5	*	10	$263,881	10	$335,587
Ophthalmology: Retina	7	*	8	*	21	$548,544	14	$588,682
Orthopedic (Nonsurgical)	3	*	7	*	5	*	24	$201,806
Orthopedic Surgery: General	65	$387,252	143	$464,232	294	$479,990	350	$410,717
Orthopedic Surgery: Foot & Ankle	8	*	13	$539,678	29	$488,019	11	$490,526
Orthopedic Surgery: Hand	8	*	24	$487,280	59	$450,742	46	$417,532
Orthopedic Surgery: Hip & Joint	7	*	14	$715,547	39	$597,685	54	$556,627
Orthopedic Surgery: Pediatric	1	*	5	*	18	$489,279	12	$445,552
Orthopedic Surgery: Spine	14	$370,949	25	$545,629	56	$670,251	31	$391,354
Orthopedic Surgery: Trauma	4	*	11	$882,535	11	$477,483	9	*
Orthopedic Surgery: Sports Med	12	$406,540	34	$561,739	63	$597,849	64	$561,907

Table 9A: Physician Compensation by Years in Specialty (continued)

	1 to 2 years		3 to 7 years		8 to 17 years		18 years or more	
	Phys	Median	Phys	Median	Phys	Median	Phys	Median
Otorhinolaryngology	34	$287,428	92	$349,013	151	$386,394	156	$350,558
Pathology: Anatomic and Clinical	15	$282,917	32	$303,972	35	$327,865	58	$354,103
Pathology: Anatomic	2	*	10	$296,322	5	*	12	$275,707
Pathology: Clinical	*	*	6	*	14	$239,000	13	$264,156
Pediatrics: General	152	$145,258	469	$183,114	848	$193,162	803	$201,395
Pediatrics: Adolescent Medicine	1	*	4	*	9	*	4	*
Pediatrics: Allergy/Immunology	*	*	1	*	2	*	3	*
Pediatrics: Cardiology	3	*	7	*	9	*	17	$329,348
Pediatrics: Child Development	*	*	1	*	2	*	4	*
Pediatrics: Critical Care/Intensivist	5	*	16	$250,578	22	$289,200	10	$281,241
Pediatrics: Emergency Medicine	3	*	12	$220,886	17	$212,060	12	$230,900
Pediatrics: Endocrinology	3	*	7	*	7	*	9	*
Pediatrics: Gastroenterology	2	*	7	*	11	$247,479	11	$266,920
Pediatrics: Genetics	1	*	*	*	1	*	5	*
Pediatrics: Hematology/Oncology	9	*	16	$181,756	19	$229,100	15	$237,506
Pediatrics: Infectious Disease	*	*	3	*	5	*	5	*
Pediatrics: Neonatal Medicine	4	*	30	$261,903	35	$333,950	40	$305,000
Pediatrics: Nephrology	0	*	*	*	4	*	6	*
Pediatrics: Neurology	3	*	13	$235,785	19	$202,004	19	$187,056
Pediatrics: Pulmonology	1	*	3	*	4	*	14	$268,364
Pediatrics: Rheumatology	*	*	*	*	6	*	3	*
Physiatry (Phys Med & Rehab)	36	$213,701	55	$241,613	67	$252,831	41	$234,377
Podiatry: General	7	*	24	$179,576	48	$197,977	37	$190,163
Podiatry: Surg-Foot & Ankle	14	$188,395	36	$227,175	26	$244,306	35	$250,896
Podiatry: Surg-Forefoot Only	*	*	1	*	2	*	1	*
Psychiatry: General	34	$200,412	93	$217,993	106	$190,000	100	$185,274
Psychiatry: Child & Adolescent	8	*	26	$238,289	31	$263,599	11	$208,737
Psychiatry: Geriatric	*	*	*	*	3	*	3	*
Pulmonary Medicine	14	$241,073	33	$266,575	47	$292,334	66	$264,851
Pulmonary Medicine: Critical Care	1	*	10	$265,910	27	$330,000	21	$317,257
Pulmonary Med: Gen & Crit Care	18	$238,685	37	$268,487	58	$286,419	42	$335,519
Radiation Oncology	13	$355,479	27	$411,483	51	$540,000	29	$434,803
Radiology: Diagnostic-Inv	29	$310,071	78	$488,170	113	$514,669	85	$503,000
Radiology: Diagnostic-Noninv	69	$362,763	146	$427,338	261	$478,988	259	$436,948
Radiology: Nuclear Medicine	4	*	9	*	12	$357,390	18	$400,555
Rheumatology	14	$208,392	47	$213,553	57	$245,692	95	$232,376
Sleep Medicine	3	*	10	$368,694	12	$313,653	21	$259,176
Surgery: General	58	$263,552	164	$316,031	295	$343,481	297	$314,411
Surgery: Bariatric	1	*	2	*	4	*	3	*
Surgery: Cardiovascular	16	$320,000	34	$504,516	87	$474,850	55	$460,193
Surgery: Colon and Rectal	2	*	4	*	11	$353,814	13	$352,000
Surgery: Neurological	14	$694,004	35	$700,962	66	$706,208	55	$642,574
Surgery: Oncology	*	*	3	*	4	*	4	*
Surgery: Oral	3	*	3	*	10	$398,283	10	$348,673
Surgery: Pediatric	3	*	8	*	14	$564,946	19	$397,983
Surgery: Plastic & Reconstruction	14	$310,440	24	$356,637	38	$397,020	35	$380,305
Surgery: Plastic & Recon-Hand	1	*	4	*	4	*	1	*
Surgery: Thoracic (primary)	5	*	6	*	13	$477,807	19	$412,895
Surgery: Transplant	2	*	5	*	12	$400,000	5	*
Surgery: Trauma	8	*	9	*	20	$371,507	10	$313,538
Surgery: Trauma-Burn	1	*	2	*	1	*	*	*
Surgery: Vascular (primary)	10	$306,630	36	$381,020	51	$412,281	50	$341,698
Urgent Care	20	$199,117	70	$222,289	104	$222,062	123	$202,056
Urology	33	$322,318	81	$366,949	150	$425,212	190	$388,064
Urology: Pediatric	1	*	3	*	4	*	4	*

Table 9B: Physician Compensation by 1–2 Years in Specialty

	Phys	Med Pracs	Mean	Std. Dev.	25th %tile	Median	75th %tile	90th %tile
Allergy/Immunology	9	8	*	*	*	*	*	*
Anesthesiology	215	46	$336,633	$119,936	$265,000	$327,525	$438,549	$482,408
Anesthesiology: Pain Management	5	5	*	*	*	*	*	*
Anesthesiology: Pediatric	15	6	$335,281	$98,751	$320,237	$359,168	$398,597	$416,813
Cardiology: Electrophysiology	16	13	$299,155	$132,983	$237,446	$292,228	$321,066	$530,229
Cardiology: Invasive	32	20	$384,483	$121,566	$294,050	$342,438	$434,672	$623,314
Cardiology: Inv-Intvl	27	17	$350,213	$100,557	$294,519	$357,515	$417,810	$461,297
Cardiology: Noninvasive	27	14	$334,065	$97,229	$303,729	$343,769	$400,000	$433,173
Critical Care: Intensivist	11	5	$236,521	$22,191	$224,048	$237,854	$243,149	$278,531
Dentistry	4	3	*	*	*	*	*	*
Dermatology	19	12	$324,842	$95,408	$259,443	$331,706	$364,291	$434,074
Dermatology: Mohs Surgery	5	4	*	*	*	*	*	*
Emergency Medicine	67	15	$221,052	$55,039	$191,030	$235,554	$251,076	$273,819
Endocrinology/Metabolism	20	15	$177,606	$30,532	$172,692	$189,118	$198,847	$208,324
Family Practice (w/ OB)	35	25	$151,571	$42,734	$124,843	$149,922	$178,488	$200,442
Family Practice (w/o OB)	304	126	$158,418	$50,893	$125,516	$147,456	$190,685	$206,950
FP: Amb Only (no inpatient work)	14	4	$161,386	$13,786	$157,735	$163,568	$171,997	$175,451
Family Practice: Sports Med	8	8	*	*	*	*	*	*
Family Practice: Urgent Care	4	2	*	*	*	*	*	*
Gastroenterology	57	29	$350,775	$141,682	$294,115	$347,120	$378,212	$490,924
Geriatrics	3	3	*	*	*	*	*	*
Hematology/Oncology	35	19	$317,713	$151,850	$256,691	$269,699	$300,000	$573,901
Hematology/Oncology: Onc (only)	82	2	*	*	*	*	*	*
Hospice/Palliative Care	1	1	*	*	*	*	*	*
Hospitalist: Family Practice	4	3	*	*	*	*	*	*
Hospitalist: Internal Medicine	142	52	$194,633	$51,773	$169,623	$189,185	$212,452	$270,086
Hospitalist: IM-Pediatrics	1	1	*	*	*	*	*	*
Hospitalist: Pediatrics	3	3	*	*	*	*	*	*
Infectious Disease	14	10	$164,732	$34,517	$140,049	$154,209	$197,805	$224,027
Internal Medicine: General	236	84	$166,719	$42,789	$137,918	$179,406	$192,920	$205,872
Internal Med: Pediatrics	9	6	*	*	*	*	*	*
Nephrology	25	12	$198,921	$39,570	$158,730	$195,140	$231,502	$250,089
Neurology	49	26	$225,090	$88,383	$167,226	$219,210	$246,515	$328,953
Obstetrics/Gynecology: General	159	68	$229,865	$54,124	$198,134	$231,766	$261,057	$292,154
OB/GYN: Gynecology (only)	1	1	*	*	*	*	*	*
OB/GYN: Gyn Oncology	2	2	*	*	*	*	*	*
OB/GYN: Maternal & Fetal Med	3	3	*	*	*	*	*	*
OB/GYN: Repro Endocrinology	4	2	*	*	*	*	*	*
OB/GYN: Urogynecology	1	1	*	*	*	*	*	*
Occupational Medicine	7	5	*	*	*	*	*	*
Ophthalmology	34	16	$240,166	$49,363	$225,749	$236,476	$255,419	$284,022
Ophthalmology: Pediatric	2	2	*	*	*	*	*	*
Ophthalmology: Retina	7	3	*	*	*	*	*	*
Orthopedic (Nonsurgical)	3	3	*	*	*	*	*	*
Orthopedic Surgery: General	65	36	$408,475	$138,098	$334,702	$387,252	$432,735	$611,733
Orthopedic Surgery: Foot & Ankle	8	8	*	*	*	*	*	*
Orthopedic Surgery: Hand	8	8	*	*	*	*	*	*
Orthopedic Surgery: Hip & Joint	7	6	*	*	*	*	*	*
Orthopedic Surgery: Pediatric	1	1	*	*	*	*	*	*
Orthopedic Surgery: Spine	14	13	$447,161	$194,600	$308,775	$370,949	$612,606	$761,137
Orthopedic Surgery: Trauma	4	3	*	*	*	*	*	*
Orthopedic Surgery: Sports Med	12	12	$414,607	$149,350	$277,859	$406,540	$556,096	$642,975

Table 9B: Physician Compensation by 1–2 Years in Specialty (continued)

	Phys	Med Pracs	Mean	Std. Dev.	25th %tile	Median	75th %tile	90th %tile
Otorhinolaryngology	34	14	$290,803	$66,426	$259,907	$287,428	$306,526	$352,954
Pathology: Anatomic and Clinical	15	5	$264,346	$59,035	$218,750	$282,917	$310,346	$312,860
Pathology: Anatomic	2	1	*	*	*	*	*	*
Pediatrics: General	152	63	$147,813	$43,354	$119,047	$145,258	$167,172	$195,240
Pediatrics: Adolescent Medicine	1	1	*	*	*	*	*	*
Pediatrics: Cardiology	3	3	*	*	*	*	*	*
Pediatrics: Critical Care/Intensivist	5	5	*	*	*	*	*	*
Pediatrics: Emergency Medicine	3	2	*	*	*	*	*	*
Pediatrics: Endocrinology	3	3	*	*	*	*	*	*
Pediatrics: Gastroenterology	2	2	*	*	*	*	*	*
Pediatrics: Genetics	1	1	*	*	*	*	*	*
Pediatrics: Hematology/Oncology	9	3	*	*	*	*	*	*
Pediatrics: Neonatal Medicine	4	4	*	*	*	*	*	*
Pediatrics: Nephrology	0	*	*	*	*	*	*	*
Pediatrics: Neurology	3	3	*	*	*	*	*	*
Pediatrics: Pulmonology	1	1	*	*	*	*	*	*
Physiatry (Phys Med & Rehab)	36	16	$221,164	$42,433	$205,543	$213,701	$224,258	$293,080
Podiatry: General	7	7	*	*	*	*	*	*
Podiatry: Surg-Foot & Ankle	14	5	$181,049	$33,617	$162,665	$188,395	$196,652	$229,090
Psychiatry: General	34	11	$190,103	$34,963	$174,137	$200,412	$209,298	$226,621
Psychiatry: Child & Adolescent	8	2	*	*	*	*	*	*
Pulmonary Medicine	14	10	$255,942	$94,552	$192,323	$241,073	$309,124	$422,330
Pulmonary Medicine: Critical Care	1	1	*	*	*	*	*	*
Pulmonary Med: Gen & Crit Care	18	9	$233,431	$53,654	$203,565	$238,685	$264,236	$310,179
Radiation Oncology	13	5	$433,597	$189,690	$339,057	$355,479	$568,268	$804,685
Radiology: Diagnostic-Inv	29	14	$308,518	$149,506	$184,022	$310,071	$406,484	$456,774
Radiology: Diagnostic-Noninv	69	18	$380,695	$103,315	$327,144	$362,763	$416,195	$490,574
Radiology: Nuclear Medicine	4	2	*	*	*	*	*	*
Rheumatology	14	10	$202,364	$21,765	$188,854	$208,392	$214,872	$229,517
Sleep Medicine	3	3	*	*	*	*	*	*
Surgery: General	58	32	$274,176	$89,357	$221,463	$263,552	$310,736	$385,099
Surgery: Bariatric	1	1	*	*	*	*	*	*
Surgery: Cardiovascular	16	9	$357,984	$93,678	$301,298	$320,000	$450,601	$497,490
Surgery: Colon and Rectal	2	2	*	*	*	*	*	*
Surgery: Neurological	14	9	$700,613	$327,460	$530,725	$694,004	$813,420	$1,300,127
Surgery: Oral	3	1	*	*	*	*	*	*
Surgery: Pediatric	3	3	*	*	*	*	*	*
Surgery: Plastic & Reconstruction	14	7	$351,686	$106,416	$293,718	$310,440	$356,933	$588,121
Surgery: Plastic & Recon-Hand	1	1	*	*	*	*	*	*
Surgery: Thoracic (primary)	5	1	*	*	*	*	*	*
Surgery: Transplant	2	2	*	*	*	*	*	*
Surgery: Trauma	8	6	*	*	*	*	*	*
Surgery: Trauma-Burn	1	1	*	*	*	*	*	*
Surgery: Vascular (primary)	10	3	$308,015	$69,668	$273,781	$306,630	$345,271	$417,874
Urgent Care	20	11	$199,920	$49,991	$163,971	$199,117	$231,566	$255,080
Urology	33	17	$350,002	$100,458	$303,853	$322,318	$360,392	$428,829
Urology: Pediatric	1	1	*	*	*	*	*	*

Table 10: Physician Compensation by Gender

	Male			Female		
	Phys	Med Pracs	Median	Phys	Med Pracs	Median
Allergy/Immunology	123	62	$272,298	42	30	$223,068
Anesthesiology	2,292	139	$390,789	483	101	$310,861
Anesthesiology: Pain Management	148	53	$500,000	18	12	$368,307
Anesthesiology: Pediatric	57	7	$412,706	38	7	$397,008
Cardiology: Electrophysiology	185	89	$500,939	14	13	$393,584
Cardiology: Invasive	448	131	$432,798	50	32	$384,673
Cardiology: Inv-Intvl	589	154	$490,000	23	17	$350,000
Cardiology: Noninvasive	435	127	$421,965	65	43	$363,881
Critical Care: Intensivist	71	19	$282,907	22	8	$268,562
Dentistry	41	15	$131,875	14	8	$115,167
Dermatology	197	96	$375,871	142	66	$302,057
Dermatology: Mohs Surgery	20	15	$745,190	11	9	$484,844
Emergency Medicine	683	53	$261,707	173	42	$236,912
Endocrinology/Metabolism	178	102	$204,715	89	66	$185,400
Family Practice (w/ OB)	468	116	$201,148	280	92	$167,260
Family Practice (w/o OB)	3,776	562	$187,409	1,630	427	$145,018
FP: Amb Only (no inpatient work)	145	23	$160,320	58	15	$135,254
Family Practice: Sports Med	31	24	$207,692	3	3	*
Family Practice: Urgent Care	79	23	$203,000	30	16	$145,803
Gastroenterology	754	177	$426,356	108	55	$331,130
Gastroenterology: Hepatology	8	6	*	2	2	*
Genetics	4	2	*	5	2	*
Geriatrics	43	22	$181,649	43	19	$159,943
Hematology/Oncology	331	101	$383,870	110	57	$321,227
Hematology/Oncology: Onc (only)	216	28	$248,659	82	4	$233,605
Hospice/Palliative Care	7	7	*	3	3	*
Hospitalist: Family Practice	37	14	$212,414	6	5	*
Hospitalist: Internal Medicine	715	128	$203,131	324	103	$181,662
Hospitalist: IM-Pediatrics	5	4	*	3	2	*
Hospitalist: Pediatrics	30	11	$161,777	39	14	$161,000
Infectious Disease	134	53	$202,434	64	29	$156,952
Internal Medicine: General	3,061	405	$205,535	1,381	307	$159,833
IM: Amb Only (no inpatient work)	29	11	$193,339	10	9	$166,940
Internal Med: Pediatrics	75	37	$199,139	51	25	$164,358
Nephrology	208	69	$314,847	56	30	$225,996
Neurology	457	157	$241,071	147	85	$206,950
Obstetrics/Gynecology: General	976	269	$303,534	919	241	$262,410
OB/GYN: Gynecology (only)	103	64	$195,719	65	42	$200,000
OB/GYN: Gyn Oncology	35	22	$365,000	15	12	$318,313
OB/GYN: Maternal & Fetal Med	57	27	$475,959	38	21	$303,731
OB/GYN: Repro Endocrinology	15	8	$462,983	5	5	*
OB/GYN: Urogynecology	8	4	*	5	3	*
Occupational Medicine	109	47	$226,311	23	13	$215,220
Ophthalmology	443	127	$324,784	102	58	$269,757
Ophthalmology: Pediatric	23	18	$314,842	10	8	$188,591
Ophthalmology: Retina	57	30	$485,572	4	3	*
Orthopedic (Nonsurgical)	39	33	$189,751	7	6	*
Orthopedic Surgery: General	905	224	$445,267	39	18	$425,913
Orthopedic Surgery: Foot & Ankle	58	43	$478,021	5	5	*
Orthopedic Surgery: Hand	139	76	$449,000	10	9	$379,769
Orthopedic Surgery: Hip & Joint	128	63	$545,904	*	*	*
Orthopedic Surgery: Pediatric	30	15	$483,515	4	4	*
Orthopedic Surgery: Spine	129	75	$586,116	2	1	*
Orthopedic Surgery: Trauma	35	20	$488,627	5	5	*
Orthopedic Surgery: Sports Med	186	79	$557,276	4	4	*

Table 10: Physician Compensation by Gender (continued)

	Male			Female		
	Phys	Med Pracs	Median	Phys	Med Pracs	Median
Otorhinolaryngology	441	143	$352,407	60	33	$286,663
Pathology: Anatomic and Clinical	133	23	$330,517	58	16	$314,541
Pathology: Anatomic	17	8	$282,000	16	6	$273,786
Pathology: Clinical	39	13	$240,000	8	5	*
Pediatrics: General	1,332	280	$205,583	1,336	295	$162,004
Pediatrics: Adolescent Medicine	25	6	$198,403	44	8	$147,075
Pediatrics: Allergy/Immunology	6	4	*	0	*	*
Pediatrics: Cardiology	44	15	$282,468	9	7	*
Pediatrics: Child Development	4	3	*	7	5	*
Pediatrics: Critical Care/Intensivist	49	20	$269,145	22	13	$240,029
Pediatrics: Emergency Medicine	26	6	$258,821	18	3	$195,000
Pediatrics: Endocrinology	17	13	$191,027	15	11	$163,183
Pediatrics: Gastroenterology	25	12	$252,000	6	5	*
Pediatrics: Genetics	4	4	*	13	10	$155,557
Pediatrics: Hematology/Oncology	45	20	$189,516	22	10	$191,859
Pediatrics: Infectious Disease	8	3	*	7	6	*
Pediatrics: Neonatal Medicine	86	20	$294,499	48	17	$263,698
Pediatrics: Nephrology	10	7	$225,338	1	1	*
Pediatrics: Neurology	39	22	$233,792	17	14	$174,718
Pediatrics: Pulmonology	21	13	$266,289	3	2	*
Pediatrics: Rheumatology	7	5	*	2	2	*
Physiatry (Phys Med & Rehab)	166	77	$247,757	69	33	$206,650
Podiatry: General	106	67	$192,255	25	22	$169,421
Podiatry: Surg-Foot & Ankle	107	26	$246,149	15	10	$202,382
Podiatry: Surg-Forefoot Only	5	3	*	*	*	*
Psychiatry: General	304	77	$199,163	139	51	$176,924
Psychiatry: Child & Adolescent	44	19	$212,484	45	18	$246,869
Psychiatry: Geriatric	7	3	*	*	*	*
Pulmonary Medicine	197	90	$284,143	39	28	$257,822
Pulmonary Medicine: Critical Care	73	19	$307,565	11	9	$265,139
Pulmonary Med: Gen & Crit Care	140	44	$306,912	27	17	$250,000
Radiation Oncology	107	35	$480,520	31	17	$434,802
Radiology: Diagnostic-Inv	289	48	$508,628	36	16	$446,319
Radiology: Diagnostic-Noninv	663	74	$467,680	180	45	$401,807
Radiology: Nuclear Medicine	46	20	$416,744	5	4	*
Rheumatology	184	101	$235,187	87	61	$187,515
Sleep Medicine	47	27	$297,346	7	5	*
Surgery: General	808	235	$322,537	126	69	$281,566
Surgery: Bariatric	21	13	$395,543	2	2	*
Surgery: Cardiovascular	214	65	$463,168	7	6	*
Surgery: Colon and Rectal	40	19	$377,030	5	5	*
Surgery: Neurological	194	68	$651,878	12	10	$689,416
Surgery: Oncology	13	10	$433,342	4	2	*
Surgery: Oral	22	11	$351,399	4	3	*
Surgery: Pediatric	39	20	$466,875	10	10	$490,079
Surgery: Plastic & Reconstruction	111	47	$385,490	21	16	$288,207
Surgery: Plastic & Recon-Hand	9	6	*	1	1	*
Surgery: Thoracic (primary)	47	18	$421,511	8	3	*
Surgery: Transplant	28	10	$410,822	3	3	*
Surgery: Trauma	58	16	$372,455	6	5	*
Surgery: Trauma-Burn	2	2	*	2	1	*
Surgery: Vascular (primary)	169	64	$378,894	15	10	$333,969
Urgent Care	289	71	$216,452	99	41	$170,000
Urology	492	138	$394,242	36	23	$329,191
Urology: Pediatric	8	6	*	5	4	*

Table 11: Physician Compensation by Clinical Service Hours Worked per Week

	Fewer than 40 hours		40 hours or more	
	Phys	**Median**	**Phys**	**Median**
Allergy/Immunology	54	$225,000	56	$268,974
Anesthesiology	374	$313,195	2,489	$403,600
Anesthesiology: Pain Management	27	$461,140	128	$489,311
Anesthesiology: Pediatric	23	$348,863	54	$409,775
Cardiology: Electrophysiology	29	$491,619	137	$491,231
Cardiology: Invasive	82	$429,074	291	$439,489
Cardiology: Inv-Intvl	107	$452,000	393	$489,450
Cardiology: Noninvasive	117	$388,151	297	$431,582
Critical Care: Intensivist	15	$261,025	11	$249,868
Dentistry	26	$138,211	27	$113,000
Dermatology	132	$317,896	102	$355,987
Dermatology: Mohs Surgery	5	*	8	*
Emergency Medicine	428	$257,162	158	$242,781
Endocrinology/Metabolism	100	$203,017	88	$188,093
Family Practice (w/ OB)	300	$180,544	372	$186,387
Family Practice (w/o OB)	2,494	$165,291	1,771	$184,000
FP: Amb Only (no inpatient work)	56	$137,190	76	$149,740
Family Practice: Sports Med	9	*	13	$219,936
Family Practice: Urgent Care	58	$149,293	36	$197,436
Gastroenterology	179	$360,539	449	$457,866
Gastroenterology: Hepatology	4	*	5	*
Genetics	3	*	*	*
Geriatrics	31	$182,358	18	$187,138
Hematology/Oncology	113	$399,130	180	$430,976
Hematology/Oncology: Onc (only)	10	$358,918	26	$505,797
Hospice/Palliative Care	2	*	4	*
Hospitalist: Family Practice	24	$232,902	16	$140,301
Hospitalist: Internal Medicine	279	$197,147	479	$210,250
Hospitalist: IM-Pediatrics	4	*	4	*
Hospitalist: Pediatrics	33	$154,145	39	$155,304
Infectious Disease	105	$167,877	54	$200,295
Internal Medicine: General	1,653	$173,163	1,421	$194,480
IM: Amb Only (no inpatient work)	10	$141,978	22	$179,583
Internal Med: Pediatrics	34	$181,167	55	$195,843
Nephrology	48	$274,318	118	$311,818
Neurology	162	$220,469	301	$235,453
Obstetrics/Gynecology: General	609	$270,305	701	$291,652
OB/GYN: Gynecology (only)	99	$205,104	70	$222,153
OB/GYN: Gyn Oncology	5	*	20	$291,884
OB/GYN: Maternal & Fetal Med	24	$316,878	48	$355,014
OB/GYN: Repro Endocrinology	5	*	4	*
OB/GYN: Urogynecology	1	*	2	*
Occupational Medicine	53	$230,861	22	$205,445
Ophthalmology	162	$307,690	184	$325,666
Ophthalmology: Pediatric	9	*	13	$263,169
Ophthalmology: Retina	11	$448,071	24	$581,744
Orthopedic (Nonsurgical)	23	$164,195	19	$192,818
Orthopedic Surgery: General	199	$406,271	440	$457,857
Orthopedic Surgery: Foot & Ankle	10	$453,809	45	$467,183
Orthopedic Surgery: Hand	35	$434,203	93	$448,099
Orthopedic Surgery: Hip & Joint	30	$511,586	83	$574,918
Orthopedic Surgery: Pediatric	11	$454,146	16	$476,258
Orthopedic Surgery: Spine	26	$598,955	80	$526,774
Orthopedic Surgery: Trauma	9	*	22	$493,220
Orthopedic Surgery: Sports Med	51	$570,691	120	$553,066

Table 11: Physician Compensation by Clinical Service Hours Worked per Week (continued)

	Fewer than 40 hours		40 hours or more	
	Phys	Median	Phys	Median
Otorhinolaryngology	99	$317,491	221	$372,281
Pathology: Anatomic and Clinical	48	$348,644	65	$313,723
Pathology: Anatomic	13	$241,725	17	$278,000
Pathology: Clinical	3	*	16	$247,794
Pediatrics: General	1,138	$166,391	729	$197,322
Pediatrics: Adolescent Medicine	24	$166,731	46	$163,930
Pediatrics: Allergy/Immunology	0	*	4	*
Pediatrics: Cardiology	16	$255,104	13	$336,003
Pediatrics: Child Development	2	*	3	*
Pediatrics: Critical Care/Intensivist	14	$244,359	42	$250,000
Pediatrics: Emergency Medicine	28	$189,163	30	$213,803
Pediatrics: Endocrinology	9	*	14	$183,292
Pediatrics: Gastroenterology	12	$230,315	6	*
Pediatrics: Genetics	9	*	8	*
Pediatrics: Hematology/Oncology	21	$180,907	26	$205,567
Pediatrics: Infectious Disease	7	*	2	*
Pediatrics: Neonatal Medicine	29	$250,000	76	$308,833
Pediatrics: Nephrology	3	*	2	*
Pediatrics: Neurology	17	$195,000	17	$208,215
Pediatrics: Pulmonology	6	*	6	*
Pediatrics: Rheumatology	4	*	2	*
Physiatry (Phys Med & Rehab)	40	$244,859	97	$234,377
Podiatry: General	45	$179,252	53	$199,925
Podiatry: Surg-Foot & Ankle	21	$244,052	25	$230,000
Podiatry: Surg-Forefoot Only	*	*	2	*
Psychiatry: General	102	$170,320	168	$173,815
Psychiatry: Child & Adolescent	10	$168,742	28	$203,622
Psychiatry: Geriatric	7	*	1	*
Pulmonary Medicine	55	$285,700	104	$274,544
Pulmonary Medicine: Critical Care	4	*	34	$280,809
Pulmonary Med: Gen & Crit Care	28	$277,056	113	$304,483
Radiation Oncology	25	$737,641	68	$538,270
Radiology: Diagnostic-Inv	72	$507,995	165	$484,706
Radiology: Diagnostic-Noninv	182	$433,126	394	$469,986
Radiology: Nuclear Medicine	7	*	24	$465,500
Rheumatology	94	$202,712	89	$211,197
Sleep Medicine	14	$195,796	34	$316,247
Surgery: General	231	$306,558	417	$308,480
Surgery: Bariatric	5	*	12	$395,807
Surgery: Cardiovascular	27	$450,000	124	$449,563
Surgery: Colon and Rectal	5	*	21	$350,476
Surgery: Neurological	40	$653,531	112	$640,214
Surgery: Oncology	3	*	7	*
Surgery: Oral	8	*	4	*
Surgery: Pediatric	16	$460,979	24	$454,302
Surgery: Plastic & Reconstruction	20	$372,692	56	$406,458
Surgery: Plastic & Recon-Hand	*	*	10	$422,532
Surgery: Thoracic (primary)	13	$354,639	16	$425,000
Surgery: Transplant	8	*	17	$390,000
Surgery: Trauma	11	$359,509	38	$348,211
Surgery: Trauma-Burn	*	*	4	*
Surgery: Vascular (primary)	20	$282,888	79	$362,921
Urgent Care	176	$201,591	76	$196,307
Urology	138	$344,765	252	$412,776
Urology: Pediatric	8	*	5	*

Table 12: Physician Compensation by Weeks Worked per Year

	Fewer than 46 weeks		46 weeks or more	
	Phys	**Median**	**Phys**	**Median**
Allergy/Immunology	17	$217,115	100	$270,881
Anesthesiology	2,220	$403,600	1,077	$366,042
Anesthesiology: Pain Management	68	$403,600	100	$515,223
Anesthesiology: Pediatric	38	$397,551	42	$384,398
Cardiology: Electrophysiology	83	$492,725	94	$492,099
Cardiology: Invasive	145	$449,056	245	$442,347
Cardiology: Inv-Intvl	214	$491,045	291	$489,764
Cardiology: Noninvasive	220	$466,175	186	$377,846
Critical Care: Intensivist	14	$278,585	14	$239,934
Dentistry	8	*	22	$160,631
Dermatology	50	$377,453	182	$327,018
Dermatology: Mohs Surgery	5	*	12	$797,827
Emergency Medicine	95	$191,030	452	$258,006
Endocrinology/Metabolism	27	$180,770	167	$204,863
Family Practice (w/ OB)	90	$179,890	519	$187,432
Family Practice (w/o OB)	622	$156,834	3,727	$176,643
FP: Amb Only (no inpatient work)	20	$138,927	114	$148,038
Family Practice: Sports Med	6	*	19	$215,227
Family Practice: Urgent Care	2	*	99	$173,748
Gastroenterology	169	$448,013	500	$416,490
Gastroenterology: Hepatology	0	*	10	$351,228
Genetics	0	*	3	*
Geriatrics	5	*	55	$189,579
Hematology/Oncology	75	$365,900	231	$425,488
Hematology/Oncology: Onc (only)	5	*	35	$490,195
Hospice/Palliative Care	1	*	6	*
Hospitalist: Family Practice	12	$219,947	34	$181,108
Hospitalist: Internal Medicine	205	$206,182	583	$205,566
Hospitalist: IM-Pediatrics	1	*	3	*
Hospitalist: Pediatrics	20	$147,036	52	$159,976
Infectious Disease	29	$177,414	113	$177,248
Internal Medicine: General	408	$169,687	2,632	$188,225
IM: Amb Only (no inpatient work)	8	*	24	$175,303
Internal Med: Pediatrics	9	*	87	$186,187
Nephrology	39	$381,529	146	$277,640
Neurology	86	$231,097	380	$230,866
Obstetrics/Gynecology: General	289	$272,969	1,016	$285,418
OB/GYN: Gynecology (only)	30	$193,396	143	$213,581
OB/GYN: Gyn Oncology	3	*	24	$269,533
OB/GYN: Maternal & Fetal Med	12	$389,371	56	$355,014
OB/GYN: Repro Endocrinology	0	*	8	*
OB/GYN: Urogynecology	1	*	1	*
Occupational Medicine	10	$196,248	66	$219,629
Ophthalmology	96	$319,366	265	$315,982
Ophthalmology: Pediatric	4	*	19	$233,406
Ophthalmology: Retina	18	$527,786	19	$590,402
Orthopedic (Nonsurgical)	16	$162,791	26	$196,409
Orthopedic Surgery: General	144	$474,429	523	$436,113
Orthopedic Surgery: Foot & Ankle	13	$325,000	43	$497,844
Orthopedic Surgery: Hand	42	$429,032	87	$463,425
Orthopedic Surgery: Hip & Joint	34	$507,902	82	$576,597
Orthopedic Surgery: Pediatric	2	*	25	$488,395
Orthopedic Surgery: Spine	23	$413,482	86	$573,975
Orthopedic Surgery: Trauma	11	$283,546	22	$537,027
Orthopedic Surgery: Sports Med	38	$509,939	136	$565,904

Table 12: Physician Compensation by Weeks Worked per Year (continued)

	Fewer than 46 weeks		46 weeks or more	
	Phys	Median	Phys	Median
Otorhinolaryngology	70	$313,300	286	$352,946
Pathology: Anatomic and Clinical	57	$433,400	42	$291,549
Pathology: Anatomic	5	*	25	$275,000
Pathology: Clinical	1	*	30	$257,069
Pediatrics: General	297	$169,006	1,562	$182,216
Pediatrics: Adolescent Medicine	0	*	55	$159,450
Pediatrics: Allergy/Immunology	2	*	3	*
Pediatrics: Cardiology	2	*	25	$255,104
Pediatrics: Child Development	3	*	2	*
Pediatrics: Critical Care/Intensivist	17	$236,059	48	$253,910
Pediatrics: Emergency Medicine	3	*	24	$203,530
Pediatrics: Endocrinology	7	*	13	$174,700
Pediatrics: Gastroenterology	2	*	13	$230,315
Pediatrics: Genetics	5	*	11	$155,557
Pediatrics: Hematology/Oncology	7	*	34	$184,430
Pediatrics: Infectious Disease	0	*	5	*
Pediatrics: Neonatal Medicine	5	*	76	$308,833
Pediatrics: Nephrology	1	*	5	*
Pediatrics: Neurology	7	*	30	$191,376
Pediatrics: Pulmonology	0	*	15	$266,289
Pediatrics: Rheumatology	1	*	6	*
Physiatry (Phys Med & Rehab)	29	$282,800	121	$230,000
Podiatry: General	9	*	93	$187,070
Podiatry: Surg-Foot & Ankle	1	*	49	$231,591
Podiatry: Surg-Forefoot Only	*	*	2	*
Psychiatry: General	44	$157,092	196	$171,902
Psychiatry: Child & Adolescent	3	*	24	$169,681
Psychiatry: Geriatric	5	*	2	*
Pulmonary Medicine	18	$250,000	142	$276,108
Pulmonary Medicine: Critical Care	23	$342,783	36	$279,341
Pulmonary Med: Gen & Crit Care	27	$259,177	118	$314,371
Radiation Oncology	41	$819,162	57	$468,000
Radiology: Diagnostic-Inv	193	$498,594	55	$502,074
Radiology: Diagnostic-Noninv	398	$472,797	189	$428,072
Radiology: Nuclear Medicine	19	$481,554	13	$365,922
Rheumatology	26	$226,365	169	$213,553
Sleep Medicine	3	*	39	$295,588
Surgery: General	126	$328,969	551	$301,856
Surgery: Bariatric	5	*	11	$322,633
Surgery: Cardiovascular	66	$409,589	95	$467,468
Surgery: Colon and Rectal	3	*	24	$348,841
Surgery: Neurological	40	$675,564	107	$632,007
Surgery: Oncology	1	*	8	*
Surgery: Oral	1	*	9	*
Surgery: Pediatric	9	*	30	$450,000
Surgery: Plastic & Reconstruction	12	$374,908	65	$390,307
Surgery: Plastic & Recon-Hand	*	*	10	$422,532
Surgery: Thoracic (primary)	12	$425,000	7	*
Surgery: Transplant	*	*	23	$402,410
Surgery: Trauma	8	*	32	$360,112
Surgery: Trauma-Burn	*	*	1	*
Surgery: Vascular (primary)	43	$342,936	66	$362,500
Urgent Care	91	$196,445	172	$209,974
Urology	65	$380,000	329	$392,013
Urology: Pediatric	*	*	13	$391,500

Table 13: Physician Compensation by Partner/Shareholder in Practice

	Yes		No	
	Phys	Median	Phys	Median
Allergy/Immunology	100	$283,981	59	$219,992
Anesthesiology	2,972	$404,722	656	$312,843
Anesthesiology: Pain Management	134	$500,000	38	$377,340
Anesthesiology: Pediatric	44	$393,425	61	$405,930
Cardiology: Electrophysiology	127	$512,401	69	$424,831
Cardiology: Invasive	356	$437,204	138	$419,781
Cardiology: Inv-Intvl	458	$490,700	141	$440,000
Cardiology: Noninvasive	295	$441,080	195	$359,754
Critical Care: Intensivist	53	$308,104	37	$232,873
Dentistry	4	*	50	$130,938
Dermatology	182	$384,862	150	$308,824
Dermatology: Mohs Surgery	15	$724,441	15	$600,295
Emergency Medicine	420	$285,115	461	$237,972
Endocrinology/Metabolism	108	$218,085	152	$190,304
Family Practice (w/ OB)	326	$200,802	442	$175,074
Family Practice (w/o OB)	1,698	$201,777	3,664	$166,270
FP: Amb Only (no inpatient work)	42	$191,702	141	$153,461
Family Practice: Sports Med	8	*	25	$205,532
Family Practice: Urgent Care	30	$209,345	77	$156,645
Gastroenterology	584	$440,771	260	$362,606
Gastroenterology: Hepatology	6	*	4	*
Genetics	7	*	3	*
Geriatrics	15	$184,456	79	$170,000
Hematology/Oncology	245	$435,296	182	$300,928
Hematology/Oncology: Onc (only)	200	$252,150	99	$205,597
Hospice/Palliative Care	0	*	7	*
Hospitalist: Family Practice	10	$254,803	29	$193,247
Hospitalist: Internal Medicine	196	$235,554	766	$194,664
Hospitalist: IM-Pediatrics	1	*	3	*
Hospitalist: Pediatrics	3	*	86	$159,976
Infectious Disease	60	$250,334	129	$175,000
Internal Medicine: General	1,863	$222,576	2,488	$173,199
IM: Amb Only (no inpatient work)	3	*	36	$181,682
Internal Med: Pediatrics	51	$208,790	51	$184,013
Nephrology	173	$319,382	92	$221,032
Neurology	279	$253,601	313	$212,346
Obstetrics/Gynecology: General	1,029	$305,480	821	$250,000
OB/GYN: Gynecology (only)	82	$200,000	108	$213,971
OB/GYN: Gyn Oncology	19	$381,781	28	$335,400
OB/GYN: Maternal & Fetal Med	39	$436,441	54	$353,981
OB/GYN: Repro Endocrinology	8	*	10	$309,729
OB/GYN: Urogynecology	7	*	7	*
Occupational Medicine	72	$233,210	64	$196,215
Ophthalmology	353	$333,667	171	$261,652
Ophthalmology: Pediatric	23	$333,628	9	*
Ophthalmology: Retina	45	$548,544	14	$416,965
Orthopedic (Nonsurgical)	22	$227,480	23	$179,547
Orthopedic Surgery: General	665	$470,980	297	$396,747
Orthopedic Surgery: Foot & Ankle	51	$502,488	17	$339,874
Orthopedic Surgery: Hand	119	$493,075	33	$371,149
Orthopedic Surgery: Hip & Joint	120	$554,798	12	$285,492
Orthopedic Surgery: Pediatric	19	$488,395	15	$455,076
Orthopedic Surgery: Spine	106	$598,696	27	$483,599
Orthopedic Surgery: Trauma	23	$490,146	16	$452,803
Orthopedic Surgery: Sports Med	165	$594,588	28	$334,690

Table 13: Physician Compensation by Partner/Shareholder in Practice (continued)

	Yes		No	
	Phys	Median	Phys	Median
Otorhinolaryngology	335	$364,078	162	$297,364
Pathology: Anatomic and Clinical	103	$338,385	95	$282,829
Pathology: Anatomic	*	*	31	$276,413
Pathology: Clinical	10	$265,478	26	$239,000
Pediatrics: General	1,078	$207,023	1,601	$168,901
Pediatrics: Adolescent Medicine	32	$167,643	38	$156,201
Pediatrics: Allergy/Immunology	2	*	4	*
Pediatrics: Cardiology	12	$328,063	40	$255,104
Pediatrics: Child Development	*	*	13	$150,000
Pediatrics: Critical Care/Intensivist	9	*	73	$250,000
Pediatrics: Emergency Medicine	1	*	80	$211,913
Pediatrics: Endocrinology	4	*	32	$174,078
Pediatrics: Gastroenterology	8	*	25	$249,441
Pediatrics: Genetics	12	$163,218	6	*
Pediatrics: Hematology/Oncology	12	$235,931	62	$196,040
Pediatrics: Infectious Disease	6	*	11	$174,154
Pediatrics: Neonatal Medicine	49	$362,826	87	$250,859
Pediatrics: Nephrology	2	*	9	*
Pediatrics: Neurology	10	$191,784	47	$208,842
Pediatrics: Pulmonology	4	*	20	$262,077
Pediatrics: Rheumatology	6	*	5	*
Physiatry (Phys Med & Rehab)	71	$261,753	153	$214,717
Podiatry: General	60	$200,781	73	$171,781
Podiatry: Surg-Foot & Ankle	82	$246,154	50	$209,456
Podiatry: Surg-Forefoot Only	2	*	3	*
Psychiatry: General	129	$229,172	288	$180,510
Psychiatry: Child & Adolescent	35	$264,400	54	$207,381
Psychiatry: Geriatric	*	*	8	*
Pulmonary Medicine	120	$302,983	93	$250,000
Pulmonary Medicine: Critical Care	53	$327,431	31	$279,330
Pulmonary Med: Gen & Crit Care	119	$325,344	53	$238,506
Radiation Oncology	64	$659,595	70	$396,740
Radiology: Diagnostic-Inv	226	$514,835	105	$402,024
Radiology: Diagnostic-Noninv	545	$478,988	300	$384,393
Radiology: Nuclear Medicine	31	$415,980	19	$391,210
Rheumatology	119	$246,003	145	$202,125
Sleep Medicine	25	$306,160	29	$262,940
Surgery: General	513	$332,860	409	$303,242
Surgery: Bariatric	9	*	14	$398,035
Surgery: Cardiovascular	122	$460,991	94	$463,037
Surgery: Colon and Rectal	31	$433,411	15	$331,205
Surgery: Neurological	102	$734,446	97	$580,371
Surgery: Oncology	11	$433,342	6	*
Surgery: Oral	19	$382,324	7	*
Surgery: Pediatric	19	$548,406	31	$438,573
Surgery: Plastic & Reconstruction	59	$438,930	66	$331,490
Surgery: Plastic & Recon-Hand	4	*	7	*
Surgery: Thoracic (primary)	25	$363,173	31	$425,000
Surgery: Transplant	5	*	26	$401,205
Surgery: Trauma	6	*	58	$356,834
Surgery: Trauma-Burn	1	*	3	*
Surgery: Vascular (primary)	110	$395,393	71	$336,575
Urgent Care	155	$238,837	211	$179,174
Urology	359	$409,848	165	$333,491
Urology: Pediatric	5	*	8	*

Table 14: Physician Retirement Benefits

	Phys	Med Pracs	Mean	Std. Dev.	25th %tile	Median	75th %tile	90th %tile
Allergy/Immunology	116	66	$21,163	$9,902	$14,528	$21,274	$29,000	$30,958
Anesthesiology	3,247	157	$33,069	$10,573	$29,000	$29,500	$45,000	$45,000
Anesthesiology: Pain Management	166	51	$29,580	$11,039	$23,124	$33,000	$36,110	$41,664
Anesthesiology: Pediatric	85	7	$19,850	$12,729	$7,875	$14,062	$35,393	$35,921
Cardiology: Electrophysiology	170	81	$27,728	$10,228	$20,000	$29,500	$31,432	$45,000
Cardiology: Invasive	379	114	$28,315	$11,619	$20,500	$29,500	$31,500	$45,000
Cardiology: Inv-Intvl	531	136	$28,475	$12,262	$20,500	$29,500	$30,500	$45,000
Cardiology: Noninvasive	402	112	$27,853	$11,562	$20,000	$29,500	$33,850	$45,000
Critical Care: Intensivist	30	12	$19,348	$9,407	$13,088	$15,234	$29,500	$31,493
Dentistry	53	15	$5,878	$2,666	$3,943	$5,811	$6,750	$9,707
Dermatology	244	103	$24,991	$13,343	$15,000	$24,179	$29,500	$43,272
Dermatology: Mohs Surgery	17	13	$29,970	$17,391	$17,406	$30,893	$32,150	$53,052
Emergency Medicine	576	49	$21,868	$12,460	$11,244	$19,000	$29,161	$40,792
Endocrinology/Metabolism	182	95	$16,595	$9,187	$9,331	$14,897	$22,389	$29,500
Family Practice (w/ OB)	542	109	$15,810	$9,148	$7,636	$14,656	$23,016	$29,500
Family Practice (w/o OB)	4,134	512	$14,585	$9,861	$7,337	$11,743	$20,000	$29,500
FP: Amb Only (no inpatient work)	167	18	$15,517	$14,183	$6,290	$9,300	$20,860	$44,943
Family Practice: Sports Med	28	19	$19,886	$12,692	$9,795	$15,540	$27,409	$45,000
Family Practice: Urgent Care	88	21	$11,379	$8,267	$4,354	$9,400	$13,500	$27,601
Gastroenterology	621	155	$27,818	$14,263	$20,010	$29,000	$30,000	$45,000
Gastroenterology: Hepatology	9	6	*	*	*	*	*	*
Genetics	4	3	*	*	*	*	*	*
Geriatrics	53	23	$15,153	$13,250	$6,070	$9,796	$19,799	$41,049
Hematology/Oncology	327	86	$23,809	$11,297	$15,500	$24,480	$29,500	$32,530
Hematology/Oncology: Onc (only)	38	24	$21,773	$9,622	$10,782	$24,675	$29,500	$29,639
Hospice/Palliative Care	6	6	*	*	*	*	*	*
Hospitalist: Family Practice	30	10	$15,709	$11,136	$9,315	$13,500	$16,357	$26,506
Hospitalist: Internal Medicine	735	106	$18,032	$11,287	$10,321	$14,962	$21,800	$31,343
Hospitalist: IM-Pediatrics	8	4	*	*	*	*	*	*
Hospitalist: Pediatrics	87	16	$12,017	$9,795	$6,200	$9,115	$12,437	$34,372
Infectious Disease	89	46	$19,348	$10,817	$11,514	$17,647	$26,000	$29,500
Internal Medicine: General	2,945	363	$16,732	$11,228	$8,306	$13,959	$23,182	$30,448
IM: Amb Only (no inpatient work)	18	11	$11,687	$8,391	$6,920	$8,232	$12,306	$30,000
Internal Med: Pediatrics	92	31	$10,586	$8,120	$4,373	$8,244	$15,667	$22,389
Nephrology	187	58	$23,932	$12,999	$14,843	$24,107	$29,515	$45,000
Neurology	426	134	$19,343	$11,398	$9,908	$17,445	$29,314	$30,000
Obstetrics/Gynecology: General	1,190	242	$21,896	$12,594	$12,037	$20,768	$29,500	$41,969
OB/GYN: Gynecology (only)	150	65	$18,990	$9,999	$10,761	$17,629	$26,615	$30,893
OB/GYN: Gyn Oncology	28	18	$19,735	$11,106	$11,599	$17,296	$25,494	$39,541
OB/GYN: Maternal & Fetal Med	62	22	$26,687	$12,251	$15,274	$24,035	$39,541	$43,252
OB/GYN: Repro Endocrinology	8	5	*	*	*	*	*	*
OB/GYN: Urogynecology	5	4	*	*	*	*	*	*
Occupational Medicine	83	44	$21,494	$14,349	$10,125	$20,174	$28,996	$47,784
Ophthalmology	366	115	$22,928	$11,805	$14,843	$22,389	$29,500	$37,913
Ophthalmology: Pediatric	28	21	$21,141	$9,630	$12,072	$20,250	$29,332	$30,341
Ophthalmology: Retina	38	21	$21,089	$13,737	$9,000	$18,147	$28,000	$38,922
Orthopedic (Nonsurgical)	28	23	$29,093	$55,488	$12,542	$18,553	$24,938	$36,759
Orthopedic Surgery: General	687	195	$28,482	$13,376	$20,500	$29,500	$31,500	$45,000
Orthopedic Surgery: Foot & Ankle	53	39	$30,764	$12,080	$26,843	$29,500	$43,750	$45,000
Orthopedic Surgery: Hand	120	68	$31,473	$11,271	$27,250	$29,500	$31,500	$45,000
Orthopedic Surgery: Hip & Joint	90	51	$33,297	$9,781	$29,500	$29,500	$42,875	$45,000
Orthopedic Surgery: Pediatric	37	19	$27,170	$13,222	$15,695	$29,500	$31,166	$54,000
Orthopedic Surgery: Spine	103	64	$32,019	$13,249	$29,000	$29,500	$42,594	$45,600
Orthopedic Surgery: Trauma	28	18	$31,576	$10,651	$28,750	$29,500	$31,145	$54,000
Orthopedic Surgery: Sports Med	153	66	$33,175	$16,088	$29,485	$29,500	$42,500	$50,000

page 76

Table 14: Physician Retirement Benefits (continued)

	Phys	Med Pracs	Mean	Std. Dev.	25th %tile	Median	75th %tile	90th %tile
Otorhinolaryngology	389	131	$24,928	$12,084	$15,500	$25,750	$30,304	$44,000
Pathology: Anatomic and Clinical	129	21	$27,814	$18,811	$18,031	$29,093	$29,500	$33,750
Pathology: Anatomic	16	5	$12,709	$3,952	$10,479	$12,678	$14,843	$18,239
Pathology: Clinical	30	9	$21,734	$7,188	$14,818	$25,375	$27,988	$29,313
Pediatrics: General	2,007	285	$14,655	$9,646	$7,439	$12,356	$19,634	$29,054
Pediatrics: Adolescent Medicine	27	6	$8,859	$4,512	$5,158	$6,500	$13,000	$16,000
Pediatrics: Allergy/Immunology	6	4	*	*	*	*	*	*
Pediatrics: Cardiology	37	15	$17,532	$9,983	$10,471	$14,217	$22,616	$33,269
Pediatrics: Child Development	9	5	*	*	*	*	*	*
Pediatrics: Critical Care/Intensivist	79	18	$14,094	$9,410	$7,875	$9,960	$16,875	$31,743
Pediatrics: Emergency Medicine	43	7	$9,691	$4,283	$5,679	$10,067	$13,572	$14,962
Pediatrics: Endocrinology	25	14	$11,767	$6,618	$8,917	$10,482	$15,719	$22,265
Pediatrics: Gastroenterology	26	13	$20,415	$9,464	$14,227	$16,145	$29,500	$39,541
Pediatrics: Genetics	17	10	$12,045	$5,837	$9,342	$10,500	$13,086	$20,211
Pediatrics: Hematology/Oncology	54	17	$14,379	$9,010	$8,817	$13,108	$18,326	$26,550
Pediatrics: Infectious Disease	14	8	$11,364	$7,331	$5,629	$9,144	$17,948	$25,130
Pediatrics: Neonatal Medicine	102	18	$22,530	$11,312	$10,750	$20,000	$29,500	$41,049
Pediatrics: Nephrology	9	7	*	*	*	*	*	*
Pediatrics: Neurology	54	23	$18,617	$11,887	$9,524	$14,905	$28,060	$39,541
Pediatrics: Pulmonology	19	11	$16,531	$6,615	$12,786	$14,806	$18,600	$29,500
Pediatrics: Rheumatology	7	4	*	*	*	*	*	*
Physiatry (Phys Med & Rehab)	148	73	$19,598	$12,269	$10,153	$15,448	$28,943	$37,611
Podiatry: General	107	66	$16,188	$7,904	$10,125	$15,070	$22,180	$28,120
Podiatry: Surg-Foot & Ankle	56	23	$24,515	$13,925	$14,843	$22,343	$30,882	$52,400
Podiatry: Surg-Forefoot Only	4	2	*	*	*	*	*	*
Psychiatry: General	230	63	$16,704	$11,635	$9,237	$13,801	$19,939	$31,432
Psychiatry: Child & Adolescent	39	20	$20,099	$16,914	$8,176	$16,482	$22,389	$59,400
Psychiatry: Geriatric	6	2	*	*	*	*	*	*
Pulmonary Medicine	181	77	$19,787	$8,458	$11,117	$20,603	$27,704	$29,500
Pulmonary Medicine: Critical Care	58	16	$24,735	$10,784	$16,945	$25,452	$29,500	$45,000
Pulmonary Med: Gen & Crit Care	135	38	$27,167	$13,028	$20,000	$29,500	$31,342	$45,000
Radiation Oncology	101	31	$27,940	$9,207	$20,604	$29,500	$31,371	$39,541
Radiology: Diagnostic-Inv	275	44	$32,452	$10,118	$29,500	$31,432	$39,573	$45,000
Radiology: Diagnostic-Noninv	617	68	$28,823	$11,976	$22,389	$29,500	$31,371	$45,000
Radiology: Nuclear Medicine	36	21	$32,954	$11,572	$26,241	$31,371	$44,000	$46,677
Rheumatology	176	100	$19,256	$10,849	$10,125	$16,320	$25,969	$31,915
Sleep Medicine	41	24	$21,683	$11,175	$11,788	$20,250	$29,406	$43,059
Surgery: General	675	198	$24,120	$12,323	$14,843	$24,780	$29,500	$39,306
Surgery: Bariatric	17	9	$24,816	$12,814	$16,022	$22,389	$31,560	$46,000
Surgery: Cardiovascular	158	51	$32,758	$20,139	$20,375	$29,500	$45,000	$64,922
Surgery: Colon and Rectal	38	17	$24,196	$11,279	$17,015	$23,550	$29,313	$41,444
Surgery: Neurological	152	57	$29,209	$20,077	$13,125	$28,200	$39,885	$59,732
Surgery: Oncology	14	9	$23,982	$9,527	$15,522	$27,782	$29,500	$37,250
Surgery: Oral	20	10	$18,296	$6,571	$14,676	$15,500	$24,932	$28,700
Surgery: Pediatric	43	20	$24,390	$14,178	$9,000	$24,300	$39,541	$45,000
Surgery: Plastic & Reconstruction	91	44	$26,631	$19,372	$14,843	$21,489	$28,000	$59,207
Surgery: Plastic & Recon-Hand	4	4	*	*	*	*	*	*
Surgery: Thoracic (primary)	29	14	$23,627	$13,416	$14,344	$23,653	$31,343	$45,000
Surgery: Transplant	20	6	$26,600	$15,543	$15,300	$20,395	$31,164	$55,930
Surgery: Trauma	34	10	$12,939	$5,971	$9,087	$11,797	$14,738	$19,771
Surgery: Trauma-Burn	1	1	*	*	*	*	*	*
Surgery: Vascular (primary)	125	49	$27,346	$12,340	$16,658	$29,485	$31,342	$45,200
Urgent Care	243	58	$19,981	$11,031	$11,060	$19,000	$28,938	$33,400
Urology	366	118	$28,201	$15,474	$15,500	$29,485	$31,628	$46,269
Urology: Pediatric	10	7	$15,775	$9,340	$9,000	$10,500	$24,175	$31,724

Table 15: Physician Retirement Benefits by Group Type

	Single Specialty			Multispecialty		
	Phys	Med Pracs	Median	Phys	Med Pracs	Median
Allergy/Immunology	25	7	$18,085	91	59	$22,162
Anesthesiology	2,808	110	$30,938	439	47	$24,456
Anesthesiology: Pain Management	98	21	$33,750	68	30	$29,500
Anesthesiology: Pediatric	17	2	*	68	5	$9,000
Cardiology: Electrophysiology	126	58	$29,500	44	23	$29,288
Cardiology: Invasive	228	56	$29,500	151	58	$23,168
Cardiology: Inv-Intvl	370	76	$29,500	161	60	$27,563
Cardiology: Noninvasive	244	55	$29,500	158	57	$22,389
Critical Care: Intensivist	9	3	*	21	9	$14,623
Dentistry	13	2	*	40	13	$6,297
Dermatology	24	9	$29,500	220	94	$23,075
Dermatology: Mohs Surgery	2	2	*	15	11	$30,893
Emergency Medicine	288	15	$28,836	288	34	$15,550
Endocrinology/Metabolism	17	9	$12,840	165	86	$15,792
Family Practice (w/ OB)	77	21	$9,233	465	88	$15,781
Family Practice (w/o OB)	790	232	$9,761	3,344	280	$12,219
FP: Amb Only (no inpatient work)	12	4	$20,488	155	14	$9,000
Family Practice: Sports Med	6	6	*	22	13	$15,500
Family Practice: Urgent Care	17	2	*	71	19	$11,076
Gastroenterology	275	34	$29,500	346	121	$23,665
Gastroenterology: Hepatology	6	5	*	3	1	*
Genetics	*	*	*	4	3	*
Geriatrics	18	4	$7,537	35	19	$13,405
Hematology/Oncology	70	13	$22,375	257	73	$24,480
Hematology/Oncology: Onc (only)	8	4	*	30	20	$24,675
Hospice/Palliative Care	3	3	*	3	3	*
Hospitalist: Family Practice	2	2	*	28	8	$13,500
Hospitalist: Internal Medicine	87	13	$11,753	648	93	$15,423
Hospitalist: IM-Pediatrics	*	*	*	8	4	*
Hospitalist: Pediatrics	9	1	*	78	15	$10,015
Infectious Disease	21	9	$19,832	68	37	$17,021
Internal Medicine: General	302	73	$14,244	2,643	290	$13,820
IM: Amb Only (no inpatient work)	1	1	*	17	10	$8,232
Internal Med: Pediatrics	0	*	*	92	31	$8,244
Nephrology	62	8	$26,311	125	50	$20,860
Neurology	111	25	$12,000	315	109	$19,779
Obstetrics/Gynecology: General	351	72	$24,035	839	170	$20,250
OB/GYN: Gynecology (only)	24	14	$13,848	126	51	$17,926
OB/GYN: Gyn Oncology	5	3	*	23	15	$17,878
OB/GYN: Maternal & Fetal Med	16	5	$24,035	46	17	$29,250
OB/GYN: Repro Endocrinology	4	1	*	4	4	*
OB/GYN: Urogynecology	*	*	*	5	4	*
Occupational Medicine	0	*	*	83	44	$20,174
Ophthalmology	123	27	$23,000	243	88	$21,750
Ophthalmology: Pediatric	12	10	$25,375	16	11	$18,673
Ophthalmology: Retina	25	10	$15,482	13	11	$20,500
Orthopedic (Nonsurgical)	15	12	$22,000	13	11	$18,001
Orthopedic Surgery: General	249	73	$29,500	438	122	$26,659
Orthopedic Surgery: Foot & Ankle	35	28	$29,500	18	11	$29,500
Orthopedic Surgery: Hand	78	43	$29,500	42	25	$29,500
Orthopedic Surgery: Hip & Joint	66	38	$29,500	24	13	$29,500
Orthopedic Surgery: Pediatric	17	8	$29,500	20	11	$26,983
Orthopedic Surgery: Spine	66	44	$29,500	37	20	$29,500
Orthopedic Surgery: Trauma	21	12	$29,500	7	6	*
Orthopedic Surgery: Sports Med	98	46	$29,500	55	20	$29,500

page 78

Table 15: Physician Retirement Benefits by Group Type (continued)

	Single Specialty			Multispecialty		
	Phys	Med Pracs	Median	Phys	Med Pracs	Median
Otorhinolaryngology	108	18	$26,892	281	113	$24,750
Pathology: Anatomic and Clinical	61	5	$29,093	68	16	$20,603
Pathology: Anatomic	*	*	*	16	5	$12,678
Pathology: Clinical	1	1	*	29	8	$25,750
Pediatrics: General	519	67	$10,519	1,488	218	$13,071
Pediatrics: Adolescent Medicine	10	2	*	17	4	$5,540
Pediatrics: Allergy/Immunology	2	1	*	4	3	*
Pediatrics: Cardiology	7	3	*	30	12	$14,112
Pediatrics: Child Development	*	*	*	9	5	*
Pediatrics: Critical Care/Intensivist	6	1	*	73	17	$10,125
Pediatrics: Emergency Medicine	0	*	*	43	7	$10,067
Pediatrics: Endocrinology	4	2	*	21	12	$9,645
Pediatrics: Gastroenterology	1	1	*	25	12	$15,290
Pediatrics: Genetics	11	5	$11,414	6	5	*
Pediatrics: Hematology/Oncology	6	2	*	48	15	$13,300
Pediatrics: Infectious Disease	*	*	*	14	8	$9,144
Pediatrics: Neonatal Medicine	25	5	$27,645	77	13	$20,000
Pediatrics: Nephrology	*	*	*	9	7	*
Pediatrics: Neurology	4	2	*	50	21	$14,905
Pediatrics: Pulmonology	5	3	*	14	8	$13,400
Pediatrics: Rheumatology	*	*	*	7	4	*
Physiatry (Phys Med & Rehab)	47	20	$16,610	101	53	$14,843
Podiatry: General	4	4	*	103	62	$15,103
Podiatry: Surg-Foot & Ankle	2	2	*	54	21	$22,343
Podiatry: Surg-Forefoot Only	0	*	*	4	2	*
Psychiatry: General	22	3	$11,388	208	60	$14,461
Psychiatry: Child & Adolescent	2	1	*	37	19	$16,316
Psychiatry: Geriatric	4	1	*	2	1	*
Pulmonary Medicine	27	7	$25,314	154	70	$20,603
Pulmonary Medicine: Critical Care	7	4	*	51	12	$26,850
Pulmonary Med: Gen & Crit Care	48	9	$29,500	87	29	$29,500
Radiation Oncology	19	5	$29,500	82	26	$29,500
Radiology: Diagnostic-Inv	182	19	$33,750	93	25	$29,322
Radiology: Diagnostic-Noninv	264	20	$29,500	353	48	$27,563
Radiology: Nuclear Medicine	15	8	$44,000	21	13	$29,500
Rheumatology	12	7	$25,818	164	93	$15,723
Sleep Medicine	4	1	*	37	23	$19,572
Surgery: General	119	31	$29,500	556	167	$22,491
Surgery: Bariatric	7	3	*	10	6	$22,389
Surgery: Cardiovascular	72	18	$29,500	86	33	$29,500
Surgery: Colon and Rectal	*	*	*	38	17	$23,550
Surgery: Neurological	37	8	$45,000	115	49	$21,249
Surgery: Oncology	1	1	*	13	8	$26,393
Surgery: Oral	9	3	*	11	7	$16,012
Surgery: Pediatric	15	4	$29,500	28	16	$16,875
Surgery: Plastic & Reconstruction	13	2	*	78	42	$19,458
Surgery: Plastic & Recon-Hand	2	2	*	2	2	*
Surgery: Thoracic (primary)	8	4	*	21	10	$17,743
Surgery: Transplant	6	1	*	14	5	$27,039
Surgery: Trauma	9	3	*	25	7	$10,125
Surgery: Trauma-Burn	*	*	*	1	1	*
Surgery: Vascular (primary)	23	9	$29,500	102	40	$26,196
Urgent Care	10	3	$18,808	233	55	$19,226
Urology	133	21	$29,500	233	97	$25,810
Urology: Pediatric	3	3	*	7	4	*

Physician Productivity

Table 16: Collections for Professional Charges (TC/NPP Excluded)

	Phys	Med Pracs	Mean	Std. Dev.	25th %tile	Median	75th %tile	90th %tile
Allergy/Immunology	71	40	$639,789	$393,116	$390,203	$573,749	$713,158	$985,624
Anesthesiology	2,364	117	$572,543	$259,992	$390,266	$531,887	$692,623	$908,022
Anesthesiology: Pain Management	71	26	$708,282	$364,757	$430,309	$677,900	$972,156	$1,248,112
Anesthesiology: Pediatric	35	4	$416,174	$106,715	$344,576	$439,315	$483,776	$544,295
Cardiology: Electrophysiology	62	29	$782,775	$306,969	$583,785	$783,130	$886,890	$1,040,122
Cardiology: Invasive	157	47	$667,176	$291,554	$473,536	$629,195	$814,793	$954,058
Cardiology: Inv-Intvl	207	55	$835,374	$356,328	$583,393	$793,914	$972,989	$1,290,414
Cardiology: Noninvasive	151	44	$613,980	$268,094	$422,813	$568,695	$742,769	$986,782
Critical Care: Intensivist	21	7	$318,786	$114,343	$226,823	$282,077	$403,353	$497,369
Dentistry	9	3	*	*	*	*	*	*
Dermatology	151	64	$838,717	$386,282	$603,635	$738,110	$1,002,420	$1,414,670
Dermatology: Mohs Surgery	13	10	$1,760,227	$575,291	$1,255,927	$1,690,651	$2,114,913	$2,727,048
Emergency Medicine	280	20	$307,788	$110,699	$235,266	$302,599	$391,470	$446,732
Endocrinology/Metabolism	121	66	$366,803	$122,064	$281,378	$357,810	$419,402	$514,071
Family Practice (w/ OB)	323	65	$401,049	$168,965	$300,675	$374,925	$464,810	$609,654
Family Practice (w/o OB)	2,463	294	$370,720	$145,562	$285,507	$363,214	$449,157	$547,754
FP: Amb Only (no inpatient work)	72	9	$365,991	$150,058	$266,756	$333,154	$429,047	$573,963
Family Practice: Sports Med	22	14	$418,907	$213,715	$264,696	$360,770	$537,016	$784,590
Family Practice: Urgent Care	61	13	$457,140	$162,641	$360,776	$436,032	$518,598	$656,448
Gastroenterology	375	102	$762,298	$280,402	$587,000	$743,867	$905,751	$1,141,749
Gastroenterology: Hepatology	6	4	*	*	*	*	*	*
Genetics	3	2	*	*	*	*	*	*
Geriatrics	38	16	$218,515	$109,224	$146,460	$197,389	$313,451	$386,366
Hematology/Oncology	174	48	$688,240	$624,253	$322,184	$526,461	$798,385	$1,106,276
Hematology/Oncology: Onc (only)	20	14	$645,763	$728,306	$215,947	$427,990	$777,671	$2,204,419
Hospice/Palliative Care	4	4	*	*	*	*	*	*
Hospitalist: Family Practice	15	5	$206,629	$68,486	$171,145	$190,000	$239,657	$327,567
Hospitalist: Internal Medicine	603	84	$197,521	$82,847	$145,060	$186,528	$239,554	$311,406
Hospitalist: IM-Pediatrics	3	2	*	*	*	*	*	*
Hospitalist: Pediatrics	29	9	$106,978	$52,151	$67,740	$116,741	$139,967	$165,168
Infectious Disease	53	28	$299,631	$143,301	$187,732	$274,396	$376,731	$487,330
Internal Medicine: General	1,837	218	$351,457	$137,430	$264,273	$345,265	$423,456	$511,995
IM: Amb Only (no inpatient work)	14	7	$378,351	$386,120	$233,428	$275,808	$392,237	$1,085,961
Internal Med: Pediatrics	42	18	$396,713	$133,547	$287,097	$401,142	$505,869	$583,354
Nephrology	96	34	$429,101	$208,293	$239,282	$432,795	$546,015	$714,108
Neurology	246	83	$428,845	$195,879	$287,463	$405,408	$540,487	$712,058
Obstetrics/Gynecology: General	624	127	$615,886	$258,464	$454,517	$588,871	$739,322	$942,272
OB/GYN: Gynecology (only)	67	36	$464,869	$211,869	$336,934	$421,995	$582,317	$808,323
OB/GYN: Gyn Oncology	13	10	$492,824	$220,843	$308,100	$418,832	$624,215	$926,743
OB/GYN: Maternal & Fetal Med	23	11	$756,781	$406,945	$371,664	$734,243	$1,121,974	$1,372,500
OB/GYN: Repro Endocrinology	3	3	*	*	*	*	*	*
OB/GYN: Urogynecology	3	2	*	*	*	*	*	*
Occupational Medicine	51	22	$398,492	$178,924	$285,569	$406,671	$546,850	$623,762
Ophthalmology	168	59	$761,667	$344,151	$515,836	$669,795	$959,176	$1,247,812
Ophthalmology: Pediatric	13	8	$653,311	$271,069	$502,326	$622,006	$806,836	$1,109,288
Ophthalmology: Retina	12	11	$1,493,772	$701,722	$958,162	$1,294,669	$1,818,993	$2,922,416
Orthopedic (Nonsurgical)	22	18	$361,805	$173,393	$237,398	$348,890	$460,600	$644,242
Orthopedic Surgery: General	355	98	$815,387	$315,870	$620,382	$797,705	$1,023,055	$1,220,832
Orthopedic Surgery: Foot & Ankle	18	15	$811,799	$344,071	$594,132	$743,131	$1,079,773	$1,430,213
Orthopedic Surgery: Hand	55	30	$941,688	$389,839	$723,181	$934,638	$1,087,183	$1,507,384
Orthopedic Surgery: Hip & Joint	40	22	$915,930	$339,785	$623,917	$880,871	$1,148,212	$1,437,853
Orthopedic Surgery: Pediatric	9	6	*	*	*	*	*	*
Orthopedic Surgery: Spine	39	26	$1,070,976	$389,963	$783,730	$932,616	$1,410,487	$1,616,213
Orthopedic Surgery: Trauma	13	9	$890,335	$367,122	$571,109	$908,004	$1,243,610	$1,411,146
Orthopedic Surgery: Sports Med	53	29	$950,250	$395,245	$729,952	$946,000	$1,153,015	$1,336,863

Table 16: Collections for Professional Charges (TC/NPP Excluded) (continued)

	Phys	Med Pracs	Mean	Std. Dev.	25th %tile	Median	75th %tile	90th %tile
Otorhinolaryngology	199	75	$785,946	$323,145	$554,662	$717,891	$981,162	$1,260,965
Pathology: Anatomic and Clinical	58	9	$856,054	$795,845	$402,022	$560,156	$1,042,671	$2,229,051
Pathology: Anatomic	3	1	*	*	*	*	*	*
Pathology: Clinical	23	6	$533,913	$268,626	$330,101	$418,151	$662,784	$966,812
Pediatrics: General	1,372	166	$428,278	$172,117	$309,036	$406,865	$523,377	$652,219
Pediatrics: Adolescent Medicine	23	6	$393,354	$212,491	$123,445	$440,328	$527,556	$692,142
Pediatrics: Allergy/Immunology	2	1	*	*	*	*	*	*
Pediatrics: Cardiology	19	8	$358,174	$176,795	$200,170	$327,857	$468,821	$580,122
Pediatrics: Child Development	7	4	*	*	*	*	*	*
Pediatrics: Critical Care/Intensivist	44	12	$211,107	$121,693	$121,774	$192,514	$251,304	$448,931
Pediatrics: Emergency Medicine	18	3	$370,621	$189,571	$197,667	$342,276	$536,095	$659,809
Pediatrics: Endocrinology	14	11	$224,447	$90,171	$151,461	$234,791	$276,880	$373,784
Pediatrics: Gastroenterology	17	7	$224,731	$79,554	$208,056	$244,732	$260,559	$307,019
Pediatrics: Genetics	3	2	*	*	*	*	*	*
Pediatrics: Hematology/Oncology	28	12	$231,545	$89,671	$150,721	$213,642	$285,417	$358,786
Pediatrics: Infectious Disease	3	3	*	*	*	*	*	*
Pediatrics: Neonatal Medicine	39	9	$457,941	$185,349	$349,585	$420,696	$560,502	$699,504
Pediatrics: Nephrology	4	4	*	*	*	*	*	*
Pediatrics: Neurology	30	17	$318,905	$159,881	$188,921	$283,737	$450,215	$588,244
Pediatrics: Pulmonology	12	8	$264,087	$194,300	$143,476	$196,108	$339,570	$690,227
Pediatrics: Rheumatology	3	2	*	*	*	*	*	*
Physiatry (Phys Med & Rehab)	95	42	$443,809	$219,562	$312,473	$396,000	$518,278	$744,671
Podiatry: General	78	46	$439,722	$187,949	$322,229	$415,156	$510,720	$686,949
Podiatry: Surg-Foot & Ankle	23	13	$495,471	$197,975	$325,915	$472,836	$608,969	$846,953
Podiatry: Surg-Forefoot Only	0	*	*	*	*	*	*	*
Psychiatry: General	123	36	$196,689	$99,788	$126,364	$196,684	$250,248	$342,857
Psychiatry: Child & Adolescent	22	13	$174,203	$112,546	$49,378	$172,172	$313,251	$324,860
Psychiatry: Geriatric	7	3	*	*	*	*	*	*
Pulmonary Medicine	123	51	$475,986	$215,680	$320,204	$446,582	$587,184	$808,427
Pulmonary Medicine: Critical Care	40	10	$402,019	$114,833	$314,278	$426,919	$475,050	$552,364
Pulmonary Med: Gen & Crit Care	39	17	$547,872	$158,159	$483,485	$557,939	$618,326	$761,352
Radiation Oncology	44	14	$588,754	$224,514	$420,530	$537,285	$807,452	$876,654
Radiology: Diagnostic-Inv	108	23	$746,360	$309,722	$569,315	$685,647	$863,972	$1,109,611
Radiology: Diagnostic-Noninv	228	33	$724,536	$396,022	$509,478	$664,825	$808,334	$1,074,993
Radiology: Nuclear Medicine	17	10	$528,417	$195,375	$351,778	$569,673	$675,813	$811,023
Rheumatology	131	66	$429,864	$253,615	$273,757	$351,849	$501,442	$779,010
Sleep Medicine	25	11	$583,977	$267,159	$405,664	$571,759	$733,035	$926,497
Surgery: General	460	131	$563,673	$207,356	$423,946	$535,803	$681,082	$853,538
Surgery: Bariatric	6	4	*	*	*	*	*	*
Surgery: Cardiovascular	123	35	$598,666	$234,053	$414,483	$598,768	$789,601	$894,696
Surgery: Colon and Rectal	27	12	$817,074	$318,263	$565,539	$771,031	$998,484	$1,186,969
Surgery: Neurological	124	40	$1,010,801	$575,196	$557,710	$882,341	$1,351,656	$1,836,169
Surgery: Oncology	11	7	$616,867	$249,370	$520,082	$622,731	$725,767	$1,005,087
Surgery: Oral	12	6	$1,150,054	$643,812	$617,682	$932,715	$1,480,292	$2,354,046
Surgery: Pediatric	32	15	$529,222	$347,521	$278,205	$382,036	$773,031	$1,007,486
Surgery: Plastic & Reconstruction	56	27	$751,118	$337,446	$480,331	$689,839	$958,755	$1,211,122
Surgery: Plastic & Recon-Hand	1	1	*	*	*	*	*	*
Surgery: Thoracic (primary)	27	12	$433,455	$153,251	$331,174	$409,500	$491,863	$659,651
Surgery: Transplant	15	4	$666,466	$258,002	$428,605	$742,228	$852,483	$1,016,406
Surgery: Trauma	35	10	$342,738	$183,595	$182,450	$313,639	$428,450	$620,477
Surgery: Trauma-Burn	1	1	*	*	*	*	*	*
Surgery: Vascular (primary)	65	31	$601,325	$249,859	$415,531	$560,707	$787,583	$946,275
Urgent Care	215	35	$487,258	$167,831	$347,184	$475,370	$603,191	$709,673
Urology	236	68	$710,171	$285,037	$503,720	$662,204	$882,787	$1,102,827
Urology: Pediatric	7	2	*	*	*	*	*	*

Table 17: Collections for Professional Charges (TC/NPP Excluded) by Group Type

	Single Specialty			Multispecialty		
	Phys	Med Pracs	Median	Phys	Med Pracs	Median
Allergy/Immunology	11	4	$641,487	60	36	$554,306
Anesthesiology	2,143	93	$533,500	221	24	$502,451
Anesthesiology: Pain Management	30	10	$430,309	41	16	$944,304
Anesthesiology: Pediatric	23	2	*	12	2	*
Cardiology: Electrophysiology	39	15	$814,182	23	14	$667,594
Cardiology: Invasive	53	12	$561,555	104	35	$658,363
Cardiology: Inv-Intvl	109	21	$730,364	98	34	$817,491
Cardiology: Noninvasive	63	19	$568,695	88	25	$562,071
Critical Care: Intensivist	2	1	*	19	6	$309,858
Dentistry	0	*	*	9	3	*
Dermatology	14	5	$718,110	137	59	$745,386
Dermatology: Mohs Surgery	1	1	*	12	9	$1,647,381
Emergency Medicine	165	8	$297,642	115	12	$316,793
Endocrinology/Metabolism	9	6	*	112	60	$366,168
Family Practice (w/ OB)	37	10	$356,141	286	55	$380,933
Family Practice (w/o OB)	362	123	$365,625	2,101	171	$362,402
FP: Amb Only (no inpatient work)	7	3	*	65	6	$330,522
Family Practice: Sports Med	7	4	*	15	10	$375,474
Family Practice: Urgent Care	23	1	*	38	12	$419,575
Gastroenterology	129	18	$709,954	246	84	$755,773
Gastroenterology: Hepatology	3	3	*	3	1	*
Genetics	*	*	*	3	2	*
Geriatrics	16	3	$215,978	22	13	$191,192
Hematology/Oncology	39	4	$609,180	135	44	$502,280
Hematology/Oncology: Onc (only)	2	2	*	18	12	$361,921
Hospice/Palliative Care	2	2	*	2	2	*
Hospitalist: Family Practice	2	2	*	13	3	$187,045
Hospitalist: Internal Medicine	114	15	$228,509	489	69	$179,720
Hospitalist: IM-Pediatrics	*	*	*	3	2	*
Hospitalist: Pediatrics	9	1	*	20	8	$110,426
Infectious Disease	18	7	$323,488	35	21	$263,487
Internal Medicine: General	142	34	$309,164	1,695	184	$350,359
IM: Amb Only (no inpatient work)	0	*	*	14	7	$275,808
Internal Med: Pediatrics	0	*	*	42	18	$401,142
Nephrology	13	2	*	83	32	$459,158
Neurology	44	13	$347,809	202	70	$412,042
Obstetrics/Gynecology: General	102	27	$573,174	522	100	$589,365
OB/GYN: Gynecology (only)	3	3	*	64	33	$411,246
OB/GYN: Gyn Oncology	4	2	*	9	8	*
OB/GYN: Maternal & Fetal Med	9	4	*	14	7	$731,615
OB/GYN: Repro Endocrinology	0	*	*	3	3	*
OB/GYN: Urogynecology	*	*	*	3	2	*
Occupational Medicine	2	1	*	49	21	$414,962
Ophthalmology	34	11	$849,402	134	48	$637,084
Ophthalmology: Pediatric	2	2	*	11	6	$601,637
Ophthalmology: Retina	3	3	*	9	8	*
Orthopedic (Nonsurgical)	12	10	$308,133	10	8	$395,047
Orthopedic Surgery: General	99	27	$787,742	256	71	$803,919
Orthopedic Surgery: Foot & Ankle	13	11	$755,581	5	4	*
Orthopedic Surgery: Hand	36	16	$946,583	19	14	$821,793
Orthopedic Surgery: Hip & Joint	26	15	$817,972	14	7	$1,021,817
Orthopedic Surgery: Pediatric	5	2	*	4	4	*
Orthopedic Surgery: Spine	22	15	$873,919	17	11	$964,934
Orthopedic Surgery: Trauma	9	6	*	4	3	*
Orthopedic Surgery: Sports Med	33	19	$946,000	20	10	$957,990

Table 17: Collections for Professional Charges (TC/NPP Excluded) by Group Type (continued)

	Single Specialty			Multispecialty		
	Phys	Med Pracs	Median	Phys	Med Pracs	Median
Otorhinolaryngology	40	9	$743,476	159	66	$717,891
Pathology: Anatomic and Clinical	31	2	*	27	7	$501,770
Pathology: Anatomic	*	*	*	3	1	*
Pathology: Clinical	1	1	*	22	5	$401,083
Pediatrics: General	398	39	$444,191	974	127	$399,584
Pediatrics: Adolescent Medicine	9	2	*	14	4	$240,062
Pediatrics: Allergy/Immunology	2	1	*	0	*	*
Pediatrics: Cardiology	4	2	*	15	6	$370,859
Pediatrics: Child Development	*	*	*	7	4	*
Pediatrics: Critical Care/Intensivist	7	1	*	37	11	$212,848
Pediatrics: Emergency Medicine	0	*	*	18	3	$342,276
Pediatrics: Endocrinology	3	2	*	11	9	$181,853
Pediatrics: Gastroenterology	0	*	*	17	7	$244,732
Pediatrics: Genetics	0	*	*	3	2	*
Pediatrics: Hematology/Oncology	6	2	*	22	10	$226,041
Pediatrics: Infectious Disease	*	*	*	3	3	*
Pediatrics: Neonatal Medicine	23	5	$353,418	16	4	$436,174
Pediatrics: Nephrology	*	*	*	4	4	*
Pediatrics: Neurology	4	2	*	26	15	$299,494
Pediatrics: Pulmonology	5	3	*	7	5	*
Pediatrics: Rheumatology	*	*	*	3	2	*
Physiatry (Phys Med & Rehab)	34	12	$400,457	61	30	$380,092
Podiatry: General	3	3	*	75	43	$427,482
Podiatry: Surg-Foot & Ankle	1	1	*	22	12	$469,023
Podiatry: Surg-Forefoot Only	0	*	*	0	*	*
Psychiatry: General	16	2	*	107	34	$192,498
Psychiatry: Child & Adolescent	2	1	*	20	12	$157,072
Psychiatry: Geriatric	4	1	*	3	2	*
Pulmonary Medicine	5	2	*	118	49	$450,459
Pulmonary Medicine: Critical Care	4	2	*	36	8	$444,513
Pulmonary Med: Gen & Crit Care	9	3	*	30	14	$545,844
Radiation Oncology	14	4	$652,572	30	10	$495,194
Radiology: Diagnostic-Inv	74	11	$671,207	34	12	$749,694
Radiology: Diagnostic-Noninv	118	11	$660,508	110	22	$686,430
Radiology: Nuclear Medicine	10	5	$485,530	7	5	*
Rheumatology	13	6	$238,517	118	60	$365,550
Sleep Medicine	4	1	*	21	10	$584,786
Surgery: General	72	20	$507,099	388	111	$542,356
Surgery: Bariatric	2	1	*	4	3	*
Surgery: Cardiovascular	62	14	$668,534	61	21	$551,788
Surgery: Colon and Rectal	*	*	*	27	12	$771,031
Surgery: Neurological	39	9	$1,162,287	85	31	$859,623
Surgery: Oncology	0	*	*	11	7	$622,731
Surgery: Oral	6	2	*	6	4	*
Surgery: Pediatric	18	5	$499,657	14	10	$356,801
Surgery: Plastic & Reconstruction	5	2	*	51	25	$709,713
Surgery: Plastic & Recon-Hand	0	*	*	1	1	*
Surgery: Thoracic (primary)	12	5	$376,880	15	7	$433,540
Surgery: Transplant	7	1	*	8	3	*
Surgery: Trauma	6	2	*	29	8	$346,780
Surgery: Trauma-Burn	*	*	*	1	1	*
Surgery: Vascular (primary)	5	4	*	60	27	$570,934
Urgent Care	16	4	$306,344	199	31	$479,585
Urology	99	12	$642,660	137	56	$670,101
Urology: Pediatric	3	1	*	4	1	*

Table 18: Collections for Professional Charges (TC/NPP Excluded) by Hospital Ownership

	Hospital Owned			Not Hospital Owned		
	Phys	Med Pracs	Median	Phys	Med Pracs	Median
Allergy/Immunology	16	10	$441,931	55	30	$603,352
Anesthesiology	104	10	$403,624	2,227	106	$533,500
Anesthesiology: Pain Management	11	5	$677,900	60	21	$686,531
Anesthesiology: Pediatric	11	1	*	24	3	$461,843
Cardiology: Electrophysiology	14	8	$704,878	48	21	$786,361
Cardiology: Invasive	46	10	$697,265	111	37	$600,000
Cardiology: Inv-Intvl	45	15	$725,620	162	40	$811,840
Cardiology: Noninvasive	68	15	$528,778	83	29	$602,802
Critical Care: Intensivist	10	2	*	11	5	$329,870
Dentistry	3	1	*	6	2	*
Dermatology	46	18	$690,589	105	46	$764,026
Dermatology: Mohs Surgery	3	1	*	10	9	$1,854,586
Emergency Medicine	110	11	$282,336	170	9	$320,620
Endocrinology/Metabolism	57	28	$324,768	64	38	$372,756
Family Practice (w/ OB)	161	32	$345,404	162	33	$405,184
Family Practice (w/o OB)	1,476	184	$348,715	987	110	$391,640
FP: Amb Only (no inpatient work)	26	4	$312,275	46	5	$344,408
Family Practice: Sports Med	6	5	*	16	9	$481,413
Family Practice: Urgent Care	25	6	$396,928	36	7	$466,775
Gastroenterology	83	26	$686,927	292	76	$751,312
Gastroenterology: Hepatology	3	1	*	3	3	*
Genetics	3	2	*	0	*	*
Geriatrics	20	9	$188,824	18	7	$249,365
Hematology/Oncology	47	9	$301,753	127	39	$624,237
Hematology/Oncology: Onc (only)	4	4	*	16	10	$464,736
Hospice/Palliative Care	3	3	*	1	1	*
Hospitalist: Family Practice	11	2	*	4	3	*
Hospitalist: Internal Medicine	394	45	$178,519	209	39	$209,576
Hospitalist: IM-Pediatrics	1	1	*	2	1	*
Hospitalist: Pediatrics	29	9	$116,741	0	*	*
Infectious Disease	27	14	$195,124	26	14	$341,108
Internal Medicine: General	1,025	108	$323,740	812	110	$377,791
IM: Amb Only (no inpatient work)	12	5	$260,767	2	2	*
Internal Med: Pediatrics	18	7	$475,801	24	11	$386,291
Nephrology	25	10	$323,909	71	24	$480,583
Neurology	113	32	$346,473	133	51	$461,571
Obstetrics/Gynecology: General	271	52	$529,278	353	75	$627,297
OB/GYN: Gynecology (only)	24	12	$362,175	43	24	$471,616
OB/GYN: Gyn Oncology	10	7	$416,885	3	3	*
OB/GYN: Maternal & Fetal Med	21	9	$728,001	2	2	*
OB/GYN: Repro Endocrinology	3	3	*	0	*	*
OB/GYN: Urogynecology	3	2	*	0	*	*
Occupational Medicine	16	9	$326,415	35	13	$425,850
Ophthalmology	42	13	$657,798	126	46	$679,832
Ophthalmology: Pediatric	4	3	*	9	5	*
Ophthalmology: Retina	5	4	*	7	7	*
Orthopedic (Nonsurgical)	3	2	*	19	16	$314,572
Orthopedic Surgery: General	97	26	$678,757	258	72	$854,086
Orthopedic Surgery: Foot & Ankle	2	1	*	16	14	$759,495
Orthopedic Surgery: Hand	4	4	*	51	26	$945,746
Orthopedic Surgery: Hip & Joint	4	2	*	36	20	$899,402
Orthopedic Surgery: Pediatric	7	4	*	2	2	*
Orthopedic Surgery: Spine	6	3	*	33	23	$932,616
Orthopedic Surgery: Trauma	2	2	*	11	7	$986,330
Orthopedic Surgery: Sports Med	10	5	$661,339	43	24	$1,003,502

Table 18: Collections for Professional Charges (TC/NPP Excluded) by Hospital Ownership (continued)

	Hospital Owned			Not Hospital Owned		
	Phys	Med Pracs	Median	Phys	Med Pracs	Median
Otorhinolaryngology	54	19	$623,524	145	56	$753,740
Pathology: Anatomic and Clinical	19	3	$430,623	39	6	$836,154
Pathology: Anatomic	0	*	*	3	1	*
Pathology: Clinical	4	1	*	19	5	$380,178
Pediatrics: General	779	75	$398,490	593	91	$418,561
Pediatrics: Adolescent Medicine	12	2	*	11	4	$527,556
Pediatrics: Allergy/Immunology	0	*	*	2	1	*
Pediatrics: Cardiology	18	7	$324,294	1	1	*
Pediatrics: Child Development	5	3	*	2	1	*
Pediatrics: Critical Care/Intensivist	32	9	$145,694	12	3	$346,705
Pediatrics: Emergency Medicine	18	3	$342,276	0	*	*
Pediatrics: Endocrinology	11	8	$239,278	3	3	*
Pediatrics: Gastroenterology	15	6	$246,539	2	1	*
Pediatrics: Genetics	0	*	*	3	2	*
Pediatrics: Hematology/Oncology	22	9	$203,534	6	3	*
Pediatrics: Infectious Disease	3	3	*	0	*	*
Pediatrics: Neonatal Medicine	27	7	$397,724	12	2	*
Pediatrics: Nephrology	3	3	*	1	1	*
Pediatrics: Neurology	21	12	$259,027	9	5	*
Pediatrics: Pulmonology	9	6	*	3	2	*
Pediatrics: Rheumatology	1	1	*	2	1	*
Physiatry (Phys Med & Rehab)	49	16	$340,513	46	26	$442,600
Podiatry: General	21	9	$396,787	57	37	$427,482
Podiatry: Surg-Foot & Ankle	8	2	*	15	11	$499,338
Podiatry: Surg-Forefoot Only	*	*	*	0	*	*
Psychiatry: General	101	25	$186,759	22	11	$266,951
Psychiatry: Child & Adolescent	18	9	$172,172	4	4	*
Psychiatry: Geriatric	3	2	*	4	1	*
Pulmonary Medicine	42	16	$367,498	81	35	$496,040
Pulmonary Medicine: Critical Care	15	4	$270,997	25	6	$463,263
Pulmonary Med: Gen & Crit Care	2	2	*	37	15	$560,003
Radiation Oncology	27	8	$454,341	17	6	$741,601
Radiology: Diagnostic-Inv	12	4	$733,969	96	19	$675,550
Radiology: Diagnostic-Noninv	48	6	$605,019	180	27	$675,618
Radiology: Nuclear Medicine	5	3	*	12	7	$485,530
Rheumatology	70	25	$342,725	61	41	$354,137
Sleep Medicine	7	5	*	18	6	$549,505
Surgery: General	166	42	$472,850	294	89	$561,242
Surgery: Bariatric	1	1	*	5	3	*
Surgery: Cardiovascular	42	13	$405,764	81	22	$700,227
Surgery: Colon and Rectal	3	2	*	24	10	$807,063
Surgery: Neurological	41	17	$640,618	83	23	$1,100,662
Surgery: Oncology	5	3	*	6	4	*
Surgery: Oral	2	1	*	10	5	$972,277
Surgery: Pediatric	14	9	$316,325	18	6	$687,506
Surgery: Plastic & Reconstruction	25	10	$560,632	31	17	$776,363
Surgery: Plastic & Recon-Hand	*	*	*	1	1	*
Surgery: Thoracic (primary)	14	6	$406,885	13	6	$409,500
Surgery: Transplant	15	4	$742,228	0	*	*
Surgery: Trauma	32	8	$279,673	3	2	*
Surgery: Trauma-Burn	1	1	*	*	*	*
Surgery: Vascular (primary)	20	6	$549,336	45	25	$560,707
Urgent Care	74	11	$434,554	141	24	$499,112
Urology	48	18	$589,854	188	50	$692,924
Urology: Pediatric	4	1	*	3	1	*

Table 19: Collections for Professional Charges (TC/NPP Excluded) by Geographic Section for All Practices

	Eastern		Midwest		Southern		Western	
	Phys	Median	Phys	Median	Phys	Median	Phys	Median
Allergy/Immunology	6	*	25	$467,527	16	$503,602	24	$676,000
Anesthesiology	624	$543,720	532	$508,095	561	$743,773	647	$370,000
Anesthesiology: Pain Management	19	$430,309	24	$730,666	24	$987,358	4	*
Anesthesiology: Pediatric	0	*	27	*	1	*	7	*
Cardiology: Electrophysiology	12	$869,622	21	$793,006	20	$781,770	9	*
Cardiology: Invasive	12	$785,052	51	$599,526	54	$632,148	40	$655,099
Cardiology: Inv-Intvl	35	$848,913	72	$801,162	56	$814,555	44	$711,608
Cardiology: Noninvasive	69	$592,342	38	$554,876	36	$568,695	8	*
Critical Care: Intensivist	10	*	5	*	0	*	6	*
Dentistry	3	*	*	*	6	*	0	*
Dermatology	23	$637,366	45	$855,369	38	$734,170	45	$716,247
Dermatology: Mohs Surgery	4	*	6	*	2	*	1	*
Emergency Medicine	74	$268,990	55	$338,032	25	*	126	$318,643
Endocrinology/Metabolism	27	$359,276	29	$339,139	44	$370,919	21	$338,776
Family Practice (w/ OB)	22	$331,354	145	$400,009	65	$360,228	91	$374,916
Family Practice (w/o OB)	447	$343,568	761	$383,126	640	$331,559	615	$389,872
FP: Amb Only (no inpatient work)	26	$312,275	1	*	42	$333,154	3	*
Family Practice: Sports Med	8	*	5	*	6	*	3	*
Family Practice: Urgent Care	14	$409,504	13	$516,360	33	$452,735	1	*
Gastroenterology	52	$683,408	140	$790,006	108	$727,054	75	$761,662
Gastroenterology: Hepatology	0	*	1	*	1	*	4	*
Genetics	0	*	3	*	0	*	0	*
Geriatrics	6	*	7	*	9	*	16	$249,365
Hematology/Oncology	40	$422,759	48	$750,641	59	$495,098	27	$490,537
Hematology/Oncology: Onc (only)	2	*	3	*	9	*	6	*
Hospice/Palliative Care	2	*	1	*	0	*	1	*
Hospitalist: Family Practice	0	*	12	*	3	*	0	*
Hospitalist: Internal Medicine	111	$193,082	140	$204,001	167	$205,901	185	$156,660
Hospitalist: IM-Pediatrics	0	*	*	*	3	*	*	*
Hospitalist: Pediatrics	4	*	7	*	10	*	8	*
Infectious Disease	21	$208,084	11	$233,026	13	$302,751	8	*
Internal Medicine: General	369	$324,828	575	$367,581	479	$335,442	414	$357,288
IM: Amb Only (no inpatient work)	6	*	2	*	5	*	1	*
Internal Med: Pediatrics	5	*	23	$467,088	13	$291,872	1	*
Nephrology	17	$415,472	25	$459,158	32	$508,991	22	$220,411
Neurology	69	$320,610	79	$461,710	49	$430,734	49	$417,412
Obstetrics/Gynecology: General	113	$474,802	221	$621,335	148	$652,492	142	$601,255
OB/GYN: Gynecology (only)	8	*	25	$569,222	24	$349,462	10	$368,719
OB/GYN: Gyn Oncology	2	*	7	*	2	*	2	*
OB/GYN: Maternal & Fetal Med	7	*	3	*	11	$559,945	2	*
OB/GYN: Repro Endocrinology	2	*	0	*	1	*	0	*
OB/GYN: Urogynecology	3	*	0	*	*	*	0	*
Occupational Medicine	2	*	14	$326,620	5	*	30	$509,829
Ophthalmology	29	$643,923	56	$698,120	48	$702,591	35	$574,183
Ophthalmology: Pediatric	3	*	0	*	5	*	5	*
Ophthalmology: Retina	2	*	5	*	3	*	2	*
Orthopedic (Nonsurgical)	5	*	7	*	6	*	4	*
Orthopedic Surgery: General	56	$765,812	109	$900,502	100	$794,987	90	$717,028
Orthopedic Surgery: Foot & Ankle	6	*	1	*	6	*	5	*
Orthopedic Surgery: Hand	15	$934,638	7	*	8	*	25	$767,613
Orthopedic Surgery: Hip & Joint	16	$796,679	10	$840,172	8	*	6	*
Orthopedic Surgery: Pediatric	1	*	2	*	6	*	0	*
Orthopedic Surgery: Spine	15	$916,225	7	*	9	*	8	*
Orthopedic Surgery: Trauma	6	*	2	*	1	*	4	*
Orthopedic Surgery: Sports Med	24	$975,951	7	*	9	*	13	$934,999

Table 19: Collections for Professional Charges (TC/NPP Excluded) by Geographic Section for All Practices (continued)

	Eastern		Midwest		Southern		Western	
	Phys	Median	Phys	Median	Phys	Median	Phys	Median
Otorhinolaryngology	37	$644,577	55	$754,507	58	$830,813	49	$717,891
Pathology: Anatomic and Clinical	17	*	4	*	32	$617,083	5	*
Pathology: Anatomic	0	*	0	*	3	*	0	*
Pathology: Clinical	5	*	6	*	12	$401,083	0	*
Pediatrics: General	210	$384,995	417	$410,465	447	$427,543	298	$400,023
Pediatrics: Adolescent Medicine	3	*	1	*	8	*	11	*
Pediatrics: Allergy/Immunology	*	*	0	*	0	*	2	*
Pediatrics: Cardiology	5	*	3	*	7	*	4	*
Pediatrics: Child Development	2	*	2	*	2	*	1	*
Pediatrics: Critical Care/Intensivist	2	*	26	$141,898	14	$247,464	2	*
Pediatrics: Emergency Medicine	1	*	17	*	0	*	0	*
Pediatrics: Endocrinology	4	*	4	*	5	*	1	*
Pediatrics: Gastroenterology	5	*	5	*	3	*	4	*
Pediatrics: Genetics	0	*	0	*	0	*	3	*
Pediatrics: Hematology/Oncology	3	*	11	$217,416	13	$234,666	1	*
Pediatrics: Infectious Disease	0	*	1	*	1	*	1	*
Pediatrics: Neonatal Medicine	8	*	12	$421,668	7	*	12	*
Pediatrics: Nephrology	1	*	2	*	0	*	1	*
Pediatrics: Neurology	3	*	17	$332,892	7	*	3	*
Pediatrics: Pulmonology	2	*	5	*	4	*	1	*
Pediatrics: Rheumatology	1	*	0	*	0	*	2	*
Physiatry (Phys Med & Rehab)	15	$427,905	25	$394,446	34	$323,770	21	$472,598
Podiatry: General	2	*	38	$424,121	20	$434,918	18	$418,780
Podiatry: Surg-Foot & Ankle	1	*	11	$608,969	0	*	11	$413,307
Podiatry: Surg-Forefoot Only	*	*	0	*	0	*	0	*
Psychiatry: General	39	$139,617	29	$214,895	34	$224,861	21	$196,764
Psychiatry: Child & Adolescent	7	*	5	*	7	*	3	*
Psychiatry: Geriatric	5	*	0	*	*	*	2	*
Pulmonary Medicine	20	$370,732	40	$513,684	38	$435,266	25	$448,979
Pulmonary Medicine: Critical Care	0	*	20	$461,457	13	$275,221	7	*
Pulmonary Med: Gen & Crit Care	7	*	13	$533,748	14	$604,691	5	*
Radiation Oncology	5	*	9	*	12	$625,743	18	$403,336
Radiology: Diagnostic-Inv	16	$673,459	13	$793,860	38	$661,182	41	$683,041
Radiology: Diagnostic-Noninv	58	$543,873	33	$627,345	96	$698,064	41	$707,037
Radiology: Nuclear Medicine	2	*	3	*	11	$569,421	1	*
Rheumatology	26	$342,725	45	$363,347	35	$338,495	25	$345,892
Sleep Medicine	1	*	0	*	18	$568,819	6	*
Surgery: General	84	$480,788	130	$662,561	119	$548,461	127	$479,707
Surgery: Bariatric	3	*	1	*	0	*	2	*
Surgery: Cardiovascular	29	$537,433	26	$673,657	43	$757,543	25	$488,580
Surgery: Colon and Rectal	10	$663,920	8	*	4	*	5	*
Surgery: Neurological	26	$869,553	23	$1,053,756	39	$865,730	36	$906,792
Surgery: Oncology	4	*	*	*	5	*	2	*
Surgery: Oral	8	*	2	*	1	*	1	*
Surgery: Pediatric	2	*	11	$276,733	16	$687,506	3	*
Surgery: Plastic & Reconstruction	11	$563,527	12	$819,715	22	$635,719	11	$846,049
Surgery: Plastic & Recon-Hand	0	*	0	*	0	*	1	*
Surgery: Thoracic (primary)	7	*	6	*	3	*	11	$423,291
Surgery: Transplant	2	*	0	*	7	*	6	*
Surgery: Trauma	12	$224,106	5	*	17	$332,309	1	*
Surgery: Trauma-Burn	0	*	*	*	1	*	*	*
Surgery: Vascular (primary)	15	$661,257	21	$578,826	21	$445,341	8	*
Urgent Care	9	*	60	$477,388	23	$446,808	123	$503,114
Urology	30	$703,225	50	$713,698	110	$648,801	46	$655,900
Urology: Pediatric	0	*	4	*	3	*	0	*

Table 20: Collections for Professional Charges (TC/NPP Excluded) by Years in Specialty

	1 to 2 years		3 to 7 years		8 to 17 years		18 years or more	
	Phys	Median	Phys	Median	Phys	Median	Phys	Median
Allergy/Immunology	4	*	8	*	17	$603,352	32	$668,091
Anesthesiology	115	$509,104	206	$481,519	973	$543,720	704	$533,500
Anesthesiology: Pain Management	3	*	26	$430,309	26	$733,275	10	$872,814
Anesthesiology: Pediatric	5	*	4	*	9	*	10	*
Cardiology: Electrophysiology	8	*	15	$814,182	20	$777,316	15	$883,662
Cardiology: Invasive	17	$606,333	33	$636,952	47	$623,756	43	$641,160
Cardiology: Inv-Intvl	7	*	28	$832,967	65	$814,793	77	$788,013
Cardiology: Noninvasive	9	*	23	$637,601	39	$624,361	64	$549,059
Critical Care: Intensivist	2	*	5	*	4	*	3	*
Dentistry	0	*	2	*	2	*	4	*
Dermatology	6	*	33	$766,215	48	$684,279	53	$791,256
Dermatology: Mohs Surgery	0	*	3	*	6	*	3	*
Emergency Medicine	14	$267,957	31	$403,387	45	$331,461	46	$263,311
Endocrinology/Metabolism	11	$290,270	26	$355,505	24	$354,453	36	$373,397
Family Practice (w/ OB)	25	$265,973	78	$359,921	111	$390,816	69	$407,803
Family Practice (w/o OB)	118	$277,970	415	$340,220	774	$363,537	748	$387,666
FP: Amb Only (no inpatient work)	1	*	12	$335,219	26	$299,039	33	$333,260
Family Practice: Sports Med	4	*	5	*	5	*	7	*
Family Practice: Urgent Care	3	*	5	*	9	*	19	$453,217
Gastroenterology	12	$698,698	51	$770,387	84	$761,331	128	$727,109
Gastroenterology: Hepatology	*	*	1	*	1	*	1	*
Genetics	*	*	0	*	0	*	2	*
Geriatrics	2	*	9	*	12	$278,642	8	*
Hematology/Oncology	15	$354,805	24	$405,991	52	$521,719	61	$521,439
Hematology/Oncology: Onc (only)	0	*	3	*	4	*	11	$392,523
Hospice/Palliative Care	1	*	1	*	1	*	1	*
Hospitalist: Family Practice	2	*	5	*	2	*	3	*
Hospitalist: Internal Medicine	78	$180,140	206	$186,418	138	$211,571	41	$172,027
Hospitalist: IM-Pediatrics	0	*	2	*	1	*	*	*
Hospitalist: Pediatrics	1	*	4	*	5	*	2	*
Infectious Disease	4	*	6	*	18	$276,961	18	$257,953
Internal Medicine: General	75	$244,875	277	$312,328	575	$359,398	577	$362,063
IM: Amb Only (no inpatient work)	*	*	*	*	1	*	6	*
Internal Med: Pediatrics	2	*	12	$407,386	25	$398,489	0	*
Nephrology	7	*	22	$408,256	25	$462,326	26	$508,546
Neurology	20	$300,366	46	$412,037	73	$420,859	77	$412,234
Obstetrics/Gynecology: General	34	$459,485	141	$544,531	218	$627,397	149	$574,649
OB/GYN: Gynecology (only)	1	*	2	*	11	$430,647	38	$390,903
OB/GYN: Gyn Oncology	1	*	2	*	6	*	2	*
OB/GYN: Maternal & Fetal Med	1	*	2	*	7	*	2	*
OB/GYN: Repro Endocrinology	0	*	*	*	1	*	0	*
OB/GYN: Urogynecology	0	*	3	*	*	*	0	*
Occupational Medicine	2	*	9	*	9	*	22	$461,235
Ophthalmology	7	*	16	$650,809	53	$723,466	64	$701,044
Ophthalmology: Pediatric	1	*	2	*	4	*	4	*
Ophthalmology: Retina	0	*	1	*	5	*	3	*
Orthopedic (Nonsurgical)	0	*	1	*	3	*	14	$298,254
Orthopedic Surgery: General	16	$689,658	56	$819,535	111	$857,111	132	$730,658
Orthopedic Surgery: Foot & Ankle	2	*	3	*	9	*	4	*
Orthopedic Surgery: Hand	2	*	8	*	28	$957,997	15	$750,000
Orthopedic Surgery: Hip & Joint	4	*	4	*	10	$962,995	20	$928,729
Orthopedic Surgery: Pediatric	1	*	2	*	3	*	2	*
Orthopedic Surgery: Spine	6	*	5	*	15	$1,247,931	10	$792,822
Orthopedic Surgery: Trauma	0	*	5	*	4	*	4	*
Orthopedic Surgery: Sports Med	4	*	13	$883,121	18	$1,025,298	18	$919,044

Table 20: Collections for Professional Charges (TC/NPP Excluded) by Years in Specialty (continued)

	1 to 2 years		3 to 7 years		8 to 17 years		18 years or more	
	Phys	Median	Phys	Median	Phys	Median	Phys	Median
Otorhinolaryngology	4	*	33	$946,305	78	$778,031	64	$652,541
Pathology: Anatomic and Clinical	4	*	9	*	13	$559,246	25	$536,656
Pathology: Anatomic	0	*	0	*	0	*	3	*
Pathology: Clinical	*	*	6	*	7	*	7	*
Pediatrics: General	74	$305,326	239	$388,794	461	$412,657	429	$432,233
Pediatrics: Adolescent Medicine	0	*	2	*	7	*	3	*
Pediatrics: Allergy/Immunology	*	*	0	*	1	*	1	*
Pediatrics: Cardiology	0	*	3	*	2	*	5	*
Pediatrics: Child Development	*	*	1	*	2	*	1	*
Pediatrics: Critical Care/Intensivist	3	*	12	$182,581	10	$184,417	5	*
Pediatrics: Emergency Medicine	1	*	6	*	6	*	5	*
Pediatrics: Endocrinology	2	*	3	*	4	*	3	*
Pediatrics: Gastroenterology	0	*	4	*	3	*	4	*
Pediatrics: Genetics	1	*	*	*	1	*	1	*
Pediatrics: Hematology/Oncology	0	*	8	*	8	*	6	*
Pediatrics: Infectious Disease	*	*	0	*	1	*	0	*
Pediatrics: Neonatal Medicine	2	*	9	*	8	*	11	$422,640
Pediatrics: Nephrology	0	*	*	*	2	*	1	*
Pediatrics: Neurology	2	*	5	*	9	*	6	*
Pediatrics: Pulmonology	0	*	1	*	5	*	5	*
Pediatrics: Rheumatology	*	*	*	*	2	*	1	*
Physiatry (Phys Med & Rehab)	7	*	20	$367,481	31	$400,372	19	$392,168
Podiatry: General	4	*	14	$363,443	26	$453,999	23	$420,760
Podiatry: Surg-Foot & Ankle	5	*	4	*	6	*	3	*
Podiatry: Surg-Forefoot Only	*	*	0	*	0	*	0	*
Psychiatry: General	5	*	16	$229,143	41	$196,684	24	$197,035
Psychiatry: Child & Adolescent	0	*	5	*	6	*	3	*
Psychiatry: Geriatric	*	*	*	*	2	*	3	*
Pulmonary Medicine	12	$315,264	15	$448,979	33	$483,806	37	$406,739
Pulmonary Medicine: Critical Care	0	*	2	*	13	$402,944	3	*
Pulmonary Med: Gen & Crit Care	2	*	8	*	12	$564,842	9	*
Radiation Oncology	2	*	9	*	20	$520,893	10	$540,742
Radiology: Diagnostic-Inv	6	*	26	$686,067	45	$724,589	25	$667,076
Radiology: Diagnostic-Noninv	14	$679,228	39	$677,157	61	$668,069	75	$567,165
Radiology: Nuclear Medicine	1	*	3	*	5	*	3	*
Rheumatology	7	*	26	$312,396	26	$403,220	54	$368,916
Sleep Medicine	1	*	5	*	5	*	14	$448,291
Surgery: General	19	$403,477	66	$533,231	140	$550,806	163	$535,615
Surgery: Bariatric	1	*	1	*	0	*	1	*
Surgery: Cardiovascular	7	*	22	$537,668	49	$685,313	35	$598,768
Surgery: Colon and Rectal	1	*	3	*	6	*	9	*
Surgery: Neurological	4	*	20	$1,031,239	39	$1,083,612	38	$782,705
Surgery: Oncology	*	*	2	*	3	*	3	*
Surgery: Oral	0	*	1	*	2	*	9	*
Surgery: Pediatric	2	*	7	*	8	*	10	$383,543
Surgery: Plastic & Reconstruction	2	*	11	$574,530	14	$881,799	16	$663,193
Surgery: Plastic & Recon-Hand	0	*	0	*	0	*	1	*
Surgery: Thoracic (primary)	0	*	3	*	3	*	12	$376,880
Surgery: Transplant	1	*	2	*	6	*	1	*
Surgery: Trauma	6	*	4	*	9	*	7	*
Surgery: Trauma-Burn	1	*	0	*	0	*	*	*
Surgery: Vascular (primary)	1	*	6	*	16	$629,733	27	$578,633
Urgent Care	15	$505,169	45	$562,662	52	$509,115	67	$446,519
Urology	13	$693,428	34	$636,132	68	$671,092	84	$644,608
Urology: Pediatric	0	*	3	*	2	*	2	*

Table 21: Collections for Professional Charges (TC/NPP Excluded) by Gender

	Male			Female		
	Phys	Med Pracs	Median	Phys	Med Pracs	Median
Allergy/Immunology	47	29	$641,487	22	18	$388,044
Anesthesiology	1,282	93	$478,393	248	65	$413,238
Anesthesiology: Pain Management	50	22	$787,357	7	6	*
Anesthesiology: Pediatric	15	2	*	13	3	$442,020
Cardiology: Electrophysiology	58	28	$786,361	4	4	*
Cardiology: Invasive	148	46	$632,148	9	9	*
Cardiology: Inv-Intvl	199	55	$801,300	8	7	*
Cardiology: Noninvasive	133	42	$572,165	18	12	$534,248
Critical Care: Intensivist	11	6	$368,941	6	3	*
Dentistry	8	3	*	1	1	*
Dermatology	88	52	$792,502	61	31	$690,747
Dermatology: Mohs Surgery	8	7	*	5	4	*
Emergency Medicine	223	20	$320,843	57	16	$265,148
Endocrinology/Metabolism	84	53	$363,681	35	29	$355,469
Family Practice (w/ OB)	202	56	$403,367	115	44	$344,475
Family Practice (w/o OB)	1,648	265	$383,236	708	199	$323,458
FP: Amb Only (no inpatient work)	55	8	$338,109	17	6	$287,681
Family Practice: Sports Med	20	13	$360,770	1	1	*
Family Practice: Urgent Care	42	11	$443,224	18	8	$429,959
Gastroenterology	324	94	$759,662	47	26	$572,910
Gastroenterology: Hepatology	5	4	*	1	1	*
Genetics	1	1	*	2	1	*
Geriatrics	20	11	$200,873	15	7	$206,336
Hematology/Oncology	139	48	$561,923	35	24	$417,463
Hematology/Oncology: Onc (only)	19	13	$463,457	1	1	*
Hospice/Palliative Care	4	4	*	0	*	*
Hospitalist: Family Practice	11	5	$191,729	3	2	*
Hospitalist: Internal Medicine	399	76	$195,769	171	58	$178,505
Hospitalist: IM-Pediatrics	2	2	*	1	1	*
Hospitalist: Pediatrics	12	6	$141,750	17	6	$76,499
Infectious Disease	38	23	$300,162	14	10	$228,061
Internal Medicine: General	1,254	196	$375,698	552	150	$288,704
IM: Amb Only (no inpatient work)	8	4	*	6	6	*
Internal Med: Pediatrics	30	17	$431,154	11	7	$291,872
Nephrology	73	32	$455,153	23	15	$301,833
Neurology	176	67	$431,264	66	44	$345,228
Obstetrics/Gynecology: General	329	115	$618,312	263	95	$563,008
OB/GYN: Gynecology (only)	42	29	$411,246	21	12	$475,954
OB/GYN: Gyn Oncology	8	7	*	5	5	*
OB/GYN: Maternal & Fetal Med	10	7	$731,122	8	5	*
OB/GYN: Repro Endocrinology	1	1	*	1	1	*
OB/GYN: Urogynecology	3	2	*	0	*	*
Occupational Medicine	39	20	$383,585	10	5	$535,219
Ophthalmology	139	56	$681,376	29	21	$637,837
Ophthalmology: Pediatric	9	7	*	4	3	*
Ophthalmology: Retina	11	11	$1,344,217	1	1	*
Orthopedic (Nonsurgical)	20	17	$348,890	2	2	*
Orthopedic Surgery: General	341	96	$806,064	6	5	*
Orthopedic Surgery: Foot & Ankle	17	15	$755,581	1	1	*
Orthopedic Surgery: Hand	50	28	$946,583	5	5	*
Orthopedic Surgery: Hip & Joint	38	21	$899,402	*	*	*
Orthopedic Surgery: Pediatric	8	5	*	1	1	*
Orthopedic Surgery: Spine	37	25	$945,511	0	*	*
Orthopedic Surgery: Trauma	11	7	$711,359	2	2	*
Orthopedic Surgery: Sports Med	52	28	$958,461	1	1	*

Table 21: Collections for Professional Charges (TC/NPP Excluded) by Gender (continued)

	Male			Female		
	Phys	Med Pracs	Median	Phys	Med Pracs	Median
Otorhinolaryngology	180	72	$744,342	16	12	$568,283
Pathology: Anatomic and Clinical	43	8	$589,689	15	6	$411,351
Pathology: Anatomic	2	1	*	1	1	*
Pathology: Clinical	17	6	$506,172	6	3	*
Pediatrics: General	667	139	$452,948	655	145	$369,917
Pediatrics: Adolescent Medicine	11	3	$323,610	12	5	$459,276
Pediatrics: Allergy/Immunology	2	1	*	0	*	*
Pediatrics: Cardiology	11	6	$313,192	4	3	*
Pediatrics: Child Development	2	1	*	3	2	*
Pediatrics: Critical Care/Intensivist	28	10	$192,514	12	7	$130,393
Pediatrics: Emergency Medicine	9	3	*	9	2	*
Pediatrics: Endocrinology	8	7	*	5	4	*
Pediatrics: Gastroenterology	9	5	*	3	2	*
Pediatrics: Genetics	0	*	*	3	2	*
Pediatrics: Hematology/Oncology	20	11	$213,078	6	4	*
Pediatrics: Infectious Disease	0	*	*	3	3	*
Pediatrics: Neonatal Medicine	24	8	$413,066	14	7	$439,247
Pediatrics: Nephrology	3	3	*	1	1	*
Pediatrics: Neurology	22	14	$313,441	6	6	*
Pediatrics: Pulmonology	12	8	$196,108	0	*	*
Pediatrics: Rheumatology	2	2	*	1	1	*
Physiatry (Phys Med & Rehab)	60	33	$426,447	31	17	$332,979
Podiatry: General	61	38	$437,804	12	12	$396,440
Podiatry: Surg-Foot & Ankle	19	11	$499,338	4	4	*
Podiatry: Surg-Forefoot Only	0	*	*	*	*	*
Psychiatry: General	82	32	$214,498	33	19	$192,152
Psychiatry: Child & Adolescent	16	10	$172,172	6	5	*
Psychiatry: Geriatric	7	3	*	*	*	*
Pulmonary Medicine	109	50	$448,979	14	12	$421,086
Pulmonary Medicine: Critical Care	27	8	$461,797	6	4	*
Pulmonary Med: Gen & Crit Care	36	17	$558,971	3	2	*
Radiation Oncology	32	13	$537,285	12	8	$557,832
Radiology: Diagnostic-Inv	97	23	$688,253	11	7	$653,876
Radiology: Diagnostic-Noninv	192	32	$690,002	36	12	$530,452
Radiology: Nuclear Medicine	16	9	$569,700	1	1	*
Rheumatology	82	50	$394,042	48	34	$318,171
Sleep Medicine	23	10	$573,107	2	2	*
Surgery: General	387	122	$544,901	50	36	$462,367
Surgery: Bariatric	5	3	*	1	1	*
Surgery: Cardiovascular	119	34	$595,269	3	3	*
Surgery: Colon and Rectal	24	12	$769,848	3	3	*
Surgery: Neurological	115	38	$873,581	3	3	*
Surgery: Oncology	6	5	*	3	1	*
Surgery: Oral	10	6	$908,909	2	2	*
Surgery: Pediatric	24	11	$372,669	7	7	*
Surgery: Plastic & Reconstruction	43	22	$739,805	11	9	$539,924
Surgery: Plastic & Recon-Hand	1	1	*	0	*	*
Surgery: Thoracic (primary)	26	11	$399,990	0	*	*
Surgery: Transplant	15	4	$742,228	0	*	*
Surgery: Trauma	30	9	$318,960	4	3	*
Surgery: Trauma-Burn	1	1	*	0	*	*
Surgery: Vascular (primary)	55	29	$598,209	5	4	*
Urgent Care	161	34	$503,114	54	19	$377,997
Urology	211	65	$675,770	22	14	$560,578
Urology: Pediatric	4	2	*	3	2	*

Table 22: Collections for Professional Charges (TC/NPP Excluded) by Clinical Service Hours Worked per Week

	Fewer than 40 hours		40 hours or more	
	Phys	**Median**	**Phys**	**Median**
Allergy/Immunology	29	$617,993	23	$535,321
Anesthesiology	213	$356,553	1,814	$543,720
Anesthesiology: Pain Management	7	*	52	$730,666
Anesthesiology: Pediatric	9	*	26	$461,843
Cardiology: Electrophysiology	16	$851,449	32	$786,361
Cardiology: Invasive	44	$633,929	67	$600,298
Cardiology: Inv-Intvl	54	$687,166	110	$794,626
Cardiology: Noninvasive	37	$615,184	83	$624,361
Critical Care: Intensivist	2	*	1	*
Dentistry	2	*	7	*
Dermatology	55	$724,176	57	$755,192
Dermatology: Mohs Surgery	3	*	2	*
Emergency Medicine	174	$292,232	47	$321,726
Endocrinology/Metabolism	37	$369,551	43	$351,097
Family Practice (w/ OB)	158	$378,663	138	$363,021
Family Practice (w/o OB)	1,177	$356,983	747	$370,056
FP: Amb Only (no inpatient work)	21	$335,534	18	$342,805
Family Practice: Sports Med	6	*	10	$409,859
Family Practice: Urgent Care	42	$428,730	13	$470,745
Gastroenterology	84	$613,922	218	$788,333
Gastroenterology: Hepatology	2	*	3	*
Genetics	3	*	*	*
Geriatrics	14	$193,605	5	*
Hematology/Oncology	57	$521,028	74	$625,408
Hematology/Oncology: Onc (only)	6	*	11	$331,318
Hospice/Palliative Care	1	*	2	*
Hospitalist: Family Practice	12	$184,970	3	*
Hospitalist: Internal Medicine	186	$165,088	231	$206,201
Hospitalist: IM-Pediatrics	0	*	3	*
Hospitalist: Pediatrics	15	$90,160	10	$127,152
Infectious Disease	16	$245,732	23	$341,100
Internal Medicine: General	790	$332,221	604	$366,535
IM: Amb Only (no inpatient work)	4	*	9	*
Internal Med: Pediatrics	5	*	27	$410,978
Nephrology	21	$297,637	48	$507,119
Neurology	66	$375,858	128	$425,525
Obstetrics/Gynecology: General	234	$550,386	248	$599,012
OB/GYN: Gynecology (only)	19	$341,066	24	$441,131
OB/GYN: Gyn Oncology	2	*	4	*
OB/GYN: Maternal & Fetal Med	7	*	7	*
OB/GYN: Repro Endocrinology	0	*	1	*
OB/GYN: Urogynecology	0	*	1	*
Occupational Medicine	36	$450,986	10	$303,850
Ophthalmology	59	$670,321	66	$667,279
Ophthalmology: Pediatric	4	*	5	*
Ophthalmology: Retina	3	*	5	*
Orthopedic (Nonsurgical)	10	$342,451	10	$304,693
Orthopedic Surgery: General	67	$646,980	173	$839,322
Orthopedic Surgery: Foot & Ankle	1	*	13	$755,581
Orthopedic Surgery: Hand	9	*	38	$935,185
Orthopedic Surgery: Hip & Joint	6	*	28	$899,402
Orthopedic Surgery: Pediatric	0	*	6	*
Orthopedic Surgery: Spine	3	*	28	$955,223
Orthopedic Surgery: Trauma	0	*	9	*
Orthopedic Surgery: Sports Med	6	*	38	$940,500

Table 22: Collections for Professional Charges (TC/NPP Excluded) by Clinical Service Hours Worked per Week (continued)

	Fewer than 40 hours		40 hours or more	
	Phys	Median	Phys	Median
Otorhinolaryngology	49	$697,862	100	$773,882
Pathology: Anatomic and Clinical	36	$851,010	10	$482,098
Pathology: Anatomic	0	*	0	*
Pathology: Clinical	1	*	8	*
Pediatrics: General	563	$374,401	393	$434,175
Pediatrics: Adolescent Medicine	20	$434,639	2	*
Pediatrics: Allergy/Immunology	0	*	2	*
Pediatrics: Cardiology	4	*	6	*
Pediatrics: Child Development	1	*	0	*
Pediatrics: Critical Care/Intensivist	7	*	21	$168,103
Pediatrics: Emergency Medicine	13	*	4	*
Pediatrics: Endocrinology	2	*	7	*
Pediatrics: Gastroenterology	9	*	0	*
Pediatrics: Genetics	3	*	0	*
Pediatrics: Hematology/Oncology	4	*	11	$239,164
Pediatrics: Infectious Disease	2	*	0	*
Pediatrics: Neonatal Medicine	5	*	30	$422,628
Pediatrics: Nephrology	1	*	1	*
Pediatrics: Neurology	7	*	13	$304,260
Pediatrics: Pulmonology	2	*	6	*
Pediatrics: Rheumatology	1	*	1	*
Physiatry (Phys Med & Rehab)	22	$366,557	43	$411,459
Podiatry: General	27	$325,161	30	$464,168
Podiatry: Surg-Foot & Ankle	6	*	12	$485,783
Podiatry: Surg-Forefoot Only	*	*	0	*
Psychiatry: General	35	$181,595	57	$198,525
Psychiatry: Child & Adolescent	5	*	13	$105,440
Psychiatry: Geriatric	6	*	1	*
Pulmonary Medicine	24	$475,689	51	$479,274
Pulmonary Medicine: Critical Care	3	*	8	*
Pulmonary Med: Gen & Crit Care	10	$562,462	19	$557,939
Radiation Oncology	10	$548,351	14	$730,815
Radiology: Diagnostic-Inv	9	*	80	$675,417
Radiology: Diagnostic-Noninv	28	$587,625	137	$704,234
Radiology: Nuclear Medicine	2	*	11	$569,421
Rheumatology	43	$375,584	47	$345,892
Sleep Medicine	1	*	18	$568,819
Surgery: General	130	$529,304	219	$539,008
Surgery: Bariatric	1	*	5	*
Surgery: Cardiovascular	3	*	82	$614,520
Surgery: Colon and Rectal	5	*	15	$722,743
Surgery: Neurological	25	$658,173	81	$1,050,987
Surgery: Oncology	2	*	4	*
Surgery: Oral	6	*	4	*
Surgery: Pediatric	12	$307,637	16	$687,506
Surgery: Plastic & Reconstruction	5	*	28	$575,994
Surgery: Plastic & Recon-Hand	*	*	0	*
Surgery: Thoracic (primary)	10	$427,802	11	$389,830
Surgery: Transplant	6	*	7	*
Surgery: Trauma	3	*	19	$234,768
Surgery: Trauma-Burn	*	*	1	*
Surgery: Vascular (primary)	6	*	34	$609,817
Urgent Care	83	$486,745	37	$373,454
Urology	88	$563,972	109	$725,900
Urology: Pediatric	5	*	2	*

Table 23: Collections for Professional Charges (TC/NPP Excluded) by Weeks Worked per Year

	Fewer than 46 weeks		46 weeks or more	
	Phys	Median	Phys	Median
Allergy/Immunology	6	*	49	$617,993
Anesthesiology	1,553	$543,720	746	$428,867
Anesthesiology: Pain Management	32	$430,309	28	$977,001
Anesthesiology: Pediatric	17	*	18	*
Cardiology: Electrophysiology	20	$818,946	34	$785,425
Cardiology: Invasive	46	$629,508	81	$600,000
Cardiology: Inv-Intvl	46	$732,712	119	$809,363
Cardiology: Noninvasive	61	$594,681	57	$635,118
Critical Care: Intensivist	3	*	2	*
Dentistry	1	*	8	*
Dermatology	25	$807,460	91	$738,110
Dermatology: Mohs Surgery	2	*	7	*
Emergency Medicine	41	$285,494	194	$300,364
Endocrinology/Metabolism	10	$379,409	75	$362,786
Family Practice (w/ OB)	48	$392,575	230	$366,894
Family Practice (w/o OB)	283	$370,667	1,696	$357,105
FP: Amb Only (no inpatient work)	0	*	39	$335,534
Family Practice: Sports Med	4	*	14	$360,770
Family Practice: Urgent Care	2	*	55	$433,573
Gastroenterology	104	$792,796	214	$722,541
Gastroenterology: Hepatology	0	*	6	*
Genetics	0	*	3	*
Geriatrics	3	*	30	$200,873
Hematology/Oncology	27	$503,953	114	$558,354
Hematology/Oncology: Onc (only)	2	*	16	$285,232
Hospice/Palliative Care	1	*	2	*
Hospitalist: Family Practice	10	*	3	*
Hospitalist: Internal Medicine	149	$179,859	314	$191,009
Hospitalist: IM-Pediatrics	1	*	2	*
Hospitalist: Pediatrics	9	*	16	$83,330
Infectious Disease	7	*	29	$263,435
Internal Medicine: General	208	$365,885	1,280	$350,366
IM: Amb Only (no inpatient work)	4	*	9	*
Internal Med: Pediatrics	4	*	32	$411,150
Nephrology	8	*	67	$445,105
Neurology	52	$432,841	154	$390,742
Obstetrics/Gynecology: General	87	$606,176	398	$561,770
OB/GYN: Gynecology (only)	8	*	43	$421,995
OB/GYN: Gyn Oncology	0	*	10	$377,531
OB/GYN: Maternal & Fetal Med	0	*	16	$731,122
OB/GYN: Repro Endocrinology	0	*	1	*
OB/GYN: Urogynecology	0	*	1	*
Occupational Medicine	8	*	37	$436,496
Ophthalmology	31	$681,376	100	$664,080
Ophthalmology: Pediatric	0	*	10	$639,623
Ophthalmology: Retina	3	*	6	*
Orthopedic (Nonsurgical)	9	*	11	$383,208
Orthopedic Surgery: General	58	$863,101	207	$760,208
Orthopedic Surgery: Foot & Ankle	5	*	8	*
Orthopedic Surgery: Hand	23	$915,000	24	$987,880
Orthopedic Surgery: Hip & Joint	12	$939,066	22	$842,017
Orthopedic Surgery: Pediatric	0	*	7	*
Orthopedic Surgery: Spine	4	*	27	$964,934
Orthopedic Surgery: Trauma	4	*	5	*
Orthopedic Surgery: Sports Med	13	$908,000	31	$970,922

Table 23: Collections for Professional Charges (TC/NPP Excluded) by Weeks Worked per Year (continued)

	Fewer than 46 weeks		46 weeks or more	
	Phys	Median	Phys	Median
Otorhinolaryngology	40	$701,035	129	$742,562
Pathology: Anatomic and Clinical	34	$627,916	10	$482,098
Pathology: Anatomic	0	*	0	*
Pathology: Clinical	0	*	17	$375,523
Pediatrics: General	163	$389,938	856	$405,237
Pediatrics: Adolescent Medicine	0	*	11	$521,304
Pediatrics: Allergy/Immunology	2	*	0	*
Pediatrics: Cardiology	2	*	6	*
Pediatrics: Child Development	1	*	2	*
Pediatrics: Critical Care/Intensivist	13	*	21	$153,697
Pediatrics: Emergency Medicine	0	*	17	*
Pediatrics: Endocrinology	2	*	8	*
Pediatrics: Gastroenterology	0	*	9	*
Pediatrics: Genetics	0	*	3	*
Pediatrics: Hematology/Oncology	1	*	17	$209,868
Pediatrics: Infectious Disease	0	*	1	*
Pediatrics: Neonatal Medicine	0	*	22	$360,060
Pediatrics: Nephrology	0	*	2	*
Pediatrics: Neurology	4	*	19	$293,990
Pediatrics: Pulmonology	1	*	9	*
Pediatrics: Rheumatology	0	*	2	*
Physiatry (Phys Med & Rehab)	13	$506,626	62	$394,084
Podiatry: General	4	*	55	$393,197
Podiatry: Surg-Foot & Ankle	0	*	19	$438,982
Podiatry: Surg-Forefoot Only	*	*	0	*
Psychiatry: General	18	$172,041	67	$224,060
Psychiatry: Child & Adolescent	1	*	11	$210,170
Psychiatry: Geriatric	4	*	2	*
Pulmonary Medicine	10	$414,153	72	$474,870
Pulmonary Medicine: Critical Care	4	*	12	$466,486
Pulmonary Med: Gen & Crit Care	2	*	29	$560,003
Radiation Oncology	12	$608,151	19	$708,611
Radiology: Diagnostic-Inv	75	$675,604	21	$696,530
Radiology: Diagnostic-Noninv	133	$670,988	50	$766,037
Radiology: Nuclear Medicine	8	*	7	*
Rheumatology	14	$510,759	87	$346,591
Sleep Medicine	0	*	21	$573,107
Surgery: General	59	$642,694	298	$532,534
Surgery: Bariatric	3	*	3	*
Surgery: Cardiovascular	43	$631,909	50	$545,646
Surgery: Colon and Rectal	4	*	15	$715,062
Surgery: Neurological	28	$1,089,618	68	$823,030
Surgery: Oncology	1	*	5	*
Surgery: Oral	0	*	8	*
Surgery: Pediatric	8	*	20	$424,702
Surgery: Plastic & Reconstruction	3	*	33	$610,029
Surgery: Plastic & Recon-Hand	*	*	0	*
Surgery: Thoracic (primary)	7	*	6	*
Surgery: Transplant	*	*	13	$763,000
Surgery: Trauma	4	*	19	$324,281
Surgery: Trauma-Burn	*	*	1	*
Surgery: Vascular (primary)	18	$540,190	31	$661,257
Urgent Care	51	$475,370	80	$484,755
Urology	38	$557,567	156	$674,998
Urology: Pediatric	*	*	7	*

Table 24: Collections for Professional Charges (NPP Excluded) with 1–10% Technical Component

	Phys	Med Pracs	Mean	Std. Dev.	25th %tile	Median	75th %tile	90th %tile
Allergy/Immunology	13	9	$648,009	$335,989	$452,120	$574,420	$795,475	$1,298,496
Anesthesiology	36	3	$367,689	$98,166	$335,000	$335,000	$411,250	$451,100
Anesthesiology: Pain Management	20	7	$695,417	$366,579	$269,225	$813,288	$1,028,851	$1,079,554
Anesthesiology: Pediatric	0	*	*	*	*	*	*	*
Cardiology: Electrophysiology	18	14	$1,062,342	$402,567	$789,999	$1,097,267	$1,338,462	$1,596,511
Cardiology: Invasive	35	17	$886,610	$495,152	$592,988	$886,777	$1,118,637	$1,660,541
Cardiology: Inv-Intvl	35	15	$879,040	$371,520	$550,066	$788,595	$1,047,900	$1,548,709
Cardiology: Noninvasive	23	15	$591,655	$302,199	$321,867	$562,910	$866,017	$984,314
Critical Care: Intensivist	1	1	*	*	*	*	*	*
Dentistry	0	*	*	*	*	*	*	*
Dermatology	36	15	$629,767	$263,720	$424,574	$597,989	$880,351	$1,017,342
Dermatology: Mohs Surgery	3	3	*	*	*	*	*	*
Emergency Medicine	24	2	*	*	*	*	*	*
Endocrinology/Metabolism	32	18	$432,520	$146,093	$338,517	$381,846	$553,446	$680,427
Family Practice (w/ OB)	96	26	$513,797	$171,554	$389,997	$495,880	$648,236	$752,231
Family Practice (w/o OB)	931	143	$429,559	$146,225	$327,235	$422,972	$524,414	$627,693
FP: Amb Only (no inpatient work)	42	5	$387,278	$144,052	$306,050	$365,164	$425,541	$495,376
Family Practice: Sports Med	6	4	*	*	*	*	*	*
Family Practice: Urgent Care	17	3	$364,005	$154,018	$250,264	$384,576	$465,553	$593,159
Gastroenterology	92	28	$789,398	$270,906	$607,170	$694,265	$944,018	$1,234,893
Gastroenterology: Hepatology	1	1	*	*	*	*	*	*
Genetics	0	*	*	*	*	*	*	*
Geriatrics	4	2	*	*	*	*	*	*
Hematology/Oncology	20	8	$461,337	$206,965	$296,596	$429,299	$657,850	$769,864
Hematology/Oncology: Onc (only)	5	3	*	*	*	*	*	*
Hospice/Palliative Care	0	*	*	*	*	*	*	*
Hospitalist: Family Practice	12	2	*	*	*	*	*	*
Hospitalist: Internal Medicine	35	5	$256,133	$104,866	$181,242	$229,419	$327,452	$413,345
Hospitalist: IM-Pediatrics	0	*	*	*	*	*	*	*
Hospitalist: Pediatrics	4	2	*	*	*	*	*	*
Infectious Disease	16	9	$295,260	$122,620	$188,230	$238,014	$418,514	$501,730
Internal Medicine: General	605	104	$441,812	$164,668	$333,681	$424,951	$525,159	$651,379
IM: Amb Only (no inpatient work)	2	2	*	*	*	*	*	*
Internal Med: Pediatrics	14	5	$426,404	$117,674	$343,307	$393,701	$515,754	$638,695
Nephrology	17	10	$476,029	$200,545	$285,047	$494,283	$612,503	$767,536
Neurology	74	32	$431,638	$145,481	$363,821	$418,671	$511,100	$658,804
Obstetrics/Gynecology: General	290	61	$651,504	$234,444	$499,361	$629,098	$778,975	$941,878
OB/GYN: Gynecology (only)	32	19	$416,471	$208,608	$269,164	$355,156	$509,261	$794,569
OB/GYN: Gyn Oncology	5	4	*	*	*	*	*	*
OB/GYN: Maternal & Fetal Med	11	4	$1,281,630	$807,659	$794,752	$1,156,384	$1,351,019	$3,123,530
OB/GYN: Repro Endocrinology	0	*	*	*	*	*	*	*
OB/GYN: Urogynecology	0	*	*	*	*	*	*	*
Occupational Medicine	8	6	*	*	*	*	*	*
Ophthalmology	95	29	$912,701	$375,538	$633,159	$835,055	$1,149,255	$1,493,622
Ophthalmology: Pediatric	7	6	*	*	*	*	*	*
Ophthalmology: Retina	19	8	$2,497,541	$1,321,427	$1,592,696	$1,965,757	$2,843,349	$5,083,623
Orthopedic (Nonsurgical)	14	10	$389,281	$190,597	$176,202	$379,850	$548,931	$673,731
Orthopedic Surgery: General	193	58	$882,156	$324,056	$660,980	$834,735	$1,073,240	$1,302,154
Orthopedic Surgery: Foot & Ankle	22	17	$932,508	$353,291	$643,920	$916,671	$1,076,239	$1,558,739
Orthopedic Surgery: Hand	48	27	$915,640	$310,443	$744,984	$862,069	$981,870	$1,409,259
Orthopedic Surgery: Hip & Joint	45	22	$1,088,782	$348,363	$801,409	$1,090,770	$1,298,815	$1,606,000
Orthopedic Surgery: Pediatric	4	4	*	*	*	*	*	*
Orthopedic Surgery: Spine	45	27	$1,024,657	$528,379	$730,925	$935,193	$1,198,174	$1,605,301
Orthopedic Surgery: Trauma	16	7	$709,903	$392,128	$409,365	$688,023	$1,034,135	$1,244,100
Orthopedic Surgery: Sports Med	66	26	$1,242,363	$582,227	$918,870	$1,169,614	$1,398,010	$2,050,265

Table 24: Collections for Professional Charges (NPP Excluded) with 1–10% Technical Component (continued)

	Phys	Med Pracs	Mean	Std. Dev.	25th %tile	Median	75th %tile	90th %tile
Otorhinolaryngology	43	15	$790,343	$266,468	$572,006	$819,413	$989,000	$1,130,386
Pathology: Anatomic and Clinical	0	*	*	*	*	*	*	*
Pathology: Anatomic	0	*	*	*	*	*	*	*
Pathology: Clinical	0	*	*	*	*	*	*	*
Pediatrics: General	302	52	$479,025	$171,458	$361,013	$454,639	$598,773	$720,827
Pediatrics: Adolescent Medicine	0	*	*	*	*	*	*	*
Pediatrics: Allergy/Immunology	0	*	*	*	*	*	*	*
Pediatrics: Cardiology	4	2	*	*	*	*	*	*
Pediatrics: Child Development	2	1	*	*	*	*	*	*
Pediatrics: Critical Care/Intensivist	3	1	*	*	*	*	*	*
Pediatrics: Emergency Medicine	0	*	*	*	*	*	*	*
Pediatrics: Endocrinology	0	*	*	*	*	*	*	*
Pediatrics: Gastroenterology	1	1	*	*	*	*	*	*
Pediatrics: Genetics	12	6	$337,729	$137,070	$245,109	$307,624	$394,693	$609,536
Pediatrics: Hematology/Oncology	10	2	*	*	*	*	*	*
Pediatrics: Infectious Disease	3	1	*	*	*	*	*	*
Pediatrics: Neonatal Medicine	11	2	*	*	*	*	*	*
Pediatrics: Nephrology	0	*	*	*	*	*	*	*
Pediatrics: Neurology	5	1	*	*	*	*	*	*
Pediatrics: Pulmonology	3	2	*	*	*	*	*	*
Pediatrics: Rheumatology	0	*	*	*	*	*	*	*
Physiatry (Phys Med & Rehab)	22	18	$669,678	$375,716	$387,881	$531,779	$903,026	$1,373,270
Podiatry: General	17	10	$408,098	$150,800	$284,083	$345,975	$529,728	$678,663
Podiatry: Surg-Foot & Ankle	12	4	$524,335	$197,857	$368,699	$464,588	$645,697	$904,544
Podiatry: Surg-Forefoot Only	3	2	*	*	*	*	*	*
Psychiatry: General	25	10	$264,035	$114,101	$217,131	$252,773	$312,250	$394,571
Psychiatry: Child & Adolescent	4	2	*	*	*	*	*	*
Psychiatry: Geriatric	0	*	*	*	*	*	*	*
Pulmonary Medicine	24	14	$470,436	$263,065	$275,830	$440,642	$644,222	$893,334
Pulmonary Medicine: Critical Care	19	5	$481,432	$193,483	$398,254	$462,235	$496,923	$873,816
Pulmonary Med: Gen & Crit Care	34	8	$478,399	$227,720	$352,180	$422,631	$497,228	$919,830
Radiation Oncology	2	2	*	*	*	*	*	*
Radiology: Diagnostic-Inv	29	6	$882,166	$444,029	$579,565	$725,000	$1,128,672	$1,450,078
Radiology: Diagnostic-Noninv	38	5	$954,188	$447,986	$618,717	$778,767	$1,211,116	$1,533,600
Radiology: Nuclear Medicine	1	1	*	*	*	*	*	*
Rheumatology	27	19	$493,540	$217,984	$328,199	$413,737	$661,881	$882,666
Sleep Medicine	3	3	*	*	*	*	*	*
Surgery: General	99	36	$598,078	$225,534	$445,727	$555,625	$759,145	$896,534
Surgery: Bariatric	6	4	*	*	*	*	*	*
Surgery: Cardiovascular	21	10	$553,644	$311,872	$315,035	$591,652	$884,560	$927,188
Surgery: Colon and Rectal	2	1	*	*	*	*	*	*
Surgery: Neurological	11	6	$698,439	$225,114	$490,811	$747,137	$894,240	$948,565
Surgery: Oncology	1	1	*	*	*	*	*	*
Surgery: Oral	5	3	*	*	*	*	*	*
Surgery: Pediatric	4	2	*	*	*	*	*	*
Surgery: Plastic & Reconstruction	15	6	$798,460	$407,694	$612,427	$672,206	$905,863	$1,622,035
Surgery: Plastic & Recon-Hand	2	2	*	*	*	*	*	*
Surgery: Thoracic (primary)	0	*	*	*	*	*	*	*
Surgery: Transplant	0	*	*	*	*	*	*	*
Surgery: Trauma	8	2	*	*	*	*	*	*
Surgery: Trauma-Burn	0	*	*	*	*	*	*	*
Surgery: Vascular (primary)	33	13	$785,545	$244,543	$634,137	$778,169	$900,014	$1,055,687
Urgent Care	35	7	$486,246	$212,463	$325,492	$477,108	$589,552	$823,641
Urology	76	22	$855,667	$308,025	$675,323	$828,215	$982,561	$1,156,461
Urology: Pediatric	2	2	*	*	*	*	*	*

Table 25: Collections for Professional Charges (NPP Excluded) with more than 10% Technical Component

	Phys	Med Pracs	Mean	Std. Dev.	25th %tile	Median	75th %tile	90th %tile
Allergy/Immunology	25	6	$901,156	$464,667	$461,264	$855,424	$1,397,513	$1,582,946
Anesthesiology	47	5	$586,452	$225,475	$450,173	$561,083	$561,083	$1,000,840
Anesthesiology: Pain Management	3	3	*	*	*	*	*	*
Anesthesiology: Pediatric	0	*	*	*	*	*	*	*
Cardiology: Electrophysiology	22	10	$801,428	$326,653	$633,869	$789,036	$992,644	$1,341,430
Cardiology: Invasive	93	27	$1,120,865	$569,465	$698,521	$1,003,355	$1,481,354	$1,856,312
Cardiology: Inv-Intvl	116	24	$1,020,254	$423,164	$675,412	$990,071	$1,283,260	$1,597,135
Cardiology: Noninvasive	68	26	$996,128	$514,135	$606,371	$937,061	$1,215,767	$2,046,948
Critical Care: Intensivist	0	*	*	*	*	*	*	*
Dentistry	0	*	*	*	*	*	*	*
Dermatology	7	5	*	*	*	*	*	*
Dermatology: Mohs Surgery	2	2	*	*	*	*	*	*
Emergency Medicine	34	5	$253,581	$100,326	$159,940	$273,126	$321,011	$380,419
Endocrinology/Metabolism	9	7	*	*	*	*	*	*
Family Practice (w/ OB)	49	15	$543,596	$206,865	$367,796	$531,344	$661,486	$759,075
Family Practice (w/o OB)	247	53	$449,689	$193,631	$328,629	$427,000	$536,661	$666,725
FP: Amb Only (no inpatient work)	28	4	$326,486	$76,129	$273,690	$332,137	$379,884	$430,854
Family Practice: Sports Med	2	2	*	*	*	*	*	*
Family Practice: Urgent Care	7	2	*	*	*	*	*	*
Gastroenterology	49	12	$897,982	$408,173	$597,353	$801,850	$1,091,898	$1,604,087
Gastroenterology: Hepatology	0	*	*	*	*	*	*	*
Genetics	0	*	*	*	*	*	*	*
Geriatrics	1	1	*	*	*	*	*	*
Hematology/Oncology	11	5	$3,319,554	$2,130,135	$464,169	$3,798,761	$4,744,149	$5,968,679
Hematology/Oncology: Onc (only)	2	2	*	*	*	*	*	*
Hospice/Palliative Care	2	2	*	*	*	*	*	*
Hospitalist: Family Practice	0	*	*	*	*	*	*	*
Hospitalist: Internal Medicine	6	3	*	*	*	*	*	*
Hospitalist: IM-Pediatrics	0	*	*	*	*	*	*	*
Hospitalist: Pediatrics	2	1	*	*	*	*	*	*
Infectious Disease	6	3	*	*	*	*	*	*
Internal Medicine: General	148	32	$468,530	$242,833	$298,249	$442,756	$591,584	$867,506
IM: Amb Only (no inpatient work)	1	1	*	*	*	*	*	*
Internal Med: Pediatrics	11	3	$405,367	$66,312	$358,786	$397,060	$446,160	$528,106
Nephrology	15	6	$663,816	$242,759	$481,900	$601,234	$751,013	$1,158,956
Neurology	32	12	$809,415	$417,166	$425,937	$791,758	$1,167,631	$1,376,460
Obstetrics/Gynecology: General	104	31	$699,205	$240,209	$523,686	$698,313	$854,831	$975,799
OB/GYN: Gynecology (only)	8	6	*	*	*	*	*	*
OB/GYN: Gyn Oncology	0	*	*	*	*	*	*	*
OB/GYN: Maternal & Fetal Med	13	3	$884,723	$223,346	$687,836	$935,923	$1,041,529	$1,196,106
OB/GYN: Repro Endocrinology	1	1	*	*	*	*	*	*
OB/GYN: Urogynecology	0	*	*	*	*	*	*	*
Occupational Medicine	6	4	*	*	*	*	*	*
Ophthalmology	32	12	$876,673	$405,944	$519,475	$853,514	$1,096,577	$1,481,665
Ophthalmology: Pediatric	3	2	*	*	*	*	*	*
Ophthalmology: Retina	3	3	*	*	*	*	*	*
Orthopedic (Nonsurgical)	1	1	*	*	*	*	*	*
Orthopedic Surgery: General	68	18	$930,160	$325,712	$678,698	$845,078	$1,145,412	$1,354,372
Orthopedic Surgery: Foot & Ankle	10	6	$963,672	$339,213	$638,600	$998,681	$1,175,698	$1,574,759
Orthopedic Surgery: Hand	12	6	$908,606	$167,404	$803,002	$910,897	$1,073,783	$1,119,358
Orthopedic Surgery: Hip & Joint	10	7	$938,854	$192,889	$749,833	$932,216	$1,121,910	$1,224,248
Orthopedic Surgery: Pediatric	6	1	*	*	*	*	*	*
Orthopedic Surgery: Spine	17	7	$1,085,700	$538,444	$767,952	$1,012,890	$1,388,985	$1,818,562
Orthopedic Surgery: Trauma	2	2	*	*	*	*	*	*
Orthopedic Surgery: Sports Med	28	10	$1,077,335	$358,751	$777,172	$1,053,163	$1,269,597	$1,573,148

Table 25: Collections for Professional Charges (NPP Excluded) with more than 10% Technical Component (continued)

	Phys	Med Pracs	Mean	Std. Dev.	25th %tile	Median	75th %tile	90th %tile
Otorhinolaryngology	14	4	$772,192	$147,265	$696,026	$769,121	$875,285	$995,681
Pathology: Anatomic and Clinical	7	1	*	*	*	*	*	*
Pathology: Anatomic	0	*	*	*	*	*	*	*
Pathology: Clinical	0	*	*	*	*	*	*	*
Pediatrics: General	121	24	$456,138	$222,673	$290,246	$458,012	$627,070	$772,302
Pediatrics: Adolescent Medicine	0	*	*	*	*	*	*	*
Pediatrics: Allergy/Immunology	0	*	*	*	*	*	*	*
Pediatrics: Cardiology	4	2	*	*	*	*	*	*
Pediatrics: Child Development	0	*	*	*	*	*	*	*
Pediatrics: Critical Care/Intensivist	5	2	*	*	*	*	*	*
Pediatrics: Emergency Medicine	3	1	*	*	*	*	*	*
Pediatrics: Endocrinology	1	1	*	*	*	*	*	*
Pediatrics: Gastroenterology	2	2	*	*	*	*	*	*
Pediatrics: Genetics	0	*	*	*	*	*	*	*
Pediatrics: Hematology/Oncology	3	1	*	*	*	*	*	*
Pediatrics: Infectious Disease	0	*	*	*	*	*	*	*
Pediatrics: Neonatal Medicine	20	1	*	*	*	*	*	*
Pediatrics: Nephrology	0	*	*	*	*	*	*	*
Pediatrics: Neurology	0	*	*	*	*	*	*	*
Pediatrics: Pulmonology	1	1	*	*	*	*	*	*
Pediatrics: Rheumatology	0	*	*	*	*	*	*	*
Physiatry (Phys Med & Rehab)	10	6	$783,644	$622,705	$183,186	$716,247	$1,325,460	$1,684,162
Podiatry: General	3	3	*	*	*	*	*	*
Podiatry: Surg-Foot & Ankle	1	1	*	*	*	*	*	*
Podiatry: Surg-Forefoot Only	0	*	*	*	*	*	*	*
Psychiatry: General	5	4	*	*	*	*	*	*
Psychiatry: Child & Adolescent	1	1	*	*	*	*	*	*
Psychiatry: Geriatric	0	*	*	*	*	*	*	*
Pulmonary Medicine	6	4	*	*	*	*	*	*
Pulmonary Medicine: Critical Care	9	2	*	*	*	*	*	*
Pulmonary Med: Gen & Crit Care	26	3	$439,628	$344,386	$253,483	$314,696	$399,039	$1,208,307
Radiation Oncology	20	3	$3,953,341	$2,149,781	$2,870,333	$3,938,797	$5,262,815	$7,368,639
Radiology: Diagnostic-Inv	7	4	*	*	*	*	*	*
Radiology: Diagnostic-Noninv	86	11	$3,449,307	$2,862,719	$1,253,023	$2,493,706	$4,973,270	$8,671,457
Radiology: Nuclear Medicine	6	2	*	*	*	*	*	*
Rheumatology	12	8	$731,866	$557,497	$430,863	$532,630	$889,998	$1,853,529
Sleep Medicine	6	6	*	*	*	*	*	*
Surgery: General	17	9	$762,309	$323,122	$482,299	$797,080	$918,792	$1,339,086
Surgery: Bariatric	0	*	*	*	*	*	*	*
Surgery: Cardiovascular	5	1	*	*	*	*	*	*
Surgery: Colon and Rectal	0	*	*	*	*	*	*	*
Surgery: Neurological	6	3	*	*	*	*	*	*
Surgery: Oncology	1	1	*	*	*	*	*	*
Surgery: Oral	0	*	*	*	*	*	*	*
Surgery: Pediatric	2	1	*	*	*	*	*	*
Surgery: Plastic & Reconstruction	0	*	*	*	*	*	*	*
Surgery: Plastic & Recon-Hand	0	*	*	*	*	*	*	*
Surgery: Thoracic (primary)	0	*	*	*	*	*	*	*
Surgery: Transplant	0	*	*	*	*	*	*	*
Surgery: Trauma	0	*	*	*	*	*	*	*
Surgery: Trauma-Burn	0	*	*	*	*	*	*	*
Surgery: Vascular (primary)	10	6	$888,752	$391,363	$585,826	$765,463	$1,166,159	$1,616,465
Urgent Care	1	1	*	*	*	*	*	*
Urology	34	8	$939,701	$314,295	$759,782	$857,886	$1,134,962	$1,369,823
Urology: Pediatric	2	1	*	*	*	*	*	*

Table 26: Physician Compensation to Collections Ratio (TC/NPP Excluded)

	Phys	Med Pracs	Mean	Std. Dev.	25th %tile	Median	75th %tile	90th %tile
Allergy/Immunology	69	38	.464	.162	.354	.465	.547	.667
Anesthesiology	1,993	110	.704	.181	.556	.742	.836	.927
Anesthesiology: Pain Management	67	24	.708	.182	.564	.700	.890	.938
Anesthesiology: Pediatric	22	3	.826	.130	.758	.836	.945	.977
Cardiology: Electrophysiology	58	27	.623	.173	.488	.589	.760	.892
Cardiology: Invasive	133	43	.671	.185	.519	.667	.814	.931
Cardiology: Inv-Intvl	189	51	.657	.152	.536	.656	.771	.870
Cardiology: Noninvasive	132	42	.672	.179	.537	.675	.796	.937
Critical Care: Intensivist	17	6	.763	.107	.657	.801	.851	.883
Dentistry	9	3	*	*	*	*	*	*
Dermatology	148	62	.532	.135	.459	.513	.589	.715
Dermatology: Mohs Surgery	13	10	.523	.148	.334	.563	.642	.717
Emergency Medicine	193	19	.702	.197	.536	.729	.867	.940
Endocrinology/Metabolism	118	64	.570	.145	.478	.581	.682	.740
Family Practice (w/ OB)	309	63	.523	.146	.429	.502	.623	.732
Family Practice (w/o OB)	2,330	290	.508	.146	.413	.487	.582	.707
FP: Amb Only (no inpatient work)	71	9	.523	.122	.423	.528	.618	.667
Family Practice: Sports Med	21	12	.567	.156	.425	.529	.688	.841
Family Practice: Urgent Care	63	14	.467	.172	.320	.480	.564	.719
Gastroenterology	357	98	.580	.151	.471	.562	.682	.792
Gastroenterology: Hepatology	6	4	*	*	*	*	*	*
Genetics	0	*	*	*	*	*	*	*
Geriatrics	28	12	.682	.177	.538	.698	.865	.916
Hematology/Oncology	107	39	.615	.214	.451	.637	.784	.883
Hematology/Oncology: Onc (only)	9	7	*	*	*	*	*	*
Hospice/Palliative Care	0	*	*	*	*	*	*	*
Hospitalist: Family Practice	6	4	*	*	*	*	*	*
Hospitalist: Internal Medicine	248	67	.813	.139	.717	.843	.930	.974
Hospitalist: IM-Pediatrics	2	1	*	*	*	*	*	*
Hospitalist: Pediatrics	4	3	*	*	*	*	*	*
Infectious Disease	43	23	.696	.163	.563	.698	.835	.892
Internal Medicine: General	1,709	212	.545	.148	.440	.527	.629	.746
IM: Amb Only (no inpatient work)	12	5	.531	.219	.385	.513	.648	.900
Internal Med: Pediatrics	45	18	.525	.172	.403	.507	.603	.785
Nephrology	69	32	.667	.189	.544	.662	.812	.948
Neurology	221	79	.602	.157	.485	.573	.697	.836
Obstetrics/Gynecology: General	603	125	.497	.135	.403	.483	.580	.671
OB/GYN: Gynecology (only)	66	35	.503	.155	.411	.466	.566	.721
OB/GYN: Gyn Oncology	10	8	.665	.148	.548	.649	.771	.949
OB/GYN: Maternal & Fetal Med	18	9	.520	.209	.350	.497	.670	.869
OB/GYN: Repro Endocrinology	3	3	*	*	*	*	*	*
OB/GYN: Urogynecology	3	2	*	*	*	*	*	*
Occupational Medicine	42	19	.498	.156	.408	.455	.567	.756
Ophthalmology	170	59	.475	.137	.374	.456	.545	.650
Ophthalmology: Pediatric	12	8	.443	.104	.342	.465	.517	.600
Ophthalmology: Retina	12	11	.457	.166	.326	.392	.602	.739
Orthopedic (Nonsurgical)	19	15	.564	.131	.467	.512	.610	.790
Orthopedic Surgery: General	343	95	.593	.142	.494	.575	.675	.791
Orthopedic Surgery: Foot & Ankle	17	15	.620	.138	.540	.646	.734	.767
Orthopedic Surgery: Hand	55	30	.580	.147	.496	.544	.648	.821
Orthopedic Surgery: Hip & Joint	38	21	.573	.131	.484	.588	.666	.780
Orthopedic Surgery: Pediatric	7	5	*	*	*	*	*	*
Orthopedic Surgery: Spine	41	26	.538	.152	.419	.513	.647	.744
Orthopedic Surgery: Trauma	12	8	.664	.127	.605	.688	.740	.832
Orthopedic Surgery: Sports Med	52	29	.586	.132	.509	.582	.638	.800

Table 26: Physician Compensation to Collections Ratio (TC/NPP Excluded) (continued)

	Phys	Med Pracs	Mean	Std. Dev.	25th %tile	Median	75th %tile	90th %tile
Otorhinolaryngology	200	73	.528	.158	.428	.508	.614	.734
Pathology: Anatomic and Clinical	42	9	.509	.247	.277	.495	.730	.847
Pathology: Anatomic	3	1	*	*	*	*	*	*
Pathology: Clinical	22	6	.642	.181	.583	.691	.731	.843
Pediatrics: General	1,338	163	.474	.147	.369	.458	.566	.657
Pediatrics: Adolescent Medicine	17	5	.332	.160	.174	.307	.413	.618
Pediatrics: Allergy/Immunology	2	1	*	*	*	*	*	*
Pediatrics: Cardiology	13	6	.575	.136	.464	.586	.694	.767
Pediatrics: Child Development	4	3	*	*	*	*	*	*
Pediatrics: Critical Care/Intensivist	9	5	*	*	*	*	*	*
Pediatrics: Emergency Medicine	15	3	.559	.243	.374	.459	.788	.973
Pediatrics: Endocrinology	11	11	.646	.218	.558	.650	.788	.900
Pediatrics: Gastroenterology	6	4	*	*	*	*	*	*
Pediatrics: Genetics	1	1	*	*	*	*	*	*
Pediatrics: Hematology/Oncology	13	8	.757	.134	.693	.730	.865	.956
Pediatrics: Infectious Disease	1	1	*	*	*	*	*	*
Pediatrics: Neonatal Medicine	31	7	.596	.166	.446	.632	.698	.808
Pediatrics: Nephrology	1	1	*	*	*	*	*	*
Pediatrics: Neurology	23	15	.715	.153	.586	.723	.864	.909
Pediatrics: Pulmonology	3	3	*	*	*	*	*	*
Pediatrics: Rheumatology	3	2	*	*	*	*	*	*
Physiatry (Phys Med & Rehab)	89	40	.553	.134	.456	.545	.639	.731
Podiatry: General	74	45	.493	.111	.402	.488	.564	.636
Podiatry: Surg-Foot & Ankle	23	13	.479	.099	.389	.486	.564	.623
Podiatry: Surg-Forefoot Only	0	*	*	*	*	*	*	*
Psychiatry: General	73	26	.714	.152	.617	.734	.830	.914
Psychiatry: Child & Adolescent	11	8	.753	.144	.628	.766	.838	.981
Psychiatry: Geriatric	2	2	*	*	*	*	*	*
Pulmonary Medicine	113	48	.616	.164	.490	.587	.753	.870
Pulmonary Medicine: Critical Care	28	8	.682	.156	.593	.680	.782	.888
Pulmonary Med: Gen & Crit Care	38	17	.613	.126	.545	.648	.688	.743
Radiation Oncology	25	12	.739	.173	.636	.738	.908	.951
Radiology: Diagnostic-Inv	96	21	.675	.179	.528	.701	.801	.926
Radiology: Diagnostic-Noninv	207	32	.640	.200	.498	.665	.789	.896
Radiology: Nuclear Medicine	12	8	.692	.136	.570	.643	.806	.919
Rheumatology	122	61	.569	.156	.474	.571	.655	.752
Sleep Medicine	20	9	.519	.158	.413	.485	.556	.824
Surgery: General	425	124	.566	.140	.466	.543	.646	.770
Surgery: Bariatric	5	3	*	*	*	*	*	*
Surgery: Cardiovascular	89	27	.664	.170	.533	.641	.809	.896
Surgery: Colon and Rectal	30	13	.540	.128	.422	.559	.613	.758
Surgery: Neurological	98	32	.660	.151	.552	.657	.756	.881
Surgery: Oncology	10	7	.592	.129	.481	.581	.723	.770
Surgery: Oral	12	6	.398	.048	.374	.374	.401	.507
Surgery: Pediatric	19	8	.588	.220	.410	.592	.822	.900
Surgery: Plastic & Reconstruction	54	27	.519	.151	.416	.504	.595	.758
Surgery: Plastic & Recon-Hand	1	1	*	*	*	*	*	*
Surgery: Thoracic (primary)	20	10	.745	.165	.617	.717	.893	.993
Surgery: Transplant	10	3	.528	.193	.317	.507	.697	.849
Surgery: Trauma	12	7	.745	.175	.603	.742	.925	.953
Surgery: Trauma-Burn	1	1	*	*	*	*	*	*
Surgery: Vascular (primary)	56	27	.564	.132	.481	.532	.666	.743
Urgent Care	215	35	.460	.130	.382	.439	.529	.612
Urology	230	65	.565	.138	.479	.556	.653	.736
Urology: Pediatric	7	2	*	*	*	*	*	*

Table 27: Physician Compensation to Collections Ratio (TC/NPP Excluded) by Group Type

	Single Specialty			Multispecialty		
	Phys	Med Pracs	Median	Phys	Med Pracs	Median
Allergy/Immunology	11	4	.397	58	34	.496
Anesthesiology	1,804	88	.742	189	22	.652
Anesthesiology: Pain Management	27	8	.938	40	16	.641
Anesthesiology: Pediatric	15	1	*	7	2	*
Cardiology: Electrophysiology	39	15	.562	19	12	.671
Cardiology: Invasive	44	11	.673	89	32	.659
Cardiology: Inv-Intvl	100	20	.628	89	31	.673
Cardiology: Noninvasive	51	18	.607	81	24	.688
Critical Care: Intensivist	2	1	*	15	5	.794
Dentistry	0	*	*	9	3	*
Dermatology	13	5	.691	135	57	.508
Dermatology: Mohs Surgery	1	1	*	12	9	.551
Emergency Medicine	117	8	.733	76	11	.722
Endocrinology/Metabolism	8	6	*	110	58	.566
Family Practice (w/ OB)	37	10	.530	272	53	.501
Family Practice (w/o OB)	361	123	.486	1,969	167	.487
FP: Amb Only (no inpatient work)	6	3	*	65	6	.531
Family Practice: Sports Med	6	3	*	15	9	.529
Family Practice: Urgent Care	23	1	*	40	13	.513
Gastroenterology	122	17	.512	235	81	.580
Gastroenterology: Hepatology	3	3	*	3	1	*
Genetics	*	*	*	0	*	*
Geriatrics	12	3	.566	16	9	.772
Hematology/Oncology	25	5	.627	82	34	.638
Hematology/Oncology: Onc (only)	3	2	*	6	5	*
Hospice/Palliative Care	0	*	*	0	*	*
Hospitalist: Family Practice	1	1	*	5	3	*
Hospitalist: Internal Medicine	60	14	.860	188	53	.838
Hospitalist: IM-Pediatrics	*	*	*	2	1	*
Hospitalist: Pediatrics	0	*	*	4	3	*
Infectious Disease	15	6	.721	28	17	.681
Internal Medicine: General	129	32	.569	1,580	180	.524
IM: Amb Only (no inpatient work)	0	*	*	12	5	.513
Internal Med: Pediatrics	0	*	*	45	18	.507
Nephrology	6	2	*	63	30	.638
Neurology	30	10	.597	191	69	.565
Obstetrics/Gynecology: General	100	27	.548	503	98	.476
OB/GYN: Gynecology (only)	2	2	*	64	33	.466
OB/GYN: Gyn Oncology	2	1	*	8	7	*
OB/GYN: Maternal & Fetal Med	7	4	*	11	5	.479
OB/GYN: Repro Endocrinology	0	*	*	3	3	*
OB/GYN: Urogynecology	*	*	*	3	2	*
Occupational Medicine	2	1	*	40	18	.453
Ophthalmology	36	12	.414	134	47	.469
Ophthalmology: Pediatric	2	2	*	10	6	.465
Ophthalmology: Retina	3	3	*	9	8	*
Orthopedic (Nonsurgical)	10	8	.608	9	7	*
Orthopedic Surgery: General	92	26	.545	251	69	.577
Orthopedic Surgery: Foot & Ankle	13	11	.646	4	4	*
Orthopedic Surgery: Hand	36	16	.562	19	14	.529
Orthopedic Surgery: Hip & Joint	26	15	.591	12	6	.535
Orthopedic Surgery: Pediatric	4	2	*	3	3	*
Orthopedic Surgery: Spine	23	15	.566	18	11	.471
Orthopedic Surgery: Trauma	9	6	*	3	2	*
Orthopedic Surgery: Sports Med	33	19	.577	19	10	.591

Table 27: Physician Compensation to Collections Ratio (TC/NPP Excluded) by Group Type (continued)

	Single Specialty			Multispecialty		
	Phys	Med Pracs	Median	Phys	Med Pracs	Median
Otorhinolaryngology	40	9	.441	160	64	.527
Pathology: Anatomic and Clinical	18	2	*	24	7	.530
Pathology: Anatomic	*	*	*	3	1	*
Pathology: Clinical	1	1	*	21	5	.692
Pediatrics: General	393	39	.503	945	124	.445
Pediatrics: Adolescent Medicine	10	2	*	7	3	*
Pediatrics: Allergy/Immunology	2	1	*	0	*	*
Pediatrics: Cardiology	0	*	*	13	6	.586
Pediatrics: Child Development	*	*	*	4	3	*
Pediatrics: Critical Care/Intensivist	0	*	*	9	5	*
Pediatrics: Emergency Medicine	0	*	*	15	3	.459
Pediatrics: Endocrinology	2	2	*	9	9	*
Pediatrics: Gastroenterology	0	*	*	6	4	*
Pediatrics: Genetics	0	*	*	1	1	*
Pediatrics: Hematology/Oncology	3	2	*	10	6	.746
Pediatrics: Infectious Disease	*	*	*	1	1	*
Pediatrics: Neonatal Medicine	17	4	.606	14	3	.633
Pediatrics: Nephrology	*	*	*	1	1	*
Pediatrics: Neurology	2	1	*	21	14	.685
Pediatrics: Pulmonology	1	1	*	2	2	*
Pediatrics: Rheumatology	*	*	*	3	2	*
Physiatry (Phys Med & Rehab)	34	12	.556	55	28	.539
Podiatry: General	3	3	*	71	42	.494
Podiatry: Surg-Foot & Ankle	1	1	*	22	12	.490
Podiatry: Surg-Forefoot Only	0	*	*	0	*	*
Psychiatry: General	15	2	*	58	24	.750
Psychiatry: Child & Adolescent	2	1	*	9	7	*
Psychiatry: Geriatric	1	1	*	1	1	*
Pulmonary Medicine	5	2	*	108	46	.576
Pulmonary Medicine: Critical Care	4	2	*	24	6	.691
Pulmonary Med: Gen & Crit Care	9	3	*	29	14	.618
Radiation Oncology	6	3	*	19	9	.741
Radiology: Diagnostic-Inv	66	9	.708	30	12	.666
Radiology: Diagnostic-Noninv	113	11	.638	94	21	.675
Radiology: Nuclear Medicine	7	5	*	5	3	*
Rheumatology	13	6	.552	109	55	.574
Sleep Medicine	1	1	*	19	8	.481
Surgery: General	71	21	.519	354	103	.550
Surgery: Bariatric	2	1	*	3	2	*
Surgery: Cardiovascular	49	12	.589	40	15	.695
Surgery: Colon and Rectal	*	*	*	30	13	.559
Surgery: Neurological	33	7	.656	65	25	.658
Surgery: Oncology	0	*	*	10	7	.581
Surgery: Oral	6	2	*	6	4	*
Surgery: Pediatric	12	3	.565	7	5	*
Surgery: Plastic & Reconstruction	5	2	*	49	25	.531
Surgery: Plastic & Recon-Hand	0	*	*	1	1	*
Surgery: Thoracic (primary)	8	4	*	12	6	.767
Surgery: Transplant	6	1	*	4	2	*
Surgery: Trauma	1	1	*	11	6	.698
Surgery: Trauma-Burn	*	*	*	1	1	*
Surgery: Vascular (primary)	4	3	*	52	24	.541
Urgent Care	16	4	.463	199	31	.439
Urology	98	12	.569	132	53	.550
Urology: Pediatric	3	1	*	4	1	*

Table 28A: Physician Compensation to Collections Ratio (TC/NPP Excluded) by Geographic Section for All Practices

	Eastern		Midwest		Southern		Western	
	Phys	Median	Phys	Median	Phys	Median	Phys	Median
Allergy/Immunology	6	*	23	.522	15	.527	25	.333
Anesthesiology	593	.742	430	.799	545	.557	425	.805
Anesthesiology: Pain Management	18	.938	23	.700	25	.598	1	*
Anesthesiology: Pediatric	0	*	21	*	1	*	0	*
Cardiology: Electrophysiology	11	.585	20	.677	20	.562	7	*
Cardiology: Invasive	11	.449	45	.813	48	.732	29	.539
Cardiology: Inv-Intvl	34	.566	69	.716	47	.683	39	.618
Cardiology: Noninvasive	63	.676	34	.674	27	.739	8	*
Critical Care: Intensivist	9	*	1	*	0	*	7	*
Dentistry	3	*	*	*	6	*	0	*
Dermatology	23	.518	44	.524	37	.533	44	.474
Dermatology: Mohs Surgery	4	*	6	*	2	*	1	*
Emergency Medicine	50	.732	39	.760	20	*	84	.722
Endocrinology/Metabolism	26	.498	28	.593	44	.589	20	.579
Family Practice (w/ OB)	22	.488	139	.517	63	.609	85	.462
Family Practice (w/o OB)	429	.480	736	.501	619	.544	546	.434
FP: Amb Only (no inpatient work)	26	.417	1	*	41	.596	3	*
Family Practice: Sports Med	7	*	5	*	6	*	3	*
Family Practice: Urgent Care	15	.496	13	.602	34	.345	1	*
Gastroenterology	46	.558	139	.547	105	.600	67	.513
Gastroenterology: Hepatology	0	*	1	*	1	*	4	*
Genetics	0	*	0	*	0	*	0	*
Geriatrics	5	*	7	*	4	*	12	*
Hematology/Oncology	19	.601	26	.646	39	.686	23	.577
Hematology/Oncology: Onc (only)	1	*	1	*	5	*	2	*
Hospice/Palliative Care	0	*	0	*	0	*	0	*
Hospitalist: Family Practice	0	*	4	*	2	*	0	*
Hospitalist: Internal Medicine	51	.791	69	.808	74	.827	54	.890
Hospitalist: IM-Pediatrics	0	*	*	*	2	*	*	*
Hospitalist: Pediatrics	2	*	0	*	1	*	1	*
Infectious Disease	13	.784	10	.776	12	.660	8	*
Internal Medicine: General	342	.492	564	.535	440	.585	363	.478
IM: Amb Only (no inpatient work)	5	*	1	*	5	*	1	*
Internal Med: Pediatrics	5	*	24	.479	15	.529	1	*
Nephrology	15	.593	21	.663	21	.691	12	.674
Neurology	57	.642	73	.581	45	.561	46	.519
Obstetrics/Gynecology: General	113	.450	218	.510	148	.509	124	.458
OB/GYN: Gynecology (only)	8	*	24	.480	24	.545	10	.371
OB/GYN: Gyn Oncology	2	*	5	*	1	*	2	*
OB/GYN: Maternal & Fetal Med	7	*	1	*	8	*	2	*
OB/GYN: Repro Endocrinology	2	*	0	*	1	*	0	*
OB/GYN: Urogynecology	3	*	0	*	*	*	0	*
Occupational Medicine	2	*	10	.548	4	*	26	.437
Ophthalmology	31	.395	58	.511	48	.417	33	.436
Ophthalmology: Pediatric	2	*	0	*	5	*	5	*
Ophthalmology: Retina	2	*	5	*	3	*	2	*
Orthopedic (Nonsurgical)	3	*	6	*	6	*	4	*
Orthopedic Surgery: General	55	.531	107	.614	98	.569	83	.586
Orthopedic Surgery: Foot & Ankle	5	*	1	*	6	*	5	*
Orthopedic Surgery: Hand	15	.596	7	*	8	*	25	.529
Orthopedic Surgery: Hip & Joint	16	.567	10	.608	6	*	6	*
Orthopedic Surgery: Pediatric	0	*	2	*	5	*	0	*
Orthopedic Surgery: Spine	15	.448	9	*	8	*	9	*
Orthopedic Surgery: Trauma	6	*	2	*	1	*	3	*
Orthopedic Surgery: Sports Med	24	.548	7	*	9	*	12	.631

Table 28A: Physician Compensation to Collections Ratio (TC/NPP Excluded) by Geographic Section for All Practices (continued)

	Eastern		Midwest		Southern		Western	
	Phys	Median	Phys	Median	Phys	Median	Phys	Median
Otorhinolaryngology	37	.559	55	.534	60	.474	48	.498
Pathology: Anatomic and Clinical	15	*	4	*	18	.328	5	*
Pathology: Anatomic	0	*	0	*	3	*	0	*
Pathology: Clinical	5	*	6	*	11	.695	0	*
Pediatrics: General	207	.455	412	.435	449	.521	270	.413
Pediatrics: Adolescent Medicine	2	*	1	*	9	*	5	*
Pediatrics: Allergy/Immunology	*	*	0	*	0	*	2	*
Pediatrics: Cardiology	4	*	2	*	5	*	2	*
Pediatrics: Child Development	1	*	0	*	2	*	1	*
Pediatrics: Critical Care/Intensivist	3	*	1	*	3	*	2	*
Pediatrics: Emergency Medicine	1	*	14	*	0	*	0	*
Pediatrics: Endocrinology	2	*	4	*	4	*	1	*
Pediatrics: Gastroenterology	0	*	2	*	3	*	1	*
Pediatrics: Genetics	0	*	0	*	0	*	1	*
Pediatrics: Hematology/Oncology	0	*	5	*	7	*	1	*
Pediatrics: Infectious Disease	0	*	1	*	0	*	0	*
Pediatrics: Neonatal Medicine	8	*	10	*	1	*	12	*
Pediatrics: Nephrology	0	*	1	*	0	*	0	*
Pediatrics: Neurology	2	*	12	.629	7	*	2	*
Pediatrics: Pulmonology	1	*	1	*	1	*	0	*
Pediatrics: Rheumatology	1	*	0	*	0	*	2	*
Physiatry (Phys Med & Rehab)	16	.464	22	.605	31	.564	20	.504
Podiatry: General	2	*	37	.529	20	.532	15	.444
Podiatry: Surg-Foot & Ankle	1	*	11	.564	0	*	11	.389
Podiatry: Surg-Forefoot Only	*	*	0	*	0	*	0	*
Psychiatry: General	16	.773	18	.760	19	.619	20	.793
Psychiatry: Child & Adolescent	0	*	5	*	4	*	2	*
Psychiatry: Geriatric	1	*	0	*	*	*	1	*
Pulmonary Medicine	19	.565	38	.612	33	.533	23	.639
Pulmonary Medicine: Critical Care	0	*	20	.700	6	*	2	*
Pulmonary Med: Gen & Crit Care	6	*	13	.661	14	.641	5	*
Radiation Oncology	5	*	8	*	5	*	7	*
Radiology: Diagnostic-Inv	13	.663	11	.639	33	.727	39	.710
Radiology: Diagnostic-Noninv	46	.606	28	.803	89	.643	44	.668
Radiology: Nuclear Medicine	1	*	2	*	8	*	1	*
Rheumatology	25	.560	42	.568	33	.641	22	.495
Sleep Medicine	1	*	0	*	14	.508	5	*
Surgery: General	78	.505	129	.539	112	.534	106	.594
Surgery: Bariatric	2	*	1	*	0	*	2	*
Surgery: Cardiovascular	19	.840	24	.712	35	.569	11	.679
Surgery: Colon and Rectal	12	.559	9	*	4	*	5	*
Surgery: Neurological	21	.639	19	.658	29	.687	29	.625
Surgery: Oncology	4	*	*	*	4	*	2	*
Surgery: Oral	8	*	2	*	1	*	1	*
Surgery: Pediatric	0	*	1	*	16	.544	2	*
Surgery: Plastic & Reconstruction	11	.434	12	.612	21	.504	10	.517
Surgery: Plastic & Recon-Hand	0	*	0	*	0	*	1	*
Surgery: Thoracic (primary)	6	*	5	*	3	*	6	*
Surgery: Transplant	0	*	0	*	6	*	4	*
Surgery: Trauma	5	*	2	*	3	*	2	*
Surgery: Trauma-Burn	0	*	*	*	1	*	*	*
Surgery: Vascular (primary)	13	.513	20	.600	16	.540	7	*
Urgent Care	9	*	60	.499	23	.450	123	.415
Urology	30	.544	49	.538	108	.589	43	.516
Urology: Pediatric	0	*	4	*	3	*	0	*

Table 28B: Physician Compensation to Collections Ratio (TC/NPP Excluded) by Geographic Section for Single-Specialty Practices

	Eastern		Midwest		Southern		Western	
	Phys	Median	Phys	Median	Phys	Median	Phys	Median
Allergy/Immunology	2	*	0	*	4	*	5	*
Anesthesiology	554	.742	393	.799	434	.555	423	.806
Anesthesiology: Pain Management	15	.938	10	.700	1	*	1	*
Anesthesiology: Pediatric	0	*	15	*	*	*	0	*
Cardiology: Electrophysiology	8	*	13	.648	15	.556	3	*
Cardiology: Invasive	5	*	18	.833	10	.624	11	.523
Cardiology: Inv-Intvl	26	.585	41	.786	21	.619	12	.594
Cardiology: Noninvasive	20	.505	11	.694	18	.664	2	*
Critical Care: Intensivist	2	*	0	*	0	*	*	*
Dentistry	*	*	*	*	0	*	0	*
Dermatology	3	*	6	*	2	*	2	*
Dermatology: Mohs Surgery	0	*	1	*	*	*	*	*
Emergency Medicine	30	.732	5	*	0	*	82	.722
Endocrinology/Metabolism	3	*	1	*	4	*	*	*
Family Practice (w/ OB)	2	*	13	*	7	*	15	.451
Family Practice (w/o OB)	122	.466	74	.483	115	.544	50	.390
FP: Amb Only (no inpatient work)	1	*	0	*	2	*	3	*
Family Practice: Sports Med	3	*	1	*	2	*	0	*
Family Practice: Urgent Care	*	*	*	*	23	*	0	*
Gastroenterology	10	.423	67	.512	36	.574	9	*
Gastroenterology: Hepatology	0	*	1	*	1	*	1	*
Geriatrics	1	*	0	*	1	*	10	*
Hematology/Oncology	2	*	2	*	14	*	7	*
Hematology/Oncology: Onc (only)	1	*	0	*	*	*	2	*
Hospice/Palliative Care	0	*	*	*	0	*	0	*
Hospitalist: Family Practice	*	*	*	*	1	*	*	*
Hospitalist: Internal Medicine	15	.947	10	.886	25	.864	10	*
Hospitalist: Pediatrics	*	*	*	*	0	*	*	*
Infectious Disease	7	*	2	*	5	*	1	*
Internal Medicine: General	33	.557	31	.495	59	.625	6	*
IM: Amb Only (no inpatient work)	0	*	*	*	*	*	*	*
Internal Med: Pediatrics	0	*	*	*	*	*	*	*
Nephrology	0	*	2	*	0	*	4	*
Neurology	20	.677	0	*	0	*	10	*
Obstetrics/Gynecology: General	31	.480	23	.542	33	.558	13	.492
OB/GYN: Gynecology (only)	0	*	0	*	2	*	0	*
OB/GYN: Gyn Oncology	*	*	2	*	0	*	*	*
OB/GYN: Maternal & Fetal Med	5	*	0	*	2	*	0	*
OB/GYN: Repro Endocrinology	*	*	*	*	0	*	*	*
Occupational Medicine	0	*	2	*	*	*	*	*
Ophthalmology	16	.355	12	.494	4	*	4	*
Ophthalmology: Pediatric	1	*	0	*	0	*	1	*
Ophthalmology: Retina	1	*	2	*	0	*	*	*
Orthopedic (Nonsurgical)	2	*	1	*	5	*	2	*
Orthopedic Surgery: General	19	.519	37	.701	24	.508	12	.635
Orthopedic Surgery: Foot & Ankle	3	*	1	*	5	*	4	*
Orthopedic Surgery: Hand	9	*	3	*	6	*	18	.543
Orthopedic Surgery: Hip & Joint	10	.565	9	*	4	*	3	*
Orthopedic Surgery: Pediatric	0	*	1	*	3	*	*	*
Orthopedic Surgery: Spine	9	*	5	*	5	*	4	*
Orthopedic Surgery: Trauma	3	*	2	*	1	*	3	*
Orthopedic Surgery: Sports Med	15	.530	2	*	8	*	8	*

Table 28B: Physician Compensation to Collections Ratio (TC/NPP Excluded) by Geographic Section for Single-Specialty Practices (continued)

	Eastern		Midwest		Southern		Western	
	Phys	Median	Phys	Median	Phys	Median	Phys	Median
Otorhinolaryngology	10	.495	0	*	21	.412	9	*
Pathology: Anatomic and Clinical	*	*	0	*	16	*	2	*
Pathology: Clinical	*	*	*	*	1	*	0	*
Pediatrics: General	52	.485	74	.416	208	.526	59	.505
Pediatrics: Adolescent Medicine	2	*	*	*	8	*	*	*
Pediatrics: Allergy/Immunology	*	*	*	*	*	*	2	*
Pediatrics: Cardiology	0	*	0	*	0	*	*	*
Pediatrics: Critical Care/Intensivist	*	*	0	*	*	*	*	*
Pediatrics: Emergency Medicine	0	*	*	*	0	*	*	*
Pediatrics: Endocrinology	*	*	*	*	1	*	1	*
Pediatrics: Gastroenterology	0	*	0	*	*	*	*	*
Pediatrics: Genetics	0	*	*	*	*	*	*	*
Pediatrics: Hematology/Oncology	*	*	*	*	2	*	1	*
Pediatrics: Neonatal Medicine	4	*	*	*	1	*	12	*
Pediatrics: Neurology	*	*	0	*	2	*	*	*
Pediatrics: Pulmonology	*	*	*	*	1	*	0	*
Physiatry (Phys Med & Rehab)	6	*	4	*	17	.540	7	*
Podiatry: General	1	*	2	*	*	*	0	*
Podiatry: Surg-Foot & Ankle	1	*	0	*	*	*	*	*
Podiatry: Surg-Forefoot Only	*	*	*	*	*	*	0	*
Psychiatry: General	6	*	0	*	9	*	*	*
Psychiatry: Child & Adolescent	*	*	0	*	2	*	*	*
Psychiatry: Geriatric	1	*	*	*	*	*	*	*
Pulmonary Medicine	3	*	0	*	2	*	*	*
Pulmonary Medicine: Critical Care	0	*	3	*	1	*	0	*
Pulmonary Med: Gen & Crit Care	0	*	0	*	7	*	2	*
Radiation Oncology	0	*	5	*	1	*	*	*
Radiology: Diagnostic-Inv	9	*	2	*	22	.740	33	.699
Radiology: Diagnostic-Noninv	31	.582	4	*	58	.639	20	.712
Radiology: Nuclear Medicine	1	*	0	*	6	*	0	*
Rheumatology	*	*	11	.552	2	*	0	*
Sleep Medicine	*	*	*	*	1	*	*	*
Surgery: General	29	.468	7	*	30	.536	5	*
Surgery: Bariatric	2	*	*	*	0	*	*	*
Surgery: Cardiovascular	15	.828	2	*	25	.539	7	*
Surgery: Neurological	*	*	3	*	13	.687	17	*
Surgery: Oncology	0	*	*	*	*	*	*	*
Surgery: Oral	6	*	*	*	0	*	*	*
Surgery: Pediatric	*	*	1	*	11	*	*	*
Surgery: Plastic & Reconstruction	0	*	1	*	4	*	*	*
Surgery: Plastic & Recon-Hand	0	*	*	*	0	*	*	*
Surgery: Thoracic (primary)	6	*	0	*	1	*	1	*
Surgery: Transplant	*	*	*	*	6	*	*	*
Surgery: Trauma	*	*	0	*	1	*	*	*
Surgery: Vascular (primary)	3	*	1	*	0	*	0	*
Urgent Care	3	*	11	*	0	*	2	*
Urology	6	*	3	*	77	.569	12	*
Urology: Pediatric	0	*	*	*	3	*	0	*

Table 28C: Physician Compensation to Collections Ratio (TC/NPP Excluded) by Geographic Section for Multispecialty Practices

	Eastern		Midwest		Southern		Western	
	Phys	Median	Phys	Median	Phys	Median	Phys	Median
Allergy/Immunology	4	*	23	.522	11	.530	20	.338
Anesthesiology	39	.743	37	.608	111	.649	2	*
Anesthesiology: Pain Management	3	*	13	.652	24	.590	0	*
Anesthesiology: Pediatric	0	*	6	*	1	*	0	*
Cardiology: Electrophysiology	3	*	7	*	5	*	4	*
Cardiology: Invasive	6	*	27	.777	38	.747	18	.556
Cardiology: Inv-Intvl	8	*	28	.696	26	.731	27	.637
Cardiology: Noninvasive	43	.707	23	.664	9	*	6	*
Critical Care: Intensivist	7	*	1	*	0	*	7	*
Dentistry	3	*	*	*	6	*	0	*
Dermatology	20	.501	38	.510	35	.524	42	.473
Dermatology: Mohs Surgery	4	*	5	*	2	*	1	*
Emergency Medicine	20	.678	34	.735	20	*	2	*
Endocrinology/Metabolism	23	.483	27	.590	40	.588	20	.579
Family Practice (w/ OB)	20	.496	126	.502	56	.613	70	.465
Family Practice (w/o OB)	307	.486	662	.506	504	.545	496	.438
FP: Amb Only (no inpatient work)	25	.423	1	*	39	*	0	*
Family Practice: Sports Med	4	*	4	*	4	*	3	*
Family Practice: Urgent Care	15	.496	13	.602	11	.544	1	*
Gastroenterology	36	.575	72	.578	69	.602	58	.546
Gastroenterology: Hepatology	*	*	*	*	*	*	3	*
Genetics	0	*	0	*	0	*	0	*
Geriatrics	4	*	7	*	3	*	2	*
Hematology/Oncology	17	.571	24	.646	25	.658	16	.622
Hematology/Oncology: Onc (only)	0	*	1	*	5	*	0	*
Hospice/Palliative Care	0	*	0	*	0	*	0	*
Hospitalist: Family Practice	0	*	4	*	1	*	0	*
Hospitalist: Internal Medicine	36	.759	59	.799	49	.811	44	.904
Hospitalist: IM-Pediatrics	0	*	*	*	2	*	*	*
Hospitalist: Pediatrics	2	*	0	*	1	*	1	*
Infectious Disease	6	*	8	*	7	*	7	*
Internal Medicine: General	309	.486	533	.539	381	.579	357	.477
IM: Amb Only (no inpatient work)	5	*	1	*	5	*	1	*
Internal Med: Pediatrics	5	*	24	.479	15	.529	1	*
Nephrology	15	.593	19	.638	21	.691	8	*
Neurology	37	.613	73	.581	45	.561	36	.552
Obstetrics/Gynecology: General	82	.449	195	.510	115	.491	111	.453
OB/GYN: Gynecology (only)	8	*	24	.480	22	.545	10	.371
OB/GYN: Gyn Oncology	2	*	3	*	1	*	2	*
OB/GYN: Maternal & Fetal Med	2	*	1	*	6	*	2	*
OB/GYN: Repro Endocrinology	2	*	0	*	1	*	0	*
OB/GYN: Urogynecology	3	*	0	*	*	*	0	*
Occupational Medicine	2	*	8	*	4	*	26	.437
Ophthalmology	15	.476	46	.524	44	.426	29	.425
Ophthalmology: Pediatric	1	*	0	*	5	*	4	*
Ophthalmology: Retina	1	*	3	*	3	*	2	*
Orthopedic (Nonsurgical)	1	*	5	*	1	*	2	*
Orthopedic Surgery: General	36	.534	70	.595	74	.581	71	.580
Orthopedic Surgery: Foot & Ankle	2	*	0	*	1	*	1	*
Orthopedic Surgery: Hand	6	*	4	*	2	*	7	*
Orthopedic Surgery: Hip & Joint	6	*	1	*	2	*	3	*
Orthopedic Surgery: Pediatric	0	*	1	*	2	*	0	*
Orthopedic Surgery: Spine	6	*	4	*	3	*	5	*
Orthopedic Surgery: Trauma	3	*	0	*	0	*	0	*
Orthopedic Surgery: Sports Med	9	*	5	*	1	*	4	*

Table 28C: Physician Compensation to Collections Ratio (TC/NPP Excluded) by Geographic Section for Multispecialty Practices (continued)

	Eastern		Midwest		Southern		Western	
	Phys	Median	Phys	Median	Phys	Median	Phys	Median
Otorhinolaryngology	27	.602	55	.534	39	.547	39	.502
Pathology: Anatomic and Clinical	15	*	4	*	2	*	3	*
Pathology: Anatomic	0	*	0	*	3	*	0	*
Pathology: Clinical	5	*	6	*	10	*	0	*
Pediatrics: General	155	.440	338	.440	241	.512	211	.396
Pediatrics: Adolescent Medicine	0	*	1	*	1	*	5	*
Pediatrics: Allergy/Immunology	*	*	0	*	0	*	0	*
Pediatrics: Cardiology	4	*	2	*	5	*	2	*
Pediatrics: Child Development	1	*	0	*	2	*	1	*
Pediatrics: Critical Care/Intensivist	3	*	1	*	3	*	2	*
Pediatrics: Emergency Medicine	1	*	14	*	0	*	0	*
Pediatrics: Endocrinology	2	*	4	*	3	*	0	*
Pediatrics: Gastroenterology	0	*	2	*	3	*	1	*
Pediatrics: Genetics	0	*	0	*	0	*	1	*
Pediatrics: Hematology/Oncology	0	*	5	*	5	*	0	*
Pediatrics: Infectious Disease	0	*	1	*	0	*	0	*
Pediatrics: Neonatal Medicine	4	*	10	*	0	*	0	*
Pediatrics: Nephrology	0	*	1	*	0	*	0	*
Pediatrics: Neurology	2	*	12	.629	5	*	2	*
Pediatrics: Pulmonology	1	*	1	*	0	*	0	*
Pediatrics: Rheumatology	1	*	0	*	0	*	2	*
Physiatry (Phys Med & Rehab)	10	.482	18	.610	14	.591	13	.445
Podiatry: General	1	*	35	.529	20	.532	15	.444
Podiatry: Surg-Foot & Ankle	0	*	11	.564	0	*	11	.389
Podiatry: Surg-Forefoot Only	*	*	0	*	0	*	*	*
Psychiatry: General	10	.729	18	.760	10	.585	20	.793
Psychiatry: Child & Adolescent	0	*	5	*	2	*	2	*
Psychiatry: Geriatric	0	*	0	*	*	*	1	*
Pulmonary Medicine	16	.542	38	.612	31	.530	23	.639
Pulmonary Medicine: Critical Care	*	*	17	.727	5	*	2	*
Pulmonary Med: Gen & Crit Care	6	*	13	.661	7	*	3	*
Radiation Oncology	5	*	3	*	4	*	7	*
Radiology: Diagnostic-Inv	4	*	9	*	11	.640	6	*
Radiology: Diagnostic-Noninv	15	*	24	.813	31	.650	24	.665
Radiology: Nuclear Medicine	0	*	2	*	2	*	1	*
Rheumatology	25	.560	31	.586	31	.641	22	.495
Sleep Medicine	1	*	0	*	13	.489	5	*
Surgery: General	49	.562	122	.533	82	.533	101	.593
Surgery: Bariatric	0	*	1	*	0	*	2	*
Surgery: Cardiovascular	4	*	22	.712	10	.590	4	*
Surgery: Colon and Rectal	12	.559	9	*	4	*	5	*
Surgery: Neurological	21	.639	16	.641	16	.691	12	.720
Surgery: Oncology	4	*	*	*	4	*	2	*
Surgery: Oral	2	*	2	*	1	*	1	*
Surgery: Pediatric	0	*	0	*	5	*	2	*
Surgery: Plastic & Reconstruction	11	.434	11	.625	17	.538	10	.517
Surgery: Plastic & Recon-Hand	*	*	0	*	0	*	1	*
Surgery: Thoracic (primary)	0	*	5	*	2	*	5	*
Surgery: Transplant	0	*	0	*	*	*	4	*
Surgery: Trauma	5	*	2	*	2	*	2	*
Surgery: Trauma-Burn	0	*	*	*	1	*	*	*
Surgery: Vascular (primary)	10	.523	19	.599	16	.540	7	*
Urgent Care	6	*	49	.506	23	.450	121	.415
Urology	24	.544	46	.547	31	.616	31	.494
Urology: Pediatric	*	*	4	*	*	*	0	*

Table 29: Physician Compensation to Collections Ratio (TC/NPP Excluded) by Clinical Service Hours Worked per Week

	Fewer than 40 hours		40 hours or more	
	Phys	Median	Phys	Median
Allergy/Immunology	29	.425	21	.496
Anesthesiology	127	.740	1,620	.742
Anesthesiology: Pain Management	6	*	52	.700
Anesthesiology: Pediatric	2	*	20	.859
Cardiology: Electrophysiology	15	.594	30	.590
Cardiology: Invasive	38	.655	57	.657
Cardiology: Inv-Intvl	50	.656	102	.700
Cardiology: Noninvasive	31	.535	74	.674
Critical Care: Intensivist	2	*	1	*
Dentistry	2	*	7	*
Dermatology	54	.486	54	.518
Dermatology: Mohs Surgery	3	*	2	*
Emergency Medicine	116	.731	32	.673
Endocrinology/Metabolism	33	.625	44	.559
Family Practice (w/ OB)	148	.493	135	.503
Family Practice (w/o OB)	1,088	.488	716	.504
FP: Amb Only (no inpatient work)	21	.400	17	.439
Family Practice: Sports Med	5	*	11	.528
Family Practice: Urgent Care	43	.474	14	.415
Gastroenterology	81	.562	208	.559
Gastroenterology: Hepatology	2	*	3	*
Genetics	0	*	*	*
Geriatrics	8	*	4	*
Hematology/Oncology	35	.630	55	.648
Hematology/Oncology: Onc (only)	4	*	2	*
Hospice/Palliative Care	0	*	0	*
Hospitalist: Family Practice	3	*	3	*
Hospitalist: Internal Medicine	59	.814	117	.828
Hospitalist: IM-Pediatrics	0	*	2	*
Hospitalist: Pediatrics	1	*	1	*
Infectious Disease	15	.645	16	.660
Internal Medicine: General	714	.518	577	.538
IM: Amb Only (no inpatient work)	4	*	8	*
Internal Med: Pediatrics	6	*	29	.490
Nephrology	16	.802	38	.589
Neurology	61	.624	114	.570
Obstetrics/Gynecology: General	213	.490	243	.510
OB/GYN: Gynecology (only)	18	.438	24	.503
OB/GYN: Gyn Oncology	1	*	3	*
OB/GYN: Maternal & Fetal Med	4	*	6	*
OB/GYN: Repro Endocrinology	0	*	1	*
OB/GYN: Urogynecology	0	*	1	*
Occupational Medicine	31	.453	7	*
Ophthalmology	58	.472	69	.474
Ophthalmology: Pediatric	4	*	5	*
Ophthalmology: Retina	3	*	5	*
Orthopedic (Nonsurgical)	10	.534	7	*
Orthopedic Surgery: General	61	.565	169	.549
Orthopedic Surgery: Foot & Ankle	1	*	13	.634
Orthopedic Surgery: Hand	9	*	38	.547
Orthopedic Surgery: Hip & Joint	6	*	28	.591
Orthopedic Surgery: Pediatric	0	*	5	*
Orthopedic Surgery: Spine	3	*	31	.518
Orthopedic Surgery: Trauma	0	*	9	*
Orthopedic Surgery: Sports Med	6	*	38	.576

Table 29: Physician Compensation to Collections Ratio (TC/NPP Excluded) by Clinical Service Hours Worked per Week (continued)

	Fewer than 40 hours		40 hours or more	
	Phys	Median	Phys	Median
Otorhinolaryngology	47	.501	103	.502
Pathology: Anatomic and Clinical	23	.429	9	*
Pathology: Anatomic	0	*	0	*
Pathology: Clinical	2	*	7	*
Pediatrics: General	537	.437	386	.451
Pediatrics: Adolescent Medicine	14	.341	2	*
Pediatrics: Allergy/Immunology	0	*	2	*
Pediatrics: Cardiology	2	*	2	*
Pediatrics: Child Development	1	*	0	*
Pediatrics: Critical Care/Intensivist	1	*	3	*
Pediatrics: Emergency Medicine	10	*	4	*
Pediatrics: Endocrinology	3	*	6	*
Pediatrics: Gastroenterology	3	*	0	*
Pediatrics: Genetics	1	*	0	*
Pediatrics: Hematology/Oncology	1	*	8	*
Pediatrics: Infectious Disease	1	*	0	*
Pediatrics: Neonatal Medicine	1	*	26	.656
Pediatrics: Nephrology	0	*	1	*
Pediatrics: Neurology	7	*	8	*
Pediatrics: Pulmonology	0	*	2	*
Pediatrics: Rheumatology	1	*	1	*
Physiatry (Phys Med & Rehab)	21	.563	43	.531
Podiatry: General	24	.431	30	.520
Podiatry: Surg-Foot & Ankle	6	*	12	.406
Podiatry: Surg-Forefoot Only	*	*	0	*
Psychiatry: General	18	.793	38	.725
Psychiatry: Child & Adolescent	4	*	4	*
Psychiatry: Geriatric	2	*	0	*
Pulmonary Medicine	23	.696	48	.514
Pulmonary Medicine: Critical Care	3	*	8	*
Pulmonary Med: Gen & Crit Care	10	.681	18	.567
Radiation Oncology	2	*	10	.787
Radiology: Diagnostic-Inv	9	*	71	.706
Radiology: Diagnostic-Noninv	31	.486	132	.641
Radiology: Nuclear Medicine	2	*	8	*
Rheumatology	43	.559	41	.560
Sleep Medicine	0	*	15	.489
Surgery: General	109	.553	213	.533
Surgery: Bariatric	1	*	4	*
Surgery: Cardiovascular	1	*	61	.624
Surgery: Colon and Rectal	6	*	16	.504
Surgery: Neurological	15	.661	67	.639
Surgery: Oncology	2	*	4	*
Surgery: Oral	6	*	4	*
Surgery: Pediatric	4	*	13	.606
Surgery: Plastic & Reconstruction	5	*	27	.464
Surgery: Plastic & Recon-Hand	*	*	0	*
Surgery: Thoracic (primary)	11	.721	4	*
Surgery: Transplant	3	*	7	*
Surgery: Trauma	3	*	2	*
Surgery: Trauma-Burn	*	*	1	*
Surgery: Vascular (primary)	5	*	32	.517
Urgent Care	83	.447	37	.532
Urology	84	.601	110	.547
Urology: Pediatric	5	*	2	*

Table 30: Physician Compensation to Collections Ratio (TC/NPP Excluded) by Years in Specialty

	1 to 2 years		3 to 7 years		8 to 17 years		18 years or more	
	Phys	Median	Phys	Median	Phys	Median	Phys	Median
Allergy/Immunology	3	*	7	*	16	.469	33	.432
Anesthesiology	100	.525	158	.735	880	.742	635	.719
Anesthesiology: Pain Management	3	*	26	.938	25	.700	9	*
Anesthesiology: Pediatric	3	*	3	*	8	*	8	*
Cardiology: Electrophysiology	8	*	14	.572	19	.682	14	.519
Cardiology: Invasive	16	.707	26	.740	37	.727	39	.587
Cardiology: Inv-Intvl	7	*	27	.654	61	.698	71	.657
Cardiology: Noninvasive	9	*	20	.656	33	.674	53	.677
Critical Care: Intensivist	2	*	5	*	5	*	2	*
Dentistry	0	*	2	*	2	*	4	*
Dermatology	6	*	32	.494	46	.513	53	.526
Dermatology: Mohs Surgery	0	*	3	*	6	*	3	*
Emergency Medicine	8	*	27	.733	37	.714	31	.688
Endocrinology/Metabolism	11	.527	26	.588	23	.555	36	.606
Family Practice (w/ OB)	25	.539	78	.469	110	.521	64	.467
Family Practice (w/o OB)	100	.468	389	.478	728	.492	714	.503
FP: Amb Only (no inpatient work)	1	*	12	.417	26	.530	32	.564
Family Practice: Sports Med	3	*	5	*	5	*	7	*
Family Practice: Urgent Care	4	*	5	*	9	*	20	.539
Gastroenterology	11	.475	49	.560	80	.592	120	.572
Gastroenterology: Hepatology	*	*	1	*	1	*	1	*
Genetics	*	*	0	*	0	*	0	*
Geriatrics	1	*	9	*	12	.643	4	*
Hematology/Oncology	9	*	14	.598	27	.638	41	.649
Hematology/Oncology: Onc (only)	0	*	2	*	1	*	4	*
Hospice/Palliative Care	0	*	0	*	0	*	0	*
Hospitalist: Family Practice	1	*	2	*	0	*	1	*
Hospitalist: Internal Medicine	36	.881	87	.861	62	.804	10	.845
Hospitalist: IM-Pediatrics	0	*	2	*	0	*	*	*
Hospitalist: Pediatrics	0	*	1	*	2	*	0	*
Infectious Disease	2	*	5	*	14	.692	16	.710
Internal Medicine: General	64	.504	266	.530	533	.533	545	.537
IM: Amb Only (no inpatient work)	*	*	*	*	1	*	4	*
Internal Med: Pediatrics	2	*	14	.551	27	.468	0	*
Nephrology	4	*	18	.661	17	.613	17	.608
Neurology	18	.597	38	.527	64	.588	70	.596
Obstetrics/Gynecology: General	30	.507	136	.481	208	.489	142	.501
OB/GYN: Gynecology (only)	1	*	2	*	11	.473	37	.446
OB/GYN: Gyn Oncology	1	*	0	*	6	*	1	*
OB/GYN: Maternal & Fetal Med	1	*	2	*	7	*	1	*
OB/GYN: Repro Endocrinology	0	*	*	*	1	*	0	*
OB/GYN: Urogynecology	0	*	3	*	*	*	0	*
Occupational Medicine	2	*	7	*	6	*	22	.457
Ophthalmology	8	*	16	.397	53	.468	63	.441
Ophthalmology: Pediatric	1	*	2	*	3	*	4	*
Ophthalmology: Retina	0	*	1	*	5	*	3	*
Orthopedic (Nonsurgical)	0	*	1	*	2	*	12	.553
Orthopedic Surgery: General	16	.527	54	.639	106	.582	127	.552
Orthopedic Surgery: Foot & Ankle	2	*	3	*	9	*	3	*
Orthopedic Surgery: Hand	2	*	8	*	28	.582	15	.549
Orthopedic Surgery: Hip & Joint	4	*	4	*	10	.605	20	.590
Orthopedic Surgery: Pediatric	1	*	2	*	3	*	0	*
Orthopedic Surgery: Spine	6	*	7	*	16	.582	10	.498
Orthopedic Surgery: Trauma	0	*	4	*	4	*	4	*
Orthopedic Surgery: Sports Med	4	*	12	.549	18	.607	18	.607

Table 30: Physician Compensation to Collections Ratio (TC/NPP Excluded) by Years in Specialty (continued)

	1 to 2 years		3 to 7 years		8 to 17 years		18 years or more	
	Phys	Median	Phys	Median	Phys	Median	Phys	Median
Otorhinolaryngology	4	*	33	.513	77	.528	66	.500
Pathology: Anatomic and Clinical	2	*	7	*	10	.530	17	.495
Pathology: Anatomic	0	*	0	*	0	*	3	*
Pathology: Clinical	*	*	6	*	7	*	6	*
Pediatrics: General	67	.416	233	.458	448	.475	421	.466
Pediatrics: Adolescent Medicine	0	*	2	*	6	*	4	*
Pediatrics: Allergy/Immunology	*	*	0	*	1	*	1	*
Pediatrics: Cardiology	0	*	1	*	2	*	3	*
Pediatrics: Child Development	*	*	1	*	0	*	0	*
Pediatrics: Critical Care/Intensivist	0	*	2	*	2	*	2	*
Pediatrics: Emergency Medicine	1	*	6	*	5	*	3	*
Pediatrics: Endocrinology	2	*	2	*	1	*	4	*
Pediatrics: Gastroenterology	0	*	0	*	1	*	0	*
Pediatrics: Genetics	1	*	*	*	0	*	0	*
Pediatrics: Hematology/Oncology	0	*	5	*	2	*	2	*
Pediatrics: Infectious Disease	*	*	0	*	1	*	0	*
Pediatrics: Neonatal Medicine	2	*	9	*	8	*	11	.606
Pediatrics: Nephrology	0	*	*	*	1	*	0	*
Pediatrics: Neurology	1	*	3	*	6	*	5	*
Pediatrics: Pulmonology	0	*	1	*	2	*	0	*
Pediatrics: Rheumatology	*	*	*	*	2	*	1	*
Physiatry (Phys Med & Rehab)	7	*	17	.498	31	.555	19	.589
Podiatry: General	4	*	14	.487	25	.529	21	.458
Podiatry: Surg-Foot & Ankle	5	*	4	*	6	*	3	*
Podiatry: Surg-Forefoot Only	*	*	0	*	0	*	0	*
Psychiatry: General	3	*	10	.761	28	.677	16	.763
Psychiatry: Child & Adolescent	0	*	2	*	1	*	2	*
Psychiatry: Geriatric	*	*	*	*	0	*	1	*
Pulmonary Medicine	11	.727	13	.513	30	.607	33	.550
Pulmonary Medicine: Critical Care	0	*	2	*	10	.671	1	*
Pulmonary Med: Gen & Crit Care	2	*	8	*	12	.567	8	*
Radiation Oncology	2	*	4	*	10	.686	5	*
Radiology: Diagnostic-Inv	5	*	23	.735	42	.688	22	.713
Radiology: Diagnostic-Noninv	13	.460	38	.708	55	.700	68	.684
Radiology: Nuclear Medicine	0	*	1	*	5	*	3	*
Rheumatology	7	*	27	.576	22	.518	50	.586
Sleep Medicine	1	*	5	*	5	*	9	*
Surgery: General	18	.602	60	.528	133	.549	150	.556
Surgery: Bariatric	0	*	1	*	0	*	1	*
Surgery: Cardiovascular	1	*	14	.614	41	.701	28	.617
Surgery: Colon and Rectal	1	*	3	*	8	*	10	.477
Surgery: Neurological	2	*	16	.619	30	.670	33	.661
Surgery: Oncology	*	*	2	*	3	*	3	*
Surgery: Oral	0	*	1	*	2	*	9	*
Surgery: Pediatric	1	*	6	*	3	*	6	*
Surgery: Plastic & Reconstruction	2	*	10	.437	14	.481	15	.499
Surgery: Plastic & Recon-Hand	0	*	0	*	0	*	1	*
Surgery: Thoracic (primary)	0	*	3	*	0	*	7	*
Surgery: Transplant	0	*	2	*	5	*	0	*
Surgery: Trauma	1	*	2	*	2	*	3	*
Surgery: Trauma-Burn	1	*	0	*	0	*	*	*
Surgery: Vascular (primary)	1	*	5	*	16	.523	25	.503
Urgent Care	15	.412	45	.416	52	.470	67	.459
Urology	12	.520	33	.497	66	.631	82	.564
Urology: Pediatric	0	*	3	*	2	*	2	*

Table 31: Physician Compensation to Collections Ratio (TC/NPP Excluded) by Hospital Ownership

	Hospital Owned			Not Hospital Owned		
	Phys	Med Pracs	Median	Phys	Med Pracs	Median
Allergy/Immunology	16	10	.528	53	28	.440
Anesthesiology	73	9	.745	1,890	100	.742
Anesthesiology: Pain Management	9	4	*	58	20	.700
Anesthesiology: Pediatric	6	1	*	16	2	*
Cardiology: Electrophysiology	13	7	.749	45	20	.564
Cardiology: Invasive	36	9	.789	97	34	.624
Cardiology: Inv-Intvl	39	13	.692	150	38	.652
Cardiology: Noninvasive	60	14	.701	72	28	.633
Critical Care: Intensivist	9	2	*	8	4	*
Dentistry	3	1	*	6	2	*
Dermatology	46	18	.502	102	44	.523
Dermatology: Mohs Surgery	3	1	*	10	9	.583
Emergency Medicine	73	10	.811	120	9	.704
Endocrinology/Metabolism	54	27	.606	64	37	.558
Family Practice (w/ OB)	146	31	.558	163	32	.470
Family Practice (w/o OB)	1,417	180	.491	913	110	.477
FP: Amb Only (no inpatient work)	26	4	.417	45	5	.583
Family Practice: Sports Med	5	4	*	16	8	.527
Family Practice: Urgent Care	27	7	.529	36	7	.345
Gastroenterology	80	24	.604	277	74	.540
Gastroenterology: Hepatology	3	1	*	3	3	*
Genetics	0	*	*	0	*	*
Geriatrics	13	7	.862	15	5	.551
Hematology/Oncology	18	5	.646	89	34	.636
Hematology/Oncology: Onc (only)	1	1	*	8	6	*
Hospice/Palliative Care	0	*	*	0	*	*
Hospitalist: Family Practice	2	1	*	4	3	*
Hospitalist: Internal Medicine	134	35	.866	114	32	.807
Hospitalist: IM-Pediatrics	0	*	*	2	1	*
Hospitalist: Pediatrics	4	3	*	0	*	*
Infectious Disease	18	10	.701	25	13	.698
Internal Medicine: General	938	104	.509	771	108	.545
IM: Amb Only (no inpatient work)	10	3	.584	2	2	*
Internal Med: Pediatrics	21	7	.539	24	11	.504
Nephrology	17	10	.697	52	22	.640
Neurology	92	30	.627	129	49	.543
Obstetrics/Gynecology: General	264	51	.502	339	74	.466
OB/GYN: Gynecology (only)	24	12	.479	42	23	.457
OB/GYN: Gyn Oncology	7	5	*	3	3	*
OB/GYN: Maternal & Fetal Med	16	7	.497	2	2	*
OB/GYN: Repro Endocrinology	3	3	*	0	*	*
OB/GYN: Urogynecology	3	2	*	0	*	*
Occupational Medicine	13	8	.516	29	11	.435
Ophthalmology	43	13	.438	127	46	.467
Ophthalmology: Pediatric	3	3	*	9	5	*
Ophthalmology: Retina	5	4	*	7	7	*
Orthopedic (Nonsurgical)	3	2	*	16	13	.528
Orthopedic Surgery: General	92	24	.648	251	71	.552
Orthopedic Surgery: Foot & Ankle	1	1	*	16	14	.640
Orthopedic Surgery: Hand	4	4	*	51	26	.543
Orthopedic Surgery: Hip & Joint	2	1	*	36	20	.589
Orthopedic Surgery: Pediatric	5	3	*	2	2	*
Orthopedic Surgery: Spine	5	3	*	36	23	.514
Orthopedic Surgery: Trauma	1	1	*	11	7	.687
Orthopedic Surgery: Sports Med	9	5	*	43	24	.560

Table 31: Physician Compensation to Collections Ratio (TC/NPP Excluded) by Hospital Ownership (continued)

	Hospital Owned			Not Hospital Owned		
	Phys	Med Pracs	Median	Phys	Med Pracs	Median
Otorhinolaryngology	53	18	.556	147	55	.495
Pathology: Anatomic and Clinical	16	3	.682	26	6	.433
Pathology: Anatomic	0	*	*	3	1	*
Pathology: Clinical	4	1	*	18	5	.662
Pediatrics: General	766	73	.474	572	90	.437
Pediatrics: Adolescent Medicine	5	1	*	12	4	.259
Pediatrics: Allergy/Immunology	0	*	*	2	1	*
Pediatrics: Cardiology	11	4	.623	2	2	*
Pediatrics: Child Development	4	3	*	0	*	*
Pediatrics: Critical Care/Intensivist	6	3	*	3	2	*
Pediatrics: Emergency Medicine	15	3	.459	0	*	*
Pediatrics: Endocrinology	9	9	*	2	2	*
Pediatrics: Gastroenterology	6	4	*	0	*	*
Pediatrics: Genetics	0	*	*	1	1	*
Pediatrics: Hematology/Oncology	10	6	.743	3	2	*
Pediatrics: Infectious Disease	1	1	*	0	*	*
Pediatrics: Neonatal Medicine	19	5	.666	12	2	*
Pediatrics: Nephrology	1	1	*	0	*	*
Pediatrics: Neurology	15	10	.745	8	5	*
Pediatrics: Pulmonology	3	3	*	0	*	*
Pediatrics: Rheumatology	1	1	*	2	1	*
Physiatry (Phys Med & Rehab)	44	15	.563	45	25	.531
Podiatry: General	20	9	.532	54	36	.473
Podiatry: Surg-Foot & Ankle	8	2	*	15	11	.519
Podiatry: Surg-Forefoot Only	*	*	*	0	*	*
Psychiatry: General	53	15	.753	20	11	.620
Psychiatry: Child & Adolescent	8	5	*	3	3	*
Psychiatry: Geriatric	1	1	*	1	1	*
Pulmonary Medicine	38	15	.648	75	33	.558
Pulmonary Medicine: Critical Care	3	2	*	25	6	.654
Pulmonary Med: Gen & Crit Care	2	2	*	36	15	.648
Radiation Oncology	15	6	.710	10	6	.744
Radiology: Diagnostic-Inv	10	4	.776	86	17	.695
Radiology: Diagnostic-Noninv	35	5	.731	172	27	.650
Radiology: Nuclear Medicine	4	2	*	8	6	*
Rheumatology	66	23	.581	56	38	.555
Sleep Medicine	6	4	*	14	5	.494
Surgery: General	141	36	.614	284	88	.528
Surgery: Bariatric	0	*	*	5	3	*
Surgery: Cardiovascular	17	9	.822	72	18	.615
Surgery: Colon and Rectal	3	2	*	27	11	.555
Surgery: Neurological	21	10	.755	77	22	.639
Surgery: Oncology	4	3	*	6	4	*
Surgery: Oral	2	1	*	10	5	.374
Surgery: Pediatric	5	3	*	14	5	.557
Surgery: Plastic & Reconstruction	23	10	.538	31	17	.460
Surgery: Plastic & Recon-Hand	*	*	*	1	1	*
Surgery: Thoracic (primary)	6	4	*	14	6	.672
Surgery: Transplant	10	3	.507	0	*	*
Surgery: Trauma	8	5	*	4	2	*
Surgery: Trauma-Burn	1	1	*	*	*	*
Surgery: Vascular (primary)	14	5	.636	42	22	.508
Urgent Care	74	11	.450	141	24	.437
Urology	45	16	.568	185	49	.552
Urology: Pediatric	4	1	*	3	1	*

Table 32: Physician Compensation to Collections Ratio (TC/NPP Excluded) by On-call Duties

	Physician had on-call duties			Physician did not have on-call duties		
	Phys	Med Pracs	Median	Phys	Med Pracs	Median
Allergy/Immunology	40	20	.428	18	13	.488
Anesthesiology	1,884	104	.742	69	26	.339
Anesthesiology: Pain Management	42	16	.641	17	5	.938
Anesthesiology: Pediatric	21	3	.856	1	1	*
Cardiology: Electrophysiology	49	22	.583	3	3	*
Cardiology: Invasive	105	34	.657	10	8	.546
Cardiology: Inv-Intvl	152	42	.659	19	5	.613
Cardiology: Noninvasive	85	31	.664	26	15	.595
Critical Care: Intensivist	5	2	*	2	1	*
Dentistry	3	1	*	6	2	*
Dermatology	85	38	.498	39	18	.508
Dermatology: Mohs Surgery	5	5	*	2	2	*
Emergency Medicine	21	2	*	155	17	.721
Endocrinology/Metabolism	74	44	.587	19	9	.557
Family Practice (w/ OB)	268	52	.493	24	8	.499
Family Practice (w/o OB)	1,476	221	.501	477	71	.468
FP: Amb Only (no inpatient work)	30	5	.430	7	3	*
Family Practice: Sports Med	8	5	*	10	6	.510
Family Practice: Urgent Care	21	7	.505	38	7	.356
Gastroenterology	284	80	.563	32	16	.481
Gastroenterology: Hepatology	6	4	*	0	*	*
Genetics	0	*	*	0	*	*
Geriatrics	19	7	.686	4	2	*
Hematology/Oncology	90	32	.638	11	7	.636
Hematology/Oncology: Onc (only)	5	4	*	0	*	*
Hospice/Palliative Care	0	*	*	*	*	*
Hospitalist: Family Practice	3	2	*	2	1	*
Hospitalist: Internal Medicine	145	44	.814	64	16	.890
Hospitalist: IM-Pediatrics	2	1	*	0	*	*
Hospitalist: Pediatrics	2	2	*	0	*	*
Infectious Disease	29	15	.656	7	4	*
Internal Medicine: General	1,167	171	.530	282	47	.516
IM: Amb Only (no inpatient work)	10	4	.584	1	1	*
Internal Med: Pediatrics	40	15	.495	0	*	*
Nephrology	53	25	.676	8	5	*
Neurology	167	63	.581	19	11	.533
Obstetrics/Gynecology: General	466	105	.490	33	11	.515
OB/GYN: Gynecology (only)	33	23	.446	13	8	.483
OB/GYN: Gyn Oncology	6	4	*	0	*	*
OB/GYN: Maternal & Fetal Med	7	5	*	0	*	*
OB/GYN: Repro Endocrinology	1	1	*	0	*	*
OB/GYN: Urogynecology	1	1	*	*	*	*
Occupational Medicine	23	8	.441	18	10	.467
Ophthalmology	109	42	.472	28	10	.433
Ophthalmology: Pediatric	5	4	*	4	1	*
Ophthalmology: Retina	6	6	*	2	2	*
Orthopedic (Nonsurgical)	2	2	*	15	11	.500
Orthopedic Surgery: General	252	79	.565	29	18	.597
Orthopedic Surgery: Foot & Ankle	15	13	.646	1	1	*
Orthopedic Surgery: Hand	47	24	.580	5	3	*
Orthopedic Surgery: Hip & Joint	30	18	.589	5	4	*
Orthopedic Surgery: Pediatric	5	3	*	0	*	*
Orthopedic Surgery: Spine	32	20	.501	3	3	*
Orthopedic Surgery: Trauma	11	7	.687	0	*	*
Orthopedic Surgery: Sports Med	43	25	.577	6	5	*

Table 32: Physician Compensation to Collections Ratio (TC/NPP Excluded) by On-call Duties (continued)

	Physician had on-call duties			Physician did not have on-call duties		
	Phys	Med Pracs	Median	Phys	Med Pracs	Median
Otorhinolaryngology	149	58	.505	18	10	.458
Pathology: Anatomic and Clinical	12	5	.723	17	2	*
Pathology: Anatomic	0	*	*	0	*	*
Pathology: Clinical	9	2	*	6	2	*
Pediatrics: General	793	133	.441	214	30	.438
Pediatrics: Adolescent Medicine	6	2	*	10	3	.341
Pediatrics: Allergy/Immunology	2	1	*	0	*	*
Pediatrics: Cardiology	3	2	*	1	1	*
Pediatrics: Child Development	1	1	*	0	*	*
Pediatrics: Critical Care/Intensivist	5	3	*	0	*	*
Pediatrics: Emergency Medicine	11	1	*	3	1	*
Pediatrics: Endocrinology	8	8	*	1	1	*
Pediatrics: Gastroenterology	2	2	*	1	1	*
Pediatrics: Genetics	1	1	*	0	*	*
Pediatrics: Hematology/Oncology	8	5	*	1	1	*
Pediatrics: Infectious Disease	0	*	*	1	1	*
Pediatrics: Neonatal Medicine	13	3	.567	9	3	*
Pediatrics: Nephrology	0	*	*	1	1	*
Pediatrics: Neurology	9	7	*	7	3	*
Pediatrics: Pulmonology	1	1	*	1	1	*
Pediatrics: Rheumatology	0	*	*	2	1	*
Physiatry (Phys Med & Rehab)	46	19	.537	26	16	.489
Podiatry: General	38	24	.481	21	15	.454
Podiatry: Surg-Foot & Ankle	11	7	.564	11	5	.404
Podiatry: Surg-Forefoot Only	0	*	*	0	*	*
Psychiatry: General	33	18	.748	22	6	.750
Psychiatry: Child & Adolescent	7	5	*	1	1	*
Psychiatry: Geriatric	2	2	*	0	*	*
Pulmonary Medicine	65	33	.558	18	8	.588
Pulmonary Medicine: Critical Care	16	7	.671	0	*	*
Pulmonary Med: Gen & Crit Care	35	16	.651	2	1	*
Radiation Oncology	12	7	.717	7	3	*
Radiology: Diagnostic-Inv	84	17	.704	5	2	*
Radiology: Diagnostic-Noninv	137	19	.647	31	15	.486
Radiology: Nuclear Medicine	7	5	*	3	2	*
Rheumatology	74	36	.575	26	16	.550
Sleep Medicine	14	6	.484	5	2	*
Surgery: General	331	104	.550	29	17	.462
Surgery: Bariatric	3	2	*	0	*	*
Surgery: Cardiovascular	72	20	.643	2	2	*
Surgery: Colon and Rectal	25	10	.555	2	2	*
Surgery: Neurological	80	26	.657	10	5	.668
Surgery: Oncology	7	5	*	0	*	*
Surgery: Oral	10	5	.374	0	*	*
Surgery: Pediatric	17	7	.606	0	*	*
Surgery: Plastic & Reconstruction	31	18	.531	7	2	*
Surgery: Plastic & Recon-Hand	1	1	*	*	*	*
Surgery: Thoracic (primary)	17	9	.689	2	1	*
Surgery: Transplant	10	3	.507	*	*	*
Surgery: Trauma	7	5	*	0	*	*
Surgery: Trauma-Burn	1	1	*	*	*	*
Surgery: Vascular (primary)	42	21	.531	4	4	*
Urgent Care	73	15	.437	119	21	.439
Urology	182	49	.561	20	13	.516
Urology: Pediatric	7	2	*	0	*	*

Table 33: Physician Gross Charges (TC/NPP Excluded)

	Phys	Med Pracs	Mean	Std. Dev.	25th %tile	Median	75th %tile	90th %tile
Allergy/Immunology	91	52	$870,831	$414,544	$582,018	$794,613	$1,012,026	$1,297,815
Anesthesiology	2,469	123	$1,319,181	$595,867	$880,504	$1,186,719	$1,754,134	$2,068,000
Anesthesiology: Pain Management	80	32	$2,020,340	$866,572	$1,490,877	$2,036,273	$2,466,616	$3,125,148
Anesthesiology: Pediatric	35	4	$763,159	$180,950	$715,918	$776,453	$848,647	$973,488
Cardiology: Electrophysiology	71	31	$2,054,827	$871,640	$1,272,334	$1,817,219	$2,958,966	$3,328,344
Cardiology: Invasive	164	51	$1,609,651	$663,055	$1,118,045	$1,497,479	$1,891,695	$2,520,093
Cardiology: Inv-Intvl	220	62	$2,171,036	$1,108,331	$1,414,134	$1,881,722	$2,680,268	$3,856,389
Cardiology: Noninvasive	184	50	$1,411,473	$632,826	$928,228	$1,306,322	$1,843,452	$2,344,156
Critical Care: Intensivist	26	8	$747,211	$338,498	$454,642	$811,106	$992,408	$1,221,795
Dentistry	12	4	$373,019	$137,372	$286,302	$305,070	$534,410	$574,236
Dermatology	182	79	$1,354,812	$655,915	$884,588	$1,207,456	$1,599,293	$2,294,104
Dermatology: Mohs Surgery	15	12	$3,277,487	$952,841	$2,686,745	$3,161,998	$4,354,822	$4,516,273
Emergency Medicine	324	25	$867,382	$319,791	$648,582	$854,009	$1,106,272	$1,290,968
Endocrinology/Metabolism	162	78	$594,076	$239,596	$438,779	$546,980	$707,529	$873,060
Family Practice (w/ OB)	417	77	$613,148	$230,895	$463,182	$585,043	$715,463	$860,664
Family Practice (w/o OB)	3,234	331	$574,847	$225,788	$431,798	$548,351	$680,798	$837,767
FP: Amb Only (no inpatient work)	79	11	$497,102	$205,596	$347,871	$452,106	$606,986	$865,252
Family Practice: Sports Med	25	17	$752,878	$403,584	$497,942	$654,183	$873,480	$1,460,645
Family Practice: Urgent Care	60	13	$642,786	$223,565	$516,845	$615,581	$749,542	$932,898
Gastroenterology	420	116	$1,686,101	$740,685	$1,147,506	$1,597,219	$2,084,385	$2,761,154
Gastroenterology: Hepatology	6	4	*	*	*	*	*	*
Genetics	3	2	*	*	*	*	*	*
Geriatrics	36	18	$388,435	$184,732	$266,466	$396,062	$506,626	$636,939
Hematology/Oncology	230	65	$1,244,321	$1,325,117	$457,378	$856,000	$1,410,384	$2,279,664
Hematology/Oncology: Onc (only)	23	16	$1,176,478	$1,279,265	$457,820	$726,629	$1,418,171	$3,718,229
Hospice/Palliative Care	4	4	*	*	*	*	*	*
Hospitalist: Family Practice	18	7	$356,301	$120,384	$296,826	$329,103	$380,700	$522,929
Hospitalist: Internal Medicine	753	95	$413,023	$151,933	$314,357	$392,982	$498,091	$599,410
Hospitalist: IM-Pediatrics	3	2	*	*	*	*	*	*
Hospitalist: Pediatrics	37	10	$228,562	$132,993	$127,428	$201,762	$305,733	$405,357
Infectious Disease	114	32	$533,873	$176,048	$385,933	$527,317	$653,291	$768,897
Internal Medicine: General	2,250	247	$560,656	$246,830	$407,088	$532,161	$667,155	$831,070
IM: Amb Only (no inpatient work)	14	7	$624,151	$729,668	$330,577	$394,835	$657,030	$1,961,159
Internal Med: Pediatrics	74	27	$567,273	$258,987	$380,952	$503,334	$698,794	$864,855
Nephrology	126	45	$857,471	$425,697	$523,667	$812,756	$1,112,640	$1,473,547
Neurology	312	100	$776,410	$412,282	$498,041	$689,827	$949,801	$1,236,544
Obstetrics/Gynecology: General	758	144	$1,053,497	$421,712	$758,192	$989,024	$1,264,363	$1,621,541
OB/GYN: Gynecology (only)	113	41	$884,330	$334,913	$632,530	$872,183	$1,071,425	$1,323,528
OB/GYN: Gyn Oncology	22	14	$1,319,356	$607,359	$738,527	$1,353,922	$1,790,445	$2,291,821
OB/GYN: Maternal & Fetal Med	27	14	$1,920,036	$1,054,479	$1,156,458	$1,937,236	$2,642,493	$3,411,733
OB/GYN: Repro Endocrinology	5	4	*	*	*	*	*	*
OB/GYN: Urogynecology	3	2	*	*	*	*	*	*
Occupational Medicine	73	30	$560,570	$235,096	$418,870	$564,431	$707,269	$773,498
Ophthalmology	213	72	$1,524,781	$766,800	$940,997	$1,317,143	$2,032,067	$2,621,713
Ophthalmology: Pediatric	14	9	$1,566,202	$650,408	$915,636	$1,780,183	$2,079,599	$2,299,994
Ophthalmology: Retina	13	12	$2,756,399	$1,099,514	$1,860,566	$2,603,694	$3,655,332	$4,467,618
Orthopedic (Nonsurgical)	25	20	$653,918	$311,926	$438,042	$624,798	$788,675	$1,019,813
Orthopedic Surgery: General	414	113	$1,817,782	$848,286	$1,202,632	$1,684,883	$2,372,217	$2,912,128
Orthopedic Surgery: Foot & Ankle	17	14	$1,863,308	$632,851	$1,208,225	$1,711,373	$2,468,423	$2,846,242
Orthopedic Surgery: Hand	52	32	$1,916,306	$884,052	$1,222,091	$1,680,896	$2,440,175	$3,393,545
Orthopedic Surgery: Hip & Joint	37	21	$2,405,204	$894,245	$1,721,287	$2,096,217	$3,277,680	$3,617,862
Orthopedic Surgery: Pediatric	12	8	$2,074,615	$843,351	$1,292,648	$2,044,122	$2,973,188	$3,256,718
Orthopedic Surgery: Spine	41	28	$3,210,847	$1,786,316	$1,809,178	$2,651,580	$4,143,566	$5,886,269
Orthopedic Surgery: Trauma	14	10	$2,024,780	$904,171	$1,254,826	$2,001,206	$2,791,619	$3,391,824
Orthopedic Surgery: Sports Med	55	32	$2,260,002	$1,076,172	$1,341,050	$2,290,886	$3,010,849	$3,866,802

Table 33: Physician Gross Charges (TC/NPP Excluded) (continued)

	Phys	Med Pracs	Mean	Std. Dev.	25th %tile	Median	75th %tile	90th %tile
Otorhinolaryngology	237	89	$1,532,776	$672,914	$1,012,951	$1,398,708	$1,979,390	$2,431,431
Pathology: Anatomic and Clinical	71	13	$1,789,319	$1,855,987	$752,537	$1,152,854	$1,879,726	$4,817,013
Pathology: Anatomic	22	5	$1,299,253	$641,160	$899,524	$1,021,274	$1,540,712	$2,496,151
Pathology: Clinical	25	7	$1,144,741	$561,970	$687,771	$890,138	$1,776,651	$1,993,190
Pediatrics: General	1,631	195	$665,915	$254,889	$487,082	$628,585	$802,991	$992,820
Pediatrics: Adolescent Medicine	27	7	$587,164	$337,350	$242,641	$635,389	$816,356	$1,043,171
Pediatrics: Allergy/Immunology	3	2	*	*	*	*	*	*
Pediatrics: Cardiology	21	11	$1,092,981	$416,522	$755,575	$1,252,500	$1,414,692	$1,575,086
Pediatrics: Child Development	10	6	$268,258	$116,954	$159,720	$311,945	$344,638	$419,118
Pediatrics: Critical Care/Intensivist	46	13	$403,876	$203,481	$230,520	$352,495	$569,364	$620,214
Pediatrics: Emergency Medicine	19	4	$461,496	$209,186	$330,426	$389,296	$592,959	$790,612
Pediatrics: Endocrinology	17	13	$459,306	$203,030	$271,005	$503,017	$638,327	$734,157
Pediatrics: Gastroenterology	19	9	$706,112	$379,988	$503,523	$584,907	$739,800	$1,400,065
Pediatrics: Genetics	4	3	*	*	*	*	*	*
Pediatrics: Hematology/Oncology	31	13	$501,916	$194,136	$379,606	$460,569	$684,151	$823,416
Pediatrics: Infectious Disease	4	4	*	*	*	*	*	*
Pediatrics: Neonatal Medicine	40	10	$895,091	$342,642	$635,367	$738,610	$1,199,472	$1,417,382
Pediatrics: Nephrology	4	4	*	*	*	*	*	*
Pediatrics: Neurology	37	20	$589,387	$247,688	$404,292	$537,934	$724,278	$981,291
Pediatrics: Pulmonology	12	8	$623,029	$452,520	$331,342	$456,941	$854,472	$1,531,409
Pediatrics: Rheumatology	3	2	*	*	*	*	*	*
Physiatry (Phys Med & Rehab)	114	48	$874,495	$610,482	$559,327	$703,393	$948,120	$1,533,187
Podiatry: General	95	54	$774,017	$324,750	$534,828	$706,236	$953,712	$1,174,806
Podiatry: Surg-Foot & Ankle	41	17	$927,693	$376,353	$709,089	$919,435	$1,039,647	$1,365,962
Podiatry: Surg-Forefoot Only	2	1	*	*	*	*	*	*
Psychiatry: General	191	47	$370,384	$158,528	$276,770	$353,499	$470,778	$575,865
Psychiatry: Child & Adolescent	30	17	$301,813	$174,309	$156,917	$272,435	$448,288	$604,373
Psychiatry: Geriatric	7	3	*	*	*	*	*	*
Pulmonary Medicine	144	59	$899,061	$404,377	$637,932	$820,336	$1,114,759	$1,445,749
Pulmonary Medicine: Critical Care	39	9	$927,256	$354,152	$661,944	$854,825	$1,248,286	$1,446,163
Pulmonary Med: Gen & Crit Care	57	20	$955,813	$277,969	$760,203	$862,217	$1,195,937	$1,355,093
Radiation Oncology	59	20	$1,792,549	$1,031,522	$867,548	$1,468,000	$2,516,655	$3,260,475
Radiology: Diagnostic-Inv	122	29	$1,978,000	$872,740	$1,428,833	$1,757,862	$2,410,159	$3,082,519
Radiology: Diagnostic-Noninv	314	40	$1,781,908	$1,036,002	$1,080,591	$1,465,268	$2,108,541	$3,251,631
Radiology: Nuclear Medicine	20	11	$1,209,757	$553,034	$887,218	$1,020,599	$1,660,675	$2,127,637
Rheumatology	164	79	$733,595	$479,261	$468,012	$602,759	$805,908	$1,283,149
Sleep Medicine	25	11	$1,173,849	$598,432	$729,652	$1,088,497	$1,414,442	$2,186,606
Surgery: General	561	155	$1,250,791	$534,560	$853,804	$1,155,305	$1,578,907	$2,002,257
Surgery: Bariatric	12	7	$1,130,629	$409,272	$812,022	$1,173,307	$1,255,432	$1,773,269
Surgery: Cardiovascular	140	41	$1,886,841	$931,444	$1,119,926	$1,762,710	$2,513,080	$3,298,646
Surgery: Colon and Rectal	35	15	$1,625,134	$1,025,639	$972,200	$1,404,614	$1,779,474	$2,724,579
Surgery: Neurological	142	46	$2,728,420	$1,711,717	$1,476,507	$2,502,722	$3,383,139	$4,858,947
Surgery: Oncology	11	7	$1,574,128	$474,993	$1,215,541	$1,621,419	$1,844,778	$2,177,899
Surgery: Oral	13	7	$1,753,683	$939,753	$977,087	$1,570,685	$2,355,522	$3,453,295
Surgery: Pediatric	35	16	$1,482,178	$941,959	$852,665	$1,149,705	$1,620,420	$3,114,742
Surgery: Plastic & Reconstruction	65	33	$1,463,829	$643,525	$1,042,219	$1,295,851	$1,742,600	$2,481,991
Surgery: Plastic & Recon-Hand	6	3	*	*	*	*	*	*
Surgery: Thoracic (primary)	30	14	$1,159,373	$597,893	$843,620	$936,314	$1,323,062	$2,037,773
Surgery: Transplant	19	6	$1,581,263	$652,710	$1,034,613	$1,642,979	$1,942,700	$2,590,916
Surgery: Trauma	43	11	$1,077,613	$525,377	$554,671	$1,062,574	$1,412,417	$1,813,596
Surgery: Trauma-Burn	1	1	*	*	*	*	*	*
Surgery: Vascular (primary)	73	35	$1,612,427	$856,585	$924,075	$1,464,866	$1,895,198	$2,875,313
Urgent Care	274	47	$672,162	$280,758	$480,997	$636,552	$807,346	$1,013,060
Urology	282	86	$1,460,202	$640,260	$963,721	$1,397,303	$1,873,927	$2,379,877
Urology: Pediatric	7	2	*	*	*	*	*	*

Table 34: Physician Gross Charges (TC/NPP Excluded) by Group Type

	Single Specialty			Multispecialty		
	Phys	**Med Pracs**	**Median**	**Phys**	**Med Pracs**	**Median**
Allergy/Immunology	10	4	$697,500	81	48	$836,350
Anesthesiology	2,089	89	$1,246,215	380	34	$876,356
Anesthesiology: Pain Management	28	9	$2,036,273	52	23	$2,161,758
Anesthesiology: Pediatric	23	2	*	12	2	*
Cardiology: Electrophysiology	38	14	$2,149,941	33	17	$1,468,067
Cardiology: Invasive	51	12	$1,472,460	113	39	$1,513,468
Cardiology: Inv-Intvl	108	21	$1,896,879	112	41	$1,847,951
Cardiology: Noninvasive	61	17	$1,309,633	123	33	$1,296,132
Critical Care: Intensivist	3	1	*	23	7	$872,126
Dentistry	0	*	*	12	4	$305,070
Dermatology	14	5	$959,934	168	74	$1,211,240
Dermatology: Mohs Surgery	1	1	*	14	11	$3,119,895
Emergency Medicine	165	8	$860,143	159	17	$824,672
Endocrinology/Metabolism	9	6	*	153	72	$552,058
Family Practice (w/ OB)	39	11	$521,780	378	66	$587,511
Family Practice (w/o OB)	391	129	$517,218	2,843	202	$552,757
FP: Amb Only (no inpatient work)	7	3	*	72	8	$440,558
Family Practice: Sports Med	7	4	*	18	13	$652,247
Family Practice: Urgent Care	23	1	*	37	12	$598,552
Gastroenterology	126	17	$1,560,600	294	99	$1,623,321
Gastroenterology: Hepatology	3	3	*	3	1	*
Genetics	*	*	*	3	2	*
Geriatrics	6	2	*	30	16	$409,411
Hematology/Oncology	44	6	$1,449,659	186	59	$745,105
Hematology/Oncology: Onc (only)	2	2	*	21	14	$677,863
Hospice/Palliative Care	2	2	*	2	2	*
Hospitalist: Family Practice	2	2	*	16	5	$329,103
Hospitalist: Internal Medicine	113	14	$453,133	640	81	$384,238
Hospitalist: IM-Pediatrics	*	*	*	3	2	*
Hospitalist: Pediatrics	9	1	*	28	9	$178,611
Infectious Disease	14	6	$567,525	100	26	$523,151
Internal Medicine: General	151	34	$437,223	2,099	213	$537,302
IM: Amb Only (no inpatient work)	0	*	*	14	7	$394,835
Internal Med: Pediatrics	0	*	*	74	27	$503,334
Nephrology	13	2	*	113	43	$843,858
Neurology	43	13	$585,275	269	87	$717,367
Obstetrics/Gynecology: General	101	27	$960,000	657	117	$996,425
OB/GYN: Gynecology (only)	2	2	*	111	39	$872,183
OB/GYN: Gyn Oncology	4	2	*	18	12	$1,423,461
OB/GYN: Maternal & Fetal Med	9	4	*	18	10	$1,820,241
OB/GYN: Repro Endocrinology	0	*	*	5	4	*
OB/GYN: Urogynecology	*	*	*	3	2	*
Occupational Medicine	2	1	*	71	29	$573,326
Ophthalmology	36	12	$1,523,878	177	60	$1,312,282
Ophthalmology: Pediatric	2	2	*	12	7	$1,780,183
Ophthalmology: Retina	3	3	*	10	9	$2,680,023
Orthopedic (Nonsurgical)	12	10	$636,348	13	10	$609,257
Orthopedic Surgery: General	93	26	$1,737,044	321	87	$1,627,543
Orthopedic Surgery: Foot & Ankle	11	9	$1,690,913	6	5	*
Orthopedic Surgery: Hand	25	15	$2,085,712	27	17	$1,477,760
Orthopedic Surgery: Hip & Joint	23	14	$2,106,421	14	7	$2,003,532
Orthopedic Surgery: Pediatric	5	2	*	7	6	*
Orthopedic Surgery: Spine	22	15	$2,630,576	19	13	$2,692,764
Orthopedic Surgery: Trauma	9	6	*	5	4	*
Orthopedic Surgery: Sports Med	33	19	$2,409,975	22	13	$1,492,054

Table 34: Physician Gross Charges (TC/NPP Excluded) by Group Type (continued)

	Single Specialty			Multispecialty		
	Phys	Med Pracs	Median	Phys	Med Pracs	Median
Otorhinolaryngology	40	9	$1,524,595	197	80	$1,347,279
Pathology: Anatomic and Clinical	31	2	*	40	11	$1,080,598
Pathology: Anatomic	*	*	*	22	5	$1,021,274
Pathology: Clinical	1	1	*	24	6	$861,481
Pediatrics: General	401	40	$689,643	1,230	155	$611,694
Pediatrics: Adolescent Medicine	10	2	*	17	5	$289,496
Pediatrics: Allergy/Immunology	2	1	*	1	1	*
Pediatrics: Cardiology	4	2	*	17	9	$1,277,750
Pediatrics: Child Development	*	*	*	10	6	$311,945
Pediatrics: Critical Care/Intensivist	7	1	*	39	12	$423,000
Pediatrics: Emergency Medicine	0	*	*	19	4	$389,296
Pediatrics: Endocrinology	3	2	*	14	11	$439,815
Pediatrics: Gastroenterology	0	*	*	19	9	$584,907
Pediatrics: Genetics	0	*	*	4	3	*
Pediatrics: Hematology/Oncology	6	2	*	25	11	$432,414
Pediatrics: Infectious Disease	*	*	*	4	4	*
Pediatrics: Neonatal Medicine	20	4	$704,756	20	6	$780,387
Pediatrics: Nephrology	*	*	*	4	4	*
Pediatrics: Neurology	4	2	*	33	18	$584,717
Pediatrics: Pulmonology	5	3	*	7	5	*
Pediatrics: Rheumatology	*	*	*	3	2	*
Physiatry (Phys Med & Rehab)	33	11	$684,668	81	37	$708,223
Podiatry: General	3	3	*	92	51	$706,971
Podiatry: Surg-Foot & Ankle	1	1	*	40	16	$916,065
Podiatry: Surg-Forefoot Only	0	*	*	2	1	*
Psychiatry: General	15	2	*	176	45	$351,045
Psychiatry: Child & Adolescent	2	1	*	28	16	$268,741
Psychiatry: Geriatric	4	1	*	3	2	*
Pulmonary Medicine	4	2	*	140	57	$829,302
Pulmonary Medicine: Critical Care	4	2	*	35	7	$861,365
Pulmonary Med: Gen & Crit Care	9	3	*	48	17	$852,916
Radiation Oncology	15	4	$2,150,000	44	16	$1,202,744
Radiology: Diagnostic-Inv	74	12	$1,639,375	48	17	$2,083,830
Radiology: Diagnostic-Noninv	128	12	$1,315,359	186	28	$1,686,079
Radiology: Nuclear Medicine	12	6	$922,631	8	5	*
Rheumatology	13	6	$482,220	151	73	$609,174
Sleep Medicine	4	1	*	21	10	$1,144,253
Surgery: General	73	20	$1,101,000	488	135	$1,160,246
Surgery: Bariatric	2	1	*	10	6	$1,144,667
Surgery: Cardiovascular	60	14	$2,130,179	80	27	$1,558,426
Surgery: Colon and Rectal	*	*	*	35	15	$1,404,614
Surgery: Neurological	40	9	$2,838,815	102	37	$2,406,404
Surgery: Oncology	0	*	*	11	7	$1,621,419
Surgery: Oral	6	2	*	7	5	*
Surgery: Pediatric	18	5	$1,456,719	17	11	$984,972
Surgery: Plastic & Reconstruction	5	2	*	60	31	$1,325,976
Surgery: Plastic & Recon-Hand	0	*	*	6	3	*
Surgery: Thoracic (primary)	12	5	$849,506	18	9	$976,811
Surgery: Transplant	7	1	*	12	5	$1,401,768
Surgery: Trauma	7	2	*	36	9	$1,121,506
Surgery: Trauma-Burn	*	*	*	1	1	*
Surgery: Vascular (primary)	5	4	*	68	31	$1,473,902
Urgent Care	16	4	$551,986	258	43	$641,072
Urology	99	12	$1,143,482	183	74	$1,494,831
Urology: Pediatric	3	1	*	4	1	*

Table 35A: Physician Gross Charges (TC/NPP Excluded) by Size of Multispecialty Practice (50 or fewer FTE Physicians)

	10 FTE or fewer		11 to 25 FTE		26 to 50 FTE	
	Phys	Median	Phys	Median	Phys	Median
Allergy/Immunology	5	*	2	*	7	*
Anesthesiology	12	$1,486,737	30	$1,552,890	5	*
Anesthesiology: Pain Management	1	*	5	*	5	*
Anesthesiology: Pediatric	*	*	*	*	11	*
Cardiology: Electrophysiology	*	*	5	*	1	*
Cardiology: Invasive	0	*	10	$1,308,670	11	$1,243,279
Cardiology: Inv-Intvl	*	*	19	$2,582,234	7	*
Cardiology: Noninvasive	1	*	4	*	33	$1,773,824
Critical Care: Intensivist	4	*	*	*	4	*
Dentistry	0	*	5	*	*	*
Dermatology	5	*	0	*	16	$1,118,811
Dermatology: Mohs Surgery	*	*	1	*	1	*
Emergency Medicine	0	*	1	*	43	$972,529
Endocrinology/Metabolism	2	*	6	*	18	$579,580
Family Practice (w/ OB)	32	$591,211	72	$580,974	42	$565,013
Family Practice (w/o OB)	100	$447,720	216	$557,293	336	$519,907
FP: Amb Only (no inpatient work)	4	*	19	*	6	*
Family Practice: Sports Med	0	*	2	*	7	*
Family Practice: Urgent Care	1	*	2	*	17	$603,290
Gastroenterology	5	*	15	$1,875,560	40	$1,410,270
Geriatrics	*	*	1	*	0	*
Hematology/Oncology	4	*	10	$1,269,076	11	$1,182,176
Hematology/Oncology: Onc (only)	1	*	3	*	4	*
Hospice/Palliative Care	1	*	*	*	*	*
Hospitalist: Family Practice	0	*	1	*	0	*
Hospitalist: Internal Medicine	10	$322,860	43	$413,675	57	$402,476
Hospitalist: IM-Pediatrics	*	*	*	*	0	*
Hospitalist: Pediatrics	*	*	0	*	3	*
Infectious Disease	0	*	0	*	2	*
Internal Medicine: General	60	$495,364	180	$490,952	275	$565,231
IM: Amb Only (no inpatient work)	0	*	5	*	5	*
Internal Med: Pediatrics	14	$375,856	10	$501,602	10	*
Nephrology	0	*	14	$878,878	12	$1,186,159
Neurology	3	*	15	$824,402	40	$771,421
Obstetrics/Gynecology: General	7	*	52	$713,186	80	$897,986
OB/GYN: Gynecology (only)	1	*	4	*	4	*
OB/GYN: Gyn Oncology	1	*	1	*	0	*
OB/GYN: Maternal & Fetal Med	0	*	1	*	0	*
OB/GYN: Repro Endocrinology	0	*	*	*	*	*
Occupational Medicine	3	*	2	*	8	*
Ophthalmology	3	*	1	*	11	$1,239,145
Ophthalmology: Pediatric	0	*	*	*	2	*
Ophthalmology: Retina	1	*	*	*	0	*
Orthopedic (Nonsurgical)	*	*	*	*	1	*
Orthopedic Surgery: General	8	*	26	$1,577,366	45	$2,001,885
Orthopedic Surgery: Foot & Ankle	0	*	2	*	0	*
Orthopedic Surgery: Hand	0	*	4	*	1	*
Orthopedic Surgery: Hip & Joint	0	*	4	*	1	*
Orthopedic Surgery: Pediatric	*	*	1	*	*	*
Orthopedic Surgery: Spine	0	*	2	*	2	*
Orthopedic Surgery: Trauma	*	*	2	*	*	*
Orthopedic Surgery: Sports Med	0	*	6	*	2	*

Table 35A: Physician Gross Charges (TC/NPP Excluded) by Size of Multispecialty Practice (50 or fewer FTE Physicians) (continued)

	10 FTE or fewer		11 to 25 FTE		26 to 50 FTE	
	Phys	Median	Phys	Median	Phys	Median
Otorhinolaryngology	7	*	3	*	28	$1,277,251
Pathology: Anatomic and Clinical	4	*	5	*	*	*
Pathology: Clinical	*	*	0	*	*	*
Pediatrics: General	51	$572,702	79	$525,419	125	$611,128
Pediatrics: Adolescent Medicine	2	*	1	*	0	*
Pediatrics: Cardiology	*	*	*	*	0	*
Pediatrics: Child Development	2	*	0	*	2	*
Pediatrics: Critical Care/Intensivist	*	*	0	*	15	$310,507
Pediatrics: Emergency Medicine	0	*	0	*	17	*
Pediatrics: Endocrinology	1	*	0	*	2	*
Pediatrics: Gastroenterology	*	*	0	*	2	*
Pediatrics: Genetics	0	*	*	*	0	*
Pediatrics: Hematology/Oncology	0	*	4	*	8	*
Pediatrics: Infectious Disease	0	*	*	*	*	*
Pediatrics: Neonatal Medicine	*	*	*	*	7	*
Pediatrics: Nephrology	*	*	*	*	1	*
Pediatrics: Neurology	0	*	*	*	7	*
Pediatrics: Pulmonology	*	*	0	*	4	*
Pediatrics: Rheumatology	0	*	*	*	*	*
Physiatry (Phys Med & Rehab)	1	*	8	*	3	*
Podiatry: General	2	*	5	*	13	$636,965
Podiatry: Surg-Foot & Ankle	0	*	2	*	1	*
Podiatry: Surg-Forefoot Only	*	*	0	*	*	*
Psychiatry: General	4	*	6	*	5	*
Psychiatry: Child & Adolescent	1	*	*	*	2	*
Pulmonary Medicine	0	*	7	*	16	$927,352
Pulmonary Medicine: Critical Care	0	*	3	*	0	*
Pulmonary Med: Gen & Crit Care	7	*	4	*	8	*
Radiation Oncology	3	*	0	*	2	*
Radiology: Diagnostic-Inv	0	*	*	*	3	*
Radiology: Diagnostic-Noninv	1	*	1	*	2	*
Radiology: Nuclear Medicine	*	*	0	*	0	*
Rheumatology	2	*	5	*	11	$946,178
Sleep Medicine	0	*	0	*	1	*
Surgery: General	25	$840,314	37	$920,217	46	$1,000,548
Surgery: Bariatric	1	*	*	*	0	*
Surgery: Cardiovascular	3	*	7	*	14	*
Surgery: Colon and Rectal	4	*	5	*	1	*
Surgery: Neurological	9	*	21	$3,199,493	4	*
Surgery: Oncology	2	*	4	*	*	*
Surgery: Oral	*	*	*	*	1	*
Surgery: Pediatric	*	*	3	*	3	*
Surgery: Plastic & Reconstruction	1	*	0	*	3	*
Surgery: Plastic & Recon-Hand	*	*	*	*	1	*
Surgery: Thoracic (primary)	*	*	1	*	2	*
Surgery: Trauma	0	*	9	*	*	*
Surgery: Vascular (primary)	3	*	4	*	15	$1,482,938
Urgent Care	0	*	7	*	13	$446,342
Urology	8	*	5	*	16	$1,439,923
Urology: Pediatric	*	*	*	*	4	*

Table 35B: Physician Gross Charges (TC/NPP Excluded) by Size of Multispecialty Practice (51 or more FTE Physicians)

	51 to 75 FTE		76 to 150 FTE		151 FTE or more	
	Phys	Median	Phys	Median	Phys	Median
Allergy/Immunology	12	$749,974	14	$811,973	41	$783,126
Anesthesiology	111	$728,297	56	$887,236	166	$1,013,266
Anesthesiology: Pain Management	13	*	10	$2,307,843	18	$1,563,688
Anesthesiology: Pediatric	1	*	0	*	0	*
Cardiology: Electrophysiology	2	*	6	*	19	$1,425,902
Cardiology: Invasive	2	*	30	$1,371,823	60	$1,789,827
Cardiology: Inv-Intvl	11	$2,718,400	28	$1,797,922	47	$1,785,100
Cardiology: Noninvasive	0	*	20	$1,175,090	65	$1,177,931
Critical Care: Intensivist	0	*	2	*	13	$894,497
Dentistry	0	*	4	*	3	*
Dermatology	23	$1,188,638	47	$1,244,203	77	$1,212,121
Dermatology: Mohs Surgery	*	*	4	*	8	*
Emergency Medicine	0	*	31	$958,352	84	$765,496
Endocrinology/Metabolism	8	*	42	$549,084	77	$559,151
Family Practice (w/ OB)	29	$586,203	64	$528,867	139	$613,135
Family Practice (w/o OB)	345	$559,205	563	$517,116	1,283	$586,170
FP: Amb Only (no inpatient work)	0	*	1	*	42	*
Family Practice: Sports Med	1	*	3	*	5	*
Family Practice: Urgent Care	4	*	9	*	4	*
Gastroenterology	23	$1,820,091	89	$1,678,170	122	$1,650,958
Gastroenterology: Hepatology	*	*	3	*	0	*
Genetics	*	*	1	*	2	*
Geriatrics	3	*	11	$356,361	15	$488,437
Hematology/Oncology	16	$1,516,290	49	$983,480	96	$564,133
Hematology/Oncology: Onc (only)	8	*	5	*	0	*
Hospice/Palliative Care	*	*	*	*	1	*
Hospitalist: Family Practice	0	*	3	*	12	*
Hospitalist: Internal Medicine	81	$367,290	114	$383,348	335	$387,651
Hospitalist: IM-Pediatrics	*	*	3	*	*	*
Hospitalist: Pediatrics	0	*	9	*	16	$127,428
Infectious Disease	0	*	11	$464,816	87	$536,875
Internal Medicine: General	227	$562,562	521	$526,133	836	$540,128
IM: Amb Only (no inpatient work)	0	*	0	*	4	*
Internal Med: Pediatrics	0	*	19	$667,400	21	$448,264
Nephrology	9	*	37	$767,370	41	$808,609
Neurology	20	$761,172	66	$722,976	125	$664,423
Obstetrics/Gynecology: General	74	$1,025,315	149	$1,003,453	295	$1,051,405
OB/GYN: Gynecology (only)	9	*	34	$925,041	59	$872,183
OB/GYN: Gyn Oncology	*	*	3	*	13	$1,490,592
OB/GYN: Maternal & Fetal Med	0	*	4	*	13	$1,817,073
OB/GYN: Repro Endocrinology	*	*	*	*	5	*
OB/GYN: Urogynecology	*	*	0	*	3	*
Occupational Medicine	2	*	9	*	47	$615,850
Ophthalmology	26	$1,665,262	47	$1,196,840	89	$1,311,477
Ophthalmology: Pediatric	0	*	6	*	4	*
Ophthalmology: Retina	0	*	2	*	7	*
Orthopedic (Nonsurgical)	2	*	4	*	6	*
Orthopedic Surgery: General	29	$1,496,939	54	$1,696,432	159	$1,528,798
Orthopedic Surgery: Foot & Ankle	*	*	1	*	3	*
Orthopedic Surgery: Hand	3	*	2	*	17	$1,264,167
Orthopedic Surgery: Hip & Joint	1	*	1	*	7	*
Orthopedic Surgery: Pediatric	0	*	1	*	5	*
Orthopedic Surgery: Spine	3	*	4	*	8	*
Orthopedic Surgery: Trauma	0	*	0	*	3	*
Orthopedic Surgery: Sports Med	1	*	2	*	11	$1,198,094

Table 35B: Physician Gross Charges (TC/NPP Excluded) by Size of Multispecialty Practice (51 or more FTE Physicians) (continued)

	51 to 75 FTE		76 to 150 FTE		151 FTE or more	
	Phys	Median	Phys	Median	Phys	Median
Otorhinolaryngology	18	$1,561,890	54	$1,326,574	87	$1,322,627
Pathology: Anatomic and Clinical	1	*	3	*	27	$1,103,380
Pathology: Anatomic	*	*	3	*	19	$1,119,388
Pathology: Clinical	*	*	18	$824,647	6	*
Pediatrics: General	166	$670,436	333	$581,021	476	$639,620
Pediatrics: Adolescent Medicine	1	*	*	*	13	*
Pediatrics: Allergy/Immunology	*	*	0	*	1	*
Pediatrics: Cardiology	0	*	5	*	12	$1,281,078
Pediatrics: Child Development	*	*	1	*	5	*
Pediatrics: Critical Care/Intensivist	7	*	6	*	11	$447,318
Pediatrics: Emergency Medicine	0	*	*	*	2	*
Pediatrics: Endocrinology	0	*	2	*	9	*
Pediatrics: Gastroenterology	1	*	3	*	13	$584,907
Pediatrics: Genetics	1	*	2	*	1	*
Pediatrics: Hematology/Oncology	0	*	4	*	9	*
Pediatrics: Infectious Disease	*	*	1	*	3	*
Pediatrics: Neonatal Medicine	0	*	3	*	10	$1,028,434
Pediatrics: Nephrology	0	*	*	*	3	*
Pediatrics: Neurology	4	*	4	*	18	$584,888
Pediatrics: Pulmonology	0	*	0	*	3	*
Pediatrics: Rheumatology	0	*	2	*	1	*
Physiatry (Phys Med & Rehab)	3	*	16	$701,015	50	$709,150
Podiatry: General	12	$593,085	21	$751,102	39	$791,087
Podiatry: Surg-Foot & Ankle	7	*	4	*	26	$941,512
Podiatry: Surg-Forefoot Only	*	*	*	*	2	*
Psychiatry: General	10	$346,442	46	$351,510	105	$347,074
Psychiatry: Child & Adolescent	1	*	5	*	19	$217,728
Psychiatry: Geriatric	*	*	2	*	1	*
Pulmonary Medicine	19	$1,143,029	37	$880,977	61	$747,282
Pulmonary Medicine: Critical Care	14	*	6	*	12	*
Pulmonary Med: Gen & Crit Care	3	*	10	$902,725	16	*
Radiation Oncology	2	*	4	*	33	$1,099,709
Radiology: Diagnostic-Inv	8	*	10	$1,899,444	27	$1,827,125
Radiology: Diagnostic-Noninv	7	*	38	$1,363,920	137	$1,688,824
Radiology: Nuclear Medicine	1	*	0	*	7	*
Rheumatology	15	$577,390	46	$646,209	72	$604,274
Sleep Medicine	3	*	11	$1,144,253	6	*
Surgery: General	39	$1,273,749	125	$1,256,151	216	$1,169,999
Surgery: Bariatric	*	*	4	*	5	*
Surgery: Cardiovascular	0	*	8	*	48	$1,184,332
Surgery: Colon and Rectal	0	*	11	$1,729,795	14	$1,555,378
Surgery: Neurological	2	*	19	$2,561,538	47	$1,774,602
Surgery: Oncology	*	*	0	*	5	*
Surgery: Oral	1	*	2	*	3	*
Surgery: Pediatric	0	*	2	*	9	*
Surgery: Plastic & Reconstruction	4	*	16	$1,389,138	36	$1,262,537
Surgery: Plastic & Recon-Hand	1	*	*	*	4	*
Surgery: Thoracic (primary)	1	*	3	*	11	$980,517
Surgery: Transplant	*	*	5	*	7	*
Surgery: Trauma	0	*	2	*	25	$1,209,390
Surgery: Trauma-Burn	*	*	*	*	1	*
Surgery: Vascular (primary)	3	*	11	$744,677	32	$1,505,290
Urgent Care	14	$554,381	64	$628,461	160	$660,903
Urology	19	$1,754,679	53	$1,436,415	82	$1,536,437
Urology: Pediatric	0	*	0	*	0	*

Table 36: Physician Gross Charges (TC/NPP Excluded) by Hospital Ownership

	Hospital Owned			Not Hospital Owned		
	Phys	Med Pracs	Median	Phys	Med Pracs	Median
Allergy/Immunology	20	14	$693,751	71	38	$829,304
Anesthesiology	143	15	$1,029,538	2,293	107	$1,200,532
Anesthesiology: Pain Management	17	8	$1,905,172	63	24	$2,036,273
Anesthesiology: Pediatric	11	1	*	24	3	$797,399
Cardiology: Electrophysiology	14	8	$2,149,941	57	23	$1,757,908
Cardiology: Invasive	45	10	$1,789,827	119	41	$1,400,000
Cardiology: Inv-Intvl	48	16	$1,654,518	172	46	$1,993,347
Cardiology: Noninvasive	70	16	$1,539,638	114	34	$1,175,090
Critical Care: Intensivist	11	2	*	15	6	$520,923
Dentistry	3	1	*	9	3	*
Dermatology	51	22	$1,181,025	131	57	$1,210,360
Dermatology: Mohs Surgery	3	1	*	12	11	$3,284,880
Emergency Medicine	129	13	$787,585	195	12	$892,588
Endocrinology/Metabolism	67	30	$552,058	95	48	$546,443
Family Practice (w/ OB)	205	38	$579,923	212	39	$592,149
Family Practice (w/o OB)	1,883	204	$522,905	1,351	127	$579,682
FP: Amb Only (no inpatient work)	34	5	$417,666	45	6	$478,054
Family Practice: Sports Med	7	6	*	18	11	$778,307
Family Practice: Urgent Care	25	6	$598,552	35	7	$638,571
Gastroenterology	92	32	$1,620,879	328	84	$1,580,455
Gastroenterology: Hepatology	3	1	*	3	3	*
Genetics	3	2	*	0	*	*
Geriatrics	25	12	$360,559	11	6	$488,437
Hematology/Oncology	57	13	$632,562	173	52	$1,086,161
Hematology/Oncology: Onc (only)	6	5	*	17	11	$841,420
Hospice/Palliative Care	3	3	*	1	1	*
Hospitalist: Family Practice	12	3	$360,115	6	4	*
Hospitalist: Internal Medicine	455	49	$384,148	298	46	$403,050
Hospitalist: IM-Pediatrics	1	1	*	2	1	*
Hospitalist: Pediatrics	27	8	$260,000	10	2	*
Infectious Disease	28	15	$497,380	86	17	$529,160
Internal Medicine: General	1,170	123	$498,747	1,080	124	$560,421
IM: Amb Only (no inpatient work)	12	5	$394,835	2	2	*
Internal Med: Pediatrics	32	11	$427,252	42	16	$579,025
Nephrology	30	13	$760,494	96	32	$841,594
Neurology	122	38	$672,932	190	62	$712,509
Obstetrics/Gynecology: General	298	60	$956,298	460	84	$1,004,881
OB/GYN: Gynecology (only)	60	14	$899,490	53	27	$838,746
OB/GYN: Gyn Oncology	12	9	$1,058,655	10	5	$1,797,899
OB/GYN: Maternal & Fetal Med	22	10	$1,820,241	5	4	*
OB/GYN: Repro Endocrinology	3	3	*	2	1	*
OB/GYN: Urogynecology	3	2	*	0	*	*
Occupational Medicine	18	11	$485,016	55	19	$614,648
Ophthalmology	41	15	$1,409,392	172	57	$1,267,258
Ophthalmology: Pediatric	4	3	*	10	6	$1,902,447
Ophthalmology: Retina	5	4	*	8	8	*
Orthopedic (Nonsurgical)	3	2	*	22	18	$617,027
Orthopedic Surgery: General	114	31	$1,321,262	300	82	$1,744,619
Orthopedic Surgery: Foot & Ankle	2	1	*	15	13	$1,690,913
Orthopedic Surgery: Hand	4	4	*	48	28	$1,680,896
Orthopedic Surgery: Hip & Joint	4	2	*	33	19	$2,096,217
Orthopedic Surgery: Pediatric	7	4	*	5	4	*
Orthopedic Surgery: Spine	7	3	*	34	25	$2,547,836
Orthopedic Surgery: Trauma	2	2	*	12	8	$2,001,206
Orthopedic Surgery: Sports Med	10	6	$1,271,620	45	26	$2,409,975

Table 36: Physician Gross Charges (TC/NPP Excluded) by Hospital Ownership (continued)

	Hospital Owned			Not Hospital Owned		
	Phys	Med Pracs	Median	Phys	Med Pracs	Median
Otorhinolaryngology	61	22	$1,515,058	176	67	$1,373,471
Pathology: Anatomic and Clinical	28	5	$1,030,708	43	8	$1,476,418
Pathology: Anatomic	3	1	*	19	4	$1,119,388
Pathology: Clinical	4	1	*	21	6	$816,470
Pediatrics: General	871	90	$620,542	760	105	$634,493
Pediatrics: Adolescent Medicine	15	3	$249,631	12	4	$776,533
Pediatrics: Allergy/Immunology	0	*	*	3	2	*
Pediatrics: Cardiology	18	8	$1,236,480	3	3	*
Pediatrics: Child Development	7	4	*	3	2	*
Pediatrics: Critical Care/Intensivist	31	9	$267,825	15	4	$475,706
Pediatrics: Emergency Medicine	18	3	$421,949	1	1	*
Pediatrics: Endocrinology	11	8	$503,017	6	5	*
Pediatrics: Gastroenterology	14	6	$581,706	5	3	*
Pediatrics: Genetics	0	*	*	4	3	*
Pediatrics: Hematology/Oncology	22	9	$496,597	9	4	*
Pediatrics: Infectious Disease	3	3	*	1	1	*
Pediatrics: Neonatal Medicine	27	8	$688,045	13	2	*
Pediatrics: Nephrology	3	3	*	1	1	*
Pediatrics: Neurology	21	12	$539,801	16	8	$511,318
Pediatrics: Pulmonology	9	6	*	3	2	*
Pediatrics: Rheumatology	1	1	*	2	1	*
Physiatry (Phys Med & Rehab)	54	18	$666,086	60	30	$710,402
Podiatry: General	28	13	$646,069	67	41	$734,499
Podiatry: Surg-Foot & Ankle	13	3	$824,098	28	14	$962,027
Podiatry: Surg-Forefoot Only	*	*	*	2	1	*
Psychiatry: General	111	29	$340,642	80	18	$381,872
Psychiatry: Child & Adolescent	21	10	$293,347	9	7	*
Psychiatry: Geriatric	3	2	*	4	1	*
Pulmonary Medicine	49	18	$718,013	95	41	$925,929
Pulmonary Medicine: Critical Care	15	4	$660,619	24	5	$1,159,657
Pulmonary Med: Gen & Crit Care	3	2	*	54	18	$859,433
Radiation Oncology	30	10	$992,252	29	10	$1,999,583
Radiology: Diagnostic-Inv	17	6	$1,951,885	105	23	$1,703,750
Radiology: Diagnostic-Noninv	63	8	$1,509,377	251	32	$1,464,899
Radiology: Nuclear Medicine	9	5	*	11	6	$904,023
Rheumatology	77	27	$546,483	87	52	$627,470
Sleep Medicine	6	4	*	19	7	$1,018,641
Surgery: General	207	55	$1,153,807	354	100	$1,155,477
Surgery: Bariatric	3	2	*	9	5	*
Surgery: Cardiovascular	42	14	$1,139,597	98	27	$1,976,704
Surgery: Colon and Rectal	3	2	*	32	13	$1,353,621
Surgery: Neurological	45	18	$2,047,386	97	28	$2,630,842
Surgery: Oncology	5	3	*	6	4	*
Surgery: Oral	2	1	*	11	6	$1,570,685
Surgery: Pediatric	14	9	$957,326	21	7	$1,532,356
Surgery: Plastic & Reconstruction	25	11	$1,258,838	40	22	$1,442,793
Surgery: Plastic & Recon-Hand	*	*	*	6	3	*
Surgery: Thoracic (primary)	13	6	$856,302	17	8	$973,104
Surgery: Transplant	15	4	$1,716,200	4	2	*
Surgery: Trauma	33	8	$994,496	10	3	$1,230,113
Surgery: Trauma-Burn	1	1	*	*	*	*
Surgery: Vascular (primary)	20	7	$1,832,632	53	28	$1,324,632
Urgent Care	83	15	$576,653	191	32	$660,294
Urology	55	23	$1,219,502	227	63	$1,409,123
Urology: Pediatric	4	1	*	3	1	*

Table 37: Physician Gross Charges (TC/NPP Excluded) by Geographic Section for All Practices

	Eastern		Midwest		Southern		Western	
	Phys	Median	Phys	Median	Phys	Median	Phys	Median
Allergy/Immunology	10	$806,856	39	$760,299	17	$914,376	25	$850,924
Anesthesiology	664	$1,651,429	574	$1,111,615	561	$1,470,365	670	$893,007
Anesthesiology: Pain Management	21	$2,036,273	31	$1,580,000	25	$2,168,274	3	*
Anesthesiology: Pediatric	0	*	27	*	1	*	7	*
Cardiology: Electrophysiology	16	$1,989,445	26	$1,698,263	20	$2,958,966	9	*
Cardiology: Invasive	16	$1,496,586	55	$1,712,531	53	$1,541,069	40	$1,301,683
Cardiology: Inv-Intvl	36	$1,828,886	81	$1,991,346	56	$2,348,199	47	$1,382,640
Cardiology: Noninvasive	77	$1,550,760	64	$1,103,299	35	$1,309,633	8	*
Critical Care: Intensivist	11	*	8	*	0	*	7	*
Dentistry	6	*	*	*	6	*	0	*
Dermatology	29	$1,091,431	60	$1,212,162	38	$1,355,170	55	$1,185,612
Dermatology: Mohs Surgery	5	*	7	*	1	*	2	*
Emergency Medicine	85	$789,971	88	$855,544	25	*	126	$903,964
Endocrinology/Metabolism	33	$532,955	50	$535,909	47	$595,998	32	$493,292
Family Practice (w/ OB)	26	$500,609	230	$585,962	64	$591,791	97	$577,761
Family Practice (w/o OB)	499	$499,791	1,298	$563,489	689	$507,854	748	$598,865
FP: Amb Only (no inpatient work)	26	$417,666	9	*	40	$452,386	4	*
Family Practice: Sports Med	8	*	6	*	6	*	5	*
Family Practice: Urgent Care	15	$607,920	10	$787,256	33	$620,310	2	*
Gastroenterology	62	$1,480,894	160	$1,607,053	112	$1,670,485	86	$1,597,219
Gastroenterology: Hepatology	0	*	1	*	1	*	4	*
Genetics	0	*	3	*	0	*	0	*
Geriatrics	7	*	15	$474,558	9	*	5	*
Hematology/Oncology	51	$505,998	77	$1,002,092	60	$1,007,857	42	$779,456
Hematology/Oncology: Onc (only)	2	*	6	*	9	*	6	*
Hospice/Palliative Care	2	*	1	*	0	*	1	*
Hospitalist: Family Practice	1	*	12	*	5	*	0	*
Hospitalist: Internal Medicine	118	$399,167	240	$388,561	168	$441,692	227	$370,272
Hospitalist: IM-Pediatrics	0	*	*	*	3	*	*	*
Hospitalist: Pediatrics	4	*	8	*	10	*	15	*
Infectious Disease	25	$381,528	71	$546,214	10	$527,530	8	*
Internal Medicine: General	437	$484,009	788	$540,502	494	$533,369	531	$558,982
IM: Amb Only (no inpatient work)	6	*	2	*	5	*	1	*
Internal Med: Pediatrics	13	$390,581	35	$547,741	15	$382,652	11	$552,544
Nephrology	21	$827,404	39	$825,282	39	$939,075	27	$659,122
Neurology	86	$570,734	104	$722,976	61	$721,802	61	$758,626
Obstetrics/Gynecology: General	125	$825,303	305	$989,237	156	$1,138,572	172	$965,407
OB/GYN: Gynecology (only)	15	$841,419	63	$1,017,689	23	$623,785	12	$577,222
OB/GYN: Gyn Oncology	4	*	9	*	2	*	7	*
OB/GYN: Maternal & Fetal Med	7	*	5	*	11	$1,156,458	4	*
OB/GYN: Repro Endocrinology	2	*	2	*	1	*	0	*
OB/GYN: Urogynecology	3	*	0	*	*	*	0	*
Occupational Medicine	2	*	30	$461,680	5	*	36	$679,025
Ophthalmology	41	$1,200,000	82	$1,360,876	48	$1,456,434	42	$1,040,199
Ophthalmology: Pediatric	3	*	1	*	5	*	5	*
Ophthalmology: Retina	3	*	5	*	3	*	2	*
Orthopedic (Nonsurgical)	5	*	9	*	6	*	5	*
Orthopedic Surgery: General	65	$1,901,412	145	$1,741,390	99	$1,847,269	105	$1,375,505
Orthopedic Surgery: Foot & Ankle	6	*	1	*	5	*	5	*
Orthopedic Surgery: Hand	18	$1,842,560	11	$1,492,358	7	*	16	$1,473,671
Orthopedic Surgery: Hip & Joint	16	$2,636,541	9	*	7	*	5	*
Orthopedic Surgery: Pediatric	1	*	3	*	6	*	2	*
Orthopedic Surgery: Spine	16	$3,608,056	7	*	10	$2,188,856	8	*
Orthopedic Surgery: Trauma	6	*	2	*	1	*	5	*
Orthopedic Surgery: Sports Med	25	$2,868,382	8	*	9	*	13	$2,171,318

Table 37: Physician Gross Charges (TC/NPP Excluded) by Geographic Section for All Practices (continued)

	Eastern		Midwest		Southern		Western	
	Phys	Median	Phys	Median	Phys	Median	Phys	Median
Otorhinolaryngology	43	$1,330,880	74	$1,448,117	61	$1,846,350	59	$1,120,336
Pathology: Anatomic and Clinical	20	$1,100,297	14	$808,967	32	$1,508,633	5	*
Pathology: Anatomic	7	*	13	$903,778	2	*	0	*
Pathology: Clinical	7	*	6	*	12	$869,839	0	*
Pediatrics: General	225	$581,796	580	$615,241	463	$674,294	363	$634,110
Pediatrics: Adolescent Medicine	3	*	3	*	9	*	12	*
Pediatrics: Allergy/Immunology	*	*	1	*	0	*	2	*
Pediatrics: Cardiology	4	*	6	*	7	*	4	*
Pediatrics: Child Development	2	*	5	*	2	*	1	*
Pediatrics: Critical Care/Intensivist	2	*	27	$279,695	16	$546,955	1	*
Pediatrics: Emergency Medicine	1	*	17	*	0	*	1	*
Pediatrics: Endocrinology	4	*	7	*	5	*	1	*
Pediatrics: Gastroenterology	5	*	5	*	3	*	6	*
Pediatrics: Genetics	0	*	0	*	0	*	4	*
Pediatrics: Hematology/Oncology	3	*	11	$397,509	13	$628,628	4	*
Pediatrics: Infectious Disease	0	*	2	*	1	*	1	*
Pediatrics: Neonatal Medicine	7	*	17	$741,412	7	*	9	*
Pediatrics: Nephrology	1	*	2	*	0	*	1	*
Pediatrics: Neurology	4	*	18	$512,252	7	*	8	*
Pediatrics: Pulmonology	2	*	5	*	4	*	1	*
Pediatrics: Rheumatology	1	*	0	*	0	*	2	*
Physiatry (Phys Med & Rehab)	15	$1,083,188	43	$638,818	34	$662,351	22	$762,281
Podiatry: General	5	*	43	$681,649	24	$765,455	23	$763,659
Podiatry: Surg-Foot & Ankle	2	*	27	$999,820	0	*	12	$728,343
Podiatry: Surg-Forefoot Only	*	*	2	*	0	*	0	*
Psychiatry: General	47	$258,707	86	$383,837	34	$510,692	24	$320,848
Psychiatry: Child & Adolescent	7	*	12	$301,263	7	*	4	*
Psychiatry: Geriatric	5	*	0	*	*	*	2	*
Pulmonary Medicine	19	$831,667	53	$929,158	43	$778,307	29	$774,703
Pulmonary Medicine: Critical Care	0	*	20	$1,218,131	12	$678,192	7	*
Pulmonary Med: Gen & Crit Care	17	$837,751	20	$832,504	13	$1,200,797	7	*
Radiation Oncology	8	*	17	$2,150,000	13	$2,458,299	21	$835,908
Radiology: Diagnostic-Inv	19	$1,493,082	23	$1,752,616	36	$1,947,816	44	$1,622,469
Radiology: Diagnostic-Noninv	87	$1,380,055	80	$1,640,706	102	$1,653,449	45	$1,369,059
Radiology: Nuclear Medicine	2	*	6	*	11	$904,023	1	*
Rheumatology	29	$577,390	60	$630,240	39	$636,921	36	$542,103
Sleep Medicine	1	*	1	*	16	$983,612	7	*
Surgery: General	101	$1,054,000	198	$1,424,924	120	$1,225,713	142	$939,764
Surgery: Bariatric	3	*	7	*	0	*	2	*
Surgery: Cardiovascular	31	$1,665,545	35	$1,928,205	45	$2,206,973	29	$1,180,246
Surgery: Colon and Rectal	17	$1,119,916	10	$1,628,234	4	*	4	*
Surgery: Neurological	30	$2,787,437	33	$2,303,333	39	$2,665,645	40	$2,406,404
Surgery: Oncology	4	*	*	*	5	*	2	*
Surgery: Oral	8	*	3	*	1	*	1	*
Surgery: Pediatric	2	*	11	$852,665	16	$1,617,978	6	*
Surgery: Plastic & Reconstruction	16	$1,202,068	15	$1,563,353	22	$1,310,839	12	$1,293,769
Surgery: Plastic & Recon-Hand	0	*	4	*	0	*	2	*
Surgery: Thoracic (primary)	8	*	9	*	2	*	11	$856,302
Surgery: Transplant	5	*	1	*	7	*	6	*
Surgery: Trauma	12	$469,835	11	$1,091,828	18	$1,177,249	2	*
Surgery: Trauma-Burn	0	*	*	*	1	*	*	*
Surgery: Vascular (primary)	17	$1,255,051	28	$1,434,283	20	$1,736,522	8	*
Urgent Care	9	*	83	$621,311	22	$580,187	160	$659,360
Urology	45	$1,599,510	66	$1,649,623	115	$1,141,074	56	$1,281,542
Urology: Pediatric	0	*	4	*	3	*	0	*

Table 38A: Physician Gross Charges (TC/NPP Excluded) by Method of Compensation (more than Two Years in Specialty)

	100% prod less allocated overhead		1–99% prod less allocated overhead		100% prod-based share of prac comp pool		1–99% prod-based share of prac comp pool	
	Phys	Median	Phys	Median	Phys	Median	Phys	Median
Allergy/Immunology	18	$854,325	5	*	11	$914,376	9	*
Anesthesiology	287	$1,128,964	53	$1,152,168	276	$1,013,642	34	$815,580
Anesthesiology: Pain Management	23	$1,835,421	1	*	10	$1,818,637	0	*
Anesthesiology: Pediatric	0	*	*	*	8	*	*	*
Cardiology: Electrophysiology	20	$1,929,181	0	*	4	*	7	*
Cardiology: Invasive	49	$1,476,682	1	*	15	$1,789,827	17	$1,541,069
Cardiology: Inv-Intvl	80	$1,972,943	5	*	19	$1,952,224	25	$2,331,689
Cardiology: Noninvasive	21	$1,169,658	8	*	19	$1,514,572	21	$1,199,602
Critical Care: Intensivist	5	*	*	*	0	*	2	*
Dentistry	6	*	*	*	*	*	*	*
Dermatology	30	$1,419,237	14	$1,214,908	19	$1,188,638	25	$1,145,642
Dermatology: Mohs Surgery	1	*	0	*	2	*	2	*
Emergency Medicine	20	*	17	*	21	*	9	*
Endocrinology/Metabolism	31	$675,917	8	*	18	$618,004	15	$508,256
Family Practice (w/ OB)	59	$593,958	36	$749,086	74	$584,351	37	$558,537
Family Practice (w/o OB)	832	$602,775	202	$539,408	346	$583,340	287	$564,678
FP: Amb Only (no inpatient work)	7	*	0	*	7	*	29	*
Family Practice: Sports Med	5	*	2	*	2	*	*	*
Family Practice: Urgent Care	6	*	5	*	2	*	3	*
Gastroenterology	89	$1,935,234	22	$1,822,096	29	$2,239,158	57	$1,697,650
Gastroenterology: Hepatology	1	*	1	*	*	*	0	*
Geriatrics	5	*	0	*	2	*	2	*
Hematology/Oncology	42	$955,920	3	*	28	$1,083,710	44	$1,154,836
Hematology/Oncology: Onc (only)	3	*	4	*	3	*	1	*
Hospitalist: Family Practice	*	*	0	*	0	*	*	*
Hospitalist: Internal Medicine	67	$457,426	6	*	30	$597,624	46	$356,294
Hospitalist: IM-Pediatrics	2	*	*	*	*	*	*	*
Hospitalist: Pediatrics	*	*	0	*	2	*	*	*
Infectious Disease	11	$673,395	3	*	2	*	61	$548,622
Internal Medicine: General	462	$596,312	120	$561,279	265	$584,718	124	$485,606
IM: Amb Only (no inpatient work)	2	*	*	*	1	*	0	*
Internal Med: Pediatrics	24	$515,155	1	*	11	$356,456	0	*
Nephrology	20	$942,451	11	$368,495	15	$1,106,566	11	$1,445,204
Neurology	55	$779,128	34	$824,108	21	$927,343	19	$605,913
Obstetrics/Gynecology: General	145	$949,058	54	$1,067,518	71	$1,131,691	90	$1,020,677
OB/GYN: Gynecology (only)	54	$873,860	2	*	9	*	6	*
OB/GYN: Gyn Oncology	6	*	0	*	0	*	2	*
OB/GYN: Maternal & Fetal Med	5	*	1	*	0	*	*	*
OB/GYN: Repro Endocrinology	*	*	*	*	0	*	*	*
Occupational Medicine	9	*	2	*	5	*	3	*
Ophthalmology	57	$1,361,355	13	$1,476,023	19	$1,683,008	34	$1,220,097
Ophthalmology: Pediatric	4	*	3	*	0	*	0	*
Ophthalmology: Retina	3	*	1	*	0	*	1	*
Orthopedic (Nonsurgical)	9	*	1	*	1	*	3	*
Orthopedic Surgery: General	151	$1,997,700	23	$1,597,915	40	$1,923,318	46	$1,608,173
Orthopedic Surgery: Foot & Ankle	8	*	1	*	2	*	1	*
Orthopedic Surgery: Hand	16	$1,941,049	5	*	3	*	4	*
Orthopedic Surgery: Hip & Joint	4	*	11	$1,928,433	2	*	4	*
Orthopedic Surgery: Pediatric	3	*	1	*	0	*	*	*
Orthopedic Surgery: Spine	14	$2,540,913	6	*	3	*	2	*
Orthopedic Surgery: Trauma	5	*	1	*	1	*	1	*
Orthopedic Surgery: Sports Med	21	$2,409,975	8	*	1	*	4	*

Table 38A: Physician Gross Charges (TC/NPP Excluded) by Method of Compensation (more than Two Years in Specialty) (continued)

	100% prod less allocated overhead		1–99% prod less allocated overhead		100% prod-based share of prac comp pool		1–99% prod-based share of prac comp pool	
	Phys	Median	Phys	Median	Phys	Median	Phys	Median
Otorhinolaryngology	85	$1,659,956	24	$1,482,797	24	$1,227,391	20	$1,313,043
Pathology: Anatomic and Clinical	1	*	4	*	5	*	0	*
Pathology: Anatomic	*	*	*	*	0	*	9	*
Pathology: Clinical	9	*	0	*	0	*	*	*
Pediatrics: General	278	$629,576	120	$710,301	179	$608,594	209	$633,982
Pediatrics: Adolescent Medicine	0	*	*	*	*	*	1	*
Pediatrics: Allergy/Immunology	0	*	2	*	0	*	*	*
Pediatrics: Cardiology	1	*	0	*	0	*	*	*
Pediatrics: Critical Care/Intensivist	0	*	*	*	0	*	*	*
Pediatrics: Endocrinology	1	*	1	*	0	*	*	*
Pediatrics: Gastroenterology	2	*	1	*	0	*	*	*
Pediatrics: Genetics	*	*	2	*	*	*	*	*
Pediatrics: Hematology/Oncology	0	*	0	*	0	*	*	*
Pediatrics: Infectious Disease	0	*	0	*	0	*	*	*
Pediatrics: Neonatal Medicine	4	*	0	*	6	*	*	*
Pediatrics: Nephrology	0	*	*	*	0	*	*	*
Pediatrics: Neurology	9	*	3	*	2	*	*	*
Pediatrics: Pulmonology	0	*	1	*	0	*	0	*
Pediatrics: Rheumatology	0	*	2	*	*	*	*	*
Physiatry (Phys Med & Rehab)	12	$733,391	3	*	18	$660,494	13	$802,866
Podiatry: General	34	$793,420	9	*	10	$628,196	6	*
Podiatry: Surg-Foot & Ankle	8	*	1	*	1	*	11	*
Psychiatry: General	20	$404,667	11	$120,129	16	$320,848	29	$349,521
Psychiatry: Child & Adolescent	2	*	6	*	3	*	1	*
Psychiatry: Geriatric	*	*	1	*	*	*	0	*
Pulmonary Medicine	30	$901,093	5	*	15	$1,049,689	19	$663,357
Pulmonary Medicine: Critical Care	0	*	2	*	2	*	5	*
Pulmonary Med: Gen & Crit Care	18	$1,170,649	4	*	4	*	6	*
Radiation Oncology	10	$2,150,000	*	*	0	*	2	*
Radiology: Diagnostic-Inv	17	$1,941,929	0	*	6	*	2	*
Radiology: Diagnostic-Noninv	34	$1,883,954	0	*	25	$1,080,591	4	*
Radiology: Nuclear Medicine	2	*	*	*	2	*	*	*
Rheumatology	26	$661,364	14	$461,863	14	$717,243	20	$600,062
Sleep Medicine	11	$1,144,253	0	*	3	*	3	*
Surgery: General	136	$1,403,853	34	$1,239,446	59	$1,133,056	56	$972,055
Surgery: Bariatric	*	*	2	*	*	*	0	*
Surgery: Cardiovascular	15	$2,318,343	*	*	2	*	23	$2,245,758
Surgery: Colon and Rectal	10	$1,567,205	1	*	5	*	*	*
Surgery: Neurological	36	$3,193,662	21	$3,193,748	13	$2,403,424	3	*
Surgery: Oncology	0	*	1	*	1	*	3	*
Surgery: Oral	6	*	1	*	*	*	3	*
Surgery: Pediatric	6	*	0	*	0	*	*	*
Surgery: Plastic & Reconstruction	19	$1,356,101	2	*	1	*	10	$1,169,022
Surgery: Plastic & Recon-Hand	1	*	1	*	*	*	4	*
Surgery: Thoracic (primary)	2	*	5	*	0	*	*	*
Surgery: Transplant	*	*	*	*	0	*	*	*
Surgery: Trauma	0	*	*	*	*	*	6	*
Surgery: Vascular (primary)	11	$744,677	1	*	7	*	3	*
Urgent Care	20	$583,010	17	$911,395	26	$713,710	63	$646,045
Urology	45	$1,616,514	31	$1,820,277	12	$1,457,744	32	$1,368,413
Urology: Pediatric	0	*	0	*	0	*	*	*

Table 38B: Physician Gross Charges (TC/NPP Excluded) by Method of Compensation (more than Two Years in Specialty)

	100% straight/guaranteed salary		1–99% base salary plus incentive		100% equal share of prac comp pool	
	Phys	Median	Phys	Median	Phys	Median
Allergy/Immunology	4	*	3	*	4	*
Anesthesiology	304	$1,879,644	241	$1,205,096	547	$1,445,004
Anesthesiology: Pain Management	18	$2,036,273	3	*	3	*
Anesthesiology: Pediatric	0	*	0	*	0	*
Cardiology: Electrophysiology	6	*	13	$1,244,400	6	*
Cardiology: Invasive	8	*	12	$937,535	21	$1,781,488
Cardiology: Inv-Intvl	5	*	20	$2,512,601	23	$1,732,740
Cardiology: Noninvasive	18	$859,856	41	$2,012,685	10	$1,357,845
Critical Care: Intensivist	3	*	6	*	0	*
Dentistry	4	*	0	*	*	*
Dermatology	9	*	15	$1,352,629	1	*
Dermatology: Mohs Surgery	*	*	4	*	*	*
Emergency Medicine	28	$667,011	46	$1,040,519	*	*
Endocrinology/Metabolism	9	*	11	$586,256	*	*
Family Practice (w/ OB)	11	$394,531	52	$589,525	1	*
Family Practice (w/o OB)	98	$398,750	319	$514,595	4	*
FP: Amb Only (no inpatient work)	11	$440,238	12	*	*	*
Family Practice: Sports Med	0	*	8	*	*	*
Family Practice: Urgent Care	4	*	11	$611,602	*	*
Gastroenterology	24	$1,079,784	29	$1,697,078	8	*
Gastroenterology: Hepatology	0	*	1	*	*	*
Genetics	*	*	0	*	*	*
Geriatrics	3	*	5	*	*	*
Hematology/Oncology	18	$451,335	15	$374,025	9	*
Hematology/Oncology: Onc (only)	2	*	3	*	0	*
Hospice/Palliative Care	1	*	2	*	*	*
Hospitalist: Family Practice	0	*	2	*	9	*
Hospitalist: Internal Medicine	81	$375,236	208	$381,274	*	*
Hospitalist: IM-Pediatrics	*	*	1	*	*	*
Hospitalist: Pediatrics	10	*	5	*	*	*
Infectious Disease	5	*	9	*	*	*
Internal Medicine: General	126	$355,754	296	$533,786	3	*
IM: Amb Only (no inpatient work)	0	*	4	*	*	*
Internal Med: Pediatrics	1	*	10	$462,733	*	*
Nephrology	11	$577,433	9	*	0	*
Neurology	35	$575,315	44	$560,043	*	*
Obstetrics/Gynecology: General	37	$729,017	91	$976,074	18	$1,460,339
OB/GYN: Gynecology (only)	8	*	6	*	*	*
OB/GYN: Gyn Oncology	5	*	4	*	*	*
OB/GYN: Maternal & Fetal Med	0	*	5	*	*	*
OB/GYN: Repro Endocrinology	*	*	1	*	*	*
OB/GYN: Urogynecology	*	*	3	*	*	*
Occupational Medicine	9	*	7	*	*	*
Ophthalmology	12	*	8	*	*	*
Ophthalmology: Pediatric	*	*	2	*	*	*
Ophthalmology: Retina	*	*	3	*	*	*
Orthopedic (Nonsurgical)	1	*	4	*	*	*
Orthopedic Surgery: General	25	$1,345,949	24	$1,801,059	1	*
Orthopedic Surgery: Foot & Ankle	2	*	1	*	1	*
Orthopedic Surgery: Hand	4	*	4	*	3	*
Orthopedic Surgery: Hip & Joint	1	*	3	*	3	*
Orthopedic Surgery: Pediatric	3	*	2	*	*	*
Orthopedic Surgery: Spine	1	*	4	*	1	*
Orthopedic Surgery: Trauma	1	*	3	*	1	*
Orthopedic Surgery: Sports Med	3	*	5	*	4	*

Table 38B: Physician Gross Charges (TC/NPP Excluded) by Method of Compensation (more than Two Years in Specialty) (continued)

	100% straight/guaranteed salary		1–99% base salary plus incentive		100% equal share of prac comp pool	
	Phys	Median	Phys	Median	Phys	Median
Otorhinolaryngology	8	*	16	$1,219,747	*	*
Pathology: Anatomic and Clinical	7	*	11	*	22	*
Pathology: Anatomic	7	*	0	*	*	*
Pathology: Clinical	8	*	0	*	4	*
Pediatrics: General	69	$553,568	254	$673,004	0	*
Pediatrics: Adolescent Medicine	6	*	4	*	*	*
Pediatrics: Cardiology	3	*	4	*	0	*
Pediatrics: Child Development	2	*	2	*	*	*
Pediatrics: Critical Care/Intensivist	17	$249,634	9	*	*	*
Pediatrics: Emergency Medicine	18	$421,949	0	*	*	*
Pediatrics: Endocrinology	3	*	4	*	*	*
Pediatrics: Gastroenterology	3	*	6	*	*	*
Pediatrics: Genetics	0	*	1	*	*	*
Pediatrics: Hematology/Oncology	10	$533,591	12	$437,687	*	*
Pediatrics: Infectious Disease	*	*	0	*	*	*
Pediatrics: Neonatal Medicine	14	$757,093	5	*	*	*
Pediatrics: Nephrology	*	*	2	*	*	*
Pediatrics: Neurology	5	*	5	*	0	*
Pediatrics: Pulmonology	4	*	5	*	*	*
Pediatrics: Rheumatology	*	*	1	*	*	*
Physiatry (Phys Med & Rehab)	6	*	16	$638,853	*	*
Podiatry: General	4	*	1	*	*	*
Podiatry: Surg-Foot & Ankle	0	*	2	*	*	*
Psychiatry: General	16	$314,815	16	$338,633	*	*
Psychiatry: Child & Adolescent	5	*	4	*	*	*
Psychiatry: Geriatric	*	*	4	*	*	*
Pulmonary Medicine	3	*	7	*	*	*
Pulmonary Medicine: Critical Care	0	*	0	*	3	*
Pulmonary Med: Gen & Crit Care	10	*	3	*	0	*
Radiation Oncology	22	$887,915	10	$1,971,517	7	*
Radiology: Diagnostic-Inv	27	$1,561,403	15	$1,951,885	35	$1,963,724
Radiology: Diagnostic-Noninv	49	$1,284,636	54	$1,862,807	59	$1,661,437
Radiology: Nuclear Medicine	0	*	3	*	6	*
Rheumatology	15	$452,546	15	$546,483	*	*
Sleep Medicine	0	*	2	*	1	*
Surgery: General	38	$853,351	70	$1,088,557	10	$1,144,974
Surgery: Bariatric	*	*	0	*	*	*
Surgery: Cardiovascular	31	$1,161,447	15	$1,904,340	18	$2,392,404
Surgery: Colon and Rectal	5	*	3	*	1	*
Surgery: Neurological	16	$1,581,707	16	$2,417,985	0	*
Surgery: Oncology	1	*	2	*	*	*
Surgery: Oral	0	*	3	*	*	*
Surgery: Pediatric	8	*	11	$2,823,351	3	*
Surgery: Plastic & Reconstruction	5	*	8	*	*	*
Surgery: Plastic & Recon-Hand	0	*	*	*	*	*
Surgery: Thoracic (primary)	7	*	4	*	1	*
Surgery: Transplant	11	$1,347,199	2	*	*	*
Surgery: Trauma	4	*	12	$1,060,529	5	*
Surgery: Vascular (primary)	7	*	10	$960,474	13	$1,482,938
Urgent Care	26	$537,550	19	$734,281	*	*
Urology	25	$1,028,060	21	$1,699,010	2	*
Urology: Pediatric	5	*	*	*	*	*

Table 39: Physician Gross Charges (TC/NPP Excluded) by Years in Specialty

	1 to 2 years		3 to 7 years		8 to 17 years		18 years or more	
	Phys	Median	Phys	Median	Phys	Median	Phys	Median
Allergy/Immunology	5	*	12	$751,788	18	$859,248	38	$848,352
Anesthesiology	122	$1,136,276	229	$1,029,538	957	$1,418,492	717	$1,200,532
Anesthesiology: Pain Management	4	*	27	$2,036,273	28	$1,808,446	12	$1,982,012
Anesthesiology: Pediatric	5	*	4	*	9	*	10	*
Cardiology: Electrophysiology	8	*	16	$2,262,294	25	$1,757,908	15	$2,348,265
Cardiology: Invasive	17	$1,662,683	33	$1,789,827	53	$1,562,567	47	$1,341,369
Cardiology: Inv-Intvl	8	*	31	$2,370,678	67	$1,896,776	82	$1,852,476
Cardiology: Noninvasive	13	$1,000,715	27	$1,402,985	48	$1,448,391	68	$1,399,669
Critical Care: Intensivist	3	*	5	*	7	*	4	*
Dentistry	1	*	3	*	2	*	5	*
Dermatology	9	*	39	$1,255,133	54	$1,183,319	60	$1,221,825
Dermatology: Mohs Surgery	2	*	4	*	5	*	3	*
Emergency Medicine	14	$651,943	38	$914,754	57	$783,580	59	$711,073
Endocrinology/Metabolism	14	$501,429	35	$500,237	33	$618,587	49	$577,236
Family Practice (w/ OB)	27	$418,948	91	$564,199	142	$594,585	99	$607,848
Family Practice (w/o OB)	162	$456,826	553	$546,417	968	$553,658	938	$564,088
FP: Amb Only (no inpatient work)	1	*	12	$465,034	26	$410,085	32	$450,608
Family Practice: Sports Med	6	*	5	*	7	*	6	*
Family Practice: Urgent Care	4	*	5	*	9	*	18	$589,427
Gastroenterology	14	$1,523,476	59	$1,887,212	93	$1,788,034	140	$1,585,895
Gastroenterology: Hepatology	*	*	1	*	1	*	1	*
Genetics	*	*	0	*	0	*	2	*
Geriatrics	2	*	6	*	7	*	8	*
Hematology/Oncology	18	$585,691	34	$702,295	62	$1,016,901	78	$897,876
Hematology/Oncology: Onc (only)	0	*	3	*	5	*	12	$702,246
Hospice/Palliative Care	1	*	1	*	1	*	1	*
Hospitalist: Family Practice	2	*	7	*	2	*	4	*
Hospitalist: Internal Medicine	105	$381,668	252	$395,685	191	$417,818	48	$361,553
Hospitalist: IM-Pediatrics	0	*	2	*	1	*	*	*
Hospitalist: Pediatrics	1	*	6	*	9	*	2	*
Infectious Disease	10	$430,596	22	$537,490	41	$540,800	31	$513,963
Internal Medicine: General	90	$391,631	350	$511,530	684	$550,564	686	$546,989
IM: Amb Only (no inpatient work)	*	*	*	*	1	*	6	*
Internal Med: Pediatrics	6	*	16	$469,348	38	$485,181	1	*
Nephrology	8	*	30	$751,217	35	$816,902	30	$981,372
Neurology	26	$503,823	62	$719,950	90	$681,122	94	$682,944
Obstetrics/Gynecology: General	39	$773,456	161	$971,780	264	$1,026,702	170	$990,258
OB/GYN: Gynecology (only)	2	*	16	$908,284	28	$833,256	48	$832,971
OB/GYN: Gyn Oncology	1	*	2	*	9	*	8	*
OB/GYN: Maternal & Fetal Med	1	*	2	*	8	*	4	*
OB/GYN: Repro Endocrinology	1	*	*	*	1	*	1	*
OB/GYN: Urogynecology	0	*	3	*	*	*	0	*
Occupational Medicine	4	*	11	$443,364	12	$661,498	29	$608,184
Ophthalmology	10	$758,428	20	$1,351,425	74	$1,316,769	70	$1,362,448
Ophthalmology: Pediatric	1	*	2	*	4	*	4	*
Ophthalmology: Retina	1	*	1	*	5	*	2	*
Orthopedic (Nonsurgical)	1	*	3	*	3	*	14	$564,204
Orthopedic Surgery: General	21	$1,380,675	61	$1,769,745	127	$1,841,294	144	$1,581,044
Orthopedic Surgery: Foot & Ankle	1	*	2	*	10	$1,672,439	4	*
Orthopedic Surgery: Hand	3	*	5	*	26	$1,932,041	13	$2,047,863
Orthopedic Surgery: Hip & Joint	4	*	5	*	9	*	17	$1,988,436
Orthopedic Surgery: Pediatric	1	*	2	*	5	*	3	*
Orthopedic Surgery: Spine	5	*	5	*	16	$3,295,955	11	$2,207,450
Orthopedic Surgery: Trauma	0	*	5	*	4	*	5	*
Orthopedic Surgery: Sports Med	4	*	13	$2,231,569	20	$2,320,990	17	$1,914,162

Table 39: Physician Gross Charges (TC/NPP Excluded) by Years in Specialty (continued)

	1 to 2 years		3 to 7 years		8 to 17 years		18 years or more	
	Phys	Median	Phys	Median	Phys	Median	Phys	Median
Otorhinolaryngology	7	*	37	$1,731,600	87	$1,616,618	74	$1,216,277
Pathology: Anatomic and Clinical	4	*	11	$1,103,380	16	$1,325,369	28	$1,258,783
Pathology: Anatomic	2	*	6	*	2	*	8	*
Pathology: Clinical	*	*	6	*	9	*	7	*
Pediatrics: General	90	$484,036	278	$616,055	527	$629,549	494	$656,554
Pediatrics: Adolescent Medicine	0	*	2	*	7	*	4	*
Pediatrics: Allergy/Immunology	*	*	0	*	1	*	2	*
Pediatrics: Cardiology	0	*	3	*	3	*	4	*
Pediatrics: Child Development	*	*	1	*	2	*	1	*
Pediatrics: Critical Care/Intensivist	3	*	13	$306,896	12	$366,438	6	*
Pediatrics: Emergency Medicine	1	*	6	*	6	*	6	*
Pediatrics: Endocrinology	2	*	3	*	4	*	4	*
Pediatrics: Gastroenterology	0	*	2	*	4	*	7	*
Pediatrics: Genetics	1	*	*	*	1	*	2	*
Pediatrics: Hematology/Oncology	0	*	8	*	9	*	8	*
Pediatrics: Infectious Disease	*	*	0	*	1	*	0	*
Pediatrics: Neonatal Medicine	1	*	11	$793,109	8	*	10	$732,226
Pediatrics: Nephrology	0	*	*	*	2	*	1	*
Pediatrics: Neurology	2	*	6	*	12	$461,487	9	*
Pediatrics: Pulmonology	0	*	1	*	5	*	5	*
Pediatrics: Rheumatology	*	*	*	*	2	*	1	*
Physiatry (Phys Med & Rehab)	8	*	22	$764,068	34	$732,299	23	$611,000
Podiatry: General	4	*	19	$706,236	31	$718,867	27	$681,649
Podiatry: Surg-Foot & Ankle	5	*	10	$992,316	10	$1,034,193	5	*
Podiatry: Surg-Forefoot Only	*	*	1	*	0	*	1	*
Psychiatry: General	5	*	30	$401,749	52	$322,060	41	$350,198
Psychiatry: Child & Adolescent	0	*	10	$268,741	7	*	4	*
Psychiatry: Geriatric	*	*	*	*	2	*	3	*
Pulmonary Medicine	12	$672,156	18	$910,735	32	$820,336	41	$804,382
Pulmonary Medicine: Critical Care	0	*	2	*	13	$823,303	3	*
Pulmonary Med: Gen & Crit Care	2	*	15	$802,239	18	$926,645	12	$844,648
Radiation Oncology	3	*	13	$2,301,603	22	$1,216,371	16	$1,069,462
Radiology: Diagnostic-Inv	7	*	29	$1,822,668	49	$1,771,539	27	$1,763,107
Radiology: Diagnostic-Noninv	15	$1,326,351	47	$1,779,585	91	$1,522,329	104	$1,544,050
Radiology: Nuclear Medicine	1	*	3	*	7	*	5	*
Rheumatology	8	*	33	$547,169	32	$627,612	65	$609,174
Sleep Medicine	2	*	4	*	5	*	14	$893,436
Surgery: General	27	$841,457	87	$1,220,789	173	$1,247,586	187	$1,078,709
Surgery: Bariatric	1	*	1	*	0	*	2	*
Surgery: Cardiovascular	14	$981,138	25	$1,327,661	51	$2,090,286	38	$2,049,431
Surgery: Colon and Rectal	1	*	3	*	9	*	14	$1,145,515
Surgery: Neurological	6	*	22	$3,003,123	46	$2,728,386	41	$2,263,997
Surgery: Oncology	*	*	2	*	3	*	3	*
Surgery: Oral	0	*	2	*	2	*	9	*
Surgery: Pediatric	2	*	7	*	8	*	13	$1,057,548
Surgery: Plastic & Reconstruction	4	*	13	$1,170,096	14	$1,520,041	18	$1,259,168
Surgery: Plastic & Recon-Hand	0	*	2	*	3	*	1	*
Surgery: Thoracic (primary)	0	*	3	*	5	*	13	$856,302
Surgery: Transplant	1	*	3	*	9	*	1	*
Surgery: Trauma	6	*	6	*	13	$974,162	8	*
Surgery: Trauma-Burn	1	*	0	*	0	*	*	*
Surgery: Vascular (primary)	1	*	9	*	17	$1,570,326	28	$1,443,319
Urgent Care	16	$640,013	53	$716,753	73	$650,247	92	$572,408
Urology	14	$1,666,374	43	$1,222,419	80	$1,604,682	96	$1,180,812
Urology: Pediatric	0	*	3	*	2	*	2	*

Table 40: Physician Professional Gross Charges (TC/NPP Excluded) by Clinical Service Hours Worked per Week

	Fewer than 40 hours			40 hours or more		
	Phys	Med Pracs	Median	Phys	Med Pracs	Median
Allergy/Immunology	34	21	$788,555	28	21	$769,663
Anesthesiology	275	38	$853,905	1,869	94	$1,283,707
Anesthesiology: Pain Management	10	5	$1,310,176	56	20	$2,036,273
Anesthesiology: Pediatric	9	3	*	26	3	$767,973
Cardiology: Electrophysiology	15	7	$2,049,193	36	15	$2,206,049
Cardiology: Invasive	45	12	$1,712,531	70	26	$1,380,353
Cardiology: Inv-Intvl	55	14	$1,733,700	117	35	$2,068,602
Cardiology: Noninvasive	39	10	$1,368,195	99	31	$1,312,706
Critical Care: Intensivist	2	1	*	2	2	*
Dentistry	3	2	*	9	3	*
Dermatology	62	29	$1,116,539	69	39	$1,180,563
Dermatology: Mohs Surgery	3	3	*	3	3	*
Emergency Medicine	175	14	$855,110	76	13	$809,616
Endocrinology/Metabolism	60	32	$574,028	48	30	$528,585
Family Practice (w/ OB)	165	38	$584,186	180	38	$564,284
Family Practice (w/o OB)	1,570	212	$555,755	913	158	$533,377
FP: Amb Only (no inpatient work)	21	6	$583,145	27	8	$400,777
Family Practice: Sports Med	6	4	*	11	8	$763,233
Family Practice: Urgent Care	42	8	$615,956	13	5	$591,520
Gastroenterology	90	40	$1,354,377	233	59	$1,709,688
Gastroenterology: Hepatology	2	1	*	3	3	*
Genetics	3	2	*	*	*	*
Geriatrics	15	8	$356,361	10	7	$269,144
Hematology/Oncology	65	21	$1,182,176	93	32	$952,542
Hematology/Oncology: Onc (only)	6	6	*	13	7	$676,708
Hospice/Palliative Care	1	1	*	2	2	*
Hospitalist: Family Practice	12	3	$360,115	4	3	*
Hospitalist: Internal Medicine	219	34	$372,950	316	50	$425,730
Hospitalist: IM-Pediatrics	0	*	*	3	2	*
Hospitalist: Pediatrics	13	4	$201,762	10	5	$301,110
Infectious Disease	75	15	$518,831	22	14	$454,454
Internal Medicine: General	955	141	$505,195	717	122	$548,382
IM: Amb Only (no inpatient work)	4	4	*	9	4	*
Internal Med: Pediatrics	9	6	*	43	16	$448,264
Nephrology	27	12	$677,836	55	24	$936,923
Neurology	90	41	$699,414	150	53	$702,745
Obstetrics/Gynecology: General	272	60	$965,123	295	82	$956,465
OB/GYN: Gynecology (only)	57	19	$841,481	29	17	$838,746
OB/GYN: Gyn Oncology	3	3	*	7	5	*
OB/GYN: Maternal & Fetal Med	7	4	*	8	5	*
OB/GYN: Repro Endocrinology	0	*	*	1	1	*
OB/GYN: Urogynecology	0	*	*	1	1	*
Occupational Medicine	43	18	$615,850	11	8	$366,201
Ophthalmology	70	30	$1,261,141	87	33	$1,319,749
Ophthalmology: Pediatric	4	1	*	5	4	*
Ophthalmology: Retina	2	2	*	6	6	*
Orthopedic (Nonsurgical)	11	10	$609,257	12	9	$618,727
Orthopedic Surgery: General	86	36	$1,592,144	190	60	$1,740,898
Orthopedic Surgery: Foot & Ankle	1	1	*	12	11	$1,780,377
Orthopedic Surgery: Hand	9	7	*	31	18	$1,881,289
Orthopedic Surgery: Hip & Joint	5	2	*	27	16	$2,325,125
Orthopedic Surgery: Pediatric	0	*	*	6	3	*
Orthopedic Surgery: Spine	3	3	*	28	19	$2,630,576
Orthopedic Surgery: Trauma	0	*	*	9	6	*
Orthopedic Surgery: Sports Med	6	6	*	39	22	$2,290,886

Table 40: Physician Professional Gross Charges (TC/NPP Excluded) by Clinical Service Hours Worked per Week (continued)

	Fewer than 40 hours			40 hours or more		
	Phys	Med Pracs	Median	Phys	Med Pracs	Median
Otorhinolaryngology	54	29	$1,173,079	113	45	$1,563,307
Pathology: Anatomic and Clinical	36	4	$1,638,927	23	8	$808,789
Pathology: Anatomic	9	2	*	10	3	$974,602
Pathology: Clinical	1	1	*	10	3	$789,881
Pediatrics: General	693	120	$588,881	445	94	$684,181
Pediatrics: Adolescent Medicine	24	5	$583,182	2	1	*
Pediatrics: Allergy/Immunology	0	*	*	2	1	*
Pediatrics: Cardiology	4	2	*	6	4	*
Pediatrics: Child Development	1	1	*	2	1	*
Pediatrics: Critical Care/Intensivist	5	3	*	22	4	$325,852
Pediatrics: Emergency Medicine	13	2	*	4	1	*
Pediatrics: Endocrinology	2	2	*	7	6	*
Pediatrics: Gastroenterology	7	5	*	0	*	*
Pediatrics: Genetics	3	2	*	0	*	*
Pediatrics: Hematology/Oncology	4	2	*	11	5	$551,878
Pediatrics: Infectious Disease	2	2	*	0	*	*
Pediatrics: Neonatal Medicine	4	1	*	28	6	$732,502
Pediatrics: Nephrology	1	1	*	1	1	*
Pediatrics: Neurology	7	6	*	14	8	$503,559
Pediatrics: Pulmonology	2	2	*	6	4	*
Pediatrics: Rheumatology	1	1	*	1	1	*
Physiatry (Phys Med & Rehab)	22	15	$566,787	50	21	$732,836
Podiatry: General	32	19	$689,796	36	26	$761,051
Podiatry: Surg-Foot & Ankle	10	4	$1,009,621	17	8	$824,098
Podiatry: Surg-Forefoot Only	*	*	*	0	*	*
Psychiatry: General	61	21	$350,892	73	25	$349,521
Psychiatry: Child & Adolescent	7	5	*	13	5	$162,960
Psychiatry: Geriatric	6	2	*	1	1	*
Pulmonary Medicine	33	18	$774,703	54	28	$893,042
Pulmonary Medicine: Critical Care	3	2	*	8	4	*
Pulmonary Med: Gen & Crit Care	14	5	$818,866	31	12	$841,656
Radiation Oncology	14	5	$2,060,855	19	8	$1,263,053
Radiology: Diagnostic-Inv	12	5	$1,657,031	82	18	$1,679,854
Radiology: Diagnostic-Noninv	42	14	$1,361,376	167	23	$1,389,281
Radiology: Nuclear Medicine	2	2	*	13	7	$904,023
Rheumatology	61	32	$635,898	50	33	$576,676
Sleep Medicine	2	2	*	17	6	$1,088,497
Surgery: General	160	55	$1,158,452	256	83	$1,124,233
Surgery: Bariatric	1	1	*	5	3	*
Surgery: Cardiovascular	5	4	*	89	28	$1,782,972
Surgery: Colon and Rectal	6	5	*	20	6	$1,301,758
Surgery: Neurological	25	9	$1,730,269	90	29	$2,564,060
Surgery: Oncology	2	2	*	4	2	*
Surgery: Oral	6	2	*	4	3	*
Surgery: Pediatric	12	7	$992,895	16	6	$1,617,978
Surgery: Plastic & Reconstruction	6	6	*	34	18	$1,259,168
Surgery: Plastic & Recon-Hand	*	*	*	5	2	*
Surgery: Thoracic (primary)	11	4	$914,551	11	6	$853,534
Surgery: Transplant	6	2	*	10	4	$1,495,089
Surgery: Trauma	5	4	*	25	6	$974,162
Surgery: Trauma-Burn	*	*	*	1	1	*
Surgery: Vascular (primary)	6	4	*	38	20	$1,443,319
Urgent Care	97	19	$658,978	52	18	$554,381
Urology	101	26	$983,613	127	47	$1,626,000
Urology: Pediatric	5	2	*	2	1	*

Table 41: Physician Gross Charges (NPP Excluded) with 1–10% Technical Component

	Phys	Med Pracs	Mean	Std. Dev.	25th %tile	Median	75th %tile	90th %tile
Allergy/Immunology	15	12	$839,804	$508,622	$507,003	$846,044	$1,286,136	$1,598,015
Anesthesiology	41	4	$7,130,818	$7,275,015	$898,089	$1,430,000	$15,660,000	$15,660,000
Anesthesiology: Pain Management	24	8	$2,663,367	$1,272,661	$1,533,695	$2,360,500	$3,702,902	$4,500,245
Anesthesiology: Pediatric	0	*	*	*	*	*	*	*
Cardiology: Electrophysiology	17	14	$2,437,260	$1,152,281	$1,312,913	$2,492,600	$3,464,462	$4,105,291
Cardiology: Invasive	37	19	$1,923,899	$1,023,908	$1,501,396	$1,835,327	$2,547,592	$3,712,762
Cardiology: Inv-Intvl	36	16	$2,096,567	$914,145	$1,429,825	$1,909,609	$2,540,637	$3,857,813
Cardiology: Noninvasive	27	17	$1,209,300	$914,940	$473,303	$1,021,266	$1,867,141	$2,554,118
Critical Care: Intensivist	3	2	*	*	*	*	*	*
Dentistry	0	*	*	*	*	*	*	*
Dermatology	47	19	$1,023,986	$570,130	$721,217	$964,208	$1,361,503	$1,626,555
Dermatology: Mohs Surgery	3	3	*	*	*	*	*	*
Emergency Medicine	24	2	*	*	*	*	*	*
Endocrinology/Metabolism	38	20	$703,771	$370,115	$472,719	$673,914	$942,255	$1,159,411
Family Practice (w/ OB)	104	28	$743,990	$244,844	$549,734	$726,270	$886,842	$1,104,517
Family Practice (w/o OB)	992	147	$678,377	$300,612	$472,051	$632,171	$866,945	$1,084,591
FP: Amb Only (no inpatient work)	44	6	$529,087	$186,449	$401,108	$506,433	$590,373	$717,392
Family Practice: Sports Med	6	4	*	*	*	*	*	*
Family Practice: Urgent Care	17	3	$582,222	$258,328	$355,437	$624,493	$770,891	$941,621
Gastroenterology	108	32	$1,810,044	$770,603	$1,443,449	$1,702,412	$2,160,034	$2,874,087
Gastroenterology: Hepatology	1	1	*	*	*	*	*	*
Genetics	0	*	*	*	*	*	*	*
Geriatrics	4	2	*	*	*	*	*	*
Hematology/Oncology	25	9	$628,420	$459,376	$270,925	$515,518	$992,483	$1,359,271
Hematology/Oncology: Onc (only)	6	4	*	*	*	*	*	*
Hospice/Palliative Care	0	*	*	*	*	*	*	*
Hospitalist: Family Practice	12	2	*	*	*	*	*	*
Hospitalist: Internal Medicine	68	11	$421,468	$211,958	$333,709	$423,537	$514,966	$717,171
Hospitalist: IM-Pediatrics	0	*	*	*	*	*	*	*
Hospitalist: Pediatrics	4	2	*	*	*	*	*	*
Infectious Disease	21	13	$487,930	$245,846	$317,391	$429,216	$697,303	$896,299
Internal Medicine: General	642	107	$727,340	$327,551	$510,443	$685,439	$925,254	$1,168,597
IM: Amb Only (no inpatient work)	2	2	*	*	*	*	*	*
Internal Med: Pediatrics	15	6	$664,798	$218,487	$526,142	$593,230	$851,296	$1,049,832
Nephrology	24	11	$929,751	$389,002	$680,122	$914,603	$1,155,388	$1,514,097
Neurology	81	35	$764,933	$312,869	$615,325	$743,834	$874,032	$1,169,243
Obstetrics/Gynecology: General	326	67	$1,106,010	$414,002	$864,193	$1,100,369	$1,336,462	$1,604,830
OB/GYN: Gynecology (only)	32	19	$885,364	$542,640	$541,435	$727,432	$1,080,775	$1,532,035
OB/GYN: Gyn Oncology	6	5	*	*	*	*	*	*
OB/GYN: Maternal & Fetal Med	11	4	$2,937,583	$2,000,716	$1,615,794	$2,857,253	$3,216,333	$7,450,950
OB/GYN: Repro Endocrinology	0	*	*	*	*	*	*	*
OB/GYN: Urogynecology	0	*	*	*	*	*	*	*
Occupational Medicine	9	7	*	*	*	*	*	*
Ophthalmology	109	33	$1,740,885	$886,451	$1,104,198	$1,610,927	$2,365,003	$3,153,000
Ophthalmology: Pediatric	7	6	*	*	*	*	*	*
Ophthalmology: Retina	19	8	$3,813,713	$1,956,978	$2,506,025	$3,006,862	$4,950,362	$8,129,698
Orthopedic (Nonsurgical)	13	10	$623,355	$260,727	$408,290	$568,378	$884,520	$1,025,058
Orthopedic Surgery: General	205	62	$1,969,883	$994,169	$1,301,949	$1,793,559	$2,581,603	$3,535,075
Orthopedic Surgery: Foot & Ankle	20	15	$2,288,468	$877,220	$1,465,136	$2,164,676	$2,881,745	$3,309,158
Orthopedic Surgery: Hand	48	27	$2,196,270	$1,033,484	$1,450,676	$2,040,283	$2,669,193	$3,532,218
Orthopedic Surgery: Hip & Joint	45	23	$3,105,651	$1,756,465	$2,001,419	$2,542,939	$3,675,535	$6,127,680
Orthopedic Surgery: Pediatric	4	4	*	*	*	*	*	*
Orthopedic Surgery: Spine	41	24	$3,072,962	$1,615,672	$1,947,705	$2,744,231	$3,688,528	$6,104,934
Orthopedic Surgery: Trauma	16	7	$2,059,614	$1,123,088	$1,315,368	$1,875,935	$2,820,380	$3,908,768
Orthopedic Surgery: Sports Med	66	27	$3,272,076	$1,578,959	$2,208,410	$2,810,728	$4,285,207	$5,270,934

Table 41: Physician Gross Charges (NPP Excluded) with 1–10% Technical Component (continued)

	Phys	Med Pracs	Mean	Std. Dev.	25th %tile	Median	75th %tile	90th %tile
Otorhinolaryngology	62	19	$1,446,713	$702,942	$1,041,081	$1,440,918	$1,997,903	$2,422,205
Pathology: Anatomic and Clinical	0	*	*	*	*	*	*	*
Pathology: Anatomic	0	*	*	*	*	*	*	*
Pathology: Clinical	2	1	*	*	*	*	*	*
Pediatrics: General	325	56	$712,570	$288,383	$542,554	$700,629	$893,457	$1,090,312
Pediatrics: Adolescent Medicine	0	*	*	*	*	*	*	*
Pediatrics: Allergy/Immunology	0	*	*	*	*	*	*	*
Pediatrics: Cardiology	4	2	*	*	*	*	*	*
Pediatrics: Child Development	2	1	*	*	*	*	*	*
Pediatrics: Critical Care/Intensivist	3	1	*	*	*	*	*	*
Pediatrics: Emergency Medicine	0	*	*	*	*	*	*	*
Pediatrics: Endocrinology	0	*	*	*	*	*	*	*
Pediatrics: Gastroenterology	1	1	*	*	*	*	*	*
Pediatrics: Genetics	12	6	$758,109	$297,938	$559,356	$699,717	$928,468	$1,325,077
Pediatrics: Hematology/Oncology	10	2	*	*	*	*	*	*
Pediatrics: Infectious Disease	3	1	*	*	*	*	*	*
Pediatrics: Neonatal Medicine	12	3	$1,018,073	$426,330	$596,623	$922,427	$1,377,715	$1,733,654
Pediatrics: Nephrology	0	*	*	*	*	*	*	*
Pediatrics: Neurology	5	1	*	*	*	*	*	*
Pediatrics: Pulmonology	3	2	*	*	*	*	*	*
Pediatrics: Rheumatology	3	1	*	*	*	*	*	*
Physiatry (Phys Med & Rehab)	23	19	$1,575,999	$1,120,233	$868,275	$1,300,799	$1,935,830	$3,817,298
Podiatry: General	21	12	$638,129	$359,815	$490,252	$679,498	$863,989	$1,033,780
Podiatry: Surg-Foot & Ankle	14	5	$1,059,284	$379,285	$691,252	$1,089,596	$1,299,161	$1,720,979
Podiatry: Surg-Forefoot Only	3	2	*	*	*	*	*	*
Psychiatry: General	28	11	$542,262	$160,857	$436,065	$502,668	$605,206	$680,822
Psychiatry: Child & Adolescent	5	3	*	*	*	*	*	*
Psychiatry: Geriatric	0	*	*	*	*	*	*	*
Pulmonary Medicine	25	15	$815,985	$469,641	$495,635	$772,905	$1,162,182	$1,424,736
Pulmonary Medicine: Critical Care	17	5	$867,107	$374,081	$644,152	$748,508	$975,795	$1,376,408
Pulmonary Med: Gen & Crit Care	42	9	$813,796	$336,915	$597,950	$742,050	$967,281	$1,410,854
Radiation Oncology	3	3	*	*	*	*	*	*
Radiology: Diagnostic-Inv	29	6	$2,357,784	$1,067,907	$1,925,000	$2,210,966	$2,631,054	$2,883,364
Radiology: Diagnostic-Noninv	44	7	$2,281,510	$1,221,666	$1,630,839	$2,172,044	$3,081,601	$3,962,202
Radiology: Nuclear Medicine	1	1	*	*	*	*	*	*
Rheumatology	29	21	$1,085,085	$895,585	$548,294	$884,630	$1,253,734	$2,074,742
Sleep Medicine	4	4	*	*	*	*	*	*
Surgery: General	104	39	$1,443,266	$704,225	$921,750	$1,371,348	$1,894,550	$2,446,464
Surgery: Bariatric	6	4	*	*	*	*	*	*
Surgery: Cardiovascular	21	10	$1,586,790	$990,486	$959,803	$1,321,717	$2,405,474	$3,135,802
Surgery: Colon and Rectal	2	1	*	*	*	*	*	*
Surgery: Neurological	15	8	$2,394,642	$1,092,446	$1,895,026	$2,427,138	$2,838,200	$3,955,562
Surgery: Oncology	1	1	*	*	*	*	*	*
Surgery: Oral	5	3	*	*	*	*	*	*
Surgery: Pediatric	4	2	*	*	*	*	*	*
Surgery: Plastic & Reconstruction	16	8	$1,204,313	$529,905	$946,556	$1,354,463	$1,599,332	$1,683,616
Surgery: Plastic & Recon-Hand	2	2	*	*	*	*	*	*
Surgery: Thoracic (primary)	0	*	*	*	*	*	*	*
Surgery: Transplant	0	*	*	*	*	*	*	*
Surgery: Trauma	8	2	*	*	*	*	*	*
Surgery: Trauma-Burn	0	*	*	*	*	*	*	*
Surgery: Vascular (primary)	33	13	$2,440,148	$1,019,188	$1,629,228	$2,227,810	$2,928,935	$4,008,369
Urgent Care	39	9	$692,403	$305,726	$503,799	$657,050	$915,255	$1,126,019
Urology	81	25	$2,146,178	$953,641	$1,552,455	$2,034,915	$2,735,314	$3,429,671
Urology: Pediatric	2	2	*	*	*	*	*	*

Table 42: Physician Gross Charges (NPP Excluded) with 1–10% Technical Component by Group Type

	Single Specialty			Multispecialty		
	Phys	Med Pracs	Median	Phys	Med Pracs	Median
Allergy/Immunology	0	*	*	15	12	$846,044
Anesthesiology	29	2	*	12	2	*
Anesthesiology: Pain Management	18	5	$2,885,344	6	3	*
Anesthesiology: Pediatric	0	*	*	0	*	*
Cardiology: Electrophysiology	13	11	$2,428,948	4	3	*
Cardiology: Invasive	19	8	$1,981,497	18	11	$1,594,600
Cardiology: Inv-Intvl	24	9	$1,852,146	12	7	$2,381,089
Cardiology: Noninvasive	6	3	*	21	14	$919,772
Critical Care: Intensivist	0	*	*	3	2	*
Dentistry	0	*	*	0	*	*
Dermatology	13	4	$890,572	34	15	$1,044,087
Dermatology: Mohs Surgery	1	1	*	2	2	*
Emergency Medicine	0	*	*	24	2	*
Endocrinology/Metabolism	7	3	*	31	17	$657,068
Family Practice (w/ OB)	31	9	$806,222	73	19	$648,944
Family Practice (w/o OB)	290	85	$748,077	702	62	$599,769
FP: Amb Only (no inpatient work)	5	2	*	39	4	$504,367
Family Practice: Sports Med	1	1	*	5	3	*
Family Practice: Urgent Care	7	1	*	10	2	*
Gastroenterology	48	7	$1,702,412	60	25	$1,662,569
Gastroenterology: Hepatology	1	1	*	0	*	*
Genetics	*	*	*	0	*	*
Geriatrics	0	*	*	4	2	*
Hematology/Oncology	7	3	*	18	6	$488,676
Hematology/Oncology: Onc (only)	0	*	*	6	4	*
Hospice/Palliative Care	0	*	*	0	*	*
Hospitalist: Family Practice	0	*	*	12	2	*
Hospitalist: Internal Medicine	0	*	*	68	11	$423,537
Hospitalist: IM-Pediatrics	*	*	*	0	*	*
Hospitalist: Pediatrics	0	*	*	4	2	*
Infectious Disease	1	1	*	20	12	$408,867
Internal Medicine: General	122	41	$771,678	520	66	$675,882
IM: Amb Only (no inpatient work)	1	1	*	1	1	*
Internal Med: Pediatrics	0	*	*	15	6	$593,230
Nephrology	8	2	*	16	9	$873,720
Neurology	44	13	$697,000	37	22	$820,350
Obstetrics/Gynecology: General	205	36	$1,178,119	121	31	$989,947
OB/GYN: Gynecology (only)	19	10	$983,886	13	9	$636,090
OB/GYN: Gyn Oncology	1	1	*	5	4	*
OB/GYN: Maternal & Fetal Med	4	2	*	7	2	*
OB/GYN: Repro Endocrinology	0	*	*	0	*	*
OB/GYN: Urogynecology	*	*	*	0	*	*
Occupational Medicine	1	1	*	8	6	*
Ophthalmology	60	12	$1,844,213	49	21	$1,421,422
Ophthalmology: Pediatric	6	5	*	1	1	*
Ophthalmology: Retina	18	7	$3,030,319	1	1	*
Orthopedic (Nonsurgical)	10	7	$540,597	3	3	*
Orthopedic Surgery: General	116	35	$1,950,485	89	27	$1,636,863
Orthopedic Surgery: Foot & Ankle	14	9	$2,597,734	6	6	*
Orthopedic Surgery: Hand	30	18	$2,099,573	18	9	$1,895,381
Orthopedic Surgery: Hip & Joint	32	16	$2,533,075	13	7	$2,726,463
Orthopedic Surgery: Pediatric	4	4	*	0	*	*
Orthopedic Surgery: Spine	26	17	$2,787,520	15	7	$2,498,098
Orthopedic Surgery: Trauma	10	5	$1,643,303	6	2	*
Orthopedic Surgery: Sports Med	43	19	$3,102,288	23	8	$2,719,484

Table 42: Physician Gross Charges (NPP Excluded) with 1–10% Technical Component by Group Type (continued)

	Single Specialty			Multispecialty		
	Phys	Med Pracs	Median	Phys	Med Pracs	Median
Otorhinolaryngology	23	3	$1,744,581	39	16	$1,211,223
Pathology: Anatomic and Clinical	0	*	*	0	*	*
Pathology: Anatomic	*	*	*	0	*	*
Pathology: Clinical	0	*	*	2	1	*
Pediatrics: General	120	19	$820,045	205	37	$641,617
Pediatrics: Adolescent Medicine	0	*	*	0	*	*
Pediatrics: Allergy/Immunology	0	*	*	0	*	*
Pediatrics: Cardiology	2	1	*	2	1	*
Pediatrics: Child Development	*	*	*	2	1	*
Pediatrics: Critical Care/Intensivist	0	*	*	3	1	*
Pediatrics: Emergency Medicine	0	*	*	0	*	*
Pediatrics: Endocrinology	0	*	*	0	*	*
Pediatrics: Gastroenterology	1	1	*	0	*	*
Pediatrics: Genetics	11	5	$712,300	1	1	*
Pediatrics: Hematology/Oncology	0	*	*	10	2	*
Pediatrics: Infectious Disease	*	*	*	3	1	*
Pediatrics: Neonatal Medicine	0	*	*	12	3	$922,427
Pediatrics: Nephrology	*	*	*	0	*	*
Pediatrics: Neurology	0	*	*	5	1	*
Pediatrics: Pulmonology	0	*	*	3	2	*
Pediatrics: Rheumatology	*	*	*	3	1	*
Physiatry (Phys Med & Rehab)	6	5	*	17	14	$928,685
Podiatry: General	2	2	*	19	10	$650,174
Podiatry: Surg-Foot & Ankle	0	*	*	14	5	$1,089,596
Podiatry: Surg-Forefoot Only	1	1	*	2	1	*
Psychiatry: General	6	1	*	22	10	$506,314
Psychiatry: Child & Adolescent	0	*	*	5	3	*
Psychiatry: Geriatric	0	*	*	0	*	*
Pulmonary Medicine	6	1	*	19	14	$797,436
Pulmonary Medicine: Critical Care	1	1	*	16	4	$745,067
Pulmonary Med: Gen & Crit Care	3	2	*	39	7	$755,539
Radiation Oncology	0	*	*	3	3	*
Radiology: Diagnostic-Inv	9	2	*	20	4	$2,361,697
Radiology: Diagnostic-Noninv	3	3	*	41	4	$2,208,125
Radiology: Nuclear Medicine	1	1	*	0	*	*
Rheumatology	1	1	*	28	20	$797,762
Sleep Medicine	0	*	*	4	4	*
Surgery: General	32	8	$1,639,323	72	31	$1,136,218
Surgery: Bariatric	4	2	*	2	2	*
Surgery: Cardiovascular	11	5	$2,087,913	10	5	$1,001,843
Surgery: Colon and Rectal	*	*	*	2	1	*
Surgery: Neurological	1	1	*	14	7	$2,417,991
Surgery: Oncology	0	*	*	1	1	*
Surgery: Oral	3	1	*	2	2	*
Surgery: Pediatric	0	*	*	4	2	*
Surgery: Plastic & Reconstruction	6	1	*	10	7	$1,229,272
Surgery: Plastic & Recon-Hand	2	2	*	0	*	*
Surgery: Thoracic (primary)	0	*	*	0	*	*
Surgery: Transplant	0	*	*	0	*	*
Surgery: Trauma	3	1	*	5	1	*
Surgery: Trauma-Burn	*	*	*	0	*	*
Surgery: Vascular (primary)	10	3	$2,315,199	23	10	$2,227,810
Urgent Care	0	*	*	39	9	$657,050
Urology	52	9	$2,286,337	29	16	$1,718,680
Urology: Pediatric	2	2	*	0	*	*

Table 43: Physician Gross Charges (NPP Excluded) with more than 10% Technical Component

	Phys	Med Pracs	Mean	Std. Dev.	25th %tile	Median	75th %tile	90th %tile
Allergy/Immunology	23	6	$1,179,574	$562,663	$743,881	$1,069,529	$1,765,132	$2,012,085
Anesthesiology	43	4	$1,501,823	$510,946	$1,243,068	$1,243,068	$1,610,000	$2,493,200
Anesthesiology: Pain Management	3	3	*	*	*	*	*	*
Anesthesiology: Pediatric	0	*	*	*	*	*	*	*
Cardiology: Electrophysiology	22	10	$1,975,862	$856,087	$1,194,089	$1,833,799	$2,701,341	$3,452,772
Cardiology: Invasive	87	27	$2,302,838	$1,161,620	$1,306,497	$2,046,560	$3,348,500	$3,914,331
Cardiology: Inv-Intvl	109	26	$2,375,556	$1,126,155	$1,402,516	$2,246,936	$3,263,334	$3,909,210
Cardiology: Noninvasive	63	24	$2,116,305	$1,143,705	$1,305,798	$1,918,661	$2,714,232	$3,724,818
Critical Care: Intensivist	0	*	*	*	*	*	*	*
Dentistry	0	*	*	*	*	*	*	*
Dermatology	7	5	*	*	*	*	*	*
Dermatology: Mohs Surgery	2	2	*	*	*	*	*	*
Emergency Medicine	34	5	$629,741	$221,325	$482,846	$587,237	$811,502	$942,564
Endocrinology/Metabolism	9	7	*	*	*	*	*	*
Family Practice (w/ OB)	49	16	$755,250	$307,746	$558,907	$695,305	$835,511	$979,776
Family Practice (w/o OB)	259	56	$672,322	$273,369	$489,405	$621,348	$783,175	$1,010,447
FP: Amb Only (no inpatient work)	29	5	$449,611	$123,833	$354,096	$429,090	$520,142	$674,518
Family Practice: Sports Med	2	2	*	*	*	*	*	*
Family Practice: Urgent Care	7	2	*	*	*	*	*	*
Gastroenterology	52	13	$1,859,624	$770,084	$1,276,738	$1,778,449	$2,192,007	$3,036,819
Gastroenterology: Hepatology	0	*	*	*	*	*	*	*
Genetics	0	*	*	*	*	*	*	*
Geriatrics	1	1	*	*	*	*	*	*
Hematology/Oncology	15	6	$4,158,967	$3,918,848	$595,977	$4,880,044	$7,285,416	$10,072,065
Hematology/Oncology: Onc (only)	2	2	*	*	*	*	*	*
Hospice/Palliative Care	2	2	*	*	*	*	*	*
Hospitalist: Family Practice	0	*	*	*	*	*	*	*
Hospitalist: Internal Medicine	7	4	*	*	*	*	*	*
Hospitalist: IM-Pediatrics	0	*	*	*	*	*	*	*
Hospitalist: Pediatrics	2	1	*	*	*	*	*	*
Infectious Disease	6	3	*	*	*	*	*	*
Internal Medicine: General	155	34	$781,224	$353,729	$518,857	$735,324	$972,762	$1,221,253
IM: Amb Only (no inpatient work)	1	1	*	*	*	*	*	*
Internal Med: Pediatrics	11	3	$625,348	$111,869	$538,706	$608,550	$715,778	$818,305
Nephrology	15	6	$1,573,015	$660,474	$1,081,655	$1,379,398	$1,872,201	$2,852,825
Neurology	30	11	$1,393,641	$751,380	$834,831	$1,233,075	$1,803,027	$2,659,158
Obstetrics/Gynecology: General	118	35	$1,185,315	$469,473	$794,492	$1,184,228	$1,522,104	$1,680,621
OB/GYN: Gynecology (only)	8	6	*	*	*	*	*	*
OB/GYN: Gyn Oncology	0	*	*	*	*	*	*	*
OB/GYN: Maternal & Fetal Med	13	3	$1,581,630	$277,222	$1,422,010	$1,570,743	$1,755,003	$2,055,543
OB/GYN: Repro Endocrinology	1	1	*	*	*	*	*	*
OB/GYN: Urogynecology	0	*	*	*	*	*	*	*
Occupational Medicine	6	4	*	*	*	*	*	*
Ophthalmology	31	12	$1,704,131	$876,620	$995,968	$1,277,617	$2,418,913	$2,886,760
Ophthalmology: Pediatric	3	2	*	*	*	*	*	*
Ophthalmology: Retina	3	3	*	*	*	*	*	*
Orthopedic (Nonsurgical)	1	1	*	*	*	*	*	*
Orthopedic Surgery: General	68	19	$1,896,643	$789,662	$1,225,816	$1,732,517	$2,482,457	$3,019,871
Orthopedic Surgery: Foot & Ankle	10	6	$2,167,880	$986,102	$1,305,165	$1,926,470	$2,915,754	$3,940,787
Orthopedic Surgery: Hand	11	5	$1,949,271	$343,739	$1,627,805	$1,985,420	$2,259,333	$2,358,261
Orthopedic Surgery: Hip & Joint	10	7	$2,734,326	$644,924	$2,221,747	$2,687,015	$3,323,622	$3,749,970
Orthopedic Surgery: Pediatric	6	1	*	*	*	*	*	*
Orthopedic Surgery: Spine	15	7	$2,665,351	$1,303,914	$2,022,213	$2,378,097	$3,424,820	$4,845,107
Orthopedic Surgery: Trauma	1	1	*	*	*	*	*	*
Orthopedic Surgery: Sports Med	28	10	$2,274,039	$758,435	$1,868,681	$2,271,387	$2,815,351	$3,364,798

Table 43: Physician Gross Charges (NPP Excluded) with more than 10% Technical Component (continued)

	Phys	Med Pracs	Mean	Std. Dev.	25th %tile	Median	75th %tile	90th %tile
Otorhinolaryngology	14	4	$1,587,475	$290,054	$1,382,281	$1,621,178	$1,827,636	$1,942,819
Pathology: Anatomic and Clinical	7	1	*	*	*	*	*	*
Pathology: Anatomic	0	*	*	*	*	*	*	*
Pathology: Clinical	0	*	*	*	*	*	*	*
Pediatrics: General	121	25	$718,180	$299,182	$508,557	$651,878	$909,403	$1,089,393
Pediatrics: Adolescent Medicine	0	*	*	*	*	*	*	*
Pediatrics: Allergy/Immunology	0	*	*	*	*	*	*	*
Pediatrics: Cardiology	4	2	*	*	*	*	*	*
Pediatrics: Child Development	0	*	*	*	*	*	*	*
Pediatrics: Critical Care/Intensivist	5	2	*	*	*	*	*	*
Pediatrics: Emergency Medicine	3	1	*	*	*	*	*	*
Pediatrics: Endocrinology	1	1	*	*	*	*	*	*
Pediatrics: Gastroenterology	2	2	*	*	*	*	*	*
Pediatrics: Genetics	0	*	*	*	*	*	*	*
Pediatrics: Hematology/Oncology	3	1	*	*	*	*	*	*
Pediatrics: Infectious Disease	0	*	*	*	*	*	*	*
Pediatrics: Neonatal Medicine	20	1	*	*	*	*	*	*
Pediatrics: Nephrology	0	*	*	*	*	*	*	*
Pediatrics: Neurology	0	*	*	*	*	*	*	*
Pediatrics: Pulmonology	1	1	*	*	*	*	*	*
Pediatrics: Rheumatology	0	*	*	*	*	*	*	*
Physiatry (Phys Med & Rehab)	10	6	$1,794,234	$1,630,812	$320,431	$1,503,095	$3,035,225	$4,843,316
Podiatry: General	3	3	*	*	*	*	*	*
Podiatry: Surg-Foot & Ankle	1	1	*	*	*	*	*	*
Podiatry: Surg-Forefoot Only	0	*	*	*	*	*	*	*
Psychiatry: General	5	4	*	*	*	*	*	*
Psychiatry: Child & Adolescent	1	1	*	*	*	*	*	*
Psychiatry: Geriatric	0	*	*	*	*	*	*	*
Pulmonary Medicine	7	5	*	*	*	*	*	*
Pulmonary Medicine: Critical Care	9	2	*	*	*	*	*	*
Pulmonary Med: Gen & Crit Care	26	3	$761,820	$697,040	$419,893	$466,634	$658,229	$2,334,607
Radiation Oncology	18	3	$5,949,514	$2,988,973	$3,937,162	$5,800,730	$7,211,469	$10,713,542
Radiology: Diagnostic-Inv	6	3	*	*	*	*	*	*
Radiology: Diagnostic-Noninv	90	12	$5,273,087	$3,409,659	$2,784,159	$4,201,426	$8,123,666	$10,811,543
Radiology: Nuclear Medicine	6	2	*	*	*	*	*	*
Rheumatology	12	8	$1,196,600	$926,592	$522,932	$974,833	$1,600,955	$3,126,410
Sleep Medicine	6	6	*	*	*	*	*	*
Surgery: General	21	11	$1,330,626	$455,937	$985,500	$1,293,824	$1,513,212	$2,040,266
Surgery: Bariatric	0	*	*	*	*	*	*	*
Surgery: Cardiovascular	5	1	*	*	*	*	*	*
Surgery: Colon and Rectal	0	*	*	*	*	*	*	*
Surgery: Neurological	6	3	*	*	*	*	*	*
Surgery: Oncology	1	1	*	*	*	*	*	*
Surgery: Oral	0	*	*	*	*	*	*	*
Surgery: Pediatric	2	1	*	*	*	*	*	*
Surgery: Plastic & Reconstruction	0	*	*	*	*	*	*	*
Surgery: Plastic & Recon-Hand	0	*	*	*	*	*	*	*
Surgery: Thoracic (primary)	0	*	*	*	*	*	*	*
Surgery: Transplant	0	*	*	*	*	*	*	*
Surgery: Trauma	0	*	*	*	*	*	*	*
Surgery: Trauma-Burn	0	*	*	*	*	*	*	*
Surgery: Vascular (primary)	10	6	$1,919,754	$789,233	$1,335,468	$1,831,761	$2,277,334	$3,465,423
Urgent Care	1	1	*	*	*	*	*	*
Urology	35	9	$2,281,858	$855,259	$1,622,912	$2,091,531	$3,000,054	$3,536,563
Urology: Pediatric	2	1	*	*	*	*	*	*

Table 44: Physician Gross Charges (NPP Excluded) with more than 10% Technical Component by Group Type

	Single Specialty			Multispecialty		
	Phys	Med Pracs	Median	Phys	Med Pracs	Median
Allergy/Immunology	20	3	$1,089,847	3	3	*
Anesthesiology	41	3	$1,243,068	2	1	*
Anesthesiology: Pain Management	1	1	*	2	2	*
Anesthesiology: Pediatric	0	*	*	0	*	*
Cardiology: Electrophysiology	19	8	$1,838,527	3	2	*
Cardiology: Invasive	74	21	$2,095,007	13	6	$1,746,068
Cardiology: Inv-Intvl	94	21	$2,255,098	15	5	$1,642,009
Cardiology: Noninvasive	44	14	$2,133,150	19	10	$1,600,377
Critical Care: Intensivist	0	*	*	0	*	*
Dentistry	0	*	*	0	*	*
Dermatology	1	1	*	6	4	*
Dermatology: Mohs Surgery	0	*	*	2	2	*
Emergency Medicine	17	1	*	17	4	$674,604
Endocrinology/Metabolism	1	1	*	8	6	*
Family Practice (w/ OB)	11	4	$771,324	38	12	$658,274
Family Practice (w/o OB)	85	27	$706,580	174	29	$573,093
FP: Amb Only (no inpatient work)	4	1	*	25	4	$413,159
Family Practice: Sports Med	1	1	*	1	1	*
Family Practice: Urgent Care	0	*	*	7	2	*
Gastroenterology	41	6	$1,944,446	11	7	$1,126,311
Gastroenterology: Hepatology	0	*	*	0	*	*
Genetics	*	*	*	0	*	*
Geriatrics	1	1	*	0	*	*
Hematology/Oncology	4	2	*	11	4	$5,646,600
Hematology/Oncology: Onc (only)	0	*	*	2	2	*
Hospice/Palliative Care	1	1	*	1	1	*
Hospitalist: Family Practice	0	*	*	0	*	*
Hospitalist: Internal Medicine	1	1	*	6	3	*
Hospitalist: IM-Pediatrics	*	*	*	0	*	*
Hospitalist: Pediatrics	0	*	*	2	1	*
Infectious Disease	0	*	*	6	3	*
Internal Medicine: General	58	11	$869,702	97	23	$667,706
IM: Amb Only (no inpatient work)	0	*	*	1	1	*
Internal Med: Pediatrics	0	*	*	11	3	$608,550
Nephrology	7	1	*	8	5	*
Neurology	6	2	*	24	9	$1,025,708
Obstetrics/Gynecology: General	44	12	$1,235,382	74	23	$1,067,738
OB/GYN: Gynecology (only)	5	3	*	3	3	*
OB/GYN: Gyn Oncology	0	*	*	0	*	*
OB/GYN: Maternal & Fetal Med	6	1	*	7	2	*
OB/GYN: Repro Endocrinology	0	*	*	1	1	*
OB/GYN: Urogynecology	*	*	*	0	*	*
Occupational Medicine	0	*	*	6	4	*
Ophthalmology	24	7	$1,900,366	7	5	*
Ophthalmology: Pediatric	3	2	*	0	*	*
Ophthalmology: Retina	2	2	*	1	1	*
Orthopedic (Nonsurgical)	1	1	*	0	*	*
Orthopedic Surgery: General	17	9	$2,101,717	51	10	$1,564,213
Orthopedic Surgery: Foot & Ankle	6	5	*	4	1	*
Orthopedic Surgery: Hand	9	4	*	2	1	*
Orthopedic Surgery: Hip & Joint	9	6	*	1	1	*
Orthopedic Surgery: Pediatric	0	*	*	6	1	*
Orthopedic Surgery: Spine	11	6	$2,378,097	4	1	*
Orthopedic Surgery: Trauma	1	1	*	0	*	*
Orthopedic Surgery: Sports Med	13	9	$2,302,537	15	1	*

Table 44: Physician Gross Charges (NPP Excluded) with more than 10% Technical Component by Group Type (continued)

	Single Specialty			Multispecialty		
	Phys	Med Pracs	Median	Phys	Med Pracs	Median
Otorhinolaryngology	9	1	*	5	3	*
Pathology: Anatomic and Clinical	7	1	*	0	*	*
Pathology: Anatomic	*	*	*	0	*	*
Pathology: Clinical	0	*	*	0	*	*
Pediatrics: General	37	6	$875,368	84	19	$567,854
Pediatrics: Adolescent Medicine	0	*	*	0	*	*
Pediatrics: Allergy/Immunology	0	*	*	0	*	*
Pediatrics: Cardiology	0	*	*	4	2	*
Pediatrics: Child Development	*	*	*	0	*	*
Pediatrics: Critical Care/Intensivist	0	*	*	5	2	*
Pediatrics: Emergency Medicine	0	*	*	3	1	*
Pediatrics: Endocrinology	0	*	*	1	1	*
Pediatrics: Gastroenterology	0	*	*	2	2	*
Pediatrics: Genetics	0	*	*	0	*	*
Pediatrics: Hematology/Oncology	0	*	*	3	1	*
Pediatrics: Infectious Disease	*	*	*	0	*	*
Pediatrics: Neonatal Medicine	0	*	*	20	1	*
Pediatrics: Nephrology	*	*	*	0	*	*
Pediatrics: Neurology	0	*	*	0	*	*
Pediatrics: Pulmonology	0	*	*	1	1	*
Pediatrics: Rheumatology	*	*	*	0	*	*
Physiatry (Phys Med & Rehab)	8	4	*	2	2	*
Podiatry: General	0	*	*	3	3	*
Podiatry: Surg-Foot & Ankle	1	1	*	0	*	*
Podiatry: Surg-Forefoot Only	0	*	*	0	*	*
Psychiatry: General	0	*	*	5	4	*
Psychiatry: Child & Adolescent	0	*	*	1	1	*
Psychiatry: Geriatric	0	*	*	0	*	*
Pulmonary Medicine	2	1	*	5	4	*
Pulmonary Medicine: Critical Care	0	*	*	9	2	*
Pulmonary Med: Gen & Crit Care	26	3	$466,634	0	*	*
Radiation Oncology	2	1	*	16	2	*
Radiology: Diagnostic-Inv	5	2	*	1	1	*
Radiology: Diagnostic-Noninv	27	4	$2,695,572	63	8	$4,592,755
Radiology: Nuclear Medicine	1	1	*	5	1	*
Rheumatology	1	1	*	11	7	$838,412
Sleep Medicine	0	*	*	6	6	*
Surgery: General	1	1	*	20	10	$1,314,017
Surgery: Bariatric	0	*	*	0	*	*
Surgery: Cardiovascular	5	1	*	0	*	*
Surgery: Colon and Rectal	*	*	*	0	*	*
Surgery: Neurological	3	1	*	3	2	*
Surgery: Oncology	1	1	*	0	*	*
Surgery: Oral	0	*	*	0	*	*
Surgery: Pediatric	0	*	*	2	1	*
Surgery: Plastic & Reconstruction	0	*	*	0	*	*
Surgery: Plastic & Recon-Hand	0	*	*	0	*	*
Surgery: Thoracic (primary)	0	*	*	0	*	*
Surgery: Transplant	0	*	*	0	*	*
Surgery: Trauma	0	*	*	0	*	*
Surgery: Trauma-Burn	*	*	*	0	*	*
Surgery: Vascular (primary)	5	3	*	5	3	*
Urgent Care	0	*	*	1	1	*
Urology	19	2	*	16	7	$2,348,907
Urology: Pediatric	0	*	*	2	1	*

Table 45: Physician Ambulatory Encounters (NPP Excluded)

	Phys	Med Pracs	Mean	Std. Dev.	25th %tile	Median	75th %tile	90th %tile
Allergy/Immunology	104	54	3,645	2,780	1,906	2,925	4,264	6,127
Anesthesiology	726	51	327	327	58	223	583	740
Anesthesiology: Pain Management	85	34	2,681	1,977	919	2,103	4,242	5,624
Anesthesiology: Pediatric	1	1	*	*	*	*	*	*
Cardiology: Electrophysiology	86	44	1,799	1,387	928	1,317	2,032	3,966
Cardiology: Invasive	238	71	2,644	1,674	1,441	2,257	3,421	5,181
Cardiology: Inv-Intvl	297	84	2,481	1,665	1,291	2,030	3,157	5,052
Cardiology: Noninvasive	242	78	2,658	1,698	1,430	2,260	3,347	5,125
Critical Care: Intensivist	15	6	261	504	5	32	270	1,466
Dentistry	26	6	2,401	892	1,816	2,475	2,820	3,449
Dermatology	208	85	4,671	1,914	3,357	4,276	5,775	7,334
Dermatology: Mohs Surgery	18	15	3,154	1,388	2,082	3,163	4,055	5,205
Emergency Medicine	340	25	2,611	888	2,110	2,621	3,077	3,593
Endocrinology/Metabolism	183	88	2,917	1,158	2,154	2,774	3,491	4,472
Family Practice (w/ OB)	634	114	4,159	2,254	2,906	3,764	4,844	6,150
Family Practice (w/o OB)	4,206	505	4,140	1,446	3,188	4,055	4,954	5,946
FP: Amb Only (no inpatient work)	129	20	4,458	1,844	3,004	4,336	5,384	6,928
Family Practice: Sports Med	30	22	3,198	1,476	2,103	3,074	3,685	5,174
Family Practice: Urgent Care	86	18	4,981	2,134	3,593	4,523	6,179	7,651
Gastroenterology	491	135	1,415	754	870	1,293	1,785	2,460
Gastroenterology: Hepatology	3	3	*	*	*	*	*	*
Genetics	2	1	*	*	*	*	*	*
Geriatrics	37	19	2,308	994	1,906	2,348	2,847	3,631
Hematology/Oncology	227	66	3,122	1,638	1,928	2,711	4,070	5,304
Hematology/Oncology: Onc (only)	28	19	3,458	1,778	1,925	3,144	4,855	6,487
Hospice/Palliative Care	6	6	*	*	*	*	*	*
Hospitalist: Family Practice	25	6	486	455	140	439	629	1,143
Hospitalist: Internal Medicine	469	64	631	967	39	116	764	2,295
Hospitalist: IM-Pediatrics	1	1	*	*	*	*	*	*
Hospitalist: Pediatrics	28	7	43	39	4	36	72	96
Infectious Disease	78	41	1,183	994	488	859	1,573	2,536
Internal Medicine: General	2,874	336	3,481	1,418	2,629	3,434	4,307	5,159
IM: Amb Only (no inpatient work)	28	12	3,812	2,162	2,346	3,479	4,203	6,576
Internal Med: Pediatrics	92	35	3,922	1,291	2,907	4,133	4,917	5,421
Nephrology	106	44	1,760	1,131	885	1,508	2,372	3,075
Neurology	383	122	2,186	1,263	1,459	2,023	2,641	3,559
Obstetrics/Gynecology: General	1,064	212	2,982	1,280	2,063	2,939	3,754	4,646
OB/GYN: Gynecology (only)	140	58	2,784	1,084	2,064	2,655	3,471	3,967
OB/GYN: Gyn Oncology	24	17	1,565	734	947	1,301	2,089	2,833
OB/GYN: Maternal & Fetal Med	34	14	1,721	1,017	802	1,467	2,669	3,394
OB/GYN: Repro Endocrinology	6	5	*	*	*	*	*	*
OB/GYN: Urogynecology	4	3	*	*	*	*	*	*
Occupational Medicine	78	36	3,387	1,896	1,921	3,158	4,469	6,348
Ophthalmology	264	85	5,060	1,736	3,846	4,856	6,099	7,295
Ophthalmology: Pediatric	21	15	4,104	1,841	2,567	4,018	4,826	6,557
Ophthalmology: Retina	28	16	7,383	3,421	4,159	7,053	8,810	12,783
Orthopedic (Nonsurgical)	33	25	2,790	964	1,949	2,707	3,448	4,150
Orthopedic Surgery: General	563	153	3,018	1,122	2,187	2,891	3,699	4,533
Orthopedic Surgery: Foot & Ankle	40	29	3,698	1,330	2,827	3,606	4,528	5,635
Orthopedic Surgery: Hand	105	52	3,604	1,248	2,727	3,445	4,458	5,456
Orthopedic Surgery: Hip & Joint	78	38	2,910	848	2,291	2,827	3,481	3,976
Orthopedic Surgery: Pediatric	13	10	3,716	1,022	2,648	3,700	4,739	5,127
Orthopedic Surgery: Spine	77	45	2,513	1,085	1,655	2,444	3,342	4,141
Orthopedic Surgery: Trauma	27	14	2,460	1,205	1,757	2,283	3,157	3,945
Orthopedic Surgery: Sports Med	126	52	3,788	1,564	2,773	3,599	4,457	5,792

Table 45: Physician Ambulatory Encounters (NPP Excluded) (continued)

	Phys	Med Pracs	Mean	Std. Dev.	25th %tile	Median	75th %tile	90th %tile
Otorhinolaryngology	284	95	3,404	1,253	2,540	3,236	4,252	5,036
Pathology: Anatomic and Clinical	7	2	*	*	*	*	*	*
Pathology: Anatomic	1	1	*	*	*	*	*	*
Pathology: Clinical	2	1	*	*	*	*	*	*
Pediatrics: General	1,964	260	4,606	1,785	3,373	4,348	5,564	6,861
Pediatrics: Adolescent Medicine	54	6	3,709	1,697	2,946	4,285	4,905	5,396
Pediatrics: Allergy/Immunology	1	1	*	*	*	*	*	*
Pediatrics: Cardiology	38	13	1,565	859	909	1,328	1,754	3,280
Pediatrics: Child Development	7	4	*	*	*	*	*	*
Pediatrics: Critical Care/Intensivist	20	7	33	19	21	31	46	62
Pediatrics: Emergency Medicine	18	3	2,946	933	2,431	2,758	4,178	4,191
Pediatrics: Endocrinology	23	15	1,891	810	1,488	1,770	2,392	3,336
Pediatrics: Gastroenterology	20	10	1,723	705	1,154	1,374	2,372	2,938
Pediatrics: Genetics	16	10	2,825	1,458	1,603	2,798	4,161	4,791
Pediatrics: Hematology/Oncology	43	14	1,175	576	819	1,020	1,355	1,679
Pediatrics: Infectious Disease	12	6	401	375	139	302	601	1,162
Pediatrics: Neonatal Medicine	31	6	20	17	6	12	32	45
Pediatrics: Nephrology	7	6	*	*	*	*	*	*
Pediatrics: Neurology	46	21	1,898	779	1,335	1,729	2,325	3,071
Pediatrics: Pulmonology	18	11	2,020	984	1,305	1,837	2,573	3,706
Pediatrics: Rheumatology	5	3	*	*	*	*	*	*
Physiatry (Phys Med & Rehab)	123	62	1,877	1,311	932	1,783	2,516	3,261
Podiatry: General	102	57	2,849	1,037	2,174	2,479	3,452	4,408
Podiatry: Surg-Foot & Ankle	52	21	3,629	1,167	2,907	3,588	4,441	5,203
Podiatry: Surg-Forefoot Only	5	3	*	*	*	*	*	*
Psychiatry: General	166	50	1,901	1,138	941	1,888	2,737	3,515
Psychiatry: Child & Adolescent	34	17	1,685	835	1,085	1,593	1,996	3,121
Psychiatry: Geriatric	5	2	*	*	*	*	*	*
Pulmonary Medicine	156	69	2,115	1,236	1,253	1,793	2,855	3,772
Pulmonary Medicine: Critical Care	32	10	1,718	1,208	1,011	1,575	2,035	3,816
Pulmonary Med: Gen & Crit Care	89	22	1,243	627	662	1,074	1,741	2,173
Radiation Oncology	55	17	1,244	991	556	808	1,891	2,581
Radiology: Diagnostic-Inv	78	18	6,461	6,222	776	5,419	10,234	15,522
Radiology: Diagnostic-Noninv	86	20	8,821	5,963	2,504	9,019	13,646	17,850
Radiology: Nuclear Medicine	14	9	5,254	4,983	1,217	3,977	8,973	13,528
Rheumatology	180	90	3,209	1,462	2,295	2,997	3,804	4,951
Sleep Medicine	33	21	2,409	925	1,661	2,094	3,095	3,872
Surgery: General	604	174	1,601	757	1,075	1,488	2,021	2,649
Surgery: Bariatric	15	10	1,249	552	836	1,288	1,698	2,069
Surgery: Cardiovascular	113	40	405	270	222	321	479	768
Surgery: Colon and Rectal	29	13	1,410	722	747	1,267	1,916	2,512
Surgery: Neurological	135	49	1,425	715	927	1,317	1,842	2,485
Surgery: Oncology	13	9	2,249	1,675	1,001	1,824	3,360	5,522
Surgery: Oral	8	6	*	*	*	*	*	*
Surgery: Pediatric	32	17	1,126	616	746	932	1,205	2,293
Surgery: Plastic & Reconstruction	67	37	1,877	942	1,100	1,738	2,333	3,257
Surgery: Plastic & Recon-Hand	3	3	*	*	*	*	*	*
Surgery: Thoracic (primary)	28	11	519	572	234	320	588	1,023
Surgery: Transplant	6	4	*	*	*	*	*	*
Surgery: Trauma	40	11	670	438	416	582	816	1,252
Surgery: Trauma-Burn	4	2	*	*	*	*	*	*
Surgery: Vascular (primary)	92	43	1,969	1,099	1,042	1,829	2,807	3,535
Urgent Care	273	47	5,008	1,904	3,671	4,700	6,078	7,559
Urology	347	98	2,932	1,116	2,204	2,733	3,578	4,445
Urology: Pediatric	12	6	5,758	4,808	2,035	2,881	11,532	13,047

Table 46: Physician Ambulatory Encounters (NPP Excluded) by Group Type

	Single Specialty			Multispecialty		
	Phys	Med Pracs	Median	Phys	Med Pracs	Median
Allergy/Immunology	28	6	3,011	76	48	2,925
Anesthesiology	605	36	300	121	15	46
Anesthesiology: Pain Management	43	13	1,400	42	21	3,435
Anesthesiology: Pediatric	0	*	*	1	1	*
Cardiology: Electrophysiology	54	26	1,187	32	18	1,586
Cardiology: Invasive	115	27	2,142	123	44	2,497
Cardiology: Inv-Intvl	170	39	1,811	127	45	2,516
Cardiology: Noninvasive	97	28	2,443	145	50	2,153
Critical Care: Intensivist	1	1	*	14	5	61
Dentistry	12	1	*	14	5	2,210
Dermatology	24	7	3,656	184	78	4,296
Dermatology: Mohs Surgery	2	2	*	16	13	2,802
Emergency Medicine	178	8	2,556	162	17	2,723
Endocrinology/Metabolism	15	8	3,071	168	80	2,722
Family Practice (w/ OB)	91	24	3,913	543	90	3,759
Family Practice (w/o OB)	770	240	4,291	3,436	265	4,009
FP: Amb Only (no inpatient work)	14	5	4,549	115	15	4,320
Family Practice: Sports Med	9	6	*	21	16	3,173
Family Practice: Urgent Care	29	2	*	57	16	4,494
Gastroenterology	173	23	1,309	318	112	1,270
Gastroenterology: Hepatology	3	3	*	0	*	*
Genetics	*	*	*	2	1	*
Geriatrics	7	3	*	30	16	2,368
Hematology/Oncology	41	7	2,592	186	59	2,731
Hematology/Oncology: Onc (only)	4	2	*	24	17	3,546
Hospice/Palliative Care	2	2	*	4	4	*
Hospitalist: Family Practice	1	1	*	24	5	432
Hospitalist: Internal Medicine	28	6	26	441	58	135
Hospitalist: IM-Pediatrics	*	*	*	1	1	*
Hospitalist: Pediatrics	0	*	*	28	7	36
Infectious Disease	7	4	*	71	37	913
Internal Medicine: General	318	79	3,758	2,556	257	3,409
IM: Amb Only (no inpatient work)	1	1	*	27	11	3,366
Internal Med: Pediatrics	0	*	*	92	35	4,133
Nephrology	12	2	*	94	42	1,682
Neurology	87	22	1,743	296	100	2,092
Obstetrics/Gynecology: General	273	59	3,366	791	153	2,821
OB/GYN: Gynecology (only)	23	12	2,882	117	46	2,631
OB/GYN: Gyn Oncology	5	3	*	19	14	1,328
OB/GYN: Maternal & Fetal Med	12	5	1,590	22	9	1,274
OB/GYN: Repro Endocrinology	0	*	*	6	5	*
OB/GYN: Urogynecology	*	*	*	4	3	*
Occupational Medicine	3	2	*	75	34	3,158
Ophthalmology	77	15	5,894	187	70	4,554
Ophthalmology: Pediatric	7	6	*	14	9	3,750
Ophthalmology: Retina	18	7	8,336	10	9	4,946
Orthopedic (Nonsurgical)	18	13	2,541	15	12	2,988
Orthopedic Surgery: General	170	50	3,113	393	103	2,820
Orthopedic Surgery: Foot & Ankle	26	20	3,333	14	9	3,910
Orthopedic Surgery: Hand	64	29	3,505	41	23	3,382
Orthopedic Surgery: Hip & Joint	52	26	2,837	26	12	2,744
Orthopedic Surgery: Pediatric	3	3	*	10	7	3,255
Orthopedic Surgery: Spine	41	28	2,202	36	17	2,618
Orthopedic Surgery: Trauma	17	9	2,277	10	5	2,605
Orthopedic Surgery: Sports Med	62	33	3,574	64	19	3,647

Table 46: Physician Ambulatory Encounters (NPP Excluded) by Group Type (continued)

	Single Specialty			Multispecialty		
	Phys	Med Pracs	Median	Phys	Med Pracs	Median
Otorhinolaryngology	62	10	3,564	222	85	3,175
Pathology: Anatomic and Clinical	0	*	*	7	2	*
Pathology: Anatomic	*	*	*	1	1	*
Pathology: Clinical	0	*	*	2	1	*
Pediatrics: General	545	64	4,546	1,419	196	4,283
Pediatrics: Adolescent Medicine	1	1	*	53	5	4,161
Pediatrics: Allergy/Immunology	0	*	*	1	1	*
Pediatrics: Cardiology	4	2	*	34	11	1,317
Pediatrics: Child Development	*	*	*	7	4	*
Pediatrics: Critical Care/Intensivist	7	1	*	13	6	33
Pediatrics: Emergency Medicine	0	*	*	18	3	2,758
Pediatrics: Endocrinology	0	*	*	23	15	1,770
Pediatrics: Gastroenterology	0	*	*	20	10	1,374
Pediatrics: Genetics	10	5	3,828	6	5	*
Pediatrics: Hematology/Oncology	0	*	*	43	14	1,020
Pediatrics: Infectious Disease	*	*	*	12	6	302
Pediatrics: Neonatal Medicine	10	2	*	21	4	23
Pediatrics: Nephrology	*	*	*	7	6	*
Pediatrics: Neurology	4	2	*	42	19	1,690
Pediatrics: Pulmonology	1	1	*	17	10	1,840
Pediatrics: Rheumatology	*	*	*	5	3	*
Physiatry (Phys Med & Rehab)	32	15	1,506	91	47	1,795
Podiatry: General	3	3	*	99	54	2,495
Podiatry: Surg-Foot & Ankle	1	1	*	51	20	3,626
Podiatry: Surg-Forefoot Only	1	1	*	4	2	*
Psychiatry: General	12	2	*	154	48	1,888
Psychiatry: Child & Adolescent	0	*	*	34	17	1,593
Psychiatry: Geriatric	4	1	*	1	1	*
Pulmonary Medicine	12	4	422	144	65	1,982
Pulmonary Medicine: Critical Care	3	2	*	29	8	1,574
Pulmonary Med: Gen & Crit Care	33	6	953	56	16	1,326
Radiation Oncology	14	2	*	41	15	753
Radiology: Diagnostic-Inv	35	5	9,456	43	13	894
Radiology: Diagnostic-Noninv	29	4	11,968	57	16	8,786
Radiology: Nuclear Medicine	7	4	*	7	5	*
Rheumatology	14	7	2,466	166	83	3,047
Sleep Medicine	0	*	*	33	21	2,094
Surgery: General	87	24	1,501	517	150	1,483
Surgery: Bariatric	5	3	*	10	7	1,198
Surgery: Cardiovascular	42	13	332	71	27	321
Surgery: Colon and Rectal	*	*	*	29	13	1,267
Surgery: Neurological	34	8	1,135	101	41	1,349
Surgery: Oncology	1	1	*	12	8	1,746
Surgery: Oral	0	*	*	8	6	*
Surgery: Pediatric	11	4	942	21	13	921
Surgery: Plastic & Reconstruction	5	2	*	62	35	1,828
Surgery: Plastic & Recon-Hand	1	1	*	2	2	*
Surgery: Thoracic (primary)	11	4	294	17	7	342
Surgery: Transplant	0	*	*	6	4	*
Surgery: Trauma	6	2	*	34	9	630
Surgery: Trauma-Burn	*	*	*	4	2	*
Surgery: Vascular (primary)	9	6	*	83	37	1,726
Urgent Care	15	4	4,088	258	43	4,744
Urology	150	15	2,979	197	83	2,641
Urology: Pediatric	5	3	*	7	3	*

Table 47: Physician Ambulatory Encounters (NPP Excluded) by Hospital Ownership

	Hospital Owned			Not Hospital Owned		
	Phys	Med Pracs	Median	Phys	Med Pracs	Median
Allergy/Immunology	20	15	2,184	84	39	3,120
Anesthesiology	39	9	250	687	42	223
Anesthesiology: Pain Management	14	8	1,679	71	26	2,314
Anesthesiology: Pediatric	0	*	*	1	1	*
Cardiology: Electrophysiology	19	11	1,451	67	33	1,218
Cardiology: Invasive	64	18	2,409	174	53	2,232
Cardiology: Inv-Intvl	66	22	2,101	231	62	2,026
Cardiology: Noninvasive	90	25	1,683	152	53	2,649
Critical Care: Intensivist	11	4	98	4	2	*
Dentistry	3	1	*	23	5	2,436
Dermatology	60	29	4,718	148	56	4,145
Dermatology: Mohs Surgery	7	5	*	11	10	3,732
Emergency Medicine	166	13	2,625	174	12	2,618
Endocrinology/Metabolism	95	42	2,614	88	46	2,892
Family Practice (w/ OB)	292	56	3,734	342	58	3,902
Family Practice (w/o OB)	2,501	318	4,086	1,705	187	4,012
FP: Amb Only (no inpatient work)	109	12	4,183	20	8	5,257
Family Practice: Sports Med	13	10	3,080	17	12	3,067
Family Practice: Urgent Care	36	8	4,455	50	10	4,523
Gastroenterology	120	43	1,386	371	92	1,232
Gastroenterology: Hepatology	0	*	*	3	3	*
Genetics	2	1	*	0	*	*
Geriatrics	23	11	1,988	14	8	2,806
Hematology/Oncology	73	21	2,653	154	45	2,822
Hematology/Oncology: Onc (only)	10	7	2,291	18	12	3,626
Hospice/Palliative Care	4	4	*	2	2	*
Hospitalist: Family Practice	9	1	*	16	5	445
Hospitalist: Internal Medicine	344	37	125	125	27	109
Hospitalist: IM-Pediatrics	1	1	*	0	*	*
Hospitalist: Pediatrics	18	5	47	10	2	*
Infectious Disease	44	20	632	34	21	1,462
Internal Medicine: General	1,548	182	3,409	1,326	154	3,463
IM: Amb Only (no inpatient work)	25	9	3,366	3	3	*
Internal Med: Pediatrics	40	15	4,283	52	20	3,680
Nephrology	35	17	1,277	71	27	1,703
Neurology	174	55	1,704	209	67	2,240
Obstetrics/Gynecology: General	436	95	2,894	628	117	2,966
OB/GYN: Gynecology (only)	79	25	2,676	61	33	2,561
OB/GYN: Gyn Oncology	18	13	1,208	6	4	*
OB/GYN: Maternal & Fetal Med	24	10	1,734	10	4	714
OB/GYN: Repro Endocrinology	3	3	*	3	2	*
OB/GYN: Urogynecology	4	3	*	0	*	*
Occupational Medicine	21	13	3,867	57	23	3,026
Ophthalmology	60	22	4,535	204	63	4,973
Ophthalmology: Pediatric	4	3	*	17	12	4,018
Ophthalmology: Retina	5	4	*	23	12	7,845
Orthopedic (Nonsurgical)	4	3	*	29	22	2,707
Orthopedic Surgery: General	150	47	2,497	413	106	3,060
Orthopedic Surgery: Foot & Ankle	3	2	*	37	27	3,649
Orthopedic Surgery: Hand	5	5	*	100	47	3,460
Orthopedic Surgery: Hip & Joint	2	1	*	76	37	2,837
Orthopedic Surgery: Pediatric	7	4	*	6	6	*
Orthopedic Surgery: Spine	5	3	*	72	42	2,446
Orthopedic Surgery: Trauma	2	2	*	25	12	2,306
Orthopedic Surgery: Sports Med	12	7	2,862	114	45	3,713

Table 47: Physician Ambulatory Encounters (NPP Excluded) by Hospital Ownership (continued)

	Hospital Owned			Not Hospital Owned		
	Phys	Med Pracs	Median	Phys	Med Pracs	Median
Otorhinolaryngology	69	27	3,175	215	68	3,245
Pathology: Anatomic and Clinical	4	1	*	3	1	*
Pathology: Anatomic	0	*	*	1	1	*
Pathology: Clinical	2	1	*	0	*	*
Pediatrics: General	1,104	130	4,458	860	130	4,178
Pediatrics: Adolescent Medicine	13	3	589	41	3	4,486
Pediatrics: Allergy/Immunology	0	*	*	1	1	*
Pediatrics: Cardiology	24	7	1,228	14	6	1,636
Pediatrics: Child Development	4	2	*	3	2	*
Pediatrics: Critical Care/Intensivist	18	6	31	2	1	*
Pediatrics: Emergency Medicine	18	3	2,758	0	*	*
Pediatrics: Endocrinology	14	10	1,713	9	5	*
Pediatrics: Gastroenterology	14	6	1,274	6	4	*
Pediatrics: Genetics	12	7	3,444	4	3	*
Pediatrics: Hematology/Oncology	28	10	948	15	4	1,140
Pediatrics: Infectious Disease	8	4	*	4	2	*
Pediatrics: Neonatal Medicine	18	4	17	13	2	*
Pediatrics: Nephrology	4	4	*	3	2	*
Pediatrics: Neurology	27	12	1,545	19	9	1,984
Pediatrics: Pulmonology	13	8	1,460	5	3	*
Pediatrics: Rheumatology	1	1	*	4	2	*
Physiatry (Phys Med & Rehab)	56	20	1,157	67	42	2,208
Podiatry: General	41	21	2,462	61	36	2,537
Podiatry: Surg-Foot & Ankle	14	4	4,118	38	17	3,525
Podiatry: Surg-Forefoot Only	*	*	*	5	3	*
Psychiatry: General	106	32	1,416	60	18	2,693
Psychiatry: Child & Adolescent	26	11	1,593	8	6	*
Psychiatry: Geriatric	1	1	*	4	1	*
Pulmonary Medicine	64	25	1,517	92	44	2,085
Pulmonary Medicine: Critical Care	6	2	*	26	8	1,760
Pulmonary Med: Gen & Crit Care	13	6	1,191	76	16	1,031
Radiation Oncology	31	10	717	24	7	1,686
Radiology: Diagnostic-Inv	9	4	*	69	14	7,376
Radiology: Diagnostic-Noninv	17	4	1,910	69	16	10,611
Radiology: Nuclear Medicine	4	2	*	10	7	3,977
Rheumatology	86	35	2,855	94	55	3,066
Sleep Medicine	10	9	2,002	23	12	2,411
Surgery: General	233	70	1,296	371	104	1,602
Surgery: Bariatric	3	3	*	12	7	1,485
Surgery: Cardiovascular	52	20	299	61	20	367
Surgery: Colon and Rectal	3	2	*	26	11	1,299
Surgery: Neurological	50	24	1,209	85	25	1,388
Surgery: Oncology	5	3	*	8	6	*
Surgery: Oral	2	1	*	6	5	*
Surgery: Pediatric	18	11	896	14	6	1,011
Surgery: Plastic & Reconstruction	31	15	1,645	36	22	1,915
Surgery: Plastic & Recon-Hand	*	*	*	3	3	*
Surgery: Thoracic (primary)	12	5	331	16	6	310
Surgery: Transplant	5	3	*	1	1	*
Surgery: Trauma	34	8	562	6	3	*
Surgery: Trauma-Burn	4	2	*	*	*	*
Surgery: Vascular (primary)	24	12	1,186	68	31	2,025
Urgent Care	91	16	4,610	182	31	4,749
Urology	64	30	2,385	283	68	2,784
Urology: Pediatric	5	2	*	7	4	*

Table 48: Physician Ambulatory Encounters (NPP Excluded) by Geographic Section for All Practices

	Eastern		Midwest		Southern		Western	
	Phys	Median	Phys	Median	Phys	Median	Phys	Median
Allergy/Immunology	14	3,422	38	3,016	28	2,761	24	2,684
Anesthesiology	220	114	243	162	170	331	93	740
Anesthesiology: Pain Management	26	374	24	2,518	24	4,515	11	1,895
Anesthesiology: Pediatric	0	*	0	*	1	*	0	*
Cardiology: Electrophysiology	14	1,486	31	1,215	28	1,216	13	1,503
Cardiology: Invasive	12	1,529	77	2,172	97	2,429	52	2,207
Cardiology: Inv-Intvl	35	1,437	87	1,971	104	2,174	71	2,124
Cardiology: Noninvasive	81	1,800	76	2,513	62	2,669	23	2,361
Critical Care: Intensivist	10	118	4	*	0	*	1	*
Dentistry	6	*	*	*	6	*	14	*
Dermatology	34	4,315	60	4,622	41	4,458	73	3,694
Dermatology: Mohs Surgery	5	*	9	*	1	*	3	*
Emergency Medicine	120	2,685	73	2,906	19	*	128	2,470
Endocrinology/Metabolism	39	2,815	52	2,391	51	3,086	41	2,635
Family Practice (w/ OB)	77	3,935	298	3,605	128	4,765	131	3,371
Family Practice (w/o OB)	864	4,110	1,451	3,985	1,076	4,314	815	3,836
FP: Amb Only (no inpatient work)	28	4,666	32	4,305	42	4,716	27	2,827
Family Practice: Sports Med	7	*	8	*	6	*	9	*
Family Practice: Urgent Care	18	3,711	22	4,709	43	5,051	3	*
Gastroenterology	71	1,272	188	1,198	126	1,481	106	1,283
Gastroenterology: Hepatology	0	*	1	*	1	*	1	*
Genetics	0	*	2	*	0	*	0	*
Geriatrics	7	*	14	2,097	11	2,589	5	*
Hematology/Oncology	45	1,893	68	2,838	64	3,195	50	2,557
Hematology/Oncology: Onc (only)	6	*	8	*	5	*	9	*
Hospice/Palliative Care	3	*	1	*	1	*	1	*
Hospitalist: Family Practice	0	*	14	321	11	602	0	*
Hospitalist: Internal Medicine	125	115	139	1,173	98	91	107	57
Hospitalist: IM-Pediatrics	0	*	*	*	1	*	*	*
Hospitalist: Pediatrics	4	*	6	*	10	*	8	*
Infectious Disease	24	501	27	939	7	*	20	1,177
Internal Medicine: General	592	3,416	883	3,333	750	3,664	649	3,399
IM: Amb Only (no inpatient work)	18	3,176	2	*	6	*	2	*
Internal Med: Pediatrics	16	4,782	45	4,250	22	3,701	9	*
Nephrology	17	1,077	41	1,510	20	2,265	28	1,464
Neurology	125	1,747	112	2,070	79	2,215	67	2,340
Obstetrics/Gynecology: General	204	2,743	374	2,787	247	3,477	239	2,794
OB/GYN: Gynecology (only)	25	2,598	69	2,820	31	2,504	15	1,929
OB/GYN: Gyn Oncology	4	*	9	*	9	*	2	*
OB/GYN: Maternal & Fetal Med	9	*	8	*	11	970	6	*
OB/GYN: Repro Endocrinology	3	*	2	*	1	*	0	*
OB/GYN: Urogynecology	4	*	0	*	*	*	0	*
Occupational Medicine	4	*	30	2,036	10	3,696	34	3,600
Ophthalmology	45	5,239	101	4,856	78	5,192	40	3,746
Ophthalmology: Pediatric	4	*	4	*	8	*	5	*
Ophthalmology: Retina	2	*	18	8,625	6	*	2	*
Orthopedic (Nonsurgical)	4	*	16	2,609	9	*	4	*
Orthopedic Surgery: General	70	2,882	195	2,831	116	3,236	182	2,790
Orthopedic Surgery: Foot & Ankle	7	*	10	3,554	10	3,333	13	3,649
Orthopedic Surgery: Hand	19	4,126	30	3,249	18	4,215	38	3,096
Orthopedic Surgery: Hip & Joint	22	2,739	28	3,375	11	2,895	17	2,675
Orthopedic Surgery: Pediatric	1	*	4	*	7	*	1	*
Orthopedic Surgery: Spine	17	2,447	26	2,290	12	3,184	22	2,233
Orthopedic Surgery: Trauma	8	*	4	*	8	*	7	*
Orthopedic Surgery: Sports Med	34	3,528	22	3,691	35	4,304	35	3,085

Table 48: Physician Ambulatory Encounters (NPP Excluded) by Geographic Section for All Practices (continued)

	Eastern		Midwest		Southern		Western	
	Phys	Median	Phys	Median	Phys	Median	Phys	Median
Otorhinolaryngology	42	3,969	84	3,142	87	3,879	71	2,656
Pathology: Anatomic and Clinical	7	*	0	*	0	*	0	*
Pathology: Anatomic	0	*	1	*	0	*	0	*
Pathology: Clinical	0	*	0	*	2	*	0	*
Pediatrics: General	301	4,191	661	4,337	618	5,012	384	3,878
Pediatrics: Adolescent Medicine	3	*	1	*	39	*	11	*
Pediatrics: Allergy/Immunology	*	*	1	*	0	*	0	*
Pediatrics: Cardiology	7	*	8	*	11	*	12	1,412
Pediatrics: Child Development	4	*	3	*	0	*	0	*
Pediatrics: Critical Care/Intensivist	4	*	9	*	7	*	0	*
Pediatrics: Emergency Medicine	1	*	17	*	0	*	0	*
Pediatrics: Endocrinology	7	*	8	*	5	*	3	*
Pediatrics: Gastroenterology	8	*	4	*	3	*	5	*
Pediatrics: Genetics	11	3,614	0	*	1	*	4	*
Pediatrics: Hematology/Oncology	6	*	8	*	17	951	12	*
Pediatrics: Infectious Disease	0	*	2	*	6	*	4	*
Pediatrics: Neonatal Medicine	9	*	13	*	0	*	9	*
Pediatrics: Nephrology	1	*	2	*	1	*	3	*
Pediatrics: Neurology	5	*	19	2,117	13	1,764	9	*
Pediatrics: Pulmonology	4	*	5	*	7	*	2	*
Pediatrics: Rheumatology	1	*	0	*	0	*	4	*
Physiatry (Phys Med & Rehab)	23	2,353	48	1,416	30	1,506	22	2,291
Podiatry: General	5	*	45	2,638	26	3,060	26	2,372
Podiatry: Surg-Foot & Ankle	11	3,395	27	3,882	1	*	13	2,695
Podiatry: Surg-Forefoot Only	*	*	2	*	2	*	1	*
Psychiatry: General	50	941	78	2,110	16	2,016	22	1,780
Psychiatry: Child & Adolescent	8	*	15	1,647	9	*	2	*
Psychiatry: Geriatric	5	*	0	*	*	*	0	*
Pulmonary Medicine	28	2,251	48	2,006	44	1,518	36	1,910
Pulmonary Medicine: Critical Care	0	*	12	1,472	7	*	13	1,109
Pulmonary Med: Gen & Crit Care	15	1,706	29	921	30	1,060	15	1,144
Radiation Oncology	5	*	12	939	18	1,350	20	582
Radiology: Diagnostic-Inv	9	*	20	1,004	10	10,736	39	7,705
Radiology: Diagnostic-Noninv	28	5,098	18	9,736	18	7,061	22	9,675
Radiology: Nuclear Medicine	2	*	3	*	8	*	1	*
Rheumatology	30	2,948	61	3,142	40	3,660	49	2,374
Sleep Medicine	1	*	4	*	19	1,909	9	*
Surgery: General	111	1,337	213	1,559	131	1,690	149	1,416
Surgery: Bariatric	5	*	5	*	2	*	3	*
Surgery: Cardiovascular	16	458	33	404	44	248	20	361
Surgery: Colon and Rectal	11	748	9	*	3	*	6	*
Surgery: Neurological	32	1,562	33	1,468	27	1,362	43	1,009
Surgery: Oncology	7	*	*	*	3	*	3	*
Surgery: Oral	2	*	3	*	2	*	1	*
Surgery: Pediatric	5	*	9	*	11	894	7	*
Surgery: Plastic & Reconstruction	10	1,610	20	2,158	17	1,594	20	1,706
Surgery: Plastic & Recon-Hand	0	*	0	*	2	*	1	*
Surgery: Thoracic (primary)	6	*	9	*	1	*	12	339
Surgery: Transplant	4	*	1	*	0	*	1	*
Surgery: Trauma	15	509	5	*	18	767	2	*
Surgery: Trauma-Burn	3	*	*	*	1	*	*	*
Surgery: Vascular (primary)	24	1,274	32	2,371	19	2,407	17	1,504
Urgent Care	10	5,232	93	5,197	24	4,935	146	4,333
Urology	47	2,798	78	2,598	156	2,878	66	2,301
Urology: Pediatric	1	*	4	*	3	*	4	*

Table 49: Physician Ambulatory Encounters (NPP Excluded) by Years in Specialty

	1 to 2 years		3 to 7 years		8 to 17 years		18 years or more	
	Phys	Median	Phys	Median	Phys	Median	Phys	Median
Allergy/Immunology	4	*	16	2,167	24	3,573	41	3,216
Anesthesiology	22	110	59	198	294	301	342	114
Anesthesiology: Pain Management	4	*	29	1,100	27	3,646	13	2,108
Anesthesiology: Pediatric	0	*	1	*	0	*	0	*
Cardiology: Electrophysiology	9	*	24	949	27	1,503	21	1,383
Cardiology: Invasive	17	2,463	45	2,341	82	2,425	69	1,877
Cardiology: Inv-Intvl	9	*	41	1,741	100	2,221	108	2,048
Cardiology: Noninvasive	12	1,539	38	2,329	59	2,347	98	2,307
Critical Care: Intensivist	3	*	3	*	4	*	2	*
Dentistry	2	*	3	*	2	*	6	*
Dermatology	10	4,109	42	4,410	68	4,161	55	4,314
Dermatology: Mohs Surgery	1	*	4	*	7	*	3	*
Emergency Medicine	24	2,614	69	2,743	90	2,665	55	2,384
Endocrinology/Metabolism	14	2,662	34	2,361	39	2,937	53	2,890
Family Practice (w/ OB)	30	3,046	130	3,637	195	3,786	148	3,998
Family Practice (w/o OB)	178	3,365	702	4,028	1,238	4,118	1,207	4,251
FP: Amb Only (no inpatient work)	2	*	13	4,866	26	3,039	30	4,389
Family Practice: Sports Med	7	*	7	*	6	*	6	*
Family Practice: Urgent Care	4	*	4	*	16	3,773	21	4,613
Gastroenterology	22	978	72	1,392	111	1,355	158	1,351
Gastroenterology: Hepatology	*	*	1	*	1	*	1	*
Genetics	*	*	0	*	0	*	2	*
Geriatrics	1	*	7	*	9	*	8	*
Hematology/Oncology	17	2,549	37	2,631	57	3,187	61	3,222
Hematology/Oncology: Onc (only)	0	*	4	*	2	*	16	3,802
Hospice/Palliative Care	1	*	2	*	2	*	1	*
Hospitalist: Family Practice	4	*	12	409	4	*	3	*
Hospitalist: Internal Medicine	73	95	165	93	120	177	28	114
Hospitalist: IM-Pediatrics	0	*	0	*	1	*	*	*
Hospitalist: Pediatrics	2	*	6	*	12	33	6	*
Infectious Disease	2	*	14	812	24	862	18	752
Internal Medicine: General	101	2,651	400	3,148	823	3,610	844	3,557
IM: Amb Only (no inpatient work)	*	*	*	*	1	*	8	*
Internal Med: Pediatrics	4	*	20	4,254	43	4,200	1	*
Nephrology	8	*	25	1,503	25	1,506	27	1,983
Neurology	23	1,215	74	2,058	92	1,979	118	2,191
Obstetrics/Gynecology: General	53	2,355	180	2,886	369	3,043	245	2,903
OB/GYN: Gynecology (only)	2	*	19	3,204	33	2,820	59	2,490
OB/GYN: Gyn Oncology	1	*	3	*	7	*	5	*
OB/GYN: Maternal & Fetal Med	1	*	4	*	11	1,783	8	*
OB/GYN: Repro Endocrinology	1	*	*	*	2	*	1	*
OB/GYN: Urogynecology	0	*	4	*	*	*	0	*
Occupational Medicine	2	*	10	2,256	17	3,428	31	3,628
Ophthalmology	10	4,152	20	4,831	83	4,702	100	5,114
Ophthalmology: Pediatric	1	*	4	*	7	*	5	*
Ophthalmology: Retina	1	*	3	*	13	6,921	5	*
Orthopedic (Nonsurgical)	1	*	4	*	3	*	20	2,822
Orthopedic Surgery: General	28	2,962	80	2,999	171	3,060	203	2,898
Orthopedic Surgery: Foot & Ankle	5	*	8	*	19	3,562	7	*
Orthopedic Surgery: Hand	8	*	16	3,244	41	3,552	31	3,515
Orthopedic Surgery: Hip & Joint	7	*	8	*	17	2,721	38	2,992
Orthopedic Surgery: Pediatric	0	*	2	*	7	*	3	*
Orthopedic Surgery: Spine	10	2,231	11	2,320	34	2,462	19	2,014
Orthopedic Surgery: Trauma	3	*	9	*	5	*	5	*
Orthopedic Surgery: Sports Med	8	*	21	3,703	38	3,691	45	3,471

Table 49: Physician Ambulatory Encounters (NPP Excluded) by Years in Specialty (continued)

	1 to 2 years		3 to 7 years		8 to 17 years		18 years or more	
	Phys	Median	Phys	Median	Phys	Median	Phys	Median
Otorhinolaryngology	6	*	46	3,428	88	3,440	86	3,170
Pathology: Anatomic and Clinical	0	*	3	*	3	*	1	*
Pathology: Anatomic	0	*	0	*	0	*	0	*
Pathology: Clinical	*	*	0	*	2	*	0	*
Pediatrics: General	90	3,917	338	4,364	655	4,349	572	4,544
Pediatrics: Adolescent Medicine	0	*	2	*	2	*	0	*
Pediatrics: Allergy/Immunology	*	*	0	*	0	*	1	*
Pediatrics: Cardiology	2	*	6	*	7	*	9	*
Pediatrics: Child Development	*	*	1	*	2	*	1	*
Pediatrics: Critical Care/Intensivist	0	*	6	*	5	*	4	*
Pediatrics: Emergency Medicine	1	*	6	*	6	*	5	*
Pediatrics: Endocrinology	2	*	6	*	5	*	6	*
Pediatrics: Gastroenterology	1	*	5	*	6	*	7	*
Pediatrics: Genetics	1	*	*	*	0	*	4	*
Pediatrics: Hematology/Oncology	6	*	12	1,024	10	991	8	*
Pediatrics: Infectious Disease	*	*	1	*	6	*	2	*
Pediatrics: Neonatal Medicine	2	*	9	*	12	10	8	*
Pediatrics: Nephrology	0	*	*	*	3	*	3	*
Pediatrics: Neurology	4	*	11	1,342	14	1,856	12	1,509
Pediatrics: Pulmonology	0	*	3	*	2	*	11	2,152
Pediatrics: Rheumatology	*	*	*	*	4	*	1	*
Physiatry (Phys Med & Rehab)	9	*	24	1,845	34	1,951	25	1,341
Podiatry: General	5	*	18	2,294	32	2,978	31	2,388
Podiatry: Surg-Foot & Ankle	5	*	14	3,446	10	4,517	10	2,614
Podiatry: Surg-Forefoot Only	*	*	1	*	2	*	1	*
Psychiatry: General	5	*	23	1,945	45	1,626	38	1,518
Psychiatry: Child & Adolescent	2	*	10	1,672	8	*	7	*
Psychiatry: Geriatric	*	*	*	*	2	*	3	*
Pulmonary Medicine	13	1,409	19	1,657	41	2,204	42	2,355
Pulmonary Medicine: Critical Care	0	*	3	*	15	1,388	7	*
Pulmonary Med: Gen & Crit Care	10	780	22	1,061	26	904	20	1,589
Radiation Oncology	4	*	9	*	25	808	11	1,042
Radiology: Diagnostic-Inv	6	*	12	1,350	30	6,905	20	7,180
Radiology: Diagnostic-Noninv	5	*	7	*	24	5,568	28	8,897
Radiology: Nuclear Medicine	0	*	2	*	5	*	2	*
Rheumatology	7	*	32	2,641	37	3,566	64	3,082
Sleep Medicine	2	*	8	*	5	*	13	2,964
Surgery: General	23	945	99	1,636	194	1,553	194	1,506
Surgery: Bariatric	1	*	2	*	3	*	3	*
Surgery: Cardiovascular	9	*	18	298	38	298	30	433
Surgery: Colon and Rectal	1	*	3	*	7	*	8	*
Surgery: Neurological	5	*	25	1,239	40	1,384	39	1,306
Surgery: Oncology	*	*	3	*	4	*	5	*
Surgery: Oral	0	*	1	*	2	*	5	*
Surgery: Pediatric	1	*	4	*	8	*	12	951
Surgery: Plastic & Reconstruction	5	*	16	1,402	16	2,220	16	1,476
Surgery: Plastic & Recon-Hand	0	*	0	*	2	*	0	*
Surgery: Thoracic (primary)	0	*	3	*	5	*	11	300
Surgery: Transplant	1	*	1	*	3	*	1	*
Surgery: Trauma	2	*	7	*	14	457	5	*
Surgery: Trauma-Burn	1	*	2	*	1	*	*	*
Surgery: Vascular (primary)	1	*	14	2,114	29	2,068	26	1,545
Urgent Care	17	4,938	57	5,162	74	4,832	78	4,398
Urology	13	2,374	44	2,323	98	2,906	134	2,815
Urology: Pediatric	1	*	3	*	3	*	4	*

Table 50: Physician Ambulatory Encounters (NPP Excluded) by Gender

	Male			Female		
	Phys	Med Pracs	Median	Phys	Med Pracs	Median
Allergy/Immunology	74	42	3,222	27	20	2,795
Anesthesiology	401	41	220	91	28	99
Anesthesiology: Pain Management	61	30	3,504	2	2	*
Anesthesiology: Pediatric	0	*	*	1	1	*
Cardiology: Electrophysiology	78	41	1,254	6	6	*
Cardiology: Invasive	209	68	2,159	18	17	2,797
Cardiology: Inv-Intvl	283	83	2,090	11	9	1,046
Cardiology: Noninvasive	211	73	2,274	28	21	1,962
Critical Care: Intensivist	11	6	14	4	2	*
Dentistry	19	6	2,436	7	4	*
Dermatology	114	66	4,819	91	46	3,716
Dermatology: Mohs Surgery	11	10	2,622	7	6	*
Emergency Medicine	267	23	2,682	73	19	2,492
Endocrinology/Metabolism	113	68	2,932	59	47	2,573
Family Practice (w/ OB)	380	97	4,320	238	79	3,308
Family Practice (w/o OB)	2,791	458	4,253	1,130	337	3,492
FP: Amb Only (no inpatient work)	88	18	4,600	41	10	3,543
Family Practice: Sports Med	26	20	3,127	3	3	*
Family Practice: Urgent Care	62	15	4,612	23	12	4,518
Gastroenterology	431	125	1,272	52	35	1,305
Gastroenterology: Hepatology	3	3	*	0	*	*
Genetics	0	*	*	2	1	*
Geriatrics	21	12	2,348	14	11	2,197
Hematology/Oncology	171	64	2,853	54	33	2,269
Hematology/Oncology: Onc (only)	27	18	3,183	1	1	*
Hospice/Palliative Care	5	5	*	1	1	*
Hospitalist: Family Practice	20	6	473	4	3	*
Hospitalist: Internal Medicine	275	58	100	127	42	71
Hospitalist: IM-Pediatrics	1	1	*	0	*	*
Hospitalist: Pediatrics	17	5	34	11	5	49
Infectious Disease	53	32	939	24	18	697
Internal Medicine: General	1,962	308	3,628	832	228	2,929
IM: Amb Only (no inpatient work)	18	7	3,860	10	9	2,496
Internal Med: Pediatrics	55	29	4,257	35	20	3,577
Nephrology	80	38	1,689	23	17	1,220
Neurology	286	101	2,089	91	61	1,754
Obstetrics/Gynecology: General	575	191	3,016	465	169	2,810
OB/GYN: Gynecology (only)	67	46	2,502	38	25	2,463
OB/GYN: Gyn Oncology	17	14	1,209	7	6	*
OB/GYN: Maternal & Fetal Med	22	10	1,624	12	8	1,073
OB/GYN: Repro Endocrinology	3	3	*	3	3	*
OB/GYN: Urogynecology	3	2	*	1	1	*
Occupational Medicine	62	31	2,952	12	8	4,088
Ophthalmology	222	80	4,954	41	29	4,719
Ophthalmology: Pediatric	13	11	4,130	8	7	*
Ophthalmology: Retina	26	16	6,493	2	2	*
Orthopedic (Nonsurgical)	30	24	2,848	3	3	*
Orthopedic Surgery: General	528	146	2,902	17	12	2,491
Orthopedic Surgery: Foot & Ankle	37	28	3,739	3	3	*
Orthopedic Surgery: Hand	96	51	3,484	9	7	*
Orthopedic Surgery: Hip & Joint	78	38	2,827	*	*	*
Orthopedic Surgery: Pediatric	12	9	3,734	1	1	*
Orthopedic Surgery: Spine	75	45	2,447	2	1	*
Orthopedic Surgery: Trauma	24	12	2,295	3	3	*
Orthopedic Surgery: Sports Med	122	51	3,594	4	4	*

Table 50: Physician Ambulatory Encounters (NPP Excluded) by Gender (continued)

	Male			Female		
	Phys	Med Pracs	Median	Phys	Med Pracs	Median
Otorhinolaryngology	246	89	3,341	30	21	2,616
Pathology: Anatomic and Clinical	4	2	*	3	2	*
Pathology: Anatomic	1	1	*	0	*	*
Pathology: Clinical	2	1	*	0	*	*
Pediatrics: General	942	211	4,765	949	219	4,021
Pediatrics: Adolescent Medicine	20	3	3,891	34	5	4,478
Pediatrics: Allergy/Immunology	1	1	*	0	*	*
Pediatrics: Cardiology	34	12	1,328	3	2	*
Pediatrics: Child Development	3	2	*	4	3	*
Pediatrics: Critical Care/Intensivist	13	7	30	7	4	*
Pediatrics: Emergency Medicine	9	3	*	9	2	*
Pediatrics: Endocrinology	11	9	2,036	12	10	1,573
Pediatrics: Gastroenterology	16	8	1,306	3	3	*
Pediatrics: Genetics	4	4	*	12	9	2,798
Pediatrics: Hematology/Oncology	28	14	1,018	15	8	1,020
Pediatrics: Infectious Disease	6	3	*	6	5	*
Pediatrics: Neonatal Medicine	20	6	12	11	5	12
Pediatrics: Nephrology	6	5	*	1	1	*
Pediatrics: Neurology	33	17	1,820	13	11	1,444
Pediatrics: Pulmonology	15	11	2,152	3	2	*
Pediatrics: Rheumatology	4	3	*	1	1	*
Physiatry (Phys Med & Rehab)	79	49	1,931	41	23	1,211
Podiatry: General	80	47	2,635	16	15	2,412
Podiatry: Surg-Foot & Ankle	38	16	3,719	9	9	*
Podiatry: Surg-Forefoot Only	5	3	*	*	*	*
Psychiatry: General	107	43	2,017	50	30	1,602
Psychiatry: Child & Adolescent	17	9	1,669	15	10	1,467
Psychiatry: Geriatric	5	2	*	*	*	*
Pulmonary Medicine	134	66	1,903	22	17	1,506
Pulmonary Medicine: Critical Care	26	10	1,565	6	5	*
Pulmonary Med: Gen & Crit Care	74	21	1,109	13	8	1,232
Radiation Oncology	41	15	808	14	9	838
Radiology: Diagnostic-Inv	71	18	4,664	7	4	*
Radiology: Diagnostic-Noninv	76	20	9,222	10	6	5,098
Radiology: Nuclear Medicine	14	9	3,977	0	*	*
Rheumatology	119	74	3,263	55	37	2,485
Sleep Medicine	30	18	2,003	3	3	*
Surgery: General	506	164	1,516	72	52	1,273
Surgery: Bariatric	14	9	1,356	0	*	*
Surgery: Cardiovascular	111	40	318	2	2	*
Surgery: Colon and Rectal	25	13	1,330	4	4	*
Surgery: Neurological	121	44	1,306	8	8	*
Surgery: Oncology	9	8	*	4	2	*
Surgery: Oral	8	6	*	0	*	*
Surgery: Pediatric	24	14	964	8	8	*
Surgery: Plastic & Reconstruction	55	33	1,933	12	10	1,172
Surgery: Plastic & Recon-Hand	3	3	*	0	*	*
Surgery: Thoracic (primary)	26	11	310	2	2	*
Surgery: Transplant	6	4	*	0	*	*
Surgery: Trauma	36	11	613	4	3	*
Surgery: Trauma-Burn	2	2	*	2	1	*
Surgery: Vascular (primary)	84	40	1,772	7	7	*
Urgent Care	205	43	4,834	66	28	4,049
Urology	313	92	2,756	26	17	2,540
Urology: Pediatric	7	5	*	5	4	*

Table 51: Physician Hospital Encounters (NPP Excluded)

	Phys	Med Pracs	Mean	Std. Dev.	25th %tile	Median	75th %tile	90th %tile
Allergy/Immunology	15	10	75	141	13	22	73	320
Anesthesiology	1,024	61	475	418	160	336	774	942
Anesthesiology: Pain Management	58	22	716	938	24	148	1,902	2,247
Anesthesiology: Pediatric	14	2	*	*	*	*	*	*
Cardiology: Electrophysiology	84	43	802	508	406	766	1,107	1,510
Cardiology: Invasive	223	61	1,491	1,034	729	1,264	1,975	3,222
Cardiology: Inv-Intvl	280	76	1,463	1,143	654	1,182	1,765	3,046
Cardiology: Noninvasive	223	64	1,149	819	602	970	1,501	2,202
Critical Care: Intensivist	21	7	1,234	369	944	1,202	1,488	1,762
Dentistry	3	1	*	*	*	*	*	*
Dermatology	44	31	33	29	13	21	45	77
Dermatology: Mohs Surgery	9	6	*	*	*	*	*	*
Emergency Medicine	54	5	61	58	10	40	96	150
Endocrinology/Metabolism	109	57	462	445	109	332	660	1,161
Family Practice (w/ OB)	437	85	344	231	164	308	493	666
Family Practice (w/o OB)	1,807	273	374	405	88	258	524	838
FP: Amb Only (no inpatient work)	17	2	*	*	*	*	*	*
Family Practice: Sports Med	10	7	126	143	17	67	200	425
Family Practice: Urgent Care	3	2	*	*	*	*	*	*
Gastroenterology	430	104	646	502	237	538	903	1,344
Gastroenterology: Hepatology	2	2	*	*	*	*	*	*
Genetics	2	1	*	*	*	*	*	*
Geriatrics	15	9	581	539	70	375	932	1,541
Hematology/Oncology	211	56	722	511	336	619	982	1,355
Hematology/Oncology: Onc (only)	23	15	998	889	346	641	1,347	2,678
Hospice/Palliative Care	6	6	*	*	*	*	*	*
Hospitalist: Family Practice	26	6	2,099	771	1,540	1,917	2,552	3,283
Hospitalist: Internal Medicine	594	83	2,157	1,006	1,433	2,005	2,863	3,538
Hospitalist: IM-Pediatrics	1	1	*	*	*	*	*	*
Hospitalist: Pediatrics	51	13	1,337	533	986	1,367	1,670	1,957
Infectious Disease	75	37	2,282	1,408	1,373	1,998	2,908	4,831
Internal Medicine: General	1,755	230	796	877	209	521	1,012	1,840
IM: Amb Only (no inpatient work)	3	3	*	*	*	*	*	*
Internal Med: Pediatrics	66	25	456	426	162	335	648	1,069
Nephrology	105	40	1,536	976	841	1,436	1,881	2,725
Neurology	316	92	589	475	242	418	905	1,323
Obstetrics/Gynecology: General	475	112	48	25	26	43	69	87
OB/GYN: Gynecology (only)	47	34	60	175	3	7	37	168
OB/GYN: Gyn Oncology	21	14	158	127	36	137	273	368
OB/GYN: Maternal & Fetal Med	27	11	393	226	196	347	557	732
OB/GYN: Repro Endocrinology	4	3	*	*	*	*	*	*
OB/GYN: Urogynecology	4	3	*	*	*	*	*	*
Occupational Medicine	5	5	*	*	*	*	*	*
Ophthalmology	166	61	23	58	3	9	16	45
Ophthalmology: Pediatric	10	7	158	139	56	100	290	421
Ophthalmology: Retina	14	6	65	59	24	42	93	187
Orthopedic (Nonsurgical)	6	5	*	*	*	*	*	*
Orthopedic Surgery: General	368	106	134	150	43	88	151	312
Orthopedic Surgery: Foot & Ankle	28	20	84	51	34	88	128	151
Orthopedic Surgery: Hand	50	30	68	62	26	49	83	170
Orthopedic Surgery: Hip & Joint	42	21	112	80	58	89	158	220
Orthopedic Surgery: Pediatric	10	8	128	65	92	121	170	240
Orthopedic Surgery: Spine	50	29	129	99	53	108	181	272
Orthopedic Surgery: Trauma	22	12	139	83	59	149	200	245
Orthopedic Surgery: Sports Med	80	32	80	55	43	66	104	149

Table 51: Physician Hospital Encounters (NPP Excluded) (continued)

	Phys	Med Pracs	Mean	Std. Dev.	25th %tile	Median	75th %tile	90th %tile
Otorhinolaryngology	192	69	107	127	40	63	126	229
Pathology: Anatomic and Clinical	6	2	*	*	*	*	*	*
Pathology: Anatomic	1	1	*	*	*	*	*	*
Pathology: Clinical	2	1	*	*	*	*	*	*
Pediatrics: General	1,576	201	283	228	126	227	377	555
Pediatrics: Adolescent Medicine	43	4	222	220	80	135	267	659
Pediatrics: Allergy/Immunology	1	1	*	*	*	*	*	*
Pediatrics: Cardiology	34	10	602	369	310	524	856	1,159
Pediatrics: Child Development	4	2	*	*	*	*	*	*
Pediatrics: Critical Care/Intensivist	49	13	944	541	554	750	1,119	1,935
Pediatrics: Emergency Medicine	4	2	*	*	*	*	*	*
Pediatrics: Endocrinology	19	13	320	320	115	223	452	982
Pediatrics: Gastroenterology	20	9	501	336	248	357	808	1,008
Pediatrics: Genetics	6	4	*	*	*	*	*	*
Pediatrics: Hematology/Oncology	39	11	1,027	470	612	908	1,470	1,664
Pediatrics: Infectious Disease	12	6	1,621	744	1,057	1,387	2,316	2,837
Pediatrics: Neonatal Medicine	72	13	1,924	799	1,421	1,978	2,416	2,991
Pediatrics: Nephrology	7	6	*	*	*	*	*	*
Pediatrics: Neurology	38	18	482	330	251	426	643	917
Pediatrics: Pulmonology	15	9	1,478	1,127	355	1,275	2,398	3,620
Pediatrics: Rheumatology	5	3	*	*	*	*	*	*
Physiatry (Phys Med & Rehab)	34	19	278	284	50	165	443	761
Podiatry: General	25	19	71	55	31	44	80	183
Podiatry: Surg-Foot & Ankle	14	9	118	102	48	81	146	320
Podiatry: Surg-Forefoot Only	3	2	*	*	*	*	*	*
Psychiatry: General	102	31	1,009	1,011	199	588	1,565	2,526
Psychiatry: Child & Adolescent	23	13	483	396	93	450	711	1,185
Psychiatry: Geriatric	5	2	*	*	*	*	*	*
Pulmonary Medicine	123	51	1,673	1,275	550	1,470	2,499	3,525
Pulmonary Medicine: Critical Care	37	11	1,589	916	1,027	1,354	2,141	2,967
Pulmonary Med: Gen & Crit Care	87	22	2,286	1,402	1,214	2,097	2,905	4,396
Radiation Oncology	45	13	63	44	29	51	87	116
Radiology: Diagnostic-Inv	51	11	2,189	1,510	724	2,321	3,325	4,435
Radiology: Diagnostic-Noninv	128	14	8,131	10,388	13	282	16,933	26,008
Radiology: Nuclear Medicine	3	2	*	*	*	*	*	*
Rheumatology	99	57	119	89	46	104	154	277
Sleep Medicine	22	12	433	339	127	434	667	864
Surgery: General	498	138	361	269	160	300	499	740
Surgery: Bariatric	15	9	339	172	196	261	523	596
Surgery: Cardiovascular	112	37	295	287	126	221	358	507
Surgery: Colon and Rectal	27	13	259	271	65	165	322	777
Surgery: Neurological	128	43	396	313	164	338	581	774
Surgery: Oncology	9	8	*	*	*	*	*	*
Surgery: Oral	4	3	*	*	*	*	*	*
Surgery: Pediatric	32	17	541	384	199	558	784	1,094
Surgery: Plastic & Reconstruction	11	8	161	46	126	160	198	244
Surgery: Plastic & Recon-Hand	1	1	*	*	*	*	*	*
Surgery: Thoracic (primary)	28	11	230	155	123	176	303	488
Surgery: Transplant	13	5	1,215	808	481	1,116	2,045	2,236
Surgery: Trauma	38	10	1,519	698	1,120	1,323	2,099	2,668
Surgery: Trauma-Burn	4	2	*	*	*	*	*	*
Surgery: Vascular (primary)	79	34	465	325	241	389	588	907
Urgent Care	26	12	64	124	2	6	30	317
Urology	291	72	240	205	81	167	357	553
Urology: Pediatric	7	4	*	*	*	*	*	*

Table 52: Physician Hospital Encounters (NPP Excluded) by Group Type

	Single Specialty			Multispecialty		
	Phys	Med Pracs	Median	Phys	Med Pracs	Median
Allergy/Immunology	2	1	*	13	9	35
Anesthesiology	878	49	413	146	12	143
Anesthesiology: Pain Management	21	7	2,247	37	15	37
Anesthesiology: Pediatric	13	1	*	1	1	*
Cardiology: Electrophysiology	53	25	812	31	18	608
Cardiology: Invasive	115	27	1,227	108	34	1,295
Cardiology: Inv-Intvl	165	38	1,215	115	38	1,076
Cardiology: Noninvasive	94	25	1,197	129	39	914
Critical Care: Intensivist	3	1	*	18	6	1,176
Dentistry	0	*	*	3	1	*
Dermatology	1	1	*	43	30	22
Dermatology: Mohs Surgery	1	1	*	8	5	*
Emergency Medicine	0	*	*	54	5	40
Endocrinology/Metabolism	6	5	*	103	52	363
Family Practice (w/ OB)	72	18	398	365	67	298
Family Practice (w/o OB)	238	88	205	1,569	185	268
FP: Amb Only (no inpatient work)	0	*	*	17	2	*
Family Practice: Sports Med	3	2	*	7	5	*
Family Practice: Urgent Care	0	*	*	3	2	*
Gastroenterology	172	20	695	258	84	448
Gastroenterology: Hepatology	2	2	*	0	*	*
Genetics	*	*	*	2	1	*
Geriatrics	2	2	*	13	7	375
Hematology/Oncology	49	10	796	162	46	559
Hematology/Oncology: Onc (only)	3	2	*	20	13	675
Hospice/Palliative Care	2	2	*	4	4	*
Hospitalist: Family Practice	0	*	*	26	6	1,917
Hospitalist: Internal Medicine	104	13	2,856	490	70	1,847
Hospitalist: IM-Pediatrics	*	*	*	1	1	*
Hospitalist: Pediatrics	9	1	*	42	12	1,310
Infectious Disease	8	5	*	67	32	2,058
Internal Medicine: General	172	38	538	1,583	192	520
IM: Amb Only (no inpatient work)	0	*	*	3	3	*
Internal Med: Pediatrics	0	*	*	66	25	335
Nephrology	21	4	1,542	84	36	1,353
Neurology	76	20	399	240	72	432
Obstetrics/Gynecology: General	93	27	39	382	85	44
OB/GYN: Gynecology (only)	10	8	26	37	26	7
OB/GYN: Gyn Oncology	5	3	*	16	11	143
OB/GYN: Maternal & Fetal Med	8	3	*	19	8	419
OB/GYN: Repro Endocrinology	0	*	*	4	3	*
OB/GYN: Urogynecology	*	*	*	4	3	*
Occupational Medicine	0	*	*	5	5	*
Ophthalmology	42	11	9	124	50	9
Ophthalmology: Pediatric	1	1	*	9	6	*
Ophthalmology: Retina	11	4	55	3	2	*
Orthopedic (Nonsurgical)	2	2	*	4	3	*
Orthopedic Surgery: General	97	33	100	271	73	77
Orthopedic Surgery: Foot & Ankle	15	12	46	13	8	122
Orthopedic Surgery: Hand	25	15	30	25	15	64
Orthopedic Surgery: Hip & Joint	26	14	72	16	7	131
Orthopedic Surgery: Pediatric	2	2	*	8	6	*
Orthopedic Surgery: Spine	20	16	88	30	13	120
Orthopedic Surgery: Trauma	12	7	91	10	5	174
Orthopedic Surgery: Sports Med	34	20	63	46	12	76

Table 52: Physician Hospital Encounters (NPP Excluded) by Group Type (continued)

	Single Specialty			Multispecialty		
	Phys	Med Pracs	Median	Phys	Med Pracs	Median
Otorhinolaryngology	41	8	79	151	61	61
Pathology: Anatomic and Clinical	0	*	*	6	2	*
Pathology: Anatomic	*	*	*	1	1	*
Pathology: Clinical	0	*	*	2	1	*
Pediatrics: General	437	45	200	1,139	156	239
Pediatrics: Adolescent Medicine	2	1	*	41	3	128
Pediatrics: Allergy/Immunology	0	*	*	1	1	*
Pediatrics: Cardiology	1	1	*	33	9	529
Pediatrics: Child Development	*	*	*	4	2	*
Pediatrics: Critical Care/Intensivist	7	1	*	42	12	797
Pediatrics: Emergency Medicine	0	*	*	4	2	*
Pediatrics: Endocrinology	0	*	*	19	13	223
Pediatrics: Gastroenterology	0	*	*	20	9	357
Pediatrics: Genetics	0	*	*	6	4	*
Pediatrics: Hematology/Oncology	0	*	*	39	11	908
Pediatrics: Infectious Disease	*	*	*	12	6	1,387
Pediatrics: Neonatal Medicine	16	3	2,002	56	10	1,950
Pediatrics: Nephrology	*	*	*	7	6	*
Pediatrics: Neurology	2	1	*	36	17	438
Pediatrics: Pulmonology	0	*	*	15	9	1,275
Pediatrics: Rheumatology	*	*	*	5	3	*
Physiatry (Phys Med & Rehab)	8	4	*	26	15	131
Podiatry: General	1	1	*	24	18	50
Podiatry: Surg-Foot & Ankle	0	*	*	14	9	81
Podiatry: Surg-Forefoot Only	0	*	*	3	2	*
Psychiatry: General	6	1	*	96	30	538
Psychiatry: Child & Adolescent	0	*	*	23	13	450
Psychiatry: Geriatric	4	1	*	1	1	*
Pulmonary Medicine	13	4	1,733	110	47	1,192
Pulmonary Medicine: Critical Care	4	2	*	33	9	1,281
Pulmonary Med: Gen & Crit Care	34	6	1,941	53	16	2,114
Radiation Oncology	15	3	61	30	10	47
Radiology: Diagnostic-Inv	28	5	3,220	23	6	724
Radiology: Diagnostic-Noninv	54	6	19,733	74	8	23
Radiology: Nuclear Medicine	0	*	*	3	2	*
Rheumatology	5	4	*	94	53	104
Sleep Medicine	0	*	*	22	12	434
Surgery: General	83	19	485	415	119	262
Surgery: Bariatric	6	3	*	9	6	*
Surgery: Cardiovascular	49	14	209	63	23	229
Surgery: Colon and Rectal	*	*	*	27	13	165
Surgery: Neurological	35	9	441	93	34	317
Surgery: Oncology	1	1	*	8	7	*
Surgery: Oral	0	*	*	4	3	*
Surgery: Pediatric	10	4	612	22	13	505
Surgery: Plastic & Reconstruction	0	*	*	11	8	160
Surgery: Plastic & Recon-Hand	0	*	*	1	1	*
Surgery: Thoracic (primary)	11	4	181	17	7	171
Surgery: Transplant	7	1	*	6	4	*
Surgery: Trauma	5	2	*	33	8	1,341
Surgery: Trauma-Burn	*	*	*	4	2	*
Surgery: Vascular (primary)	8	5	*	71	29	371
Urgent Care	0	*	*	26	12	6
Urology	149	15	203	142	57	151
Urology: Pediatric	4	2	*	3	2	*

Table 53: Physician Surgery/Anesthesia Cases (NPP Excluded)

	Phys	Med Pracs	Mean	Std. Dev.	25th %tile	Median	75th %tile	90th %tile
Allergy/Immunology	9	9	*	*	*	*	*	*
Anesthesiology	2,382	113	1,145	939	796	1,010	1,252	1,700
Anesthesiology: Pain Management	59	20	2,067	1,428	735	1,844	3,846	3,997
Anesthesiology: Pediatric	24	3	1,064	286	693	1,145	1,304	1,412
Cardiology: Electrophysiology	37	23	252	123	155	249	342	404
Cardiology: Invasive	76	34	133	133	36	82	213	333
Cardiology: Inv-Intvl	128	46	245	255	68	138	327	684
Cardiology: Noninvasive	20	14	168	153	63	138	181	482
Critical Care: Intensivist	10	5	87	61	21	107	140	160
Dentistry	0	*	*	*	*	*	*	*
Dermatology	125	54	3,210	1,908	1,809	2,872	4,275	5,531
Dermatology: Mohs Surgery	10	9	3,293	2,565	1,389	2,216	6,545	7,311
Emergency Medicine	52	7	260	206	120	190	393	506
Endocrinology/Metabolism	65	36	291	477	51	98	223	1,303
Family Practice (w/ OB)	232	45	274	193	126	243	383	584
Family Practice (w/o OB)	1,841	219	373	526	92	173	364	1,105
FP: Amb Only (no inpatient work)	13	3	25	23	5	18	41	67
Family Practice: Sports Med	14	9	732	568	180	612	1,272	1,617
Family Practice: Urgent Care	21	7	202	107	121	202	275	371
Gastroenterology	312	91	1,566	690	1,166	1,456	1,862	2,283
Gastroenterology: Hepatology	2	2	*	*	*	*	*	*
Genetics	2	1	*	*	*	*	*	*
Geriatrics	12	6	24	27	2	14	49	71
Hematology/Oncology	73	33	266	415	54	92	226	922
Hematology/Oncology: Onc (only)	10	7	116	67	59	114	150	241
Hospice/Palliative Care	0	*	*	*	*	*	*	*
Hospitalist: Family Practice	18	2	*	*	*	*	*	*
Hospitalist: Internal Medicine	43	17	26	20	14	20	31	64
Hospitalist: IM-Pediatrics	0	*	*	*	*	*	*	*
Hospitalist: Pediatrics	8	5	*	*	*	*	*	*
Infectious Disease	14	10	130	163	26	71	170	486
Internal Medicine: General	1,054	136	417	719	45	107	301	1,664
IM: Amb Only (no inpatient work)	5	3	*	*	*	*	*	*
Internal Med: Pediatrics	56	21	336	556	48	87	283	1,619
Nephrology	30	15	292	409	36	65	533	1,027
Neurology	116	52	171	183	38	92	239	446
Obstetrics/Gynecology: General	711	143	545	363	296	488	717	966
OB/GYN: Gynecology (only)	49	32	366	216	187	343	447	681
OB/GYN: Gyn Oncology	11	9	307	130	204	285	385	557
OB/GYN: Maternal & Fetal Med	24	9	840	489	513	988	1,229	1,375
OB/GYN: Repro Endocrinology	3	3	*	*	*	*	*	*
OB/GYN: Urogynecology	3	2	*	*	*	*	*	*
Occupational Medicine	44	17	118	106	59	84	147	238
Ophthalmology	236	68	583	418	296	469	766	1,154
Ophthalmology: Pediatric	17	12	439	254	218	388	692	812
Ophthalmology: Retina	24	15	459	439	127	242	779	1,067
Orthopedic (Nonsurgical)	13	10	832	835	269	626	1,257	2,470
Orthopedic Surgery: General	437	117	798	526	422	649	1,005	1,555
Orthopedic Surgery: Foot & Ankle	35	26	615	386	382	516	684	1,239
Orthopedic Surgery: Hand	92	46	714	505	411	590	761	1,285
Orthopedic Surgery: Hip & Joint	75	38	529	269	358	456	626	908
Orthopedic Surgery: Pediatric	5	5	*	*	*	*	*	*
Orthopedic Surgery: Spine	71	41	448	375	225	327	457	944
Orthopedic Surgery: Trauma	22	13	647	546	359	418	657	1,710
Orthopedic Surgery: Sports Med	114	47	687	503	396	529	797	1,379

Table 53: Physician Surgery/Anesthesia Cases (NPP Excluded) (continued)

	Phys	Med Pracs	Mean	Std. Dev.	25th %tile	Median	75th %tile	90th %tile
Otorhinolaryngology	201	67	938	597	428	919	1,291	1,809
Pathology: Anatomic and Clinical	2	1	*	*	*	*	*	*
Pathology: Anatomic	1	1	*	*	*	*	*	*
Pathology: Clinical	7	1	*	*	*	*	*	*
Pediatrics: General	776	111	207	242	62	110	239	561
Pediatrics: Adolescent Medicine	8	2	*	*	*	*	*	*
Pediatrics: Allergy/Immunology	0	*	*	*	*	*	*	*
Pediatrics: Cardiology	7	4	*	*	*	*	*	*
Pediatrics: Child Development	0	*	*	*	*	*	*	*
Pediatrics: Critical Care/Intensivist	17	4	16	11	8	14	22	41
Pediatrics: Emergency Medicine	1	1	*	*	*	*	*	*
Pediatrics: Endocrinology	1	1	*	*	*	*	*	*
Pediatrics: Gastroenterology	5	4	*	*	*	*	*	*
Pediatrics: Genetics	0	*	*	*	*	*	*	*
Pediatrics: Hematology/Oncology	14	5	87	49	46	75	137	161
Pediatrics: Infectious Disease	2	2	*	*	*	*	*	*
Pediatrics: Neonatal Medicine	37	5	46	40	9	33	80	111
Pediatrics: Nephrology	1	1	*	*	*	*	*	*
Pediatrics: Neurology	7	6	*	*	*	*	*	*
Pediatrics: Pulmonology	6	5	*	*	*	*	*	*
Pediatrics: Rheumatology	1	1	*	*	*	*	*	*
Physiatry (Phys Med & Rehab)	46	28	542	508	104	384	1,101	1,373
Podiatry: General	63	33	1,803	941	1,025	1,881	2,388	2,967
Podiatry: Surg-Foot & Ankle	32	15	1,458	861	1,011	1,403	1,883	2,845
Podiatry: Surg-Forefoot Only	2	1	*	*	*	*	*	*
Psychiatry: General	8	4	*	*	*	*	*	*
Psychiatry: Child & Adolescent	4	2	*	*	*	*	*	*
Psychiatry: Geriatric	0	*	*	*	*	*	*	*
Pulmonary Medicine	92	36	195	149	85	149	259	418
Pulmonary Medicine: Critical Care	16	6	202	144	89	174	283	445
Pulmonary Med: Gen & Crit Care	59	15	166	147	62	107	221	409
Radiation Oncology	17	4	16	20	2	6	29	49
Radiology: Diagnostic-Inv	79	15	668	605	260	489	914	1,860
Radiology: Diagnostic-Noninv	135	23	213	321	30	83	254	641
Radiology: Nuclear Medicine	5	4	*	*	*	*	*	*
Rheumatology	105	55	663	628	249	469	886	1,486
Sleep Medicine	11	4	653	437	29	828	997	1,078
Surgery: General	446	130	689	328	469	637	863	1,143
Surgery: Bariatric	13	7	585	175	528	633	696	781
Surgery: Cardiovascular	81	32	348	155	248	306	416	603
Surgery: Colon and Rectal	31	13	1,218	526	901	1,261	1,634	1,802
Surgery: Neurological	113	35	403	260	243	325	476	724
Surgery: Oncology	11	8	1,186	918	396	892	1,929	2,854
Surgery: Oral	7	5	*	*	*	*	*	*
Surgery: Pediatric	24	12	650	356	374	525	847	1,252
Surgery: Plastic & Reconstruction	42	24	654	371	391	537	845	1,226
Surgery: Plastic & Recon-Hand	1	1	*	*	*	*	*	*
Surgery: Thoracic (primary)	23	10	250	205	110	249	331	388
Surgery: Transplant	10	3	257	103	174	280	356	388
Surgery: Trauma	30	9	295	191	196	237	339	490
Surgery: Trauma-Burn	1	1	*	*	*	*	*	*
Surgery: Vascular (primary)	72	33	685	396	384	665	971	1,240
Urgent Care	204	30	459	324	204	382	663	966
Urology	287	70	1,388	824	843	1,316	1,814	2,438
Urology: Pediatric	6	3	*	*	*	*	*	*

Table 54: Physician Surgery/Anesthesia Cases (NPP Excluded) by Group Type

	Single Specialty			Multispecialty		
	Phys	Med Pracs	Median	Phys	Med Pracs	Median
Allergy/Immunology	0	*	*	9	9	*
Anesthesiology	2,142	95	1,015	240	18	851
Anesthesiology: Pain Management	38	11	2,194	21	9	1,581
Anesthesiology: Pediatric	23	2	*	1	1	*
Cardiology: Electrophysiology	21	13	284	16	10	199
Cardiology: Invasive	26	12	74	50	22	82
Cardiology: Inv-Intvl	52	18	135	76	28	153
Cardiology: Noninvasive	2	2	*	18	12	138
Critical Care: Intensivist	0	*	*	10	5	107
Dentistry	0	*	*	0	*	*
Dermatology	19	4	2,556	106	50	2,941
Dermatology: Mohs Surgery	1	1	*	9	8	*
Emergency Medicine	0	*	*	52	7	190
Endocrinology/Metabolism	5	4	*	60	32	101
Family Practice (w/ OB)	36	8	283	196	37	222
Family Practice (w/o OB)	280	94	133	1,561	125	185
FP: Amb Only (no inpatient work)	1	1	*	12	2	*
Family Practice: Sports Med	4	3	*	10	6	612
Family Practice: Urgent Care	0	*	*	21	7	202
Gastroenterology	105	17	1,463	207	74	1,453
Gastroenterology: Hepatology	2	2	*	0	*	*
Genetics	*	*	*	2	1	*
Geriatrics	0	*	*	12	6	14
Hematology/Oncology	4	2	*	69	31	97
Hematology/Oncology: Onc (only)	0	*	*	10	7	114
Hospice/Palliative Care	0	*	*	0	*	*
Hospitalist: Family Practice	0	*	*	18	2	*
Hospitalist: Internal Medicine	1	1	*	42	16	21
Hospitalist: IM-Pediatrics	*	*	*	0	*	*
Hospitalist: Pediatrics	0	*	*	8	5	*
Infectious Disease	1	1	*	13	9	94
Internal Medicine: General	82	23	87	972	113	109
IM: Amb Only (no inpatient work)	0	*	*	5	3	*
Internal Med: Pediatrics	0	*	*	56	21	87
Nephrology	0	*	*	30	15	65
Neurology	21	9	153	95	43	79
Obstetrics/Gynecology: General	196	44	377	515	99	545
OB/GYN: Gynecology (only)	12	7	285	37	25	363
OB/GYN: Gyn Oncology	1	1	*	10	8	278
OB/GYN: Maternal & Fetal Med	6	2	*	18	7	988
OB/GYN: Repro Endocrinology	0	*	*	3	3	*
OB/GYN: Urogynecology	*	*	*	3	2	*
Occupational Medicine	0	*	*	44	17	84
Ophthalmology	100	19	462	136	49	469
Ophthalmology: Pediatric	8	7	*	9	5	*
Ophthalmology: Retina	18	9	242	6	6	*
Orthopedic (Nonsurgical)	6	4	*	7	6	*
Orthopedic Surgery: General	153	47	556	284	70	731
Orthopedic Surgery: Foot & Ankle	21	17	516	14	9	498
Orthopedic Surgery: Hand	59	29	538	33	17	679
Orthopedic Surgery: Hip & Joint	52	28	445	23	10	497
Orthopedic Surgery: Pediatric	3	3	*	2	2	*
Orthopedic Surgery: Spine	40	28	327	31	13	327
Orthopedic Surgery: Trauma	12	7	411	10	6	441
Orthopedic Surgery: Sports Med	60	32	582	54	15	506

Table 54: Physician Surgery/Anesthesia Cases (NPP Excluded) by Group Type (continued)

	Single Specialty			Multispecialty		
	Phys	Med Pracs	Median	Phys	Med Pracs	Median
Otorhinolaryngology	59	9	481	142	58	1,064
Pathology: Anatomic and Clinical	0	*	*	2	1	*
Pathology: Anatomic	*	*	*	1	1	*
Pathology: Clinical	0	*	*	7	1	*
Pediatrics: General	93	18	63	683	93	120
Pediatrics: Adolescent Medicine	0	*	*	8	2	*
Pediatrics: Allergy/Immunology	0	*	*	0	*	*
Pediatrics: Cardiology	2	1	*	5	3	*
Pediatrics: Child Development	*	*	*	0	*	*
Pediatrics: Critical Care/Intensivist	6	1	*	11	3	14
Pediatrics: Emergency Medicine	0	*	*	1	1	*
Pediatrics: Endocrinology	0	*	*	1	1	*
Pediatrics: Gastroenterology	0	*	*	5	4	*
Pediatrics: Genetics	0	*	*	0	*	*
Pediatrics: Hematology/Oncology	0	*	*	14	5	75
Pediatrics: Infectious Disease	*	*	*	2	2	*
Pediatrics: Neonatal Medicine	4	1	*	33	4	28
Pediatrics: Nephrology	*	*	*	1	1	*
Pediatrics: Neurology	2	1	*	5	5	*
Pediatrics: Pulmonology	0	*	*	6	5	*
Pediatrics: Rheumatology	*	*	*	1	1	*
Physiatry (Phys Med & Rehab)	15	7	210	31	21	447
Podiatry: General	1	1	*	62	32	1,893
Podiatry: Surg-Foot & Ankle	2	2	*	30	13	1,464
Podiatry: Surg-Forefoot Only	0	*	*	2	1	*
Psychiatry: General	0	*	*	8	4	*
Psychiatry: Child & Adolescent	0	*	*	4	2	*
Psychiatry: Geriatric	0	*	*	0	*	*
Pulmonary Medicine	11	3	175	81	33	143
Pulmonary Medicine: Critical Care	1	1	*	15	5	142
Pulmonary Med: Gen & Crit Care	26	4	67	33	11	186
Radiation Oncology	8	1	*	9	3	*
Radiology: Diagnostic-Inv	31	3	515	48	12	459
Radiology: Diagnostic-Noninv	14	3	794	121	20	62
Radiology: Nuclear Medicine	0	*	*	5	4	*
Rheumatology	4	4	*	101	51	474
Sleep Medicine	0	*	*	11	4	828
Surgery: General	93	24	588	353	106	655
Surgery: Bariatric	6	3	*	7	4	*
Surgery: Cardiovascular	38	12	309	43	20	289
Surgery: Colon and Rectal	*	*	*	31	13	1,261
Surgery: Neurological	34	8	334	79	27	319
Surgery: Oncology	1	1	*	10	7	842
Surgery: Oral	0	*	*	7	5	*
Surgery: Pediatric	11	4	534	13	8	378
Surgery: Plastic & Reconstruction	5	2	*	37	22	528
Surgery: Plastic & Recon-Hand	1	1	*	0	*	*
Surgery: Thoracic (primary)	10	4	184	13	6	255
Surgery: Transplant	7	1	*	3	2	*
Surgery: Trauma	6	2	*	24	7	229
Surgery: Trauma-Burn	*	*	*	1	1	*
Surgery: Vascular (primary)	9	6	*	63	27	608
Urgent Care	2	1	*	202	29	384
Urology	153	16	1,433	134	54	1,132
Urology: Pediatric	4	2	*	2	1	*

Table 55: Total RVUs (CMS RBRVS Method) (TC/NPP Excluded)

	Phys	Med Pracs	Mean	Std. Dev.	25th %tile	Median	75th %tile	90th %tile
Allergy/Immunology	39	20	11,722	5,439	7,490	10,479	13,192	20,862
Anesthesiology	1,957	90	13,417	6,177	9,488	13,625	15,782	21,730
Anesthesiology: Pain Management	27	15	20,002	10,069	10,183	19,503	28,329	34,276
Anesthesiology: Pediatric	23	3	8,114	3,841	3,826	6,888	12,732	13,210
Cardiology: Electrophysiology	40	18	20,664	9,275	13,365	19,962	24,213	37,025
Cardiology: Invasive	118	29	20,738	10,292	14,182	18,419	26,688	33,660
Cardiology: Inv-Intvl	139	33	24,159	14,066	16,148	20,364	26,295	45,684
Cardiology: Noninvasive	128	26	19,562	11,094	10,122	18,056	25,768	35,826
Critical Care: Intensivist	4	2	*	*	*	*	*	*
Dentistry	6	2	*	*	*	*	*	*
Dermatology	123	46	20,231	16,599	11,310	16,414	23,146	33,333
Dermatology: Mohs Surgery	9	8	*	*	*	*	*	*
Emergency Medicine	185	14	8,274	2,892	6,445	8,155	10,074	11,800
Endocrinology/Metabolism	99	50	9,560	5,624	6,586	8,791	11,106	14,694
Family Practice (w/ OB)	225	37	9,631	3,170	7,489	9,194	11,453	13,880
Family Practice (w/o OB)	1,652	142	9,298	4,696	6,920	8,830	10,874	12,928
FP: Amb Only (no inpatient work)	17	2	*	*	*	*	*	*
Family Practice: Sports Med	14	9	11,842	8,509	5,544	9,968	16,408	28,463
Family Practice: Urgent Care	18	5	8,505	3,283	6,656	7,317	9,711	13,288
Gastroenterology	256	60	18,185	7,268	12,968	17,218	22,499	27,055
Gastroenterology: Hepatology	1	1	*	*	*	*	*	*
Genetics	2	1	*	*	*	*	*	*
Geriatrics	24	10	5,696	2,583	4,269	5,627	7,629	9,538
Hematology/Oncology	136	34	14,275	7,990	7,954	14,399	17,884	22,834
Hematology/Oncology: Onc (only)	11	6	39,660	47,586	11,883	18,652	78,732	141,057
Hospice/Palliative Care	1	1	*	*	*	*	*	*
Hospitalist: Family Practice	11	2	*	*	*	*	*	*
Hospitalist: Internal Medicine	480	59	5,927	2,257	4,343	5,645	7,422	8,795
Hospitalist: IM-Pediatrics	0	*	*	*	*	*	*	*
Hospitalist: Pediatrics	13	5	2,078	1,688	1,105	1,878	2,330	5,585
Infectious Disease	85	17	7,600	2,640	5,919	7,212	8,500	11,205
Internal Medicine: General	1,383	120	8,406	3,830	5,845	8,251	10,456	12,770
IM: Amb Only (no inpatient work)	4	3	*	*	*	*	*	*
Internal Med: Pediatrics	34	12	8,298	2,660	6,697	8,246	10,542	11,466
Nephrology	65	26	13,849	6,030	9,112	12,146	17,129	24,537
Neurology	163	46	11,229	6,653	7,275	9,579	14,006	19,341
Obstetrics/Gynecology: General	414	67	13,260	5,747	9,567	12,625	16,076	20,559
OB/GYN: Gynecology (only)	34	21	8,869	5,497	5,406	7,384	11,077	14,247
OB/GYN: Gyn Oncology	9	4	*	*	*	*	*	*
OB/GYN: Maternal & Fetal Med	7	5	*	*	*	*	*	*
OB/GYN: Repro Endocrinology	1	1	*	*	*	*	*	*
OB/GYN: Urogynecology	0	*	*	*	*	*	*	*
Occupational Medicine	44	16	7,748	3,337	6,199	8,051	8,988	10,713
Ophthalmology	116	32	16,016	7,965	10,446	15,067	19,239	27,056
Ophthalmology: Pediatric	8	5	*	*	*	*	*	*
Ophthalmology: Retina	7	6	*	*	*	*	*	*
Orthopedic (Nonsurgical)	12	9	7,576	2,836	5,573	6,951	9,937	12,278
Orthopedic Surgery: General	191	49	16,668	7,270	11,298	15,377	20,636	27,207
Orthopedic Surgery: Foot & Ankle	6	5	*	*	*	*	*	*
Orthopedic Surgery: Hand	23	12	20,101	9,445	13,555	17,628	22,997	37,608
Orthopedic Surgery: Hip & Joint	18	7	18,951	7,879	14,571	18,039	19,943	33,709
Orthopedic Surgery: Pediatric	3	2	*	*	*	*	*	*
Orthopedic Surgery: Spine	15	9	32,969	38,037	17,522	21,679	31,952	93,481
Orthopedic Surgery: Trauma	10	6	21,179	11,824	12,120	16,758	33,407	40,803
Orthopedic Surgery: Sports Med	24	11	19,913	10,769	11,012	18,149	28,940	36,135

Table 55: Total RVUs (CMS RBRVS Method) (TC/NPP Excluded) (continued)

	Phys	Med Pracs	Mean	Std. Dev.	25th %tile	Median	75th %tile	90th %tile
Otorhinolaryngology	111	44	15,362	7,262	9,965	14,041	18,732	23,230
Pathology: Anatomic and Clinical	31	8	15,895	7,908	6,991	18,076	22,029	26,601
Pathology: Anatomic	11	2	*	*	*	*	*	*
Pathology: Clinical	11	2	*	*	*	*	*	*
Pediatrics: General	896	90	9,840	3,822	7,126	9,433	12,222	15,307
Pediatrics: Adolescent Medicine	13	2	*	*	*	*	*	*
Pediatrics: Allergy/Immunology	2	1	*	*	*	*	*	*
Pediatrics: Cardiology	4	3	*	*	*	*	*	*
Pediatrics: Child Development	1	1	*	*	*	*	*	*
Pediatrics: Critical Care/Intensivist	12	3	2,215	1,964	1,119	1,303	2,799	6,608
Pediatrics: Emergency Medicine	2	2	*	*	*	*	*	*
Pediatrics: Endocrinology	6	5	*	*	*	*	*	*
Pediatrics: Gastroenterology	5	2	*	*	*	*	*	*
Pediatrics: Genetics	4	3	*	*	*	*	*	*
Pediatrics: Hematology/Oncology	8	5	*	*	*	*	*	*
Pediatrics: Infectious Disease	4	4	*	*	*	*	*	*
Pediatrics: Neonatal Medicine	16	4	11,096	3,298	9,293	11,148	13,036	15,181
Pediatrics: Nephrology	2	2	*	*	*	*	*	*
Pediatrics: Neurology	15	8	9,894	4,404	6,488	8,655	11,348	17,464
Pediatrics: Pulmonology	2	2	*	*	*	*	*	*
Pediatrics: Rheumatology	2	1	*	*	*	*	*	*
Physiatry (Phys Med & Rehab)	60	22	10,162	4,316	7,513	9,660	11,457	15,641
Podiatry: General	45	24	9,378	3,026	6,661	8,594	11,877	13,868
Podiatry: Surg-Foot & Ankle	29	9	10,604	2,996	8,187	10,375	12,071	15,407
Podiatry: Surg-Forefoot Only	0	*	*	*	*	*	*	*
Psychiatry: General	113	23	5,021	1,812	3,737	4,850	5,898	7,784
Psychiatry: Child & Adolescent	10	8	5,620	3,709	2,542	4,350	9,257	12,368
Psychiatry: Geriatric	0	*	*	*	*	*	*	*
Pulmonary Medicine	89	33	13,237	6,192	8,735	11,538	16,351	21,918
Pulmonary Medicine: Critical Care	23	5	15,319	3,379	12,947	15,407	17,862	19,946
Pulmonary Med: Gen & Crit Care	22	10	11,165	4,266	7,653	8,441	14,650	17,193
Radiation Oncology	38	12	17,945	13,044	9,787	14,383	19,821	43,708
Radiology: Diagnostic-Inv	78	18	23,548	17,228	12,782	16,423	27,487	53,608
Radiology: Diagnostic-Noninv	187	25	26,536	18,265	12,148	20,148	36,883	52,990
Radiology: Nuclear Medicine	14	8	21,061	17,101	8,307	14,675	27,236	58,493
Rheumatology	96	42	11,084	7,045	6,921	8,820	11,765	23,697
Sleep Medicine	26	10	17,424	15,221	4,690	15,337	23,494	42,477
Surgery: General	306	77	13,117	4,916	10,331	12,811	15,592	19,721
Surgery: Bariatric	7	3	*	*	*	*	*	*
Surgery: Cardiovascular	63	21	14,050	5,652	10,310	13,539	17,896	22,828
Surgery: Colon and Rectal	19	8	13,681	8,716	5,718	14,893	19,578	22,845
Surgery: Neurological	85	23	18,407	6,566	14,143	18,023	22,660	26,526
Surgery: Oncology	6	4	*	*	*	*	*	*
Surgery: Oral	1	1	*	*	*	*	*	*
Surgery: Pediatric	7	5	*	*	*	*	*	*
Surgery: Plastic & Reconstruction	31	15	47,194	105,698	11,746	13,076	19,825	230,519
Surgery: Plastic & Recon-Hand	5	2	*	*	*	*	*	*
Surgery: Thoracic (primary)	17	5	11,932	4,150	8,872	11,707	13,965	19,164
Surgery: Transplant	11	3	11,751	4,016	7,554	11,418	14,451	18,455
Surgery: Trauma	12	2	*	*	*	*	*	*
Surgery: Trauma-Burn	1	1	*	*	*	*	*	*
Surgery: Vascular (primary)	26	15	16,622	11,363	7,377	15,178	21,448	37,215
Urgent Care	218	30	10,007	4,327	6,831	9,448	12,709	16,378
Urology	109	36	25,640	21,299	13,446	18,385	31,748	46,069
Urology: Pediatric	0	*	*	*	*	*	*	*

Table 56: Total RVUs (CMS RBRVS Method) (TC/NPP Excluded) by Group Type

	Single Specialty			Multispecialty		
	Phys	Med Pracs	Median	Phys	Med Pracs	Median
Allergy/Immunology	2	1	*	37	19	10,306
Anesthesiology	1,747	74	14,175	210	16	10,044
Anesthesiology: Pain Management	5	4	*	22	11	20,589
Anesthesiology: Pediatric	22	2	*	1	1	*
Cardiology: Electrophysiology	25	8	19,813	15	10	20,547
Cardiology: Invasive	36	7	18,421	82	22	18,419
Cardiology: Inv-Intvl	65	11	18,660	74	22	22,199
Cardiology: Noninvasive	40	9	20,433	88	17	16,619
Critical Care: Intensivist	0	*	*	4	2	*
Dentistry	0	*	*	6	2	*
Dermatology	3	2	*	120	44	16,433
Dermatology: Mohs Surgery	0	*	*	9	8	*
Emergency Medicine	105	4	8,007	80	10	9,073
Endocrinology/Metabolism	8	5	*	91	45	8,676
Family Practice (w/ OB)	27	6	8,335	198	31	9,429
Family Practice (w/o OB)	180	47	9,984	1,472	95	8,679
FP: Amb Only (no inpatient work)	0	*	*	17	2	*
Family Practice: Sports Med	4	2	*	10	7	11,825
Family Practice: Urgent Care	0	*	*	18	5	7,317
Gastroenterology	69	5	16,405	187	55	18,328
Gastroenterology: Hepatology	0	*	*	1	1	*
Genetics	*	*	*	2	1	*
Geriatrics	0	*	*	24	10	5,627
Hematology/Oncology	32	2	*	104	32	12,577
Hematology/Oncology: Onc (only)	0	*	*	11	6	18,652
Hospice/Palliative Care	1	1	*	0	*	*
Hospitalist: Family Practice	0	*	*	11	2	*
Hospitalist: Internal Medicine	70	10	7,688	410	49	5,289
Hospitalist: IM-Pediatrics	*	*	*	0	*	*
Hospitalist: Pediatrics	0	*	*	13	5	1,878
Infectious Disease	7	3	*	78	14	7,170
Internal Medicine: General	66	16	10,925	1,317	104	8,128
IM: Amb Only (no inpatient work)	0	*	*	4	3	*
Internal Med: Pediatrics	0	*	*	34	12	8,246
Nephrology	0	*	*	65	26	12,146
Neurology	7	2	*	156	44	9,625
Obstetrics/Gynecology: General	25	9	13,802	389	58	12,535
OB/GYN: Gynecology (only)	2	2	*	32	19	7,384
OB/GYN: Gyn Oncology	1	1	*	8	3	*
OB/GYN: Maternal & Fetal Med	0	*	*	7	5	*
OB/GYN: Repro Endocrinology	0	*	*	1	1	*
OB/GYN: Urogynecology	*	*	*	0	*	*
Occupational Medicine	0	*	*	44	16	8,051
Ophthalmology	8	2	*	108	30	15,248
Ophthalmology: Pediatric	1	1	*	7	4	*
Ophthalmology: Retina	1	1	*	6	5	*
Orthopedic (Nonsurgical)	4	4	*	8	5	*
Orthopedic Surgery: General	17	7	16,835	174	42	15,185
Orthopedic Surgery: Foot & Ankle	4	3	*	2	2	*
Orthopedic Surgery: Hand	8	4	*	15	8	20,857
Orthopedic Surgery: Hip & Joint	6	4	*	12	3	18,416
Orthopedic Surgery: Pediatric	0	*	*	3	2	*
Orthopedic Surgery: Spine	5	4	*	10	5	28,690
Orthopedic Surgery: Trauma	6	3	*	4	3	*
Orthopedic Surgery: Sports Med	10	5	20,326	14	6	15,499

Table 56: Total RVUs (CMS RBRVS Method) (TC/NPP Excluded) by Group Type (continued)

	Single Specialty			Multispecialty		
	Phys	Med Pracs	Median	Phys	Med Pracs	Median
Otorhinolaryngology	7	3	*	104	41	14,258
Pathology: Anatomic and Clinical	0	*	*	31	8	18,076
Pathology: Anatomic	*	*	*	11	2	*
Pathology: Clinical	0	*	*	11	2	*
Pediatrics: General	240	20	10,405	656	70	9,173
Pediatrics: Adolescent Medicine	0	*	*	13	2	*
Pediatrics: Allergy/Immunology	2	1	*	0	*	*
Pediatrics: Cardiology	0	*	*	4	3	*
Pediatrics: Child Development	*	*	*	1	1	*
Pediatrics: Critical Care/Intensivist	0	*	*	12	3	1,303
Pediatrics: Emergency Medicine	0	*	*	2	2	*
Pediatrics: Endocrinology	1	1	*	5	4	*
Pediatrics: Gastroenterology	0	*	*	5	2	*
Pediatrics: Genetics	0	*	*	4	3	*
Pediatrics: Hematology/Oncology	1	1	*	7	4	*
Pediatrics: Infectious Disease	*	*	*	4	4	*
Pediatrics: Neonatal Medicine	12	2	*	4	2	*
Pediatrics: Nephrology	*	*	*	2	2	*
Pediatrics: Neurology	0	*	*	15	8	8,655
Pediatrics: Pulmonology	1	1	*	1	1	*
Pediatrics: Rheumatology	*	*	*	2	1	*
Physiatry (Phys Med & Rehab)	20	5	9,742	40	17	9,537
Podiatry: General	1	1	*	44	23	8,694
Podiatry: Surg-Foot & Ankle	0	*	*	29	9	10,375
Podiatry: Surg-Forefoot Only	0	*	*	0	*	*
Psychiatry: General	0	*	*	113	23	4,850
Psychiatry: Child & Adolescent	0	*	*	10	8	4,350
Psychiatry: Geriatric	0	*	*	0	*	*
Pulmonary Medicine	2	1	*	87	32	11,538
Pulmonary Medicine: Critical Care	1	1	*	22	4	15,701
Pulmonary Med: Gen & Crit Care	0	*	*	22	10	8,441
Radiation Oncology	8	1	*	30	11	12,352
Radiology: Diagnostic-Inv	47	7	14,326	31	11	27,235
Radiology: Diagnostic-Noninv	62	8	14,095	125	17	29,866
Radiology: Nuclear Medicine	8	4	*	6	4	*
Rheumatology	11	4	6,833	85	38	9,157
Sleep Medicine	0	*	*	26	10	15,337
Surgery: General	32	8	12,039	274	69	12,874
Surgery: Bariatric	0	*	*	7	3	*
Surgery: Cardiovascular	16	4	15,432	47	17	12,366
Surgery: Colon and Rectal	*	*	*	19	8	14,893
Surgery: Neurological	25	4	18,745	60	19	17,478
Surgery: Oncology	0	*	*	6	4	*
Surgery: Oral	0	*	*	1	1	*
Surgery: Pediatric	0	*	*	7	5	*
Surgery: Plastic & Reconstruction	3	1	*	28	14	12,883
Surgery: Plastic & Recon-Hand	0	*	*	5	2	*
Surgery: Thoracic (primary)	10	3	12,090	7	2	*
Surgery: Transplant	7	1	*	4	2	*
Surgery: Trauma	0	*	*	12	2	*
Surgery: Trauma-Burn	*	*	*	1	1	*
Surgery: Vascular (primary)	3	2	*	23	13	15,379
Urgent Care	4	1	*	214	29	9,585
Urology	28	4	36,293	81	32	16,231
Urology: Pediatric	0	*	*	0	*	*

Table 57: Total RVUs (CMS RBRVS Method) (TC/NPP Excluded) by Hospital Ownership

	Hospital Owned			Not Hospital Owned		
	Phys	Med Pracs	Median	Phys	Med Pracs	Median
Allergy/Immunology	11	7	12,415	28	13	10,392
Anesthesiology	83	10	10,013	1,841	79	13,727
Anesthesiology: Pain Management	11	5	25,557	16	10	18,108
Anesthesiology: Pediatric	0	*	*	23	3	6,888
Cardiology: Electrophysiology	8	5	*	32	13	19,702
Cardiology: Invasive	42	9	18,097	76	20	22,234
Cardiology: Inv-Intvl	40	10	18,547	99	23	22,153
Cardiology: Noninvasive	44	8	22,510	84	18	14,245
Critical Care: Intensivist	0	*	*	4	2	*
Dentistry	3	1	*	3	1	*
Dermatology	43	19	16,276	80	27	16,693
Dermatology: Mohs Surgery	0	*	*	9	8	*
Emergency Medicine	59	8	8,155	126	6	8,154
Endocrinology/Metabolism	40	21	9,185	59	29	8,666
Family Practice (w/ OB)	121	18	9,458	104	19	8,952
Family Practice (w/o OB)	907	89	9,177	745	53	8,461
FP: Amb Only (no inpatient work)	11	1	*	6	1	*
Family Practice: Sports Med	3	2	*	11	7	6,912
Family Practice: Urgent Care	15	3	6,812	3	2	*
Gastroenterology	65	20	21,726	191	40	16,069
Gastroenterology: Hepatology	0	*	*	1	1	*
Genetics	2	1	*	0	*	*
Geriatrics	15	7	4,710	9	3	*
Hematology/Oncology	32	8	11,961	104	26	15,076
Hematology/Oncology: Onc (only)	2	2	*	9	4	*
Hospice/Palliative Care	1	1	*	0	*	*
Hospitalist: Family Practice	10	1	*	1	1	*
Hospitalist: Internal Medicine	265	28	5,681	215	31	5,620
Hospitalist: IM-Pediatrics	0	*	*	0	*	*
Hospitalist: Pediatrics	3	3	*	10	2	*
Infectious Disease	18	9	7,589	67	8	7,128
Internal Medicine: General	639	62	8,734	744	58	7,770
IM: Amb Only (no inpatient work)	3	2	*	1	1	*
Internal Med: Pediatrics	10	4	7,446	24	8	8,630
Nephrology	16	6	10,407	49	20	14,108
Neurology	61	19	8,934	102	27	9,643
Obstetrics/Gynecology: General	146	26	13,779	268	41	12,021
OB/GYN: Gynecology (only)	16	8	7,288	18	13	7,471
OB/GYN: Gyn Oncology	4	3	*	5	1	*
OB/GYN: Maternal & Fetal Med	3	2	*	4	3	*
OB/GYN: Repro Endocrinology	0	*	*	1	1	*
OB/GYN: Urogynecology	0	*	*	0	*	*
Occupational Medicine	6	5	*	38	11	8,324
Ophthalmology	30	9	17,747	86	23	14,519
Ophthalmology: Pediatric	2	2	*	6	3	*
Ophthalmology: Retina	4	3	*	3	3	*
Orthopedic (Nonsurgical)	2	1	*	10	8	6,951
Orthopedic Surgery: General	75	14	15,745	116	35	15,166
Orthopedic Surgery: Foot & Ankle	0	*	*	6	5	*
Orthopedic Surgery: Hand	2	2	*	21	10	17,628
Orthopedic Surgery: Hip & Joint	0	*	*	18	7	18,039
Orthopedic Surgery: Pediatric	1	1	*	2	1	*
Orthopedic Surgery: Spine	1	1	*	14	8	21,646
Orthopedic Surgery: Trauma	1	1	*	9	5	*
Orthopedic Surgery: Sports Med	6	3	*	18	8	20,326

Table 57: Total RVUs (CMS RBRVS Method) (TC/NPP Excluded) by Hospital Ownership (continued)

	Hospital Owned			Not Hospital Owned		
	Phys	Med Pracs	Median	Phys	Med Pracs	Median
Otorhinolaryngology	37	13	16,816	74	31	13,404
Pathology: Anatomic and Clinical	10	2	*	21	6	20,593
Pathology: Anatomic	0	*	*	11	2	*
Pathology: Clinical	4	1	*	7	1	*
Pediatrics: General	495	46	10,424	401	44	8,316
Pediatrics: Adolescent Medicine	12	1	*	1	1	*
Pediatrics: Allergy/Immunology	0	*	*	2	1	*
Pediatrics: Cardiology	4	3	*	0	*	*
Pediatrics: Child Development	0	*	*	1	1	*
Pediatrics: Critical Care/Intensivist	5	2	*	7	1	*
Pediatrics: Emergency Medicine	1	1	*	1	1	*
Pediatrics: Endocrinology	3	3	*	3	2	*
Pediatrics: Gastroenterology	0	*	*	5	2	*
Pediatrics: Genetics	0	*	*	4	3	*
Pediatrics: Hematology/Oncology	4	3	*	4	2	*
Pediatrics: Infectious Disease	3	3	*	1	1	*
Pediatrics: Neonatal Medicine	4	2	*	12	2	*
Pediatrics: Nephrology	2	2	*	0	*	*
Pediatrics: Neurology	5	4	*	10	4	8,594
Pediatrics: Pulmonology	1	1	*	1	1	*
Pediatrics: Rheumatology	0	*	*	2	1	*
Physiatry (Phys Med & Rehab)	37	9	9,801	23	13	7,971
Podiatry: General	19	9	11,441	26	15	8,259
Podiatry: Surg-Foot & Ankle	7	1	*	22	8	11,047
Podiatry: Surg-Forefoot Only	*	*	*	0	*	*
Psychiatry: General	48	14	5,300	65	9	4,566
Psychiatry: Child & Adolescent	7	5	*	3	3	*
Psychiatry: Geriatric	0	*	*	0	*	*
Pulmonary Medicine	32	11	10,840	57	22	12,401
Pulmonary Medicine: Critical Care	6	2	*	17	3	17,015
Pulmonary Med: Gen & Crit Care	3	2	*	19	8	8,306
Radiation Oncology	20	6	10,180	18	6	18,082
Radiology: Diagnostic-Inv	12	5	16,039	66	13	16,423
Radiology: Diagnostic-Noninv	44	6	14,175	143	19	22,231
Radiology: Nuclear Medicine	7	4	*	7	4	*
Rheumatology	41	15	10,257	55	27	8,377
Sleep Medicine	5	3	*	21	7	14,710
Surgery: General	119	26	12,670	187	51	12,968
Surgery: Bariatric	2	1	*	5	2	*
Surgery: Cardiovascular	27	9	13,040	36	12	14,111
Surgery: Colon and Rectal	1	1	*	18	7	14,142
Surgery: Neurological	22	9	15,961	63	14	18,711
Surgery: Oncology	1	1	*	5	3	*
Surgery: Oral	0	*	*	1	1	*
Surgery: Pediatric	3	3	*	4	2	*
Surgery: Plastic & Reconstruction	18	6	12,506	13	9	19,825
Surgery: Plastic & Recon-Hand	*	*	*	5	2	*
Surgery: Thoracic (primary)	12	4	11,473	5	1	*
Surgery: Transplant	8	2	*	3	1	*
Surgery: Trauma	6	1	*	6	1	*
Surgery: Trauma-Burn	1	1	*	*	*	*
Surgery: Vascular (primary)	5	3	*	21	12	13,072
Urgent Care	65	9	12,894	153	21	8,092
Urology	26	9	16,140	83	27	20,364
Urology: Pediatric	0	*	*	0	*	*

Table 58: Physician Compensation to Total RVUs Ratio (CMS RBRVS Method) (TC/NPP Excluded)

	Phys	Med Pracs	Mean	Std. Dev.	25th %tile	Median	75th %tile	90th %tile
Allergy/Immunology	39	20	$24.91	$7.88	$19.70	$23.39	$29.33	$33.60
Anesthesiology	1,916	86	$35.14	$21.38	$25.36	$28.81	$38.46	$54.44
Anesthesiology: Pain Management	29	17	$31.27	$15.24	$22.59	$29.20	$35.66	$65.13
Anesthesiology: Pediatric	24	3	$57.08	$26.51	$31.98	$55.70	$91.18	$91.18
Cardiology: Electrophysiology	38	17	$30.47	$13.70	$21.52	$25.55	$36.20	$53.82
Cardiology: Invasive	118	28	$30.24	$22.75	$18.21	$24.03	$35.31	$53.64
Cardiology: Inv-Intvl	139	33	$28.16	$14.02	$18.08	$24.53	$34.45	$50.12
Cardiology: Noninvasive	128	26	$29.96	$18.34	$16.66	$23.23	$43.71	$59.71
Critical Care: Intensivist	4	2	*	*	*	*	*	*
Dentistry	6	2	*	*	*	*	*	*
Dermatology	123	45	$24.36	$9.72	$18.20	$22.07	$29.33	$40.32
Dermatology: Mohs Surgery	9	8	*	*	*	*	*	*
Emergency Medicine	179	13	$32.79	$12.51	$22.54	$30.99	$41.87	$48.49
Endocrinology/Metabolism	99	49	$25.50	$10.72	$18.74	$23.56	$29.99	$37.59
Family Practice (w/ OB)	225	37	$21.73	$7.40	$17.46	$20.59	$24.77	$30.59
Family Practice (w/o OB)	1,652	142	$22.31	$9.09	$17.00	$20.71	$24.45	$32.01
FP: Amb Only (no inpatient work)	17	2	*	*	*	*	*	*
Family Practice: Sports Med	14	9	$28.47	$14.41	$19.13	$24.53	$33.33	$57.22
Family Practice: Urgent Care	20	5	$26.45	$7.74	$20.35	$28.67	$32.58	$33.85
Gastroenterology	264	61	$26.05	$8.99	$19.91	$24.29	$30.07	$40.58
Gastroenterology: Hepatology	1	1	*	*	*	*	*	*
Genetics	2	1	*	*	*	*	*	*
Geriatrics	22	9	$35.93	$11.83	$25.15	$33.47	$46.46	$51.35
Hematology/Oncology	136	34	$39.32	$19.85	$22.96	$33.82	$56.31	$68.15
Hematology/Oncology: Onc (only)	11	6	$50.37	$37.24	$23.63	$50.18	$67.15	$123.82
Hospice/Palliative Care	1	1	*	*	*	*	*	*
Hospitalist: Family Practice	11	2	*	*	*	*	*	*
Hospitalist: Internal Medicine	480	59	$40.40	$15.05	$31.49	$36.38	$45.01	$57.07
Hospitalist: IM-Pediatrics	0	*	*	*	*	*	*	*
Hospitalist: Pediatrics	13	5	$109.45	$98.72	$69.33	$88.30	$99.84	$317.61
Infectious Disease	85	17	$24.91	$6.12	$20.89	$22.66	$27.80	$35.22
Internal Medicine: General	1,383	120	$26.69	$15.08	$18.47	$22.94	$30.41	$42.13
IM: Amb Only (no inpatient work)	4	3	*	*	*	*	*	*
Internal Med: Pediatrics	32	12	$24.03	$9.91	$19.13	$22.68	$24.65	$31.73
Nephrology	67	26	$24.45	$8.14	$18.97	$24.44	$30.60	$35.63
Neurology	163	48	$26.35	$9.62	$20.65	$25.67	$31.10	$38.39
Obstetrics/Gynecology: General	414	66	$24.63	$9.46	$18.10	$22.46	$28.70	$37.75
OB/GYN: Gynecology (only)	34	19	$25.18	$10.34	$17.63	$22.84	$29.70	$47.06
OB/GYN: Gyn Oncology	9	4	*	*	*	*	*	*
OB/GYN: Maternal & Fetal Med	7	5	*	*	*	*	*	*
OB/GYN: Repro Endocrinology	1	1	*	*	*	*	*	*
OB/GYN: Urogynecology	0	*	*	*	*	*	*	*
Occupational Medicine	40	16	$31.95	$13.11	$24.92	$29.26	$33.93	$48.74
Ophthalmology	116	32	$22.65	$11.64	$15.21	$19.08	$26.48	$37.18
Ophthalmology: Pediatric	8	5	*	*	*	*	*	*
Ophthalmology: Retina	7	6	*	*	*	*	*	*
Orthopedic (Nonsurgical)	12	9	$24.19	$5.79	$20.87	$24.29	$29.73	$31.35
Orthopedic Surgery: General	197	51	$30.26	$11.40	$22.84	$28.39	$35.75	$46.63
Orthopedic Surgery: Foot & Ankle	6	5	*	*	*	*	*	*
Orthopedic Surgery: Hand	25	13	$26.94	$9.98	$23.46	$28.15	$32.97	$38.48
Orthopedic Surgery: Hip & Joint	16	7	$29.35	$9.54	$22.50	$26.55	$34.72	$46.27
Orthopedic Surgery: Pediatric	3	2	*	*	*	*	*	*
Orthopedic Surgery: Spine	15	9	$22.61	$10.98	$15.32	$17.65	$28.86	$39.49
Orthopedic Surgery: Trauma	10	6	$30.47	$11.38	$23.69	$28.58	$36.88	$54.21
Orthopedic Surgery: Sports Med	26	12	$29.65	$9.28	$21.97	$29.53	$35.14	$43.45

Table 58: Physician Compensation to Total RVUs Ratio (CMS RBRVS Method) (TC/NPP Excluded) (continued)

	Phys	Med Pracs	Mean	Std. Dev.	25th %tile	Median	75th %tile	90th %tile
Otorhinolaryngology	115	46	$26.77	$10.26	$21.26	$24.46	$31.53	$42.14
Pathology: Anatomic and Clinical	31	8	$27.90	$21.71	$14.70	$17.66	$32.38	$75.73
Pathology: Anatomic	11	2	*	*	*	*	*	*
Pathology: Clinical	11	2	*	*	*	*	*	*
Pediatrics: General	896	91	$21.91	$7.23	$16.67	$20.32	$25.05	$32.77
Pediatrics: Adolescent Medicine	13	2	*	*	*	*	*	*
Pediatrics: Allergy/Immunology	2	1	*	*	*	*	*	*
Pediatrics: Cardiology	4	3	*	*	*	*	*	*
Pediatrics: Child Development	1	1	*	*	*	*	*	*
Pediatrics: Critical Care/Intensivist	12	3	$228.15	$162.22	$89.87	$167.75	$398.70	$452.02
Pediatrics: Emergency Medicine	2	2	*	*	*	*	*	*
Pediatrics: Endocrinology	6	5	*	*	*	*	*	*
Pediatrics: Gastroenterology	5	2	*	*	*	*	*	*
Pediatrics: Genetics	4	3	*	*	*	*	*	*
Pediatrics: Hematology/Oncology	8	5	*	*	*	*	*	*
Pediatrics: Infectious Disease	4	4	*	*	*	*	*	*
Pediatrics: Neonatal Medicine	16	4	$30.09	$9.60	$20.64	$31.00	$38.36	$45.59
Pediatrics: Nephrology	2	2	*	*	*	*	*	*
Pediatrics: Neurology	17	8	$28.67	$8.25	$23.06	$28.91	$36.98	$39.44
Pediatrics: Pulmonology	2	2	*	*	*	*	*	*
Pediatrics: Rheumatology	2	1	*	*	*	*	*	*
Physiatry (Phys Med & Rehab)	60	22	$25.15	$8.39	$18.00	$22.76	$29.54	$38.27
Podiatry: General	49	24	$23.09	$8.11	$17.95	$21.32	$26.03	$34.53
Podiatry: Surg-Foot & Ankle	29	9	$22.52	$4.95	$18.99	$21.72	$26.45	$29.47
Podiatry: Surg-Forefoot Only	0	*	*	*	*	*	*	*
Psychiatry: General	113	25	$38.45	$9.82	$32.73	$37.27	$43.28	$50.16
Psychiatry: Child & Adolescent	10	8	$46.89	$13.40	$37.46	$44.00	$63.03	$66.37
Psychiatry: Geriatric	0	*	*	*	*	*	*	*
Pulmonary Medicine	89	34	$27.44	$14.12	$17.49	$23.84	$32.25	$50.88
Pulmonary Medicine: Critical Care	21	5	$24.02	$8.94	$19.87	$22.02	$25.50	$38.91
Pulmonary Med: Gen & Crit Care	24	11	$32.79	$10.25	$22.33	$32.22	$42.22	$46.46
Radiation Oncology	40	12	$41.29	$22.55	$22.04	$41.32	$56.51	$74.81
Radiology: Diagnostic-Inv	82	18	$30.76	$16.49	$16.02	$32.15	$39.95	$49.88
Radiology: Diagnostic-Noninv	187	23	$26.24	$15.45	$13.33	$24.27	$36.43	$48.07
Radiology: Nuclear Medicine	14	8	$31.43	$18.25	$14.89	$29.97	$50.25	$56.76
Rheumatology	100	43	$25.83	$11.14	$19.17	$23.91	$31.56	$43.64
Sleep Medicine	26	9	$25.83	$16.10	$13.46	$19.73	$38.88	$53.98
Surgery: General	304	77	$31.61	$26.00	$20.65	$26.50	$32.48	$47.06
Surgery: Bariatric	7	3	*	*	*	*	*	*
Surgery: Cardiovascular	61	20	$47.52	$74.86	$24.60	$35.35	$46.39	$70.90
Surgery: Colon and Rectal	14	7	$23.24	$7.23	$18.48	$20.49	$26.38	$36.74
Surgery: Neurological	85	24	$41.14	$13.95	$31.77	$37.68	$50.58	$59.44
Surgery: Oncology	6	4	*	*	*	*	*	*
Surgery: Oral	1	1	*	*	*	*	*	*
Surgery: Pediatric	7	5	*	*	*	*	*	*
Surgery: Plastic & Reconstruction	33	16	$28.07	$14.88	$21.85	$27.60	$35.53	$48.94
Surgery: Plastic & Recon-Hand	5	2	*	*	*	*	*	*
Surgery: Thoracic (primary)	17	5	$36.64	$16.34	$23.99	$35.18	$43.06	$58.81
Surgery: Transplant	11	3	$38.59	$26.29	$16.11	$29.18	$51.61	$94.69
Surgery: Trauma	12	2	*	*	*	*	*	*
Surgery: Trauma-Burn	1	1	*	*	*	*	*	*
Surgery: Vascular (primary)	23	12	$22.50	$10.37	$15.74	$19.23	$22.55	$36.15
Urgent Care	218	30	$271.28	$2,766.45	$16.35	$21.45	$29.15	$39.57
Urology	109	35	$22.22	$10.70	$16.15	$20.98	$26.83	$37.81
Urology: Pediatric	0	*	*	*	*	*	*	*

Table 59: Physician Compensation to Total RVUs Ratio (CMS RBRVS Method) (TC/NPP Excluded) by Group Type

	Single Specialty			Multispecialty		
	Phys	Med Pracs	Median	Phys	Med Pracs	Median
Allergy/Immunology	2	1	*	37	19	$23.65
Anesthesiology	1,723	72	$28.81	193	14	$36.20
Anesthesiology: Pain Management	6	5	*	23	12	$28.86
Anesthesiology: Pediatric	23	2	*	1	1	*
Cardiology: Electrophysiology	24	8	$23.82	14	9	$27.27
Cardiology: Invasive	39	7	$21.93	79	21	$26.53
Cardiology: Inv-Intvl	66	11	$27.92	73	22	$23.59
Cardiology: Noninvasive	42	9	$18.58	86	17	$25.70
Critical Care: Intensivist	0	*	*	4	2	*
Dentistry	0	*	*	6	2	*
Dermatology	3	2	*	120	43	$21.81
Dermatology: Mohs Surgery	0	*	*	9	8	*
Emergency Medicine	100	4	$32.79	79	9	$28.06
Endocrinology/Metabolism	8	5	*	91	44	$23.56
Family Practice (w/ OB)	27	6	$21.65	198	31	$20.51
Family Practice (w/o OB)	180	47	$17.96	1,472	95	$20.95
FP: Amb Only (no inpatient work)	0	*	*	17	2	*
Family Practice: Sports Med	4	2	*	10	7	$21.10
Family Practice: Urgent Care	0	*	*	20	5	$28.67
Gastroenterology	73	5	$24.76	191	56	$24.07
Gastroenterology: Hepatology	0	*	*	1	1	*
Genetics	*	*	*	2	1	*
Geriatrics	0	*	*	22	9	$33.47
Hematology/Oncology	32	2	*	104	32	$32.77
Hematology/Oncology: Onc (only)	0	*	*	11	6	$50.18
Hospice/Palliative Care	1	1	*	0	*	*
Hospitalist: Family Practice	0	*	*	11	2	*
Hospitalist: Internal Medicine	68	10	$32.07	412	49	$38.73
Hospitalist: IM-Pediatrics	*	*	*	0	*	*
Hospitalist: Pediatrics	0	*	*	13	5	$88.30
Infectious Disease	7	3	*	78	14	$22.72
Internal Medicine: General	66	16	$18.26	1,317	104	$23.12
IM: Amb Only (no inpatient work)	0	*	*	4	3	*
Internal Med: Pediatrics	0	*	*	32	12	$22.68
Nephrology	0	*	*	67	26	$24.44
Neurology	8	3	*	155	45	$25.76
Obstetrics/Gynecology: General	25	9	$19.24	389	57	$22.73
OB/GYN: Gynecology (only)	2	1	*	32	18	$22.84
OB/GYN: Gyn Oncology	1	1	*	8	3	*
OB/GYN: Maternal & Fetal Med	0	*	*	7	5	*
OB/GYN: Repro Endocrinology	0	*	*	1	1	*
OB/GYN: Urogynecology	*	*	*	0	*	*
Occupational Medicine	0	*	*	40	16	$29.26
Ophthalmology	8	2	*	108	30	$19.54
Ophthalmology: Pediatric	1	1	*	7	4	*
Ophthalmology: Retina	1	1	*	6	5	*
Orthopedic (Nonsurgical)	4	4	*	8	5	*
Orthopedic Surgery: General	17	7	$27.09	180	44	$28.49
Orthopedic Surgery: Foot & Ankle	4	3	*	2	2	*
Orthopedic Surgery: Hand	8	4	*	17	9	$25.48
Orthopedic Surgery: Hip & Joint	6	4	*	10	3	$28.40
Orthopedic Surgery: Pediatric	0	*	*	3	2	*
Orthopedic Surgery: Spine	5	4	*	10	5	$16.24
Orthopedic Surgery: Trauma	6	3	*	4	3	*
Orthopedic Surgery: Sports Med	10	5	$33.21	16	7	$28.49

Table 59: Physician Compensation to Total RVUs Ratio (CMS RBRVS Method) (TC/NPP Excluded) by Group Type (continued)

	Single Specialty			Multispecialty		
	Phys	Med Pracs	Median	Phys	Med Pracs	Median
Otorhinolaryngology	7	3	*	108	43	$24.52
Pathology: Anatomic and Clinical	0	*	*	31	8	$17.66
Pathology: Anatomic	*	*	*	11	2	*
Pathology: Clinical	0	*	*	11	2	*
Pediatrics: General	241	20	$22.63	655	71	$19.87
Pediatrics: Adolescent Medicine	0	*	*	13	2	*
Pediatrics: Allergy/Immunology	2	1	*	0	*	*
Pediatrics: Cardiology	0	*	*	4	3	*
Pediatrics: Child Development	*	*	*	1	1	*
Pediatrics: Critical Care/Intensivist	0	*	*	12	3	$167.75
Pediatrics: Emergency Medicine	0	*	*	2	2	*
Pediatrics: Endocrinology	1	1	*	5	4	*
Pediatrics: Gastroenterology	0	*	*	5	2	*
Pediatrics: Genetics	0	*	*	4	3	*
Pediatrics: Hematology/Oncology	1	1	*	7	4	*
Pediatrics: Infectious Disease	*	*	*	4	4	*
Pediatrics: Neonatal Medicine	12	2	*	4	2	*
Pediatrics: Nephrology	*	*	*	2	2	*
Pediatrics: Neurology	0	*	*	17	8	$28.91
Pediatrics: Pulmonology	1	1	*	1	1	*
Pediatrics: Rheumatology	*	*	*	2	1	*
Physiatry (Phys Med & Rehab)	20	5	$19.87	40	17	$27.67
Podiatry: General	1	1	*	48	23	$21.44
Podiatry: Surg-Foot & Ankle	0	*	*	29	9	$21.72
Podiatry: Surg-Forefoot Only	0	*	*	0	*	*
Psychiatry: General	0	*	*	113	25	$37.27
Psychiatry: Child & Adolescent	0	*	*	10	8	$44.00
Psychiatry: Geriatric	0	*	*	0	*	*
Pulmonary Medicine	2	1	*	87	33	$23.99
Pulmonary Medicine: Critical Care	1	1	*	20	4	$21.48
Pulmonary Med: Gen & Crit Care	0	*	*	24	11	$32.22
Radiation Oncology	8	1	*	32	11	$35.26
Radiology: Diagnostic-Inv	48	7	$35.67	34	11	$17.67
Radiology: Diagnostic-Noninv	62	8	$32.44	125	15	$14.86
Radiology: Nuclear Medicine	8	4	*	6	4	*
Rheumatology	11	4	$20.20	89	39	$24.55
Sleep Medicine	0	*	*	26	9	$19.73
Surgery: General	32	8	$25.46	272	69	$26.60
Surgery: Bariatric	0	*	*	7	3	*
Surgery: Cardiovascular	15	4	$32.38	46	16	$39.23
Surgery: Colon and Rectal	*	*	*	14	7	$20.49
Surgery: Neurological	26	4	$36.25	59	20	$38.84
Surgery: Oncology	0	*	*	6	4	*
Surgery: Oral	0	*	*	1	1	*
Surgery: Pediatric	0	*	*	7	5	*
Surgery: Plastic & Reconstruction	4	1	*	29	15	$29.89
Surgery: Plastic & Recon-Hand	0	*	*	5	2	*
Surgery: Thoracic (primary)	10	3	$27.51	7	2	*
Surgery: Transplant	7	1	*	4	2	*
Surgery: Trauma	0	*	*	12	2	*
Surgery: Trauma-Burn	*	*	*	1	1	*
Surgery: Vascular (primary)	3	2	*	20	10	$19.55
Urgent Care	4	1	*	214	29	$21.56
Urology	29	4	$13.07	80	31	$22.76
Urology: Pediatric	0	*	*	0	*	*

Table 60: Collections to Total RVUs Ratio (CMS RBRVS Method) (TC/NPP Excluded)

	Phys	Med Pracs	Mean	Std. Dev.	25th %tile	Median	75th %tile	90th %tile
Allergy/Immunology	22	15	$44.87	$34.22	$25.41	$34.97	$54.33	$75.04
Anesthesiology	1,796	80	$58.07	$126.23	$34.65	$37.63	$49.93	$60.23
Anesthesiology: Pain Management	21	12	$49.48	$30.87	$36.31	$41.22	$50.15	$121.05
Anesthesiology: Pediatric	24	3	$63.01	$23.46	$38.61	$67.95	$90.06	$90.06
Cardiology: Electrophysiology	34	15	$42.91	$11.28	$35.03	$39.32	$43.73	$66.77
Cardiology: Invasive	106	26	$45.06	$57.14	$23.67	$34.21	$44.78	$56.18
Cardiology: Inv-Intvl	129	28	$38.65	$14.00	$29.73	$36.80	$44.75	$62.34
Cardiology: Noninvasive	93	19	$31.04	$14.75	$17.68	$28.21	$40.11	$50.20
Critical Care: Intensivist	1	1	*	*	*	*	*	*
Dentistry	3	1	*	*	*	*	*	*
Dermatology	88	36	$42.18	$18.79	$32.98	$41.75	$49.05	$60.94
Dermatology: Mohs Surgery	4	4	*	*	*	*	*	*
Emergency Medicine	169	11	$38.95	$6.74	$35.51	$40.47	$43.81	$46.37
Endocrinology/Metabolism	72	40	$37.05	$14.87	$28.18	$36.15	$43.01	$53.45
Family Practice (w/ OB)	175	31	$38.24	$13.36	$27.20	$38.11	$45.43	$56.86
Family Practice (w/o OB)	1,267	127	$41.44	$16.48	$32.18	$40.50	$47.35	$58.59
FP: Amb Only (no inpatient work)	17	2	*	*	*	*	*	*
Family Practice: Sports Med	12	7	$40.02	$12.73	$29.93	$40.25	$44.97	$63.10
Family Practice: Urgent Care	20	5	$51.61	$12.06	$43.68	$57.29	$60.51	$62.63
Gastroenterology	210	48	$43.15	$11.81	$33.36	$42.43	$49.50	$60.12
Gastroenterology: Hepatology	0	*	*	*	*	*	*	*
Genetics	2	1	*	*	*	*	*	*
Geriatrics	14	6	$35.32	$12.44	$27.52	$34.83	$45.98	$50.71
Hematology/Oncology	96	22	$46.98	$42.92	$28.99	$32.64	$42.13	$91.29
Hematology/Oncology: Onc (only)	11	6	$31.08	$33.68	$11.89	$13.94	$38.90	$107.49
Hospice/Palliative Care	1	1	*	*	*	*	*	*
Hospitalist: Family Practice	11	2	*	*	*	*	*	*
Hospitalist: Internal Medicine	391	48	$33.45	$10.01	$29.45	$32.54	$35.90	$47.43
Hospitalist: IM-Pediatrics	0	*	*	*	*	*	*	*
Hospitalist: Pediatrics	3	3	*	*	*	*	*	*
Infectious Disease	24	14	$38.32	$12.00	$30.07	$36.84	$45.91	$53.89
Internal Medicine: General	1,001	105	$40.76	$15.24	$32.00	$39.75	$47.44	$56.29
IM: Amb Only (no inpatient work)	4	3	*	*	*	*	*	*
Internal Med: Pediatrics	19	6	$37.99	$11.28	$25.35	$39.34	$45.04	$53.83
Nephrology	50	18	$33.06	$8.42	$30.89	$32.78	$37.96	$43.76
Neurology	131	39	$40.52	$15.79	$32.00	$42.31	$49.23	$54.97
Obstetrics/Gynecology: General	275	54	$42.40	$16.59	$33.38	$40.60	$51.71	$61.40
OB/GYN: Gynecology (only)	25	15	$44.76	$11.35	$37.44	$46.07	$52.77	$60.44
OB/GYN: Gyn Oncology	4	3	*	*	*	*	*	*
OB/GYN: Maternal & Fetal Med	4	3	*	*	*	*	*	*
OB/GYN: Repro Endocrinology	0	*	*	*	*	*	*	*
OB/GYN: Urogynecology	0	*	*	*	*	*	*	*
Occupational Medicine	25	10	$70.10	$55.99	$51.48	$60.81	$69.43	$91.84
Ophthalmology	76	25	$48.12	$41.04	$34.67	$40.54	$46.42	$55.40
Ophthalmology: Pediatric	7	4	*	*	*	*	*	*
Ophthalmology: Retina	6	5	*	*	*	*	*	*
Orthopedic (Nonsurgical)	7	6	*	*	*	*	*	*
Orthopedic Surgery: General	155	39	$43.23	$15.69	$36.40	$41.19	$46.35	$67.16
Orthopedic Surgery: Foot & Ankle	6	5	*	*	*	*	*	*
Orthopedic Surgery: Hand	18	10	$43.90	$19.86	$35.71	$41.18	$52.33	$78.05
Orthopedic Surgery: Hip & Joint	13	6	$51.01	$24.31	$36.08	$39.11	$70.02	$95.35
Orthopedic Surgery: Pediatric	1	1	*	*	*	*	*	*
Orthopedic Surgery: Spine	13	8	$42.17	$27.23	$31.04	$37.67	$44.99	$94.91
Orthopedic Surgery: Trauma	9	5	*	*	*	*	*	*
Orthopedic Surgery: Sports Med	19	9	$41.88	$8.38	$34.52	$38.50	$49.52	$52.80

Table 60: Collections to Total RVUs Ratio (CMS RBRVS Method) (TC/NPP Excluded) (continued)

	Phys	Med Pracs	Mean	Std. Dev.	25th %tile	Median	75th %tile	90th %tile
Otorhinolaryngology	81	34	$49.61	$16.88	$40.17	$46.05	$53.99	$75.51
Pathology: Anatomic and Clinical	11	4	$31.92	$16.82	$22.84	$23.82	$43.32	$58.26
Pathology: Anatomic	0	*	*	*	*	*	*	*
Pathology: Clinical	11	2	*	*	*	*	*	*
Pediatrics: General	695	77	$42.31	$17.94	$34.49	$39.73	$44.73	$60.92
Pediatrics: Adolescent Medicine	13	2	*	*	*	*	*	*
Pediatrics: Allergy/Immunology	2	1	*	*	*	*	*	*
Pediatrics: Cardiology	3	2	*	*	*	*	*	*
Pediatrics: Child Development	0	*	*	*	*	*	*	*
Pediatrics: Critical Care/Intensivist	12	3	$236.65	$175.02	$26.89	$324.74	$399.23	$415.82
Pediatrics: Emergency Medicine	1	1	*	*	*	*	*	*
Pediatrics: Endocrinology	4	4	*	*	*	*	*	*
Pediatrics: Gastroenterology	2	1	*	*	*	*	*	*
Pediatrics: Genetics	3	2	*	*	*	*	*	*
Pediatrics: Hematology/Oncology	5	4	*	*	*	*	*	*
Pediatrics: Infectious Disease	3	3	*	*	*	*	*	*
Pediatrics: Neonatal Medicine	15	3	$56.36	$9.30	$50.36	$55.63	$61.10	$74.00
Pediatrics: Nephrology	2	2	*	*	*	*	*	*
Pediatrics: Neurology	12	7	$42.31	$14.83	$27.09	$44.06	$54.14	$64.75
Pediatrics: Pulmonology	2	2	*	*	*	*	*	*
Pediatrics: Rheumatology	2	1	*	*	*	*	*	*
Physiatry (Phys Med & Rehab)	47	17	$39.63	$9.71	$32.84	$39.15	$42.54	$54.52
Podiatry: General	36	18	$46.00	$21.82	$34.01	$41.56	$50.36	$88.68
Podiatry: Surg-Foot & Ankle	13	5	$46.31	$6.76	$39.56	$45.83	$52.34	$55.03
Podiatry: Surg-Forefoot Only	0	*	*	*	*	*	*	*
Psychiatry: General	54	16	$42.34	$10.73	$35.07	$42.09	$51.70	$55.67
Psychiatry: Child & Adolescent	7	5	*	*	*	*	*	*
Psychiatry: Geriatric	0	*	*	*	*	*	*	*
Pulmonary Medicine	75	29	$35.09	$11.98	$29.83	$33.76	$39.85	$46.71
Pulmonary Medicine: Critical Care	23	5	$29.17	$2.84	$26.66	$28.78	$30.52	$33.56
Pulmonary Med: Gen & Crit Care	10	6	$47.11	$17.43	$32.15	$37.81	$66.44	$72.34
Radiation Oncology	32	8	$34.43	$10.15	$32.09	$36.58	$42.08	$44.84
Radiology: Diagnostic-Inv	65	13	$42.53	$15.61	$35.10	$47.12	$52.73	$62.86
Radiology: Diagnostic-Noninv	126	19	$40.44	$20.58	$20.78	$43.27	$51.89	$65.19
Radiology: Nuclear Medicine	11	6	$33.21	$15.15	$11.53	$41.83	$45.51	$47.60
Rheumatology	68	34	$38.37	$21.67	$22.65	$36.05	$44.17	$64.69
Sleep Medicine	14	5	$31.56	$12.36	$23.41	$33.59	$42.03	$47.80
Surgery: General	249	63	$45.46	$28.66	$35.24	$41.17	$48.10	$61.10
Surgery: Bariatric	2	1	*	*	*	*	*	*
Surgery: Cardiovascular	47	16	$36.87	$8.77	$33.67	$37.24	$40.07	$43.11
Surgery: Colon and Rectal	18	8	$170.74	$237.55	$39.18	$45.33	$228.51	$704.21
Surgery: Neurological	75	19	$50.64	$18.42	$40.84	$48.20	$62.01	$74.67
Surgery: Oncology	6	4	*	*	*	*	*	*
Surgery: Oral	1	1	*	*	*	*	*	*
Surgery: Pediatric	4	4	*	*	*	*	*	*
Surgery: Plastic & Reconstruction	26	13	$43.85	$21.57	$33.95	$44.93	$54.65	$66.92
Surgery: Plastic & Recon-Hand	1	1	*	*	*	*	*	*
Surgery: Thoracic (primary)	17	5	$36.64	$5.62	$30.94	$38.38	$40.84	$44.02
Surgery: Transplant	8	2	*	*	*	*	*	*
Surgery: Trauma	6	1	*	*	*	*	*	*
Surgery: Trauma-Burn	1	1	*	*	*	*	*	*
Surgery: Vascular (primary)	21	12	$123.51	$281.45	$26.43	$36.77	$43.57	$787.29
Urgent Care	148	18	$50.80	$21.33	$34.42	$45.16	$56.66	$91.32
Urology	90	28	$35.92	$18.96	$25.81	$34.66	$43.51	$51.92
Urology: Pediatric	0	*	*	*	*	*	*	*

Table 61: Total RVUs to Total Encounters Ratio (TC/NPP Excluded)

	Phys	Med Pracs	Mean	Std. Dev.	25th %tile	Median	75th %tile	90th %tile
Allergy/Immunology	28	18	6.149	5.973	2.506	4.285	7.632	11.156
Anesthesiology	1,701	79	11.347	8.540	8.184	11.550	13.704	14.946
Anesthesiology: Pain Management	24	14	7.558	9.739	2.576	4.389	8.323	22.794
Anesthesiology: Pediatric	22	2	*	*	*	*	*	*
Cardiology: Electrophysiology	32	15	8.445	4.724	4.649	7.564	10.487	16.873
Cardiology: Invasive	103	24	4.775	2.770	2.784	3.920	6.683	8.900
Cardiology: Inv-Intvl	111	27	7.800	11.162	4.295	5.634	7.519	10.577
Cardiology: Noninvasive	103	20	6.535	3.654	3.842	5.827	8.053	10.847
Critical Care: Intensivist	1	1	*	*	*	*	*	*
Dentistry	3	1	*	*	*	*	*	*
Dermatology	90	40	3.861	4.208	2.190	2.930	3.612	4.766
Dermatology: Mohs Surgery	5	5	*	*	*	*	*	*
Emergency Medicine	153	12	3.101	.669	2.761	3.171	3.435	3.627
Endocrinology/Metabolism	79	42	11.010	55.202	2.195	2.779	3.680	5.172
Family Practice (w/ OB)	186	34	2.252	.528	1.927	2.153	2.462	2.788
Family Practice (w/o OB)	1,396	130	3.507	8.709	1.857	2.107	2.408	2.913
FP: Amb Only (no inpatient work)	11	2	*	*	*	*	*	*
Family Practice: Sports Med	13	8	3.337	1.330	2.347	3.046	4.023	5.929
Family Practice: Urgent Care	18	4	1.936	.492	1.730	1.888	1.916	2.408
Gastroenterology	226	55	7.976	4.222	5.172	7.099	9.741	12.387
Gastroenterology: Hepatology	0	*	*	*	*	*	*	*
Genetics	2	1	*	*	*	*	*	*
Geriatrics	18	8	2.285	.302	2.128	2.306	2.495	2.702
Hematology/Oncology	117	28	15.325	125.479	2.513	3.271	4.167	4.968
Hematology/Oncology: Onc (only)	8	4	*	*	*	*	*	*
Hospice/Palliative Care	1	1	*	*	*	*	*	*
Hospitalist: Family Practice	11	2	*	*	*	*	*	*
Hospitalist: Internal Medicine	374	47	36.423	407.921	2.266	2.540	2.966	3.810
Hospitalist: IM-Pediatrics	0	*	*	*	*	*	*	*
Hospitalist: Pediatrics	5	4	*	*	*	*	*	*
Infectious Disease	26	14	2.406	.563	2.056	2.287	2.692	2.982
Internal Medicine: General	1,101	105	5.634	48.271	1.878	2.211	2.567	3.412
IM: Amb Only (no inpatient work)	3	3	*	*	*	*	*	*
Internal Med: Pediatrics	31	11	3.241	5.084	1.836	2.277	2.517	4.641
Nephrology	54	20	14.433	57.065	2.996	3.942	5.516	7.504
Neurology	141	43	4.765	4.990	3.149	3.786	4.953	7.269
Obstetrics/Gynecology: General	338	63	5.402	5.282	3.560	4.104	4.970	6.772
OB/GYN: Gynecology (only)	28	17	4.387	3.943	2.886	3.595	4.562	5.778
OB/GYN: Gyn Oncology	4	3	*	*	*	*	*	*
OB/GYN: Maternal & Fetal Med	5	4	*	*	*	*	*	*
OB/GYN: Repro Endocrinology	0	*	*	*	*	*	*	*
OB/GYN: Urogynecology	0	*	*	*	*	*	*	*
Occupational Medicine	36	13	5.944	12.942	1.951	2.933	4.180	4.745
Ophthalmology	85	27	4.328	4.725	2.570	3.077	3.861	5.715
Ophthalmology: Pediatric	8	5	*	*	*	*	*	*
Ophthalmology: Retina	6	5	*	*	*	*	*	*
Orthopedic (Nonsurgical)	7	6	*	*	*	*	*	*
Orthopedic Surgery: General	171	42	5.422	2.259	4.011	4.946	6.435	8.309
Orthopedic Surgery: Foot & Ankle	6	5	*	*	*	*	*	*
Orthopedic Surgery: Hand	19	10	6.173	5.379	3.890	5.381	6.175	6.911
Orthopedic Surgery: Hip & Joint	13	6	6.099	1.433	4.974	6.781	7.264	7.764
Orthopedic Surgery: Pediatric	1	1	*	*	*	*	*	*
Orthopedic Surgery: Spine	13	8	11.287	16.836	4.066	8.038	9.745	44.256
Orthopedic Surgery: Trauma	9	5	*	*	*	*	*	*
Orthopedic Surgery: Sports Med	19	8	5.631	2.173	4.192	5.189	6.303	8.970

Table 61: Total RVUs to Total Encounters Ratio (TC/NPP Excluded) (continued)

	Phys	Med Pracs	Mean	Std. Dev.	25th %tile	Median	75th %tile	90th %tile
Otorhinolaryngology	96	38	4.348	3.369	3.076	3.741	4.467	5.701
Pathology: Anatomic and Clinical	3	1	*	*	*	*	*	*
Pathology: Anatomic	1	1	*	*	*	*	*	*
Pathology: Clinical	7	1	*	*	*	*	*	*
Pediatrics: General	754	82	3.574	12.154	1.945	2.113	2.395	3.032
Pediatrics: Adolescent Medicine	13	2	*	*	*	*	*	*
Pediatrics: Allergy/Immunology	0	*	*	*	*	*	*	*
Pediatrics: Cardiology	4	3	*	*	*	*	*	*
Pediatrics: Child Development	1	1	*	*	*	*	*	*
Pediatrics: Critical Care/Intensivist	5	2	*	*	*	*	*	*
Pediatrics: Emergency Medicine	1	1	*	*	*	*	*	*
Pediatrics: Endocrinology	5	4	*	*	*	*	*	*
Pediatrics: Gastroenterology	2	1	*	*	*	*	*	*
Pediatrics: Genetics	3	2	*	*	*	*	*	*
Pediatrics: Hematology/Oncology	4	3	*	*	*	*	*	*
Pediatrics: Infectious Disease	4	4	*	*	*	*	*	*
Pediatrics: Neonatal Medicine	16	4	5.148	.759	4.893	5.185	5.602	5.928
Pediatrics: Nephrology	2	2	*	*	*	*	*	*
Pediatrics: Neurology	12	7	4.145	1.809	2.853	3.656	5.221	7.786
Pediatrics: Pulmonology	1	1	*	*	*	*	*	*
Pediatrics: Rheumatology	2	1	*	*	*	*	*	*
Physiatry (Phys Med & Rehab)	54	20	4.364	3.598	2.324	3.459	4.867	7.593
Podiatry: General	41	22	2.669	.934	2.112	2.461	3.155	3.463
Podiatry: Surg-Foot & Ankle	17	5	2.451	.518	2.043	2.263	2.815	3.432
Podiatry: Surg-Forefoot Only	0	*	*	*	*	*	*	*
Psychiatry: General	73	21	2.450	2.348	1.762	2.020	2.280	2.841
Psychiatry: Child & Adolescent	8	6	*	*	*	*	*	*
Psychiatry: Geriatric	0	*	*	*	*	*	*	*
Pulmonary Medicine	78	31	5.925	9.956	2.692	3.723	5.059	7.718
Pulmonary Medicine: Critical Care	11	4	3.946	.806	3.156	3.914	4.662	5.218
Pulmonary Med: Gen & Crit Care	8	6	*	*	*	*	*	*
Radiation Oncology	32	9	16.706	11.621	10.370	13.013	17.533	32.831
Radiology: Diagnostic-Inv	39	13	26.145	45.905	1.222	2.749	21.120	101.389
Radiology: Diagnostic-Noninv	87	16	345.712	1,310.311	3.734	84.681	194.518	393.973
Radiology: Nuclear Medicine	10	7	125.308	216.429	2.887	6.541	265.842	603.519
Rheumatology	78	35	3.804	2.685	2.415	2.897	3.418	8.747
Sleep Medicine	15	6	9.072	9.871	4.778	5.840	6.515	30.717
Surgery: General	265	64	6.465	2.411	4.836	5.718	7.534	9.384
Surgery: Bariatric	7	3	*	*	*	*	*	*
Surgery: Cardiovascular	45	17	25.927	13.971	12.814	24.883	34.756	51.049
Surgery: Colon and Rectal	15	6	7.230	2.993	4.552	6.732	10.319	11.478
Surgery: Neurological	78	21	10.706	4.292	7.278	9.506	14.180	16.661
Surgery: Oncology	4	2	*	*	*	*	*	*
Surgery: Oral	0	*	*	*	*	*	*	*
Surgery: Pediatric	4	4	*	*	*	*	*	*
Surgery: Plastic & Reconstruction	29	14	27.690	58.007	4.717	6.188	10.279	170.161
Surgery: Plastic & Recon-Hand	0	*	*	*	*	*	*	*
Surgery: Thoracic (primary)	15	5	19.580	5.743	19.069	21.398	24.565	25.408
Surgery: Transplant	8	2	*	*	*	*	*	*
Surgery: Trauma	6	1	*	*	*	*	*	*
Surgery: Trauma-Burn	1	1	*	*	*	*	*	*
Surgery: Vascular (primary)	21	11	8.461	8.682	2.719	6.144	8.387	27.432
Urgent Care	175	26	3.137	6.291	1.741	2.008	2.367	2.704
Urology	94	30	6.294	4.197	4.028	5.050	6.499	11.571
Urology: Pediatric	0	*	*	*	*	*	*	*

Table 62: Physician Work RVUs (CMS RBRVS Method) (NPP Excluded)

	Phys	Med Pracs	Mean	Std. Dev.	25th %tile	Median	75th %tile	90th %tile
Allergy/Immunology	84	49	4,393	1,750	3,295	4,159	5,112	6,990
Anesthesiology	253	19	7,354	5,480	2,391	5,357	12,176	13,803
Anesthesiology: Pain Management	50	24	7,877	4,166	4,982	6,272	9,931	14,083
Anesthesiology: Pediatric	32	3	1,340	398	1,221	1,330	1,330	1,766
Cardiology: Electrophysiology	95	47	12,045	5,338	8,368	11,291	13,552	18,067
Cardiology: Invasive	244	68	9,409	3,366	6,837	9,256	11,332	13,562
Cardiology: Inv-Intvl	299	79	11,430	5,058	8,359	10,225	13,015	18,126
Cardiology: Noninvasive	241	70	8,005	3,767	5,352	7,274	9,849	12,847
Critical Care: Intensivist	25	9	4,742	2,001	3,848	4,980	6,119	7,263
Dentistry	6	2	*	*	*	*	*	*
Dermatology	213	78	8,224	5,120	5,306	7,113	9,458	12,755
Dermatology: Mohs Surgery	17	14	17,494	6,996	11,730	17,387	22,578	27,604
Emergency Medicine	281	25	6,686	2,447	4,939	6,516	8,403	9,716
Endocrinology/Metabolism	191	88	4,712	1,473	3,748	4,519	5,696	6,710
Family Practice (w/ OB)	552	77	4,785	1,482	3,868	4,664	5,555	6,691
Family Practice (w/o OB)	3,629	300	4,800	1,926	3,701	4,600	5,606	6,796
FP: Amb Only (no inpatient work)	77	10	4,031	1,426	3,074	3,773	4,875	5,771
Family Practice: Sports Med	25	19	4,624	2,177	3,196	3,717	5,600	7,988
Family Practice: Urgent Care	35	9	4,707	2,117	3,355	3,938	5,130	9,249
Gastroenterology	491	121	8,779	3,085	6,812	8,381	10,428	12,733
Gastroenterology: Hepatology	5	3	*	*	*	*	*	*
Genetics	3	2	*	*	*	*	*	*
Geriatrics	32	18	3,274	1,440	2,258	2,989	4,216	5,504
Hematology/Oncology	241	62	4,973	1,636	3,608	4,903	5,993	7,302
Hematology/Oncology: Onc (only)	26	16	5,179	2,897	3,104	5,141	6,576	9,597
Hospice/Palliative Care	5	5	*	*	*	*	*	*
Hospitalist: Family Practice	28	8	4,430	1,424	3,072	4,342	5,481	6,449
Hospitalist: Internal Medicine	784	98	4,091	1,550	3,000	3,943	5,017	6,293
Hospitalist: IM-Pediatrics	3	2	*	*	*	*	*	*
Hospitalist: Pediatrics	67	15	2,144	983	1,368	2,280	2,882	3,508
Infectious Disease	134	39	4,348	1,602	3,290	3,988	4,910	6,890
Internal Medicine: General	2,613	229	4,711	1,797	3,546	4,554	5,632	6,779
IM: Amb Only (no inpatient work)	21	9	3,853	1,304	2,977	3,587	4,876	5,649
Internal Med: Pediatrics	72	24	4,208	1,302	3,367	4,291	4,958	5,964
Nephrology	117	51	7,268	3,000	5,320	6,471	9,499	11,347
Neurology	376	105	5,391	2,034	4,023	5,154	6,425	8,214
Obstetrics/Gynecology: General	885	153	7,117	2,566	5,404	6,850	8,392	10,282
OB/GYN: Gynecology (only)	126	47	5,779	2,275	4,188	5,421	6,765	8,497
OB/GYN: Gyn Oncology	23	14	6,542	2,596	4,910	6,042	8,962	10,277
OB/GYN: Maternal & Fetal Med	50	15	7,760	3,123	5,801	7,107	10,432	12,045
OB/GYN: Repro Endocrinology	6	5	*	*	*	*	*	*
OB/GYN: Urogynecology	4	3	*	*	*	*	*	*
Occupational Medicine	72	37	4,476	2,242	3,071	4,275	6,031	7,620
Ophthalmology	211	70	8,288	4,143	5,871	7,655	9,627	12,220
Ophthalmology: Pediatric	13	9	7,754	3,872	4,378	6,277	11,466	13,947
Ophthalmology: Retina	12	9	13,075	2,846	11,066	12,387	14,093	19,067
Orthopedic (Nonsurgical)	23	17	4,088	1,414	3,013	3,592	5,434	6,212
Orthopedic Surgery: General	454	110	8,633	3,413	6,462	8,256	10,504	13,147
Orthopedic Surgery: Foot & Ankle	27	16	10,058	3,762	7,016	9,605	11,503	16,032
Orthopedic Surgery: Hand	66	34	9,094	3,747	6,795	8,324	10,410	15,511
Orthopedic Surgery: Hip & Joint	60	24	11,285	3,873	8,774	10,078	13,936	16,364
Orthopedic Surgery: Pediatric	21	12	9,603	4,146	5,938	9,776	12,549	16,786
Orthopedic Surgery: Spine	53	26	12,820	5,094	9,363	11,751	15,712	20,593
Orthopedic Surgery: Trauma	16	10	9,255	4,814	6,027	8,525	11,516	17,560
Orthopedic Surgery: Sports Med	100	35	10,843	4,947	7,784	10,284	13,075	17,442

Table 62: Physician Work RVUs (CMS RBRVS Method) (NPP Excluded) (continued)

	Phys	Med Pracs	Mean	Std. Dev.	25th %tile	Median	75th %tile	90th %tile
Otorhinolaryngology	231	88	7,353	2,745	5,460	7,116	8,932	11,004
Pathology: Anatomic and Clinical	73	13	5,658	2,400	3,736	5,518	7,075	8,550
Pathology: Anatomic	19	4	5,704	2,263	4,535	5,238	6,330	9,552
Pathology: Clinical	31	9	5,475	2,453	3,709	4,463	8,249	9,186
Pediatrics: General	1,598	185	5,053	1,748	3,825	4,835	6,018	7,401
Pediatrics: Adolescent Medicine	56	6	3,732	1,256	2,941	3,940	4,703	5,303
Pediatrics: Allergy/Immunology	2	2	*	*	*	*	*	*
Pediatrics: Cardiology	40	13	4,646	1,461	3,892	4,689	5,550	6,166
Pediatrics: Child Development	10	6	2,274	699	1,591	2,241	2,808	3,391
Pediatrics: Critical Care/Intensivist	37	12	4,336	2,597	2,358	3,250	5,428	8,310
Pediatrics: Emergency Medicine	9	4	*	*	*	*	*	*
Pediatrics: Endocrinology	23	15	3,504	1,287	2,848	3,347	4,251	5,517
Pediatrics: Gastroenterology	27	14	4,942	2,315	3,285	4,529	6,352	8,854
Pediatrics: Genetics	7	5	*	*	*	*	*	*
Pediatrics: Hematology/Oncology	49	14	3,710	1,472	2,767	3,898	4,555	5,084
Pediatrics: Infectious Disease	11	5	4,104	1,885	2,653	3,600	5,525	7,699
Pediatrics: Neonatal Medicine	70	12	9,788	4,220	6,853	8,437	12,685	16,433
Pediatrics: Nephrology	7	6	*	*	*	*	*	*
Pediatrics: Neurology	45	20	4,311	1,512	3,369	3,776	5,080	6,159
Pediatrics: Pulmonology	15	8	5,272	3,101	3,113	4,695	5,789	11,700
Pediatrics: Rheumatology	5	3	*	*	*	*	*	*
Physiatry (Phys Med & Rehab)	114	48	5,408	2,429	3,460	4,963	6,986	9,095
Podiatry: General	96	51	4,889	1,983	3,492	4,756	5,976	6,910
Podiatry: Surg-Foot & Ankle	59	21	5,706	1,694	4,514	5,516	6,696	7,960
Podiatry: Surg-Forefoot Only	3	2	*	*	*	*	*	*
Psychiatry: General	228	57	3,528	1,418	2,553	3,398	4,300	5,464
Psychiatry: Child & Adolescent	35	19	3,026	1,462	1,962	2,562	3,979	5,174
Psychiatry: Geriatric	7	3	*	*	*	*	*	*
Pulmonary Medicine	170	66	7,355	3,149	5,076	6,773	9,369	11,483
Pulmonary Medicine: Critical Care	46	11	8,521	2,625	6,796	8,470	10,076	11,877
Pulmonary Med: Gen & Crit Care	86	21	6,241	2,443	4,267	5,918	7,299	9,697
Radiation Oncology	78	24	9,969	4,889	6,814	8,625	12,186	15,547
Radiology: Diagnostic-Inv	154	32	11,042	4,068	8,412	10,475	13,701	16,473
Radiology: Diagnostic-Noninv	421	50	9,801	4,107	6,824	9,377	12,193	14,894
Radiology: Nuclear Medicine	24	13	8,881	4,118	5,406	7,809	12,566	14,464
Rheumatology	184	84	4,565	1,400	3,684	4,488	5,349	6,586
Sleep Medicine	41	20	7,411	3,185	4,627	7,159	9,570	11,613
Surgery: General	568	148	7,424	2,705	5,792	7,170	8,843	10,964
Surgery: Bariatric	16	10	8,406	3,460	6,256	8,217	9,949	14,799
Surgery: Cardiovascular	138	43	10,096	4,371	6,586	9,608	13,537	15,491
Surgery: Colon and Rectal	29	12	7,505	4,218	3,920	6,865	10,379	13,745
Surgery: Neurological	129	43	10,511	5,093	7,208	9,783	12,885	16,103
Surgery: Oncology	10	8	6,842	4,234	3,783	6,630	9,765	13,891
Surgery: Oral	6	4	*	*	*	*	*	*
Surgery: Pediatric	28	16	6,438	3,142	4,144	5,845	7,763	11,266
Surgery: Plastic & Reconstruction	64	34	6,804	2,816	5,044	6,280	7,899	11,576
Surgery: Plastic & Recon-Hand	6	3	*	*	*	*	*	*
Surgery: Thoracic (primary)	21	10	8,729	3,876	5,440	7,353	10,759	15,227
Surgery: Transplant	24	8	7,448	2,887	4,902	6,952	9,423	11,661
Surgery: Trauma	43	9	5,976	2,293	4,165	5,491	7,880	9,113
Surgery: Trauma-Burn	4	2	*	*	*	*	*	*
Surgery: Vascular (primary)	78	31	9,920	4,565	7,609	9,486	11,646	13,755
Urgent Care	332	52	5,397	2,150	3,798	5,015	6,657	8,476
Urology	256	84	8,604	3,126	6,437	8,222	10,417	12,848
Urology: Pediatric	4	3	*	*	*	*	*	*

Table 63: Physician Work RVUs (CMS RBRVS Method) (NPP Excluded) by Group Type

	Single Specialty			Multispecialty		
	Phys	Med Pracs	Median	Phys	Med Pracs	Median
Allergy/Immunology	9	2	*	75	47	3,972
Anesthesiology	229	10	7,161	24	9	4,746
Anesthesiology: Pain Management	11	5	6,202	39	19	6,924
Anesthesiology: Pediatric	16	1	*	16	2	*
Cardiology: Electrophysiology	54	23	11,790	41	24	10,585
Cardiology: Invasive	99	21	9,007	145	47	9,362
Cardiology: Inv-Intvl	149	27	9,784	150	52	10,896
Cardiology: Noninvasive	85	25	8,854	156	45	6,721
Critical Care: Intensivist	3	1	*	22	8	4,984
Dentistry	0	*	*	6	2	*
Dermatology	20	5	6,915	193	73	7,113
Dermatology: Mohs Surgery	1	1	*	16	13	16,506
Emergency Medicine	46	2	*	235	23	6,512
Endocrinology/Metabolism	9	6	*	182	82	4,556
Family Practice (w/ OB)	32	9	4,650	520	68	4,664
Family Practice (w/o OB)	311	98	4,657	3,318	202	4,591
FP: Amb Only (no inpatient work)	1	1	*	76	9	3,768
Family Practice: Sports Med	6	5	*	19	14	3,717
Family Practice: Urgent Care	0	*	*	35	9	3,938
Gastroenterology	136	12	8,260	355	109	8,440
Gastroenterology: Hepatology	1	1	*	4	2	*
Genetics	*	*	*	3	2	*
Geriatrics	1	1	*	31	17	3,050
Hematology/Oncology	38	5	5,096	203	57	4,852
Hematology/Oncology: Onc (only)	2	1	*	24	15	5,141
Hospice/Palliative Care	2	2	*	3	3	*
Hospitalist: Family Practice	1	1	*	27	7	4,418
Hospitalist: Internal Medicine	83	12	5,377	701	86	3,804
Hospitalist: IM-Pediatrics	*	*	*	3	2	*
Hospitalist: Pediatrics	9	1	*	58	14	1,826
Infectious Disease	8	4	*	126	35	3,973
Internal Medicine: General	155	33	4,484	2,458	196	4,563
IM: Amb Only (no inpatient work)	0	*	*	21	9	3,587
Internal Med: Pediatrics	0	*	*	72	24	4,291
Nephrology	2	1	*	115	50	6,488
Neurology	56	15	5,737	320	90	5,069
Obstetrics/Gynecology: General	115	27	6,763	770	126	6,864
OB/GYN: Gynecology (only)	11	6	8,009	115	41	5,358
OB/GYN: Gyn Oncology	2	2	*	21	12	6,753
OB/GYN: Maternal & Fetal Med	12	3	9,454	38	12	7,000
OB/GYN: Repro Endocrinology	0	*	*	6	5	*
OB/GYN: Urogynecology	*	*	*	4	3	*
Occupational Medicine	1	1	*	71	36	4,297
Ophthalmology	11	3	10,652	200	67	7,524
Ophthalmology: Pediatric	1	1	*	12	8	5,929
Ophthalmology: Retina	2	1	*	10	8	12,387
Orthopedic (Nonsurgical)	8	6	*	15	11	3,590
Orthopedic Surgery: General	88	21	8,652	366	89	8,186
Orthopedic Surgery: Foot & Ankle	14	8	10,219	13	8	9,376
Orthopedic Surgery: Hand	23	10	8,406	43	24	8,243
Orthopedic Surgery: Hip & Joint	35	15	10,794	25	9	10,001
Orthopedic Surgery: Pediatric	3	3	*	18	9	9,695
Orthopedic Surgery: Spine	23	13	10,788	30	13	12,106
Orthopedic Surgery: Trauma	10	5	8,605	6	5	*
Orthopedic Surgery: Sports Med	41	17	12,076	59	18	8,908

Table 63: Physician Work RVUs (CMS RBRVS Method) (NPP Excluded) by Group Type (continued)

	Single Specialty			Multispecialty		
	Phys	Med Pracs	Median	Phys	Med Pracs	Median
Otorhinolaryngology	15	3	7,636	216	85	7,043
Pathology: Anatomic and Clinical	19	1	*	54	12	6,043
Pathology: Anatomic	*	*	*	19	4	5,238
Pathology: Clinical	0	*	*	31	9	4,463
Pediatrics: General	252	25	5,263	1,346	160	4,804
Pediatrics: Adolescent Medicine	0	*	*	56	6	3,940
Pediatrics: Allergy/Immunology	0	*	*	2	2	*
Pediatrics: Cardiology	2	1	*	38	12	4,700
Pediatrics: Child Development	*	*	*	10	6	2,241
Pediatrics: Critical Care/Intensivist	0	*	*	37	12	3,250
Pediatrics: Emergency Medicine	0	*	*	9	4	*
Pediatrics: Endocrinology	0	*	*	23	15	3,347
Pediatrics: Gastroenterology	1	1	*	26	13	4,322
Pediatrics: Genetics	0	*	*	7	5	*
Pediatrics: Hematology/Oncology	0	*	*	49	14	3,898
Pediatrics: Infectious Disease	*	*	*	11	5	3,600
Pediatrics: Neonatal Medicine	16	3	8,253	54	9	8,533
Pediatrics: Nephrology	*	*	*	7	6	*
Pediatrics: Neurology	2	1	*	43	19	3,787
Pediatrics: Pulmonology	0	*	*	15	8	4,695
Pediatrics: Rheumatology	*	*	*	5	3	*
Physiatry (Phys Med & Rehab)	24	8	5,326	90	40	4,829
Podiatry: General	1	1	*	95	50	4,758
Podiatry: Surg-Foot & Ankle	0	*	*	59	21	5,516
Podiatry: Surg-Forefoot Only	1	1	*	2	1	*
Psychiatry: General	15	2	*	213	55	3,314
Psychiatry: Child & Adolescent	2	1	*	33	18	2,561
Psychiatry: Geriatric	4	1	*	3	2	*
Pulmonary Medicine	11	3	5,644	159	63	7,038
Pulmonary Medicine: Critical Care	1	1	*	45	10	8,433
Pulmonary Med: Gen & Crit Care	19	2	*	67	19	6,287
Radiation Oncology	14	2	*	64	22	8,191
Radiology: Diagnostic-Inv	82	11	10,454	72	21	10,641
Radiology: Diagnostic-Noninv	125	11	11,852	296	39	8,313
Radiology: Nuclear Medicine	13	6	8,910	11	7	7,077
Rheumatology	12	5	2,994	172	79	4,543
Sleep Medicine	0	*	*	41	20	7,159
Surgery: General	57	14	7,318	511	134	7,136
Surgery: Bariatric	4	2	*	12	8	7,380
Surgery: Cardiovascular	39	11	11,388	99	32	9,572
Surgery: Colon and Rectal	*	*	*	29	12	6,865
Surgery: Neurological	19	3	11,027	110	40	9,744
Surgery: Oncology	1	1	*	9	7	*
Surgery: Oral	0	*	*	6	4	*
Surgery: Pediatric	6	2	*	22	14	5,542
Surgery: Plastic & Reconstruction	1	1	*	63	33	6,296
Surgery: Plastic & Recon-Hand	0	*	*	6	3	*
Surgery: Thoracic (primary)	7	3	*	14	7	6,960
Surgery: Transplant	7	1	*	17	7	5,614
Surgery: Trauma	6	2	*	37	7	5,947
Surgery: Trauma-Burn	*	*	*	4	2	*
Surgery: Vascular (primary)	7	4	*	71	27	9,586
Urgent Care	4	1	*	328	51	5,053
Urology	64	9	9,716	192	75	7,761
Urology: Pediatric	1	1	*	3	2	*

Table 64: Physician Work RVUs (CMS RBRVS Method) (NPP Excluded) by Hospital Ownership

	Hospital Owned			Not Hospital Owned		
	Phys	Med Pracs	Median	Phys	Med Pracs	Median
Allergy/Immunology	20	15	4,443	64	34	4,121
Anesthesiology	6	4	*	247	15	5,357
Anesthesiology: Pain Management	14	6	5,504	36	18	6,517
Anesthesiology: Pediatric	15	1	*	17	2	*
Cardiology: Electrophysiology	23	13	10,980	72	34	11,726
Cardiology: Invasive	58	14	9,018	186	54	9,269
Cardiology: Inv-Intvl	67	22	9,291	232	57	10,622
Cardiology: Noninvasive	83	22	6,815	158	48	7,701
Critical Care: Intensivist	15	4	4,507	10	5	4,987
Dentistry	3	1	*	3	1	*
Dermatology	56	26	7,193	157	52	7,072
Dermatology: Mohs Surgery	5	3	*	12	11	19,615
Emergency Medicine	166	14	6,203	115	11	7,382
Endocrinology/Metabolism	92	40	4,562	99	48	4,461
Family Practice (w/ OB)	289	43	4,488	263	34	4,754
Family Practice (w/o OB)	2,248	193	4,540	1,381	107	4,736
FP: Amb Only (no inpatient work)	71	9	3,711	6	1	*
Family Practice: Sports Med	11	7	3,717	14	12	4,114
Family Practice: Urgent Care	29	6	3,625	6	3	*
Gastroenterology	114	42	8,555	377	79	8,261
Gastroenterology: Hepatology	3	1	*	2	2	*
Genetics	3	2	*	0	*	*
Geriatrics	20	12	2,759	12	6	3,281
Hematology/Oncology	76	19	4,532	165	43	5,034
Hematology/Oncology: Onc (only)	12	8	3,026	14	8	5,830
Hospice/Palliative Care	4	4	*	1	1	*
Hospitalist: Family Practice	12	3	3,377	16	5	5,168
Hospitalist: Internal Medicine	433	49	3,913	351	49	3,987
Hospitalist: IM-Pediatrics	1	1	*	2	1	*
Hospitalist: Pediatrics	41	10	1,844	26	5	2,746
Infectious Disease	47	22	4,183	87	17	3,852
Internal Medicine: General	1,286	128	4,582	1,327	101	4,519
IM: Amb Only (no inpatient work)	19	7	4,197	2	2	*
Internal Med: Pediatrics	46	14	4,139	26	10	4,693
Nephrology	36	17	6,000	81	34	7,220
Neurology	155	47	4,717	221	58	5,387
Obstetrics/Gynecology: General	365	71	6,792	520	82	6,879
OB/GYN: Gynecology (only)	68	18	5,265	58	29	5,643
OB/GYN: Gyn Oncology	12	10	5,477	11	4	7,828
OB/GYN: Maternal & Fetal Med	23	8	10,142	27	7	6,444
OB/GYN: Repro Endocrinology	3	3	*	3	2	*
OB/GYN: Urogynecology	4	3	*	0	*	*
Occupational Medicine	15	13	3,915	57	24	4,315
Ophthalmology	52	22	8,058	159	48	7,528
Ophthalmology: Pediatric	3	2	*	10	7	8,405
Ophthalmology: Retina	4	3	*	8	6	*
Orthopedic (Nonsurgical)	3	2	*	20	15	3,591
Orthopedic Surgery: General	127	35	8,041	327	75	8,302
Orthopedic Surgery: Foot & Ankle	3	2	*	24	14	9,874
Orthopedic Surgery: Hand	5	5	*	61	29	8,406
Orthopedic Surgery: Hip & Joint	2	1	*	58	23	10,127
Orthopedic Surgery: Pediatric	7	4	*	14	8	10,365
Orthopedic Surgery: Spine	6	4	*	47	22	11,241
Orthopedic Surgery: Trauma	3	3	*	13	7	8,627
Orthopedic Surgery: Sports Med	11	6	6,224	89	29	10,905

Table 64: Physician Work RVUs (CMS RBRVS Method) (NPP Excluded) by Hospital Ownership (continued)

	Hospital Owned			Not Hospital Owned		
	Phys	Med Pracs	Median	Phys	Med Pracs	Median
Otorhinolaryngology	65	27	7,491	166	61	6,877
Pathology: Anatomic and Clinical	29	5	5,200	44	8	5,571
Pathology: Anatomic	1	1	*	18	3	5,354
Pathology: Clinical	12	4	4,485	19	5	4,463
Pediatrics: General	933	105	5,098	665	80	4,608
Pediatrics: Adolescent Medicine	16	4	2,161	40	2	*
Pediatrics: Allergy/Immunology	1	1	*	1	1	*
Pediatrics: Cardiology	25	7	4,092	15	6	5,322
Pediatrics: Child Development	7	4	*	3	2	*
Pediatrics: Critical Care/Intensivist	29	9	4,242	8	3	*
Pediatrics: Emergency Medicine	8	3	*	1	1	*
Pediatrics: Endocrinology	14	10	3,717	9	5	*
Pediatrics: Gastroenterology	17	8	3,978	10	6	5,066
Pediatrics: Genetics	1	1	*	6	4	*
Pediatrics: Hematology/Oncology	29	9	3,763	20	5	4,142
Pediatrics: Infectious Disease	7	3	*	4	2	*
Pediatrics: Neonatal Medicine	34	8	7,769	36	4	9,869
Pediatrics: Nephrology	4	4	*	3	2	*
Pediatrics: Neurology	22	11	3,650	23	9	4,207
Pediatrics: Pulmonology	11	6	3,451	4	2	*
Pediatrics: Rheumatology	1	1	*	4	2	*
Physiatry (Phys Med & Rehab)	56	19	5,750	58	29	4,183
Podiatry: General	32	18	5,276	64	33	4,526
Podiatry: Surg-Foot & Ankle	18	5	5,526	41	16	5,516
Podiatry: Surg-Forefoot Only	*	*	*	3	2	*
Psychiatry: General	130	39	3,404	98	18	3,365
Psychiatry: Child & Adolescent	28	14	2,564	7	5	*
Psychiatry: Geriatric	3	2	*	4	1	*
Pulmonary Medicine	62	23	6,172	108	43	7,382
Pulmonary Medicine: Critical Care	8	3	*	38	8	8,867
Pulmonary Med: Gen & Crit Care	11	5	8,354	75	16	5,709
Radiation Oncology	37	12	8,269	41	12	10,184
Radiology: Diagnostic-Inv	25	8	8,586	129	24	10,624
Radiology: Diagnostic-Noninv	70	11	7,498	351	39	9,582
Radiology: Nuclear Medicine	10	5	5,601	14	8	10,300
Rheumatology	85	34	4,493	99	50	4,483
Sleep Medicine	8	6	*	33	14	6,386
Surgery: General	221	60	6,874	347	88	7,312
Surgery: Bariatric	5	4	*	11	6	8,836
Surgery: Cardiovascular	53	20	8,152	85	23	11,287
Surgery: Colon and Rectal	3	2	*	26	10	6,783
Surgery: Neurological	53	22	8,769	76	21	10,106
Surgery: Oncology	5	3	*	5	5	*
Surgery: Oral	2	1	*	4	3	*
Surgery: Pediatric	16	11	4,862	12	5	7,201
Surgery: Plastic & Reconstruction	26	11	6,320	38	23	6,207
Surgery: Plastic & Recon-Hand	*	*	*	6	3	*
Surgery: Thoracic (primary)	10	5	6,248	11	5	9,225
Surgery: Transplant	17	5	7,386	7	3	*
Surgery: Trauma	37	8	5,448	6	1	*
Surgery: Trauma-Burn	4	2	*	*	*	*
Surgery: Vascular (primary)	20	10	10,882	58	21	8,981
Urgent Care	109	17	5,179	223	35	4,947
Urology	51	22	7,442	205	62	8,412
Urology: Pediatric	0	*	*	4	3	*

Table 65: Physician Work RVUs (CMS RBRVS Method) (NPP Excluded) by Method of Compensation

	Productivity Based		Non-Productivity Based	
	Phys	Median	Phys	Median
Allergy/Immunology	57	4,042	17	4,633
Anesthesiology	84	10,518	131	3,651
Anesthesiology: Pain Management	33	6,924	12	5,424
Anesthesiology: Pediatric	0	*	15	*
Cardiology: Electrophysiology	45	11,981	39	10,454
Cardiology: Invasive	151	9,788	64	8,034
Cardiology: Inv-Intvl	185	11,625	89	9,140
Cardiology: Noninvasive	99	8,377	125	6,538
Critical Care: Intensivist	5	*	20	4,884
Dentistry	3	*	3	*
Dermatology	132	7,570	36	5,732
Dermatology: Mohs Surgery	10	19,615	5	*
Emergency Medicine	80	7,979	121	6,515
Endocrinology/Metabolism	118	4,763	38	4,181
Family Practice (w/ OB)	251	5,062	86	4,544
Family Practice (w/o OB)	2,131	4,759	718	4,278
FP: Amb Only (no inpatient work)	32	4,889	23	3,297
Family Practice: Sports Med	10	6,200	8	*
Family Practice: Urgent Care	17	5,011	16	3,389
Gastroenterology	330	8,858	87	6,752
Gastroenterology: Hepatology	1	*	4	*
Genetics	*	*	1	*
Geriatrics	11	3,972	14	2,909
Hematology/Oncology	145	5,197	68	4,108
Hematology/Oncology: Onc (only)	15	5,513	9	*
Hospice/Palliative Care	*	*	4	*
Hospitalist: Family Practice	12	*	14	3,377
Hospitalist: Internal Medicine	232	4,059	424	3,741
Hospitalist: IM-Pediatrics	2	*	1	*
Hospitalist: Pediatrics	7	*	46	1,736
Infectious Disease	94	4,007	25	3,310
Internal Medicine: General	1,480	4,796	636	4,068
IM: Amb Only (no inpatient work)	13	4,327	8	*
Internal Med: Pediatrics	33	4,668	11	3,660
Nephrology	57	7,607	30	5,188
Neurology	190	5,781	124	4,355
Obstetrics/Gynecology: General	476	7,051	207	6,181
OB/GYN: Gynecology (only)	95	5,358	21	5,855
OB/GYN: Gyn Oncology	9	*	8	*
OB/GYN: Maternal & Fetal Med	23	6,983	17	7,178
OB/GYN: Repro Endocrinology	1	*	3	*
OB/GYN: Urogynecology	0	*	3	*
Occupational Medicine	31	3,711	20	4,048
Ophthalmology	131	7,855	30	6,685
Ophthalmology: Pediatric	7	*	2	*
Ophthalmology: Retina	5	*	2	*
Orthopedic (Nonsurgical)	14	3,571	7	*
Orthopedic Surgery: General	333	8,252	72	7,944
Orthopedic Surgery: Foot & Ankle	19	10,294	8	*
Orthopedic Surgery: Hand	52	8,558	10	8,083
Orthopedic Surgery: Hip & Joint	44	9,966	8	*
Orthopedic Surgery: Pediatric	14	10,464	5	*
Orthopedic Surgery: Spine	45	11,751	8	*
Orthopedic Surgery: Trauma	6	*	6	*
Orthopedic Surgery: Sports Med	74	10,738	14	8,039

Table 65: Physician Work RVUs (CMS RBRVS Method) (NPP Excluded) by Method of Compensation (continued)

	Productivity Based		Non-Productivity Based	
	Phys	Median	Phys	Median
Otorhinolaryngology	153	7,317	30	6,758
Pathology: Anatomic and Clinical	9	*	56	5,231
Pathology: Anatomic	11	*	8	*
Pathology: Clinical	15	4,745	13	4,341
Pediatrics: General	931	4,825	401	4,644
Pediatrics: Adolescent Medicine	0	*	15	2,204
Pediatrics: Allergy/Immunology	1	*	*	*
Pediatrics: Cardiology	6	*	21	4,046
Pediatrics: Child Development	1	*	9	*
Pediatrics: Critical Care/Intensivist	4	*	33	3,250
Pediatrics: Emergency Medicine	*	*	9	*
Pediatrics: Endocrinology	7	*	9	*
Pediatrics: Gastroenterology	8	*	12	3,788
Pediatrics: Genetics	2	*	3	*
Pediatrics: Hematology/Oncology	19	4,205	23	3,073
Pediatrics: Infectious Disease	9	*	1	*
Pediatrics: Neonatal Medicine	42	9,846	23	7,197
Pediatrics: Nephrology	1	*	3	*
Pediatrics: Neurology	20	4,130	18	3,686
Pediatrics: Pulmonology	7	*	6	*
Pediatrics: Rheumatology	2	*	1	*
Physiatry (Phys Med & Rehab)	65	5,177	31	4,313
Podiatry: General	64	4,936	8	*
Podiatry: Surg-Foot & Ankle	42	5,482	5	*
Podiatry: Surg-Forefoot Only	1	*	*	*
Psychiatry: General	125	3,227	66	3,286
Psychiatry: Child & Adolescent	16	2,016	15	2,566
Psychiatry: Geriatric	1	*	6	*
Pulmonary Medicine	120	7,443	25	5,405
Pulmonary Medicine: Critical Care	34	8,470	4	*
Pulmonary Med: Gen & Crit Care	35	6,287	40	5,808
Radiation Oncology	19	8,112	56	8,461
Radiology: Diagnostic-Inv	37	11,425	110	10,259
Radiology: Diagnostic-Noninv	97	7,568	277	9,950
Radiology: Nuclear Medicine	5	*	16	9,759
Rheumatology	106	4,616	41	3,958
Sleep Medicine	28	8,823	6	*
Surgery: General	344	7,474	131	6,403
Surgery: Bariatric	8	*	5	*
Surgery: Cardiovascular	37	10,913	87	9,572
Surgery: Colon and Rectal	16	8,916	12	6,585
Surgery: Neurological	59	9,981	51	8,531
Surgery: Oncology	3	*	5	*
Surgery: Oral	4	*	2	*
Surgery: Pediatric	5	*	20	4,662
Surgery: Plastic & Reconstruction	39	6,264	17	6,117
Surgery: Plastic & Recon-Hand	5	*	0	*
Surgery: Thoracic (primary)	7	*	12	6,960
Surgery: Transplant	0	*	22	7,290
Surgery: Trauma	7	*	30	5,027
Surgery: Trauma-Burn	*	*	1	*
Surgery: Vascular (primary)	29	8,981	42	9,681
Urgent Care	166	5,884	98	4,203
Urology	148	8,551	75	7,964
Urology: Pediatric	3	*	0	*

Table 66: Physician Compensation to Physician Work RVUs Ratio (CMS RBRVS Method) (NPP Excluded)

	Phys	Med Pracs	Mean	Std. Dev.	25th %tile	Median	75th %tile	90th %tile
Allergy/Immunology	84	48	$70.55	$22.62	$54.37	$66.54	$79.04	$97.72
Anesthesiology	554	40	$727.71	$1,181.99	$110.32	$337.39	$842.21	$1,708.98
Anesthesiology: Pain Management	50	24	$75.24	$29.63	$57.33	$73.99	$84.10	$104.71
Anesthesiology: Pediatric	32	3	$329.93	$68.70	$296.45	$349.42	$369.26	$396.89
Cardiology: Electrophysiology	95	47	$44.55	$16.20	$35.10	$40.96	$50.52	$65.18
Cardiology: Invasive	244	69	$52.89	$18.49	$41.61	$49.23	$61.64	$80.92
Cardiology: Inv-Intvl	299	79	$50.85	$17.67	$38.78	$47.79	$61.48	$76.95
Cardiology: Noninvasive	241	70	$58.97	$27.12	$41.82	$52.07	$69.72	$93.45
Critical Care: Intensivist	23	9	$63.89	$52.69	$37.99	$45.74	$64.59	$136.85
Dentistry	6	2	*	*	*	*	*	*
Dermatology	213	77	$52.41	$17.80	$41.33	$49.31	$59.01	$75.56
Dermatology: Mohs Surgery	17	14	$46.75	$13.74	$39.08	$44.57	$56.65	$68.91
Emergency Medicine	273	25	$41.56	$19.66	$30.44	$36.55	$45.95	$59.44
Endocrinology/Metabolism	191	88	$47.24	$16.64	$37.36	$44.60	$53.02	$62.52
Family Practice (w/ OB)	552	78	$42.94	$11.64	$35.26	$40.48	$47.32	$58.49
Family Practice (w/o OB)	3,629	300	$41.99	$22.16	$32.80	$38.89	$45.58	$56.11
FP: Amb Only (no inpatient work)	77	10	$38.68	$11.36	$33.02	$38.04	$42.24	$47.29
Family Practice: Sports Med	27	19	$55.70	$24.26	$40.19	$51.08	$65.92	$85.99
Family Practice: Urgent Care	37	10	$46.74	$17.88	$34.92	$45.30	$60.29	$68.16
Gastroenterology	491	120	$53.79	$16.71	$42.25	$51.45	$61.61	$77.39
Gastroenterology: Hepatology	5	3	*	*	*	*	*	*
Genetics	3	2	*	*	*	*	*	*
Geriatrics	32	17	$63.54	$32.37	$40.03	$52.83	$73.56	$126.55
Hematology/Oncology	241	64	$91.00	$37.90	$63.38	$82.09	$111.65	$150.20
Hematology/Oncology: Onc (only)	26	16	$1,305.60	$6,114.61	$68.58	$89.91	$158.07	$226.25
Hospice/Palliative Care	5	5	*	*	*	*	*	*
Hospitalist: Family Practice	28	8	$55.38	$12.99	$43.14	$54.20	$67.93	$71.60
Hospitalist: Internal Medicine	783	98	$57.75	$23.51	$44.04	$52.74	$63.68	$83.47
Hospitalist: IM-Pediatrics	3	2	*	*	*	*	*	*
Hospitalist: Pediatrics	65	13	$94.75	$65.96	$52.75	$78.72	$114.94	$156.90
Infectious Disease	134	40	$45.81	$10.17	$39.58	$44.11	$53.50	$59.74
Internal Medicine: General	2,613	229	$45.09	$27.11	$34.59	$40.88	$49.02	$59.89
IM: Amb Only (no inpatient work)	19	8	$47.54	$16.26	$40.25	$41.67	$46.98	$79.63
Internal Med: Pediatrics	70	23	$44.83	$15.72	$37.23	$40.91	$46.97	$61.03
Nephrology	117	51	$46.21	$22.15	$34.29	$43.74	$52.27	$63.88
Neurology	376	105	$50.30	$17.23	$38.94	$47.07	$55.97	$71.74
Obstetrics/Gynecology: General	885	152	$43.35	$13.65	$34.31	$41.20	$48.55	$62.99
OB/GYN: Gynecology (only)	130	49	$43.21	$13.40	$36.97	$44.09	$48.38	$55.47
OB/GYN: Gyn Oncology	21	13	$56.17	$15.85	$45.42	$50.67	$64.42	$77.74
OB/GYN: Maternal & Fetal Med	46	14	$59.36	$18.18	$45.87	$54.75	$77.45	$83.29
OB/GYN: Repro Endocrinology	6	5	*	*	*	*	*	*
OB/GYN: Urogynecology	4	3	*	*	*	*	*	*
Occupational Medicine	70	36	$181.13	$804.51	$40.02	$48.02	$64.11	$132.12
Ophthalmology	211	69	$43.29	$16.58	$34.29	$39.18	$50.24	$59.83
Ophthalmology: Pediatric	13	9	$38.97	$12.02	$29.13	$38.85	$47.65	$58.34
Ophthalmology: Retina	12	9	$41.64	$9.15	$34.60	$39.92	$51.15	$55.06
Orthopedic (Nonsurgical)	25	18	$53.26	$15.96	$41.33	$51.65	$59.58	$76.46
Orthopedic Surgery: General	454	109	$62.06	$25.69	$45.43	$55.64	$71.42	$97.97
Orthopedic Surgery: Foot & Ankle	25	15	$58.69	$28.40	$36.48	$54.36	$69.40	$106.33
Orthopedic Surgery: Hand	68	34	$64.04	$30.66	$43.52	$60.40	$70.73	$117.30
Orthopedic Surgery: Hip & Joint	60	23	$58.05	$25.64	$40.59	$49.78	$67.10	$90.36
Orthopedic Surgery: Pediatric	21	12	$52.42	$15.04	$41.47	$49.59	$65.87	$74.09
Orthopedic Surgery: Spine	53	27	$51.68	$23.33	$34.77	$46.21	$62.47	$83.14
Orthopedic Surgery: Trauma	14	9	$60.56	$21.18	$47.25	$55.84	$61.85	$101.08
Orthopedic Surgery: Sports Med	96	34	$65.32	$29.33	$43.10	$56.44	$78.33	$114.97

Table 66: Physician Compensation to Physician Work RVUs Ratio (CMS RBRVS Method) (NPP Excluded) (continued)

	Phys	Med Pracs	Mean	Std. Dev.	25th %tile	Median	75th %tile	90th %tile
Otorhinolaryngology	231	88	$52.69	$17.71	$41.67	$49.99	$59.59	$74.24
Pathology: Anatomic and Clinical	73	14	$69.44	$45.10	$40.06	$51.66	$86.46	$126.74
Pathology: Anatomic	19	4	$57.78	$19.51	$49.53	$54.25	$62.20	$87.68
Pathology: Clinical	33	9	$65.01	$23.49	$51.71	$60.47	$73.13	$96.02
Pediatrics: General	1,598	185	$40.37	$12.63	$32.19	$38.21	$45.87	$54.99
Pediatrics: Adolescent Medicine	54	4	$53.30	$32.60	$37.54	$40.49	$51.40	$99.11
Pediatrics: Allergy/Immunology	2	2	*	*	*	*	*	*
Pediatrics: Cardiology	38	13	$71.05	$29.24	$47.06	$57.62	$91.09	$117.78
Pediatrics: Child Development	10	6	$74.44	$27.79	$53.12	$63.79	$95.04	$127.29
Pediatrics: Critical Care/Intensivist	37	12	$75.59	$30.32	$55.77	$68.73	$104.94	$123.81
Pediatrics: Emergency Medicine	9	4	*	*	*	*	*	*
Pediatrics: Endocrinology	21	13	$56.64	$21.77	$43.94	$51.27	$63.58	$76.92
Pediatrics: Gastroenterology	29	14	$70.15	$30.24	$46.62	$63.82	$89.57	$115.61
Pediatrics: Genetics	7	5	*	*	*	*	*	*
Pediatrics: Hematology/Oncology	45	14	$62.56	$27.44	$43.29	$54.76	$74.00	$108.89
Pediatrics: Infectious Disease	11	5	$46.41	$12.23	$36.57	$44.26	$54.73	$70.16
Pediatrics: Neonatal Medicine	70	12	$41.70	$19.72	$29.05	$37.13	$47.23	$72.22
Pediatrics: Nephrology	7	6	*	*	*	*	*	*
Pediatrics: Neurology	45	22	$58.91	$22.53	$44.15	$51.20	$64.95	$100.06
Pediatrics: Pulmonology	15	8	$56.34	$17.94	$49.06	$52.54	$57.43	$94.66
Pediatrics: Rheumatology	5	3	*	*	*	*	*	*
Physiatry (Phys Med & Rehab)	114	48	$51.32	$22.24	$34.94	$47.23	$63.84	$79.46
Podiatry: General	96	51	$47.22	$16.98	$35.37	$43.75	$55.25	$68.04
Podiatry: Surg-Foot & Ankle	59	21	$45.79	$10.14	$40.09	$43.67	$50.68	$59.77
Podiatry: Surg-Forefoot Only	3	2	*	*	*	*	*	*
Psychiatry: General	228	58	$70.79	$62.98	$44.73	$53.77	$62.21	$111.03
Psychiatry: Child & Adolescent	35	18	$102.47	$80.02	$54.65	$65.49	$89.86	$243.76
Psychiatry: Geriatric	7	3	*	*	*	*	*	*
Pulmonary Medicine	170	66	$44.00	$18.71	$31.95	$38.83	$50.84	$67.39
Pulmonary Medicine: Critical Care	42	10	$40.18	$12.63	$31.34	$37.07	$48.59	$57.67
Pulmonary Med: Gen & Crit Care	86	21	$52.25	$18.26	$39.79	$49.90	$65.12	$77.92
Radiation Oncology	76	24	$56.59	$23.03	$39.34	$52.24	$68.87	$91.68
Radiology: Diagnostic-Inv	150	31	$51.73	$20.98	$34.20	$50.50	$62.63	$77.48
Radiology: Diagnostic-Noninv	420	49	$52.56	$23.49	$35.10	$48.62	$64.09	$82.47
Radiology: Nuclear Medicine	24	14	$60.60	$30.08	$39.90	$50.75	$81.36	$118.21
Rheumatology	184	84	$52.86	$15.06	$41.81	$48.37	$60.18	$73.47
Sleep Medicine	41	20	$45.97	$21.79	$31.29	$39.35	$56.75	$66.35
Surgery: General	556	143	$50.27	$22.72	$37.44	$45.42	$55.72	$74.23
Surgery: Bariatric	16	10	$55.40	$22.13	$41.52	$52.02	$62.15	$96.04
Surgery: Cardiovascular	134	42	$63.81	$91.56	$35.19	$48.76	$66.74	$98.14
Surgery: Colon and Rectal	29	12	$82.29	$81.18	$35.93	$43.89	$85.14	$265.10
Surgery: Neurological	129	44	$76.43	$30.19	$57.30	$69.21	$91.46	$107.73
Surgery: Oncology	8	6	*	*	*	*	*	*
Surgery: Oral	6	4	*	*	*	*	*	*
Surgery: Pediatric	28	16	$81.95	$40.68	$55.72	$67.32	$100.67	$131.66
Surgery: Plastic & Reconstruction	62	34	$65.71	$28.11	$45.93	$58.43	$75.74	$100.88
Surgery: Plastic & Recon-Hand	6	3	*	*	*	*	*	*
Surgery: Thoracic (primary)	23	10	$53.77	$28.21	$26.98	$54.40	$74.80	$91.63
Surgery: Transplant	24	8	$70.54	$35.36	$44.80	$66.46	$87.29	$131.45
Surgery: Trauma	39	9	$64.00	$19.60	$51.25	$56.10	$69.40	$93.78
Surgery: Trauma-Burn	4	2	*	*	*	*	*	*
Surgery: Vascular (primary)	78	31	$41.63	$14.38	$34.42	$40.18	$50.67	$57.88
Urgent Care	332	52	$43.63	$16.68	$32.38	$38.73	$51.21	$65.40
Urology	256	80	$52.90	$16.13	$42.56	$49.62	$59.67	$75.81
Urology: Pediatric	4	3	*	*	*	*	*	*

Table 67: Physician Compensation to Physician Work RVUs Ratio (CMS RBRVS Method) (NPP Excluded) by Group Type

	Single Specialty			Multispecialty		
	Phys	Med Pracs	Median	Phys	Med Pracs	Median
Allergy/Immunology	9	2	*	75	46	$67.01
Anesthesiology	430	25	$292.89	124	15	$517.35
Anesthesiology: Pain Management	11	5	$74.35	39	19	$68.51
Anesthesiology: Pediatric	16	1	*	16	2	*
Cardiology: Electrophysiology	55	23	$37.12	40	24	$49.21
Cardiology: Invasive	102	21	$46.05	142	48	$52.16
Cardiology: Inv-Intvl	149	27	$44.55	150	52	$50.62
Cardiology: Noninvasive	86	25	$46.46	155	45	$53.64
Critical Care: Intensivist	3	1	*	20	8	$47.25
Dentistry	0	*	*	6	2	*
Dermatology	20	5	$49.96	193	72	$49.31
Dermatology: Mohs Surgery	1	1	*	16	13	$44.33
Emergency Medicine	46	2	*	227	23	$38.63
Endocrinology/Metabolism	9	6	*	182	82	$44.54
Family Practice (w/ OB)	32	9	$38.77	520	69	$40.52
Family Practice (w/o OB)	311	98	$36.49	3,318	202	$39.16
FP: Amb Only (no inpatient work)	1	1	*	76	9	$38.21
Family Practice: Sports Med	7	5	*	20	14	$50.66
Family Practice: Urgent Care	0	*	*	37	10	$45.30
Gastroenterology	137	12	$52.01	354	108	$51.12
Gastroenterology: Hepatology	1	1	*	4	2	*
Genetics	*	*	*	3	2	*
Geriatrics	1	1	*	31	16	$52.12
Hematology/Oncology	36	5	$124.94	205	59	$79.11
Hematology/Oncology: Onc (only)	2	1	*	24	15	$89.91
Hospice/Palliative Care	2	2	*	3	3	*
Hospitalist: Family Practice	1	1	*	27	7	$53.46
Hospitalist: Internal Medicine	80	11	$45.29	703	87	$54.04
Hospitalist: IM-Pediatrics	*	*	*	3	2	*
Hospitalist: Pediatrics	9	1	*	56	12	$90.01
Infectious Disease	7	4	*	127	36	$44.15
Internal Medicine: General	157	33	$41.93	2,456	196	$40.83
IM: Amb Only (no inpatient work)	0	*	*	19	8	$41.67
Internal Med: Pediatrics	0	*	*	70	23	$40.91
Nephrology	2	1	*	115	50	$42.88
Neurology	53	15	$40.67	323	90	$47.40
Obstetrics/Gynecology: General	114	27	$40.38	771	125	$41.34
OB/GYN: Gynecology (only)	14	7	$32.75	116	42	$44.14
OB/GYN: Gyn Oncology	2	2	*	19	11	$50.27
OB/GYN: Maternal & Fetal Med	12	3	$56.85	34	11	$54.56
OB/GYN: Repro Endocrinology	0	*	*	6	5	*
OB/GYN: Urogynecology	*	*	*	4	3	*
Occupational Medicine	0	*	*	70	36	$48.02
Ophthalmology	11	3	$31.60	200	66	$39.75
Ophthalmology: Pediatric	1	1	*	12	8	$40.01
Ophthalmology: Retina	2	1	*	10	8	$41.36
Orthopedic (Nonsurgical)	10	7	$55.21	15	11	$44.41
Orthopedic Surgery: General	87	21	$53.39	367	88	$56.10
Orthopedic Surgery: Foot & Ankle	13	7	$50.24	12	8	$61.44
Orthopedic Surgery: Hand	23	10	$53.88	45	24	$62.49
Orthopedic Surgery: Hip & Joint	34	14	$46.67	26	9	$55.75
Orthopedic Surgery: Pediatric	3	3	*	18	9	$51.33
Orthopedic Surgery: Spine	23	14	$46.21	30	13	$47.83
Orthopedic Surgery: Trauma	10	5	$54.82	4	4	*
Orthopedic Surgery: Sports Med	39	16	$55.62	57	18	$56.70

Table 67: Physician Compensation to Physician Work RVUs Ratio (CMS RBRVS Method) (NPP Excluded) by Group Type (continued)

	Single Specialty			Multispecialty		
	Phys	Med Pracs	Median	Phys	Med Pracs	Median
Otorhinolaryngology	15	3	$38.63	216	85	$50.72
Pathology: Anatomic and Clinical	19	1	*	54	13	$51.04
Pathology: Anatomic	*	*	*	19	4	$54.25
Pathology: Clinical	0	*	*	33	9	$60.47
Pediatrics: General	253	25	$45.28	1,345	160	$37.54
Pediatrics: Adolescent Medicine	0	*	*	54	4	$40.49
Pediatrics: Allergy/Immunology	0	*	*	2	2	*
Pediatrics: Cardiology	2	1	*	36	12	$55.63
Pediatrics: Child Development	*	*	*	10	6	$63.79
Pediatrics: Critical Care/Intensivist	0	*	*	37	12	$68.73
Pediatrics: Emergency Medicine	0	*	*	9	4	*
Pediatrics: Endocrinology	0	*	*	21	13	$51.27
Pediatrics: Gastroenterology	1	1	*	28	13	$63.99
Pediatrics: Genetics	0	*	*	7	5	*
Pediatrics: Hematology/Oncology	0	*	*	45	14	$54.76
Pediatrics: Infectious Disease	*	*	*	11	5	$44.26
Pediatrics: Neonatal Medicine	16	3	$37.92	54	9	$36.09
Pediatrics: Nephrology	*	*	*	7	6	*
Pediatrics: Neurology	2	1	*	43	21	$50.69
Pediatrics: Pulmonology	0	*	*	15	8	$52.54
Pediatrics: Rheumatology	*	*	*	5	3	*
Physiatry (Phys Med & Rehab)	24	8	$36.69	90	40	$50.51
Podiatry: General	1	1	*	95	50	$43.93
Podiatry: Surg-Foot & Ankle	0	*	*	59	21	$43.67
Podiatry: Surg-Forefoot Only	1	1	*	2	1	*
Psychiatry: General	14	2	*	214	56	$54.61
Psychiatry: Child & Adolescent	2	1	*	33	17	$67.66
Psychiatry: Geriatric	4	1	*	3	2	*
Pulmonary Medicine	11	3	$48.48	159	63	$38.78
Pulmonary Medicine: Critical Care	1	1	*	41	9	$36.88
Pulmonary Med: Gen & Crit Care	19	2	*	67	19	$50.82
Radiation Oncology	13	2	*	63	22	$49.49
Radiology: Diagnostic-Inv	80	11	$45.36	70	20	$59.97
Radiology: Diagnostic-Noninv	126	11	$37.50	294	38	$52.97
Radiology: Nuclear Medicine	13	6	$42.27	11	8	$58.24
Rheumatology	12	5	$46.90	172	79	$48.58
Sleep Medicine	0	*	*	41	20	$39.35
Surgery: General	57	14	$39.78	499	129	$46.06
Surgery: Bariatric	4	2	*	12	8	$52.02
Surgery: Cardiovascular	37	11	$49.95	97	31	$46.72
Surgery: Colon and Rectal	*	*	*	29	12	$43.89
Surgery: Neurological	19	3	$71.91	110	41	$68.85
Surgery: Oncology	1	1	*	7	5	*
Surgery: Oral	0	*	*	6	4	*
Surgery: Pediatric	5	2	*	23	14	$65.76
Surgery: Plastic & Reconstruction	1	1	*	61	33	$56.47
Surgery: Plastic & Recon-Hand	0	*	*	6	3	*
Surgery: Thoracic (primary)	7	3	*	16	7	$63.47
Surgery: Transplant	7	1	*	17	7	$69.09
Surgery: Trauma	4	2	*	35	7	$55.04
Surgery: Trauma-Burn	*	*	*	4	2	*
Surgery: Vascular (primary)	7	4	*	71	27	$40.35
Urgent Care	4	1	*	328	51	$38.04
Urology	65	9	$56.17	191	71	$48.68
Urology: Pediatric	1	1	*	3	2	*

Table 68: Collections to Physician Work RVUs Ratio (CMS RBRVS Method) (NPP Excluded)

	Phys	Med Pracs	Mean	Std. Dev.	25th %tile	Median	75th %tile	90th %tile
Allergy/Immunology	35	23	$122.58	$48.77	$91.32	$112.88	$170.34	$184.76
Anesthesiology	477	31	$1,542.04	$5,795.02	$137.28	$509.94	$1,209.47	$2,927.51
Anesthesiology: Pain Management	31	15	$109.09	$40.50	$85.51	$105.15	$132.03	$148.75
Anesthesiology: Pediatric	17	2	*	*	*	*	*	*
Cardiology: Electrophysiology	48	22	$65.49	$13.76	$57.43	$63.83	$74.63	$83.28
Cardiology: Invasive	125	33	$74.27	$34.82	$55.58	$64.98	$83.25	$97.80
Cardiology: Inv-Intvl	153	41	$73.62	$21.20	$59.77	$70.06	$85.71	$99.69
Cardiology: Noninvasive	127	30	$70.68	$27.71	$55.57	$64.28	$77.13	$104.52
Critical Care: Intensivist	15	5	$51.42	$6.09	$46.73	$51.51	$55.27	$61.32
Dentistry	3	1	*	*	*	*	*	*
Dermatology	116	46	$95.15	$33.26	$77.88	$95.26	$115.19	$127.63
Dermatology: Mohs Surgery	9	7	*	*	*	*	*	*
Emergency Medicine	161	14	$43.21	$11.46	$35.49	$42.71	$49.21	$57.15
Endocrinology/Metabolism	97	52	$71.67	$24.52	$61.35	$69.44	$78.87	$97.67
Family Practice (w/ OB)	241	42	$79.19	$35.55	$64.89	$72.92	$85.83	$104.47
Family Practice (w/o OB)	1,886	181	$75.97	$21.86	$64.68	$75.37	$88.68	$101.86
FP: Amb Only (no inpatient work)	32	5	$88.99	$14.62	$78.63	$83.15	$106.53	$109.27
Family Practice: Sports Med	14	9	$78.26	$26.63	$58.74	$78.07	$95.16	$123.56
Family Practice: Urgent Care	26	7	$101.57	$23.98	$82.77	$111.88	$121.86	$129.26
Gastroenterology	261	66	$92.91	$28.73	$73.35	$85.57	$111.76	$136.64
Gastroenterology: Hepatology	3	1	*	*	*	*	*	*
Genetics	3	2	*	*	*	*	*	*
Geriatrics	17	8	$54.85	$14.17	$44.35	$47.30	$69.09	$78.58
Hematology/Oncology	130	29	$111.42	$90.42	$75.00	$94.21	$111.08	$145.97
Hematology/Oncology: Onc (only)	14	8	$1,221.46	$4,242.11	$41.35	$87.39	$133.75	$8,085.56
Hospice/Palliative Care	2	2	*	*	*	*	*	*
Hospitalist: Family Practice	12	3	$56.72	$8.36	$50.02	$56.14	$61.29	$72.43
Hospitalist: Internal Medicine	494	65	$46.01	$11.21	$40.92	$44.94	$50.12	$55.84
Hospitalist: IM-Pediatrics	3	2	*	*	*	*	*	*
Hospitalist: Pediatrics	28	8	$52.73	$12.62	$46.48	$50.83	$57.52	$67.86
Infectious Disease	33	19	$56.13	$19.69	$43.37	$53.74	$65.02	$85.31
Internal Medicine: General	1,349	143	$73.05	$27.78	$59.36	$70.61	$86.13	$101.02
IM: Amb Only (no inpatient work)	9	6	*	*	*	*	*	*
Internal Med: Pediatrics	21	8	$71.83	$18.66	$53.14	$73.20	$82.43	$99.87
Nephrology	70	28	$56.71	$13.44	$49.38	$53.05	$64.42	$70.55
Neurology	195	57	$74.48	$27.70	$57.55	$72.82	$86.00	$109.80
Obstetrics/Gynecology: General	428	84	$80.89	$26.24	$68.72	$78.91	$92.98	$112.51
OB/GYN: Gynecology (only)	49	27	$85.69	$15.29	$76.19	$87.96	$96.63	$105.66
OB/GYN: Gyn Oncology	8	7	*	*	*	*	*	*
OB/GYN: Maternal & Fetal Med	12	7	$85.95	$44.28	$59.27	$70.30	$93.38	$179.33
OB/GYN: Repro Endocrinology	2	2	*	*	*	*	*	*
OB/GYN: Urogynecology	3	2	*	*	*	*	*	*
Occupational Medicine	34	17	$106.55	$76.39	$73.40	$85.47	$120.53	$175.33
Ophthalmology	93	34	$89.21	$38.86	$72.90	$81.28	$94.54	$118.84
Ophthalmology: Pediatric	8	4	*	*	*	*	*	*
Ophthalmology: Retina	5	4	*	*	*	*	*	*
Orthopedic (Nonsurgical)	8	7	*	*	*	*	*	*
Orthopedic Surgery: General	228	55	$88.78	$25.71	$74.59	$85.92	$100.17	$118.62
Orthopedic Surgery: Foot & Ankle	7	5	*	*	*	*	*	*
Orthopedic Surgery: Hand	24	15	$96.30	$31.78	$80.07	$97.69	$124.71	$135.39
Orthopedic Surgery: Hip & Joint	19	8	$85.38	$21.23	$73.00	$77.84	$88.84	$135.12
Orthopedic Surgery: Pediatric	5	5	*	*	*	*	*	*
Orthopedic Surgery: Spine	20	11	$82.41	$29.22	$68.46	$78.96	$94.67	$112.60
Orthopedic Surgery: Trauma	10	6	$77.24	$9.70	$73.42	$80.31	$84.28	$86.40
Orthopedic Surgery: Sports Med	26	11	$84.88	$17.60	$71.97	$77.90	$93.45	$114.27

Table 68: Collections to Physician Work RVUs Ratio (CMS RBRVS Method) (NPP Excluded) (continued)

	Phys	Med Pracs	Mean	Std. Dev.	25th %tile	Median	75th %tile	90th %tile
Otorhinolaryngology	111	50	$101.40	$29.48	$80.20	$96.51	$124.94	$146.01
Pathology: Anatomic and Clinical	24	6	$82.83	$34.10	$60.21	$66.24	$105.13	$142.05
Pathology: Anatomic	0	*	*	*	*	*	*	*
Pathology: Clinical	23	5	$83.39	$17.95	$72.96	$80.35	$88.12	$116.53
Pediatrics: General	943	108	$79.56	$23.23	$67.65	$78.50	$89.99	$109.00
Pediatrics: Adolescent Medicine	13	2	*	*	*	*	*	*
Pediatrics: Allergy/Immunology	0	*	*	*	*	*	*	*
Pediatrics: Cardiology	14	7	$94.96	$51.66	$59.68	$76.06	$139.94	$190.22
Pediatrics: Child Development	5	3	*	*	*	*	*	*
Pediatrics: Critical Care/Intensivist	20	7	$55.89	$16.41	$38.06	$60.10	$66.49	$79.02
Pediatrics: Emergency Medicine	8	3	*	*	*	*	*	*
Pediatrics: Endocrinology	11	8	$88.73	$123.68	$48.25	$55.27	$64.90	$381.47
Pediatrics: Gastroenterology	14	6	$63.98	$30.12	$60.75	$62.55	$77.59	$108.64
Pediatrics: Genetics	3	2	*	*	*	*	*	*
Pediatrics: Hematology/Oncology	17	7	$64.96	$17.35	$48.23	$67.15	$76.97	$91.21
Pediatrics: Infectious Disease	2	2	*	*	*	*	*	*
Pediatrics: Neonatal Medicine	32	7	$64.28	$16.88	$54.08	$61.85	$74.46	$81.85
Pediatrics: Nephrology	4	4	*	*	*	*	*	*
Pediatrics: Neurology	22	14	$70.91	$25.04	$54.18	$63.20	$93.70	$111.41
Pediatrics: Pulmonology	6	4	*	*	*	*	*	*
Pediatrics: Rheumatology	3	2	*	*	*	*	*	*
Physiatry (Phys Med & Rehab)	71	26	$81.29	$32.69	$50.86	$77.44	$105.00	$131.84
Podiatry: General	59	30	$91.56	$33.97	$73.42	$84.68	$99.34	$150.33
Podiatry: Surg-Foot & Ankle	15	7	$95.06	$16.99	$80.47	$94.00	$113.72	$118.51
Podiatry: Surg-Forefoot Only	0	*	*	*	*	*	*	*
Psychiatry: General	105	28	$55.02	$19.07	$41.43	$56.33	$69.94	$78.21
Psychiatry: Child & Adolescent	19	9	$48.61	$23.29	$24.43	$48.68	$66.54	$86.15
Psychiatry: Geriatric	7	3	*	*	*	*	*	*
Pulmonary Medicine	102	40	$63.48	$20.83	$49.89	$57.26	$69.04	$88.25
Pulmonary Medicine: Critical Care	25	6	$45.50	$5.27	$41.03	$44.41	$49.85	$54.52
Pulmonary Med: Gen & Crit Care	10	6	$81.74	$44.82	$48.98	$56.99	$126.62	$148.31
Radiation Oncology	44	13	$59.65	$13.90	$54.45	$57.80	$64.54	$69.01
Radiology: Diagnostic-Inv	102	19	$66.28	$17.74	$53.63	$64.22	$73.15	$91.34
Radiology: Diagnostic-Noninv	200	24	$76.58	$53.47	$55.13	$63.82	$73.56	$97.54
Radiology: Nuclear Medicine	16	9	$59.38	$14.24	$51.94	$60.70	$66.20	$82.93
Rheumatology	95	44	$84.68	$25.76	$67.44	$79.25	$97.09	$120.84
Sleep Medicine	18	8	$68.05	$18.70	$61.50	$67.03	$80.41	$85.25
Surgery: General	321	83	$80.66	$46.66	$62.63	$72.48	$88.17	$103.54
Surgery: Bariatric	3	2	*	*	*	*	*	*
Surgery: Cardiovascular	89	25	$58.56	$17.25	$49.90	$56.41	$62.05	$71.08
Surgery: Colon and Rectal	20	9	$191.08	$215.21	$70.23	$80.59	$237.81	$680.91
Surgery: Neurological	83	25	$87.65	$30.76	$71.04	$82.65	$111.23	$127.99
Surgery: Oncology	5	4	*	*	*	*	*	*
Surgery: Oral	5	3	*	*	*	*	*	*
Surgery: Pediatric	18	10	$62.75	$17.63	$48.85	$62.89	$73.70	$80.27
Surgery: Plastic & Reconstruction	34	18	$103.90	$27.66	$89.22	$97.39	$110.11	$146.96
Surgery: Plastic & Recon-Hand	1	1	*	*	*	*	*	*
Surgery: Thoracic (primary)	15	6	$49.94	$13.65	$31.10	$57.33	$60.88	$62.48
Surgery: Transplant	15	4	$79.54	$9.50	$76.35	$79.60	$83.75	$95.09
Surgery: Trauma	26	6	$53.72	$11.52	$45.80	$47.81	$61.42	$78.44
Surgery: Trauma-Burn	1	1	*	*	*	*	*	*
Surgery: Vascular (primary)	36	13	$68.19	$14.27	$56.56	$68.57	$74.83	$81.62
Urgent Care	187	26	$90.86	$24.51	$69.86	$87.43	$105.55	$131.62
Urology	144	46	$89.21	$28.12	$74.81	$86.34	$102.17	$115.11
Urology: Pediatric	0	*	*	*	*	*	*	*

Table 69: Work RVUs to Total Encounters Ratio (CMS RBRVS Method) (NPP Excluded)

	Phys	Med Pracs	Mean	Std. Dev.	25th %tile	Median	75th %tile	90th %tile
Allergy/Immunology	42	26	1.818	.493	1.557	1.706	1.912	2.282
Anesthesiology	201	16	8.451	5.932	1.542	12.410	12.410	16.589
Anesthesiology: Pain Management	38	19	3.147	2.859	1.664	2.233	3.273	6.413
Anesthesiology: Pediatric	4	1	*	*	*	*	*	*
Cardiology: Electrophysiology	77	36	5.687	3.124	3.106	5.206	7.521	10.108
Cardiology: Invasive	184	50	2.897	1.600	1.859	2.394	3.495	5.111
Cardiology: Inv-Intvl	242	63	3.840	2.877	2.217	3.093	4.401	6.462
Cardiology: Noninvasive	190	55	2.868	1.387	1.901	2.471	3.523	4.675
Critical Care: Intensivist	17	5	3.270	1.042	2.361	3.432	3.879	5.009
Dentistry	2	1	*	*	*	*	*	*
Dermatology	110	43	1.944	1.681	1.285	1.434	1.707	3.699
Dermatology: Mohs Surgery	11	9	7.941	10.889	2.780	3.737	7.733	34.019
Emergency Medicine	199	17	2.343	.457	2.047	2.310	2.667	2.989
Endocrinology/Metabolism	139	69	5.182	24.941	1.234	1.504	1.697	2.427
Family Practice (w/ OB)	337	59	1.367	.798	1.119	1.231	1.375	1.580
Family Practice (w/o OB)	1,940	215	12.377	117.566	1.100	1.204	1.358	1.694
FP: Amb Only (no inpatient work)	45	6	1.188	.129	1.093	1.146	1.255	1.389
Family Practice: Sports Med	18	12	1.399	.404	1.141	1.226	1.612	2.334
Family Practice: Urgent Care	10	7	1.198	.252	1.037	1.107	1.264	1.705
Gastroenterology	383	101	3.692	2.098	2.523	3.019	4.124	5.916
Gastroenterology: Hepatology	0	*	*	*	*	*	*	*
Genetics	2	1	*	*	*	*	*	*
Geriatrics	23	13	2.394	4.474	1.243	1.513	1.628	1.977
Hematology/Oncology	165	44	2.944	11.924	1.240	1.471	1.878	2.401
Hematology/Oncology: Onc (only)	12	9	1.596	.478	1.204	1.334	2.048	2.354
Hospice/Palliative Care	4	4	*	*	*	*	*	*
Hospitalist: Family Practice	25	6	1.721	.425	1.591	1.664	1.745	1.813
Hospitalist: Internal Medicine	598	77	17.713	241.617	1.554	1.780	2.133	2.742
Hospitalist: IM-Pediatrics	1	1	*	*	*	*	*	*
Hospitalist: Pediatrics	50	12	1.782	.408	1.544	1.666	1.906	2.429
Infectious Disease	67	32	1.727	.761	1.341	1.570	1.780	2.480
Internal Medicine: General	1,607	179	2.365	10.119	1.146	1.291	1.489	1.830
IM: Amb Only (no inpatient work)	15	5	1.433	.395	1.124	1.316	1.709	2.125
Internal Med: Pediatrics	28	13	4.208	11.853	1.090	1.299	1.436	6.306
Nephrology	84	38	3.964	9.976	2.003	2.464	3.353	4.619
Neurology	285	86	2.391	1.173	1.794	2.140	2.568	3.345
Obstetrics/Gynecology: General	716	135	3.162	4.776	1.845	2.156	2.766	3.999
OB/GYN: Gynecology (only)	105	38	2.107	.902	1.640	1.906	2.261	2.900
OB/GYN: Gyn Oncology	14	10	3.386	1.450	2.119	3.108	4.645	5.550
OB/GYN: Maternal & Fetal Med	21	8	3.012	.634	2.646	2.994	3.139	3.665
OB/GYN: Repro Endocrinology	5	4	*	*	*	*	*	*
OB/GYN: Urogynecology	4	3	*	*	*	*	*	*
Occupational Medicine	42	18	2.618	4.694	1.488	1.778	2.344	2.604
Ophthalmology	144	58	2.058	1.761	1.346	1.599	2.061	3.162
Ophthalmology: Pediatric	12	8	2.067	.812	1.502	1.846	2.442	3.758
Ophthalmology: Retina	8	6	*	*	*	*	*	*
Orthopedic (Nonsurgical)	13	11	1.277	.193	1.124	1.240	1.450	1.574
Orthopedic Surgery: General	402	91	2.610	1.053	1.978	2.344	2.991	3.857
Orthopedic Surgery: Foot & Ankle	21	14	2.492	.786	1.993	2.274	2.687	4.085
Orthopedic Surgery: Hand	54	28	2.222	1.501	1.559	1.948	2.403	2.959
Orthopedic Surgery: Hip & Joint	49	20	3.049	.921	2.278	3.033	3.758	4.059
Orthopedic Surgery: Pediatric	12	9	2.029	.702	1.529	1.933	2.396	3.420
Orthopedic Surgery: Spine	42	23	5.189	2.575	3.354	4.562	6.158	9.587
Orthopedic Surgery: Trauma	14	8	4.819	5.259	2.537	2.834	4.148	15.943
Orthopedic Surgery: Sports Med	84	29	2.500	.901	1.945	2.314	2.920	3.985

Table 69: Work RVUs to Total Encounters Ratio (CMS RBRVS Method) (NPP Excluded) (continued)

	Phys	Med Pracs	Mean	Std. Dev.	25th %tile	Median	75th %tile	90th %tile
Otorhinolaryngology	184	72	2.138	1.496	1.472	1.798	2.217	3.290
Pathology: Anatomic and Clinical	5	2	*	*	*	*	*	*
Pathology: Anatomic	1	1	*	*	*	*	*	*
Pathology: Clinical	9	2	*	*	*	*	*	*
Pediatrics: General	817	129	2.104	6.575	1.073	1.156	1.292	1.607
Pediatrics: Adolescent Medicine	15	4	1.858	.733	1.068	1.805	2.550	2.841
Pediatrics: Allergy/Immunology	1	1	*	*	*	*	*	*
Pediatrics: Cardiology	38	12	2.620	1.244	1.658	2.490	3.632	4.470
Pediatrics: Child Development	6	4	*	*	*	*	*	*
Pediatrics: Critical Care/Intensivist	31	9	5.054	2.283	3.395	4.661	7.101	8.239
Pediatrics: Emergency Medicine	7	2	*	*	*	*	*	*
Pediatrics: Endocrinology	22	14	1.610	.273	1.411	1.553	1.810	2.052
Pediatrics: Gastroenterology	21	9	2.178	.446	1.888	2.024	2.582	2.924
Pediatrics: Genetics	5	3	*	*	*	*	*	*
Pediatrics: Hematology/Oncology	41	12	1.864	.443	1.599	1.774	2.117	2.541
Pediatrics: Infectious Disease	11	5	2.055	.743	1.665	1.732	2.107	3.821
Pediatrics: Neonatal Medicine	69	11	5.314	2.493	3.830	4.400	5.756	7.200
Pediatrics: Nephrology	7	6	*	*	*	*	*	*
Pediatrics: Neurology	40	18	1.944	.624	1.558	1.832	2.182	2.581
Pediatrics: Pulmonology	13	7	1.578	.397	1.289	1.468	1.834	2.307
Pediatrics: Rheumatology	5	3	*	*	*	*	*	*
Physiatry (Phys Med & Rehab)	95	40	2.380	2.746	1.428	1.725	2.337	3.147
Podiatry: General	51	30	1.543	.547	1.131	1.327	1.622	2.560
Podiatry: Surg-Foot & Ankle	36	12	1.335	.255	1.183	1.266	1.485	1.613
Podiatry: Surg-Forefoot Only	2	2	*	*	*	*	*	*
Psychiatry: General	147	43	1.762	1.252	1.275	1.496	1.709	2.319
Psychiatry: Child & Adolescent	27	12	1.610	.274	1.423	1.531	1.783	2.110
Psychiatry: Geriatric	5	2	*	*	*	*	*	*
Pulmonary Medicine	135	53	2.782	2.616	1.569	2.144	2.828	4.169
Pulmonary Medicine: Critical Care	27	8	2.481	.536	2.038	2.394	2.908	3.308
Pulmonary Med: Gen & Crit Care	53	12	2.423	.690	1.935	2.264	2.808	3.705
Radiation Oncology	53	17	10.531	6.258	6.664	9.076	14.117	18.114
Radiology: Diagnostic-Inv	52	16	23.265	68.854	2.791	6.394	20.963	34.332
Radiology: Diagnostic-Noninv	179	19	368.875	1,099.217	10.110	33.083	127.941	713.769
Radiology: Nuclear Medicine	15	9	46.092	58.311	2.724	17.606	78.623	150.510
Rheumatology	126	56	1.510	.396	1.253	1.442	1.645	1.916
Sleep Medicine	29	16	3.468	3.904	2.260	2.463	3.321	4.240
Surgery: General	469	120	3.730	2.076	2.666	3.168	4.052	5.583
Surgery: Bariatric	15	9	3.955	1.083	3.301	3.708	4.132	5.977
Surgery: Cardiovascular	104	35	16.928	10.152	9.220	15.529	21.629	31.695
Surgery: Colon and Rectal	19	8	4.133	1.660	2.733	3.949	5.858	6.407
Surgery: Neurological	106	37	6.526	5.457	3.791	5.073	7.666	9.855
Surgery: Oncology	7	5	*	*	*	*	*	*
Surgery: Oral	3	2	*	*	*	*	*	*
Surgery: Pediatric	23	12	3.604	.814	3.013	3.314	4.163	4.589
Surgery: Plastic & Reconstruction	45	24	3.573	1.949	2.251	2.935	4.358	6.026
Surgery: Plastic & Recon-Hand	1	1	*	*	*	*	*	*
Surgery: Thoracic (primary)	20	8	13.429	6.829	7.856	13.634	17.049	25.147
Surgery: Transplant	13	5	4.112	.868	3.389	4.153	4.950	5.271
Surgery: Trauma	34	8	2.700	.961	2.107	2.368	3.017	4.449
Surgery: Trauma-Burn	4	2	*	*	*	*	*	*
Surgery: Vascular (primary)	65	25	5.535	5.545	2.730	3.511	7.175	10.718
Urgent Care	154	21	2.099	3.724	1.142	1.251	1.382	1.635
Urology	208	66	2.165	.681	1.710	2.053	2.443	3.175
Urology: Pediatric	4	3	*	*	*	*	*	*

Physician Time Worked

Table 70: Physician Weeks Worked per Year

	Phys	Med Pracs	Mean	Std. Dev.	25th %tile	Median	75th %tile	90th %tile
Allergy/Immunology	115	64	47.24	2.16	46.00	48.00	48.00	49.00
Anesthesiology	3,053	154	44.42	2.76	43.00	44.00	46.00	48.00
Anesthesiology: Pain Management	170	51	45.23	3.06	43.00	46.00	48.00	48.90
Anesthesiology: Pediatric	77	8	44.55	2.45	42.00	46.00	46.00	48.00
Cardiology: Electrophysiology	168	81	45.28	2.82	44.00	46.00	48.00	48.00
Cardiology: Invasive	388	113	45.75	2.69	44.00	46.00	48.00	48.00
Cardiology: Inv-Intvl	495	134	45.43	2.78	44.00	46.00	48.00	48.00
Cardiology: Noninvasive	397	113	44.41	3.25	41.00	45.00	47.00	48.00
Critical Care: Intensivist	28	13	44.04	3.38	40.50	45.50	46.00	48.20
Dentistry	32	12	46.12	1.83	44.25	46.00	48.00	48.00
Dermatology	234	98	46.85	2.37	46.00	47.00	48.00	49.00
Dermatology: Mohs Surgery	19	16	46.51	1.56	45.00	47.00	48.00	48.00
Emergency Medicine	523	39	47.59	2.88	46.00	48.00	48.00	52.00
Endocrinology/Metabolism	195	100	47.20	1.93	46.00	47.00	48.00	49.00
Family Practice (w/ OB)	616	121	47.45	2.62	46.00	48.00	48.00	52.00
Family Practice (w/o OB)	4,314	546	46.99	2.15	46.00	47.00	48.00	49.00
FP: Amb Only (no inpatient work)	134	22	47.17	2.15	46.00	47.00	48.00	49.00
Family Practice: Sports Med	29	19	46.52	2.26	45.50	47.00	48.00	50.00
Family Practice: Urgent Care	103	24	48.06	1.98	47.00	48.00	49.00	51.00
Gastroenterology	665	159	46.32	2.86	46.00	47.00	48.00	49.00
Gastroenterology: Hepatology	10	7	47.50	1.35	46.00	48.00	49.00	49.00
Genetics	3	2	*	*	*	*	*	*
Geriatrics	60	22	46.78	1.43	46.00	47.00	48.00	48.00
Hematology/Oncology	309	86	46.43	2.54	46.00	46.00	48.00	48.20
Hematology/Oncology: Onc (only)	45	28	46.67	2.21	46.00	48.00	48.00	48.00
Hospice/Palliative Care	6	6	*	*	*	*	*	*
Hospitalist: Family Practice	46	13	47.52	3.13	44.75	48.00	48.50	52.00
Hospitalist: Internal Medicine	706	108	46.82	2.36	46.00	47.00	48.00	48.00
Hospitalist: IM-Pediatrics	3	2	*	*	*	*	*	*
Hospitalist: Pediatrics	70	14	46.26	2.73	45.00	47.00	48.00	48.00
Infectious Disease	144	43	46.70	1.90	46.00	47.00	48.00	48.50
Internal Medicine: General	3,015	389	47.15	2.16	46.00	47.00	48.00	49.00
IM: Amb Only (no inpatient work)	32	13	46.38	1.95	45.25	47.00	48.00	48.00
Internal Med: Pediatrics	92	36	47.22	1.91	46.00	48.00	48.00	49.00
Nephrology	188	58	46.62	2.09	46.00	46.00	48.00	49.00
Neurology	471	146	46.85	2.12	46.00	47.00	48.00	49.00
Obstetrics/Gynecology: General	1,289	258	46.64	2.36	46.00	47.00	48.00	49.00
OB/GYN: Gynecology (only)	173	74	46.32	2.92	46.00	46.20	48.00	48.00
OB/GYN: Gyn Oncology	26	18	47.54	2.14	46.00	48.00	48.00	52.00
OB/GYN: Maternal & Fetal Med	67	24	47.52	2.63	46.00	48.00	48.00	52.00
OB/GYN: Repro Endocrinology	8	5	*	*	*	*	*	*
OB/GYN: Urogynecology	2	2	*	*	*	*	*	*
Occupational Medicine	78	42	47.17	2.35	46.00	47.00	48.00	50.00
Ophthalmology	365	116	46.24	2.81	45.00	46.00	48.00	49.00
Ophthalmology: Pediatric	25	19	46.20	2.55	46.00	46.00	48.00	48.40
Ophthalmology: Retina	38	21	45.32	3.00	42.00	46.00	48.00	48.10
Orthopedic (Nonsurgical)	40	30	46.08	3.68	45.00	46.00	48.00	50.00
Orthopedic Surgery: General	660	198	46.79	2.55	46.00	47.00	48.00	50.00
Orthopedic Surgery: Foot & Ankle	55	39	46.48	2.69	46.00	47.00	48.00	49.00
Orthopedic Surgery: Hand	130	68	45.95	3.02	45.00	46.00	48.00	49.00
Orthopedic Surgery: Hip & Joint	117	55	46.33	2.71	45.00	46.00	48.00	50.00
Orthopedic Surgery: Pediatric	27	13	46.41	1.34	46.00	46.00	48.00	48.00
Orthopedic Surgery: Spine	112	65	46.59	2.51	46.00	47.00	48.00	50.00
Orthopedic Surgery: Trauma	29	17	46.28	3.06	45.00	46.00	48.00	52.00
Orthopedic Surgery: Sports Med	177	71	46.76	2.73	46.00	47.00	48.00	50.00

Table 70: Physician Weeks Worked per Year (continued)

	Phys	Med Pracs	Mean	Std. Dev.	25th %tile	Median	75th %tile	90th %tile
Otorhinolaryngology	350	122	46.84	2.63	46.00	48.00	48.00	49.00
Pathology: Anatomic and Clinical	102	16	44.99	2.17	44.00	44.50	46.00	48.00
Pathology: Anatomic	31	6	46.61	1.56	46.00	47.00	48.00	48.00
Pathology: Clinical	33	10	47.76	2.12	46.00	48.00	48.50	51.60
Pediatrics: General	1,829	302	46.98	2.24	46.00	47.00	48.00	49.00
Pediatrics: Adolescent Medicine	57	7	50.81	1.85	49.00	52.00	52.00	52.00
Pediatrics: Allergy/Immunology	5	3	*	*	*	*	*	*
Pediatrics: Cardiology	27	11	47.04	1.26	46.00	48.00	48.00	48.00
Pediatrics: Child Development	5	3	*	*	*	*	*	*
Pediatrics: Critical Care/Intensivist	66	14	46.14	2.18	44.00	46.00	48.00	48.00
Pediatrics: Emergency Medicine	24	3	46.58	.93	46.00	46.00	48.00	48.00
Pediatrics: Endocrinology	20	14	45.85	2.58	45.00	46.00	48.00	48.00
Pediatrics: Gastroenterology	17	11	46.29	1.57	46.00	46.00	48.00	48.00
Pediatrics: Genetics	16	9	45.25	2.93	43.00	47.00	47.00	47.00
Pediatrics: Hematology/Oncology	41	14	46.46	1.73	46.00	46.00	48.00	48.00
Pediatrics: Infectious Disease	6	4	*	*	*	*	*	*
Pediatrics: Neonatal Medicine	81	14	46.68	1.24	46.00	46.00	48.00	48.00
Pediatrics: Nephrology	6	4	*	*	*	*	*	*
Pediatrics: Neurology	39	18	46.46	1.79	46.00	46.00	48.00	50.00
Pediatrics: Pulmonology	16	11	47.50	1.67	46.00	48.00	48.00	50.00
Pediatrics: Rheumatology	7	3	*	*	*	*	*	*
Physiatry (Phys Med & Rehab)	154	76	46.80	2.35	46.00	47.50	48.00	48.50
Podiatry: General	106	70	47.62	2.14	46.00	48.00	48.00	50.30
Podiatry: Surg-Foot & Ankle	54	25	47.65	1.66	46.00	48.00	48.25	49.50
Podiatry: Surg-Forefoot Only	2	1	*	*	*	*	*	*
Psychiatry: General	245	66	46.81	2.23	46.00	47.00	48.00	49.00
Psychiatry: Child & Adolescent	27	17	46.48	1.34	46.00	46.00	48.00	48.00
Psychiatry: Geriatric	7	3	*	*	*	*	*	*
Pulmonary Medicine	163	76	47.19	1.69	46.00	48.00	48.00	49.00
Pulmonary Medicine: Critical Care	56	16	45.79	3.36	44.00	46.00	47.75	50.00
Pulmonary Med: Gen & Crit Care	141	37	46.69	3.28	46.00	48.00	48.00	50.00
Radiation Oncology	99	29	45.59	2.34	44.00	46.00	48.00	48.00
Radiology: Diagnostic-Inv	211	38	43.27	3.60	41.00	44.00	46.00	48.00
Radiology: Diagnostic-Noninv	556	63	43.84	3.72	42.00	44.00	46.00	48.00
Radiology: Nuclear Medicine	30	17	45.17	2.69	42.75	45.00	48.00	48.90
Rheumatology	202	106	46.94	1.99	46.00	47.00	48.00	48.98
Sleep Medicine	41	26	47.95	2.02	46.00	48.00	48.00	52.00
Surgery: General	683	211	46.80	2.32	46.00	47.00	48.00	50.00
Surgery: Bariatric	17	10	47.12	1.93	45.00	48.00	48.00	50.00
Surgery: Cardiovascular	164	53	45.57	2.96	44.00	46.00	48.00	48.00
Surgery: Colon and Rectal	30	12	47.17	3.06	46.00	48.00	48.25	50.00
Surgery: Neurological	145	54	46.14	3.47	45.00	47.20	48.00	50.00
Surgery: Oncology	9	7	*	*	*	*	*	*
Surgery: Oral	12	6	46.75	3.89	46.50	48.00	48.75	49.00
Surgery: Pediatric	38	18	46.11	1.66	46.00	46.00	47.25	48.00
Surgery: Plastic & Reconstruction	80	41	46.63	2.02	46.00	46.00	48.00	48.00
Surgery: Plastic & Recon-Hand	10	6	47.80	1.87	46.75	47.00	48.50	51.80
Surgery: Thoracic (primary)	17	11	45.00	2.94	42.00	44.00	48.00	48.20
Surgery: Transplant	25	6	46.88	1.01	46.00	46.00	48.00	48.00
Surgery: Trauma	39	10	46.56	2.14	46.00	47.00	48.00	49.00
Surgery: Trauma-Burn	1	1	*	*	*	*	*	*
Surgery: Vascular (primary)	106	52	45.77	2.54	43.00	46.00	48.00	48.00
Urgent Care	247	55	46.11	3.07	45.00	46.00	48.00	50.00
Urology	402	117	47.17	2.23	46.00	48.00	48.00	50.00
Urology: Pediatric	13	7	46.62	1.33	46.00	46.00	46.50	49.60

Table 71: Physician Weeks Worked per Year by Years in Specialty

	1 to 2 years		3 to 7 years		8 to 17 years		18 years or more	
	Phys	Median	Phys	Median	Phys	Median	Phys	Median
Allergy/Immunology	5	*	18	48.00	33	47.00	45	48.00
Anesthesiology	149	45.00	261	45.00	1,187	44.00	805	44.00
Anesthesiology: Pain Management	3	*	36	43.00	46	45.00	28	46.00
Anesthesiology: Pediatric	7	*	15	45.00	21	44.00	22	45.00
Cardiology: Electrophysiology	11	47.00	38	45.50	62	46.00	36	45.00
Cardiology: Invasive	23	47.00	64	46.00	146	46.00	102	46.00
Cardiology: Inv-Intvl	12	46.00	72	46.00	181	46.00	181	46.00
Cardiology: Noninvasive	17	46.00	62	44.00	107	44.00	175	45.00
Critical Care: Intensivist	2	*	3	*	5	*	6	*
Dentistry	4	*	4	*	3	*	8	*
Dermatology	10	47.50	49	47.00	72	47.25	70	46.00
Dermatology: Mohs Surgery	1	*	3	*	7	*	3	*
Emergency Medicine	18	46.00	71	48.00	78	46.50	77	46.00
Endocrinology/Metabolism	16	48.00	36	47.00	50	48.00	58	48.00
Family Practice (w/ OB)	33	48.00	128	47.00	197	48.00	133	47.00
Family Practice (w/o OB)	202	48.00	774	47.00	1,328	48.00	1,302	47.00
FP: Amb Only (no inpatient work)	3	*	18	47.00	30	47.00	46	46.00
Family Practice: Sports Med	6	*	5	*	7	*	8	*
Family Practice: Urgent Care	4	*	9	*	22	48.00	30	48.00
Gastroenterology	29	48.00	105	48.00	176	47.00	236	47.00
Gastroenterology: Hepatology	*	*	1	*	2	*	3	*
Genetics	*	*	0	*	0	*	2	*
Geriatrics	3	*	9	*	16	46.50	20	47.50
Hematology/Oncology	14	48.00	50	46.45	87	47.00	103	46.00
Hematology/Oncology: Onc (only)	1	*	7	*	9	*	21	48.00
Hospice/Palliative Care	1	*	2	*	3	*	0	*
Hospitalist: Family Practice	4	*	16	46.00	5	*	4	*
Hospitalist: Internal Medicine	94	48.00	248	48.00	159	47.00	29	48.00
Hospitalist: IM-Pediatrics	1	*	2	*	0	*	*	*
Hospitalist: Pediatrics	3	*	11	47.00	11	47.00	6	*
Infectious Disease	8	*	33	46.00	50	47.00	37	47.00
Internal Medicine: General	107	47.00	434	48.00	896	48.00	933	48.00
IM: Amb Only (no inpatient work)	*	*	*	*	3	*	11	46.00
Internal Med: Pediatrics	8	*	20	48.00	46	48.00	2	*
Nephrology	16	47.50	43	47.00	50	48.00	52	46.00
Neurology	33	46.00	90	48.00	119	48.00	154	46.00
Obstetrics/Gynecology: General	64	47.00	202	46.00	448	47.00	307	47.00
OB/GYN: Gynecology (only)	2	*	23	46.00	37	47.00	87	47.00
OB/GYN: Gyn Oncology	1	*	4	*	12	48.00	4	*
OB/GYN: Maternal & Fetal Med	1	*	10	48.00	23	46.00	13	48.00
OB/GYN: Repro Endocrinology	0	*	*	*	2	*	3	*
OB/GYN: Urogynecology	0	*	1	*	*	*	0	*
Occupational Medicine	3	*	12	46.00	16	48.00	36	47.30
Ophthalmology	15	48.00	36	47.00	117	47.00	143	46.00
Ophthalmology: Pediatric	2	*	5	*	7	*	8	*
Ophthalmology: Retina	2	*	4	*	15	45.00	11	45.00
Orthopedic (Nonsurgical)	3	*	6	*	5	*	21	46.00
Orthopedic Surgery: General	32	48.00	88	47.00	221	48.00	273	48.00
Orthopedic Surgery: Foot & Ankle	6	*	12	48.00	23	47.00	11	46.00
Orthopedic Surgery: Hand	5	*	23	46.00	50	46.00	45	46.00
Orthopedic Surgery: Hip & Joint	7	*	12	47.50	38	46.00	50	46.00
Orthopedic Surgery: Pediatric	1	*	5	*	13	46.00	8	*
Orthopedic Surgery: Spine	10	48.00	22	48.00	47	46.00	29	46.00
Orthopedic Surgery: Trauma	1	*	8	*	10	46.00	7	*
Orthopedic Surgery: Sports Med	11	48.00	31	48.00	60	46.00	60	47.00

Table 71: Physician Weeks Worked per Year by Years in Specialty (continued)

	1 to 2 years		3 to 7 years		8 to 17 years		18 years or more	
	Phys	Median	Phys	Median	Phys	Median	Phys	Median
Otorhinolaryngology	10	48.00	60	47.50	116	48.00	112	47.00
Pathology: Anatomic and Clinical	4	*	9	*	14	44.00	29	44.00
Pathology: Anatomic	2	*	10	47.00	6	*	10	48.00
Pathology: Clinical	*	*	5	*	11	46.00	14	48.00
Pediatrics: General	75	48.00	303	47.00	588	48.00	558	47.00
Pediatrics: Adolescent Medicine	2	*	4	*	8	*	4	*
Pediatrics: Allergy/Immunology	*	*	1	*	2	*	2	*
Pediatrics: Cardiology	1	*	2	*	3	*	7	*
Pediatrics: Child Development	*	*	0	*	1	*	1	*
Pediatrics: Critical Care/Intensivist	3	*	12	45.00	17	46.00	5	*
Pediatrics: Emergency Medicine	0	*	6	*	6	*	5	*
Pediatrics: Endocrinology	3	*	5	*	3	*	5	*
Pediatrics: Gastroenterology	0	*	4	*	5	*	3	*
Pediatrics: Genetics	1	*	*	*	1	*	1	*
Pediatrics: Hematology/Oncology	4	*	10	46.50	11	48.00	9	*
Pediatrics: Infectious Disease	*	*	1	*	2	*	3	*
Pediatrics: Neonatal Medicine	0	*	14	46.00	19	46.00	22	46.00
Pediatrics: Nephrology	0	*	*	*	4	*	2	*
Pediatrics: Neurology	4	*	4	*	12	47.00	13	46.00
Pediatrics: Pulmonology	0	*	2	*	4	*	8	*
Pediatrics: Rheumatology	*	*	*	*	4	*	3	*
Physiatry (Phys Med & Rehab)	12	46.00	35	48.00	49	47.00	34	48.00
Podiatry: General	6	*	20	48.00	37	48.00	31	48.00
Podiatry: Surg-Foot & Ankle	5	*	14	48.00	13	48.00	11	48.00
Podiatry: Surg-Forefoot Only	*	*	0	*	2	*	0	*
Psychiatry: General	11	48.00	42	46.70	57	47.00	60	46.45
Psychiatry: Child & Adolescent	0	*	8	*	7	*	2	*
Psychiatry: Geriatric	*	*	*	*	2	*	3	*
Pulmonary Medicine	10	46.00	26	48.00	41	48.00	55	48.00
Pulmonary Medicine: Critical Care	1	*	9	*	21	45.00	15	46.00
Pulmonary Med: Gen & Crit Care	9	*	30	48.00	52	48.00	40	47.00
Radiation Oncology	3	*	18	46.00	42	46.00	22	46.00
Radiology: Diagnostic-Inv	14	43.00	54	44.00	81	43.00	50	42.50
Radiology: Diagnostic-Noninv	23	44.00	87	45.00	197	43.00	174	43.00
Radiology: Nuclear Medicine	0	*	6	*	5	*	11	45.00
Rheumatology	8	*	32	48.00	49	48.00	69	48.00
Sleep Medicine	3	*	9	*	8	*	13	48.00
Surgery: General	32	48.00	115	48.00	223	46.00	233	47.00
Surgery: Bariatric	1	*	2	*	4	*	3	*
Surgery: Cardiovascular	16	48.00	21	46.00	67	46.00	45	45.00
Surgery: Colon and Rectal	0	*	3	*	8	*	15	48.00
Surgery: Neurological	9	*	24	48.00	50	47.00	43	48.00
Surgery: Oncology	*	*	1	*	3	*	3	*
Surgery: Oral	0	*	1	*	5	*	6	*
Surgery: Pediatric	1	*	7	*	12	46.00	12	46.00
Surgery: Plastic & Reconstruction	4	*	19	48.00	25	46.00	24	46.00
Surgery: Plastic & Recon-Hand	1	*	4	*	4	*	0	*
Surgery: Thoracic (primary)	0	*	2	*	3	*	8	*
Surgery: Transplant	0	*	2	*	11	48.00	4	*
Surgery: Trauma	7	*	6	*	15	46.00	7	*
Surgery: Trauma-Burn	1	*	0	*	0	*	*	*
Surgery: Vascular (primary)	2	*	17	48.00	37	46.00	34	46.00
Urgent Care	10	46.00	42	46.00	64	46.42	79	46.00
Urology	17	48.00	57	47.00	116	48.00	156	48.00
Urology: Pediatric	1	*	3	*	4	*	4	*

Table 72: Physician Clinical Service Hours Worked per Week

	Phys	Med Pracs	Mean	Std. Dev.	25th %tile	Median	75th %tile	90th %tile
Allergy/Immunology	113	61	37.00	7.45	32.00	38.00	40.00	47.40
Anesthesiology	2,863	137	45.91	9.87	40.00	45.00	54.00	60.00
Anesthesiology: Pain Management	159	48	47.15	10.83	40.00	45.00	60.00	60.00
Anesthesiology: Pediatric	77	7	41.37	8.37	39.19	40.00	42.52	55.00
Cardiology: Electrophysiology	166	78	45.48	10.72	40.00	40.00	50.00	61.50
Cardiology: Invasive	373	108	44.25	9.34	40.00	40.00	50.00	60.00
Cardiology: Inv-Intvl	511	136	44.91	10.31	40.00	40.00	50.00	60.00
Cardiology: Noninvasive	423	115	41.52	8.12	36.00	40.00	45.00	50.00
Critical Care: Intensivist	26	12	36.86	5.16	32.00	36.00	40.00	40.00
Dentistry	55	15	37.42	4.37	35.00	38.00	40.00	42.00
Dermatology	232	96	35.40	7.02	32.00	36.00	40.00	40.00
Dermatology: Mohs Surgery	15	13	38.20	3.53	35.00	40.00	40.00	42.00
Emergency Medicine	597	42	33.67	7.64	30.00	34.20	40.00	40.00
Endocrinology/Metabolism	190	97	36.90	9.15	32.00	36.00	40.00	46.80
Family Practice (w/ OB)	632	119	37.04	8.00	32.00	40.00	40.00	45.00
Family Practice (w/o OB)	4,287	552	36.08	7.48	32.00	36.00	40.00	40.00
FP: Amb Only (no inpatient work)	132	21	36.83	6.33	33.25	40.00	40.00	42.00
Family Practice: Sports Med	26	16	38.19	6.79	36.00	40.00	40.00	45.20
Family Practice: Urgent Care	96	21	38.10	9.83	35.00	36.00	40.00	44.00
Gastroenterology	636	150	40.12	7.29	36.00	40.00	40.00	50.00
Gastroenterology: Hepatology	9	6	*	*	*	*	*	*
Genetics	3	2	*	*	*	*	*	*
Geriatrics	49	21	37.04	3.15	36.00	38.00	40.00	40.00
Hematology/Oncology	297	81	38.68	9.19	35.00	40.00	40.00	50.00
Hematology/Oncology: Onc (only)	42	25	39.57	8.26	36.00	40.00	40.50	50.00
Hospice/Palliative Care	6	6	*	*	*	*	*	*
Hospitalist: Family Practice	40	12	37.75	4.11	36.00	36.00	40.00	40.00
Hospitalist: Internal Medicine	755	112	41.79	12.42	36.00	40.00	40.00	60.00
Hospitalist: IM-Pediatrics	8	4	*	*	*	*	*	*
Hospitalist: Pediatrics	70	13	39.73	7.81	36.00	40.00	50.00	50.00
Infectious Disease	164	49	34.93	9.92	28.50	36.00	40.00	46.50
Internal Medicine: General	3,046	383	36.43	7.41	32.00	36.00	40.00	40.00
IM: Amb Only (no inpatient work)	32	13	38.59	4.70	36.25	40.00	40.00	41.40
Internal Med: Pediatrics	88	33	39.22	6.18	36.00	40.00	40.00	50.00
Nephrology	170	57	40.49	8.21	36.00	40.00	45.00	50.00
Neurology	468	145	38.96	7.23	36.00	40.00	40.00	45.00
Obstetrics/Gynecology: General	1,292	249	37.98	7.09	34.00	40.00	40.00	45.00
OB/GYN: Gynecology (only)	175	75	35.96	7.63	32.00	36.00	40.00	40.00
OB/GYN: Gyn Oncology	22	16	36.95	7.46	39.50	40.00	40.00	40.00
OB/GYN: Maternal & Fetal Med	72	25	38.38	5.25	36.00	40.00	40.00	40.00
OB/GYN: Repro Endocrinology	9	6	*	*	*	*	*	*
OB/GYN: Urogynecology	3	3	*	*	*	*	*	*
Occupational Medicine	76	42	36.04	3.97	34.00	36.00	40.00	40.00
Ophthalmology	352	106	36.67	7.88	34.00	40.00	40.00	40.00
Ophthalmology: Pediatric	22	16	36.86	7.67	36.00	40.00	40.00	43.50
Ophthalmology: Retina	36	21	38.94	12.11	35.00	40.00	50.00	50.00
Orthopedic (Nonsurgical)	42	30	33.21	11.10	24.00	35.00	40.00	42.80
Orthopedic Surgery: General	645	189	40.58	9.88	36.00	40.00	48.00	50.00
Orthopedic Surgery: Foot & Ankle	57	40	42.81	8.64	40.00	40.00	48.00	56.00
Orthopedic Surgery: Hand	131	67	41.51	9.62	36.00	40.00	48.00	55.00
Orthopedic Surgery: Hip & Joint	115	54	42.01	11.20	36.00	40.00	50.00	55.00
Orthopedic Surgery: Pediatric	27	13	38.57	15.78	32.00	40.00	40.00	70.00
Orthopedic Surgery: Spine	110	64	42.55	11.37	39.00	40.00	50.00	60.00
Orthopedic Surgery: Trauma	31	18	42.35	7.52	36.00	40.00	50.00	55.00
Orthopedic Surgery: Sports Med	171	70	42.06	13.59	36.00	40.00	50.00	60.00

Table 72: Physician Clinical Service Hours Worked per Week (continued)

	Phys	Med Pracs	Mean	Std. Dev.	25th %tile	Median	75th %tile	90th %tile
Otorhinolaryngology	322	113	39.49	7.27	36.00	40.00	40.00	50.00
Pathology: Anatomic and Clinical	117	19	38.27	5.25	36.00	40.00	40.00	40.00
Pathology: Anatomic	31	6	35.68	5.84	32.00	40.00	40.00	40.00
Pathology: Clinical	20	7	36.90	7.24	40.00	40.00	40.00	40.00
Pediatrics: General	1,876	300	35.25	7.24	32.00	36.00	40.00	40.00
Pediatrics: Adolescent Medicine	33	9	34.97	4.40	32.00	36.00	38.00	40.00
Pediatrics: Allergy/Immunology	4	2	*	*	*	*	*	*
Pediatrics: Cardiology	30	12	40.41	10.90	36.00	37.00	40.00	67.50
Pediatrics: Child Development	5	3	*	*	*	*	*	*
Pediatrics: Critical Care/Intensivist	59	13	42.34	7.18	40.00	40.00	50.00	50.00
Pediatrics: Emergency Medicine	58	6	36.07	8.72	32.00	40.00	40.00	50.00
Pediatrics: Endocrinology	23	15	40.85	10.64	36.00	40.00	40.00	65.00
Pediatrics: Gastroenterology	20	13	36.70	4.27	33.00	36.00	40.00	40.00
Pediatrics: Genetics	19	11	35.39	5.90	32.00	36.00	40.00	40.00
Pediatrics: Hematology/Oncology	47	14	39.63	7.25	36.00	40.00	40.00	52.80
Pediatrics: Infectious Disease	10	6	32.24	5.44	28.00	30.20	37.00	40.00
Pediatrics: Neonatal Medicine	108	19	39.97	6.21	36.00	40.00	40.00	50.00
Pediatrics: Nephrology	5	4	*	*	*	*	*	*
Pediatrics: Neurology	36	18	37.73	5.64	36.00	40.00	40.00	44.00
Pediatrics: Pulmonology	14	11	41.77	10.36	35.70	40.00	45.00	60.00
Pediatrics: Rheumatology	6	3	*	*	*	*	*	*
Physiatry (Phys Med & Rehab)	140	68	40.63	9.11	36.25	40.00	44.75	53.80
Podiatry: General	99	66	37.11	5.21	34.00	40.00	40.00	40.00
Podiatry: Surg-Foot & Ankle	50	22	38.93	6.70	35.75	40.00	40.00	49.80
Podiatry: Surg-Forefoot Only	2	1	*	*	*	*	*	*
Psychiatry: General	280	69	37.37	6.58	36.00	40.00	40.00	40.00
Psychiatry: Child & Adolescent	38	19	38.87	6.76	37.50	40.00	40.00	40.00
Psychiatry: Geriatric	8	4	*	*	*	*	*	*
Pulmonary Medicine	164	74	38.97	7.37	36.00	40.00	40.00	45.00
Pulmonary Medicine: Critical Care	36	11	45.22	7.98	40.00	44.00	50.00	60.00
Pulmonary Med: Gen & Crit Care	141	36	42.07	9.22	40.00	40.00	49.00	55.00
Radiation Oncology	96	27	39.94	4.57	38.00	40.00	43.00	45.00
Radiology: Diagnostic-Invasive	237	37	40.32	9.09	37.00	40.00	45.00	50.00
Radiology: Diagnostic-Noninv	576	62	38.00	9.02	36.00	40.00	43.00	45.00
Radiology: Nuclear Medicine	30	15	38.37	10.74	39.00	40.00	45.00	45.00
Rheumatology	187	104	36.46	9.01	34.00	36.00	40.00	45.00
Sleep Medicine	45	26	37.76	7.54	35.00	40.00	40.00	45.00
Surgery: General	651	195	39.76	9.23	36.00	40.00	40.00	50.00
Surgery: Bariatric	18	11	39.37	10.51	34.75	40.00	42.00	51.00
Surgery: Cardiovascular	157	48	46.27	16.92	40.00	44.00	55.00	62.00
Surgery: Colon and Rectal	29	11	35.41	10.50	39.50	40.00	40.00	40.00
Surgery: Neurological	157	57	43.08	11.21	36.00	40.00	50.00	60.00
Surgery: Oncology	11	8	39.64	11.94	35.00	40.00	50.00	50.00
Surgery: Oral	14	7	35.00	7.05	35.50	36.00	40.00	40.00
Surgery: Pediatric	40	19	44.23	16.48	35.25	40.00	45.00	80.00
Surgery: Plastic & Reconstruction	78	39	38.65	6.13	36.00	40.00	40.00	40.00
Surgery: Plastic & Recon-Hand	9	5	*	*	*	*	*	*
Surgery: Thoracic (primary)	29	13	39.14	13.19	36.00	40.00	40.00	55.00
Surgery: Transplant	27	7	37.81	3.40	36.00	40.00	40.00	40.00
Surgery: Trauma	49	12	39.96	11.08	40.00	40.00	40.00	40.00
Surgery: Trauma-Burn	4	2	*	*	*	*	*	*
Surgery: Vascular (primary)	99	49	42.43	12.79	40.00	40.00	50.00	55.00
Urgent Care	255	55	34.98	6.37	32.00	36.00	40.00	40.00
Urology	398	116	40.14	9.22	35.75	40.00	40.00	50.00
Urology: Pediatric	13	7	37.38	7.76	32.00	36.00	40.00	52.00

Table 73: Physician Clinical Service Hours Worked per Week by Years in Specialty

	1 to 2 years		3 to 7 years		8 to 17 years		18 years or more	
	Phys	Median	Phys	Median	Phys	Median	Phys	Median
Allergy/Immunology	6	*	18	39.00	26	38.00	44	39.00
Anesthesiology	132	46.50	220	41.66	1,031	50.00	741	45.00
Anesthesiology: Pain Management	1	*	34	46.50	40	45.00	25	40.00
Anesthesiology: Pediatric	8	*	15	40.00	21	40.00	24	40.00
Cardiology: Electrophysiology	12	40.00	38	40.00	61	45.00	37	40.00
Cardiology: Invasive	22	50.00	57	45.00	146	45.00	108	40.00
Cardiology: Inv-Intvl	15	47.00	71	40.00	179	45.00	190	40.00
Cardiology: Noninvasive	19	40.00	60	40.00	111	40.00	194	40.00
Critical Care: Intensivist	2	*	1	*	5	*	6	*
Dentistry	4	*	7	*	7	*	11	40.00
Dermatology	6	*	48	36.00	69	36.00	76	38.00
Dermatology: Mohs Surgery	1	*	2	*	6	*	2	*
Emergency Medicine	32	38.00	89	38.00	105	36.00	98	36.00
Endocrinology/Metabolism	13	40.00	35	36.00	46	40.00	52	36.00
Family Practice (w/ OB)	35	40.00	136	40.00	196	40.00	154	40.00
Family Practice (w/o OB)	198	36.00	723	36.00	1,262	36.00	1,251	36.00
FP: Amb Only (no inpatient work)	3	*	18	40.00	29	38.00	46	36.00
Family Practice: Sports Med	5	*	5	*	7	*	7	*
Family Practice: Urgent Care	4	*	8	*	22	36.00	30	36.50
Gastroenterology	31	40.00	99	40.00	163	40.00	231	40.00
Gastroenterology: Hepatology	*	*	1	*	1	*	3	*
Genetics	*	*	0	*	0	*	2	*
Geriatrics	2	*	6	*	9	*	21	38.00
Hematology/Oncology	12	40.00	47	40.00	82	40.00	103	40.00
Hematology/Oncology: Onc (only)	1	*	7	*	9	*	19	40.00
Hospice/Palliative Care	1	*	2	*	3	*	0	*
Hospitalist: Family Practice	4	*	15	36.00	5	*	3	*
Hospitalist: Internal Medicine	108	40.00	241	40.00	188	40.00	42	40.00
Hospitalist: IM-Pediatrics	1	*	2	*	1	*	*	*
Hospitalist: Pediatrics	3	*	11	36.00	12	36.00	6	*
Infectious Disease	10	38.00	34	32.00	54	36.00	41	36.00
Internal Medicine: General	104	40.00	447	36.00	914	36.00	956	36.00
IM: Amb Only (no inpatient work)	*	*	*	*	3	*	11	40.00
Internal Med: Pediatrics	8	*	21	40.00	42	40.00	2	*
Nephrology	16	47.50	38	40.00	40	40.00	49	40.00
Neurology	29	40.00	80	40.00	120	40.00	158	40.00
Obstetrics/Gynecology: General	66	40.00	198	40.00	445	38.00	339	38.00
OB/GYN: Gynecology (only)	2	*	21	32.00	34	32.00	88	36.00
OB/GYN: Gyn Oncology	0	*	4	*	10	40.00	5	*
OB/GYN: Maternal & Fetal Med	2	*	11	40.00	24	40.00	15	40.00
OB/GYN: Repro Endocrinology	0	*	*	*	3	*	3	*
OB/GYN: Urogynecology	0	*	2	*	*	*	0	*
Occupational Medicine	2	*	8	*	16	35.00	37	36.00
Ophthalmology	15	40.00	32	40.00	112	40.00	147	40.00
Ophthalmology: Pediatric	2	*	5	*	6	*	8	*
Ophthalmology: Retina	2	*	3	*	15	40.00	12	40.00
Orthopedic (Nonsurgical)	3	*	6	*	5	*	24	30.00
Orthopedic Surgery: General	32	40.00	77	40.00	208	40.00	276	40.00
Orthopedic Surgery: Foot & Ankle	6	*	12	40.00	25	42.00	11	40.00
Orthopedic Surgery: Hand	4	*	22	40.00	52	40.00	46	40.00
Orthopedic Surgery: Hip & Joint	7	*	11	40.00	37	40.00	51	40.00
Orthopedic Surgery: Pediatric	1	*	4	*	13	36.00	8	*
Orthopedic Surgery: Spine	12	40.00	19	40.00	46	40.00	29	40.00
Orthopedic Surgery: Trauma	4	*	7	*	11	40.00	6	*
Orthopedic Surgery: Sports Med	11	50.00	29	36.00	59	44.00	61	40.00

Table 73: Physician Clinical Service Hours Worked per Week by Years in Specialty (continued)

	1 to 2 years		3 to 7 years		8 to 17 years		18 years or more	
	Phys	Median	Phys	Median	Phys	Median	Phys	Median
Otorhinolaryngology	10	40.00	55	40.00	111	40.00	116	40.00
Pathology: Anatomic and Clinical	5	*	10	38.00	16	38.00	34	37.00
Pathology: Anatomic	2	*	10	32.00	6	*	10	40.00
Pathology: Clinical	*	*	2	*	9	*	9	*
Pediatrics: General	70	38.50	303	36.00	607	36.00	560	36.00
Pediatrics: Adolescent Medicine	2	*	4	*	9	*	4	*
Pediatrics: Allergy/Immunology	*	*	1	*	2	*	1	*
Pediatrics: Cardiology	1	*	2	*	3	*	7	*
Pediatrics: Child Development	*	*	0	*	0	*	0	*
Pediatrics: Critical Care/Intensivist	2	*	9	*	15	42.00	4	*
Pediatrics: Emergency Medicine	0	*	6	*	7	*	7	*
Pediatrics: Endocrinology	3	*	4	*	2	*	6	*
Pediatrics: Gastroenterology	0	*	5	*	6	*	3	*
Pediatrics: Genetics	1	*	*	*	1	*	3	*
Pediatrics: Hematology/Oncology	4	*	9	*	8	*	7	*
Pediatrics: Infectious Disease	*	*	1	*	2	*	3	*
Pediatrics: Neonatal Medicine	1	*	18	40.00	27	40.00	30	40.00
Pediatrics: Nephrology	0	*	*	*	2	*	2	*
Pediatrics: Neurology	2	*	5	*	9	*	12	36.00
Pediatrics: Pulmonology	0	*	2	*	4	*	6	*
Pediatrics: Rheumatology	*	*	*	*	3	*	1	*
Physiatry (Phys Med & Rehab)	11	42.00	30	40.00	47	40.00	34	40.00
Podiatry: General	5	*	15	38.00	35	40.00	30	38.00
Podiatry: Surg-Foot & Ankle	5	*	14	40.00	13	36.00	11	40.00
Podiatry: Surg-Forefoot Only	*	*	0	*	2	*	0	*
Psychiatry: General	9	*	47	40.00	68	40.00	75	40.00
Psychiatry: Child & Adolescent	0	*	11	40.00	10	40.00	4	*
Psychiatry: Geriatric	*	*	*	*	3	*	3	*
Pulmonary Medicine	9	*	25	40.00	40	40.00	50	40.00
Pulmonary Medicine: Critical Care	1	*	6	*	15	40.00	12	50.00
Pulmonary Med: Gen & Crit Care	10	40.00	32	40.00	53	40.00	36	40.00
Radiation Oncology	1	*	19	40.00	41	40.00	23	40.00
Radiology: Diagnostic-Inv	19	39.00	51	41.00	86	42.00	70	40.00
Radiology: Diagnostic-Noninv	26	40.00	85	40.00	201	40.00	201	40.00
Radiology: Nuclear Medicine	0	*	7	*	4	*	13	40.00
Rheumatology	6	*	29	36.00	43	40.00	73	40.00
Sleep Medicine	2	*	10	40.00	10	40.00	19	40.00
Surgery: General	31	40.00	100	40.00	205	40.00	230	40.00
Surgery: Bariatric	1	*	2	*	5	*	3	*
Surgery: Cardiovascular	15	40.00	17	45.00	63	45.00	45	45.00
Surgery: Colon and Rectal	0	*	3	*	7	*	13	40.00
Surgery: Neurological	7	*	25	40.00	52	40.00	45	40.00
Surgery: Oncology	*	*	2	*	3	*	4	*
Surgery: Oral	0	*	1	*	6	*	7	*
Surgery: Pediatric	2	*	7	*	11	40.00	13	40.00
Surgery: Plastic & Reconstruction	4	*	17	40.00	22	40.00	26	40.00
Surgery: Plastic & Recon-Hand	1	*	4	*	4	*	0	*
Surgery: Thoracic (primary)	0	*	3	*	4	*	13	40.00
Surgery: Transplant	0	*	2	*	12	40.00	5	*
Surgery: Trauma	7	*	5	*	17	40.00	8	*
Surgery: Trauma-Burn	1	*	2	*	1	*	*	*
Surgery: Vascular (primary)	2	*	14	40.00	37	40.00	31	44.00
Urgent Care	5	*	36	36.00	65	36.00	82	36.00
Urology	14	40.00	53	40.00	113	40.00	160	40.00
Urology: Pediatric	1	*	3	*	4	*	4	*

Summary Tables

For each of the specialties listed, you will find four tables as follows:

Table *.A:
Compensation
Overall (aggregate)
Group Type
Geographic Section (All Practices)

Table *.B:
Collections for Professional Charges (TC/NPP Excluded)
Overall (aggregate)
Group Type
Geographic Section (All Practices)

Table *.C:
Compensation to Collections Ratio (TC/NPP Excluded)
Overall (aggregate)
Group Type
Geographic Section (All Practices)

Table *.D:
Physician Work RVUs (CMS RBRVS Method) (NPP Excluded)
Overall (aggregate)
Group Type
Geographic Section (All Practices)

Allergy/Immunology

Table 74A: Compensation

	Phys	Med Pracs	Mean	Std. Dev.	25th %tile	Median	75th %tile	90th %tile
Overall	175	85	$295,873	$136,255	$208,263	$267,688	$340,967	$539,160
Group Type								
Single Specialty	36	9	$313,900	$163,046	$191,250	$263,548	$400,092	$607,931
Multispecialty	139	76	$291,205	$128,684	$208,895	$267,688	$329,994	$477,136
Geographic Section (All Pracs)								
Eastern	21	11	$342,666	$135,644	$256,830	$329,994	$398,281	$598,787
Midwest	56	33	$296,952	$132,256	$200,972	$273,542	$347,920	$500,939
Southern	37	17	$305,181	$153,613	$183,325	$272,298	$396,111	$580,312
Western	61	24	$273,129	$127,152	$211,170	$237,857	$280,828	$475,905

Table 74B: Collections for Professional Charges (TC/NPP Excluded)

	Phys	Med Pracs	Mean	Std. Dev.	25th %tile	Median	75th %tile	90th %tile
Overall	71	40	$639,789	$393,116	$390,203	$573,749	$713,158	$985,624
Group Type								
Single Specialty	11	4	$575,756	$185,375	$501,463	$641,487	$680,000	$800,000
Multispecialty	60	36	$651,528	$420,266	$370,056	$554,306	$734,622	$1,163,341
Geographic Section (All Pracs)								
Eastern	6	4	*	*	*	*	*	*
Midwest	25	15	$543,948	$244,371	$349,066	$467,527	$709,237	$953,195
Southern	16	11	$536,864	$230,641	$325,925	$503,602	$751,391	$864,547
Western	24	10	$833,681	$555,815	$461,704	$676,000	$926,120	$1,861,398

Table 74C: Compensation to Collections Ratio (TC/NPP Excluded)

	Phys	Med Pracs	Mean	Std. Dev.	25th %tile	Median	75th %tile	90th %tile
Overall	69	38	.464	.162	.354	.465	.547	.667
Group Type								
Single Specialty	11	4	.398	.109	.331	.397	.522	.553
Multispecialty	58	34	.476	.168	.379	.496	.584	.669
Geographic Section (All Pracs)								
Eastern	6	4	*	*	*	*	*	*
Midwest	23	14	.537	.099	.448	.522	.615	.659
Southern	15	10	.509	.150	.405	.527	.546	.755
Western	25	10	.345	.150	.265	.333	.412	.588

Table 74D: Physician Work RVUs (CMS RBRVS Method) (NPP Excluded)

	Phys	Med Pracs	Mean	Std. Dev.	25th %tile	Median	75th %tile	90th %tile
Overall	84	49	4,393	1,750	3,295	4,159	5,112	6,990
Group Type								
Single Specialty	9	2	*	*	*	*	*	*
Multispecialty	75	47	4,155	1,601	3,160	3,972	4,837	6,377
Geographic Section (All Pracs)								
Eastern	17	7	5,411	1,780	4,297	5,033	6,529	8,471
Midwest	30	19	4,219	1,877	2,614	3,813	5,163	7,038
Southern	11	8	5,091	1,891	3,748	4,518	6,313	8,823
Western	26	15	3,634	1,030	2,675	3,700	4,411	5,073

Anesthesiology

Table 75A: Compensation

	Phys	Med Pracs	Mean	Std. Dev.	25th %tile	Median	75th %tile	90th %tile
Overall	3,903	184	$399,222	$127,132	$324,679	$398,925	$453,692	$558,712
Group Type								
Single Specialty	3,211	128	$406,727	$132,882	$325,773	$403,600	$465,038	$582,019
Multispecialty	692	56	$364,400	$88,117	$322,106	$362,095	$414,089	$454,340
Geographic Section (All Pracs)								
Eastern	912	42	$424,447	$150,090	$365,000	$403,600	$454,000	$696,604
Midwest	731	50	$421,183	$121,641	$350,413	$412,694	$498,000	$566,355
Southern	857	49	$422,892	$128,574	$346,816	$433,990	$499,265	$588,100
Western	1,403	43	$356,925	$98,739	$299,556	$358,252	$410,070	$476,109

Table 75B: Collections for Professional Charges (TC/NPP Excluded)

	Phys	Med Pracs	Mean	Std. Dev.	25th %tile	Median	75th %tile	90th %tile
Overall	2,364	117	$572,543	$259,992	$390,266	$531,887	$692,623	$908,022
Group Type								
Single Specialty	2,143	93	$576,609	$261,433	$393,323	$533,500	$707,227	$933,430
Multispecialty	221	24	$533,116	$242,621	$372,599	$502,451	$617,647	$830,740
Geographic Section (All Pracs)								
Eastern	624	26	$650,131	$241,867	$516,568	$543,720	$758,213	$1,173,057
Midwest	532	33	$516,973	$188,889	$383,451	$508,095	$630,436	$767,094
Southern	561	32	$751,648	$303,909	$533,500	$743,773	$796,356	$1,325,800
Western	647	26	$388,107	$105,662	$328,560	$370,000	$457,761	$517,970

Table 75C: Compensation to Collections Ratio (TC/NPP Excluded)

	Phys	Med Pracs	Mean	Std. Dev.	25th %tile	Median	75th %tile	90th %tile
Overall	1,993	110	.704	.181	.556	.742	.836	.927
Group Type								
Single Specialty	1,804	88	.709	.180	.558	.742	.840	.928
Multispecialty	189	22	.655	.182	.550	.652	.800	.892
Geographic Section (All Pracs)								
Eastern	593	25	.669	.170	.509	.742	.746	.816
Midwest	430	31	.764	.160	.675	.799	.889	.930
Southern	545	32	.622	.197	.475	.557	.800	.894
Western	425	22	.795	.123	.694	.805	.882	.962

Table 75D: Physician Work RVUs (CMS RBRVS Method) (NPP Excluded)

	Phys	Med Pracs	Mean	Std. Dev.	25th %tile	Median	75th %tile	90th %tile
Overall	253	19	7,354	5,480	2,391	5,357	12,176	13,803
Group Type								
Single Specialty	229	10	7,705	5,620	2,391	7,161	12,176	14,306
Multispecialty	24	9	4,012	1,746	2,270	4,746	5,357	5,357
Geographic Section (All Pracs)								
Eastern	52	6	6,437	5,299	3,651	3,651	9,534	14,944
Midwest	56	3	2,386	1,467	1,515	1,515	2,780	5,357
Southern	47	6	10,291	6,905	2,036	12,176	12,176	22,000
Western	98	4	9,272	4,101	6,671	10,071	12,401	14,172

Anesthesiology: Pain Management

Table 76A: Compensation

	Phys	Med Pracs	Mean	Std. Dev.	25th %tile	Median	75th %tile	90th %tile
Overall	191	62	$481,595	$166,135	$380,000	$457,604	$561,833	$660,002
Group Type								
Single Specialty	116	27	$473,776	$140,461	$385,466	$461,140	$546,134	$632,000
Multispecialty	75	35	$493,689	$199,907	$360,305	$440,059	$561,833	$760,297
Geographic Section (All Pracs)								
Eastern	46	11	$456,379	$113,996	$403,600	$403,600	$561,833	$632,000
Midwest	75	22	$491,788	$164,260	$384,533	$472,496	$551,329	$691,281
Southern	50	19	$512,883	$195,020	$380,000	$494,413	$593,308	$819,732
Western	20	10	$423,150	$184,228	$269,387	$459,372	$461,140	$799,043

Table 76B: Collections for Professional Charges (TC/NPP Excluded)

	Phys	Med Pracs	Mean	Std. Dev.	25th %tile	Median	75th %tile	90th %tile
Overall	71	26	$708,282	$364,757	$430,309	$677,900	$972,156	$1,248,112
Group Type								
Single Specialty	30	10	$480,914	$211,916	$430,309	$430,309	$622,069	$808,463
Multispecialty	41	16	$874,649	$364,874	$564,056	$944,304	$1,108,052	$1,344,031
Geographic Section (All Pracs)								
Eastern	19	4	$446,337	$121,543	$430,309	$430,309	$430,309	$677,900
Midwest	24	11	$738,742	$337,619	$474,646	$730,666	$893,303	$1,283,129
Southern	24	8	$957,737	$314,165	$780,516	$987,358	$1,120,823	$1,381,696
Western	4	3	*	*	*	*	*	*

Table 76C: Compensation to Collections Ratio (TC/NPP Excluded)

	Phys	Med Pracs	Mean	Std. Dev.	25th %tile	Median	75th %tile	90th %tile
Overall	67	24	.708	.182	.564	.700	.890	.938
Group Type								
Single Specialty	27	8	.834	.142	.700	.938	.938	.938
Multispecialty	40	16	.623	.155	.535	.641	.742	.827
Geographic Section (All Pracs)								
Eastern	18	4	.881	.135	.926	.938	.938	.938
Midwest	23	10	.661	.143	.613	.700	.772	.836
Southern	25	9	.619	.157	.536	.598	.750	.820
Western	1	1	*	*	*	*	*	*

Table 76D: Physician Work RVUs (CMS RBRVS Method) (NPP Excluded)

	Phys	Med Pracs	Mean	Std. Dev.	25th %tile	Median	75th %tile	90th %tile
Overall	50	24	7,877	4,166	4,982	6,272	9,931	14,083
Group Type								
Single Specialty	11	5	7,496	4,523	6,202	6,202	6,320	18,126
Multispecialty	39	19	7,985	4,116	4,696	6,924	10,901	14,186
Geographic Section (All Pracs)								
Eastern	7	3	*	*	*	*	*	*
Midwest	18	10	6,661	2,443	4,496	6,441	8,965	10,904
Southern	15	7	10,987	4,372	7,391	11,443	14,186	17,795
Western	10	4	6,760	4,900	5,423	6,202	6,208	18,451

Cardiology: Electrophysiology

Table 77A: Compensation

	Phys	Med Pracs	Mean	Std. Dev.	25th %tile	Median	75th %tile	90th %tile
Overall	203	96	$499,667	$183,539	$370,000	$491,231	$581,762	$760,093
Group Type								
Single Specialty	139	62	$488,558	$177,309	$362,714	$488,554	$567,299	$776,852
Multispecialty	64	34	$523,795	$195,657	$395,319	$516,985	$614,166	$733,719
Geographic Section (All Pracs)								
Eastern	41	18	$483,754	$151,736	$393,000	$469,527	$543,261	$741,131
Midwest	61	28	$518,462	$185,051	$411,885	$526,543	$578,481	$712,833
Southern	72	28	$512,735	$179,979	$369,974	$497,993	$617,732	$814,949
Western	29	22	$450,185	$224,721	$316,640	$368,802	$551,526	$776,852

Table 77B: Collections for Professional Charges (TC/NPP Excluded)

	Phys	Med Pracs	Mean	Std. Dev.	25th %tile	Median	75th %tile	90th %tile
Overall	62	29	$782,775	$306,969	$583,785	$783,130	$886,890	$1,040,122
Group Type								
Single Specialty	39	15	$816,680	$229,339	$748,017	$814,182	$899,575	$1,040,138
Multispecialty	23	14	$725,284	$406,118	$480,792	$667,594	$845,044	$1,423,097
Geographic Section (All Pracs)								
Eastern	12	6	$828,775	$319,868	$606,313	$869,622	$1,021,966	$1,331,343
Midwest	21	9	$748,660	$197,810	$552,395	$793,006	$891,619	$938,587
Southern	20	8	$770,201	$204,389	$635,618	$781,770	$814,640	$896,572
Western	9	6	*	*	*	*	*	*

Table 77C: Compensation to Collections Ratio (TC/NPP Excluded)

	Phys	Med Pracs	Mean	Std. Dev.	25th %tile	Median	75th %tile	90th %tile
Overall	58	27	.623	.173	.488	.589	.760	.892
Group Type								
Single Specialty	39	15	.586	.180	.418	.562	.682	.890
Multispecialty	19	12	.699	.132	.580	.671	.789	.914
Geographic Section (All Pracs)								
Eastern	11	5	.598	.163	.453	.585	.639	.941
Midwest	20	9	.678	.175	.543	.677	.815	.947
Southern	20	8	.601	.197	.413	.562	.779	.912
Western	7	5	*	*	*	*	*	*

Table 77D: Physician Work RVUs (CMS RBRVS Method) (NPP Excluded)

	Phys	Med Pracs	Mean	Std. Dev.	25th %tile	Median	75th %tile	90th %tile
Overall	95	47	12,045	5,338	8,368	11,291	13,552	18,067
Group Type								
Single Specialty	54	23	12,516	4,958	9,221	11,790	13,971	18,146
Multispecialty	41	24	11,425	5,804	7,334	10,585	13,170	20,907
Geographic Section (All Pracs)								
Eastern	18	9	11,854	5,593	7,450	11,261	13,111	22,532
Midwest	30	13	12,188	6,456	7,582	10,520	14,367	24,725
Southern	33	14	11,966	2,626	10,730	11,956	13,430	15,185
Western	14	11	12,170	7,416	7,323	10,049	13,947	27,751

Cardiology: Invasive

Table 78A: Compensation

	Phys	Med Pracs	Mean	Std. Dev.	25th %tile	Median	75th %tile	90th %tile
Overall	528	139	$452,970	$149,346	$352,211	$431,533	$541,442	$661,560
Group Type								
Single Specialty	243	61	$458,322	$153,873	$353,700	$434,814	$545,940	$676,577
Multispecialty	285	78	$448,406	$145,491	$351,471	$430,253	$539,910	$642,995
Geographic Section (All Pracs)								
Eastern	71	25	$461,810	$140,058	$366,000	$439,489	$543,562	$632,279
Midwest	122	36	$469,031	$144,354	$375,879	$441,140	$547,639	$690,245
Southern	172	45	$475,846	$177,534	$345,711	$466,700	$617,619	$698,832
Western	163	33	$412,958	$113,369	$347,227	$397,659	$471,765	$549,730

Table 78B: Collections for Professional Charges (TC/NPP Excluded)

	Phys	Med Pracs	Mean	Std. Dev.	25th %tile	Median	75th %tile	90th %tile
Overall	157	47	$667,176	$291,554	$473,536	$629,195	$814,793	$954,058
Group Type								
Single Specialty	53	12	$622,983	$288,500	$463,421	$561,555	$697,909	$934,037
Multispecialty	104	35	$689,697	$291,902	$508,571	$658,363	$814,793	$966,972
Geographic Section (All Pracs)								
Eastern	12	6	$884,578	$515,385	$530,879	$785,052	$1,197,431	$1,809,861
Midwest	51	15	$598,155	$192,355	$489,513	$599,526	$711,304	$798,266
Southern	54	14	$638,409	$235,292	$443,646	$632,148	$814,793	$849,633
Western	40	12	$728,791	$341,485	$483,849	$655,099	$920,226	$1,117,938

Table 78C: Compensation to Collections Ratio (TC/NPP Excluded)

	Phys	Med Pracs	Mean	Std. Dev.	25th %tile	Median	75th %tile	90th %tile
Overall	133	43	.671	.185	.519	.667	.814	.931
Group Type								
Single Specialty	44	11	.692	.175	.545	.673	.866	.947
Multispecialty	89	32	.661	.190	.508	.659	.805	.918
Geographic Section (All Pracs)								
Eastern	11	5	.482	.120	.410	.449	.591	.667
Midwest	45	15	.771	.152	.641	.813	.888	.952
Southern	48	14	.695	.164	.531	.732	.799	.938
Western	29	9	.549	.168	.452	.539	.666	.791

Table 78D: Physician Work RVUs (CMS RBRVS Method) (NPP Excluded)

	Phys	Med Pracs	Mean	Std. Dev.	25th %tile	Median	75th %tile	90th %tile
Overall	244	68	9,409	3,366	6,837	9,256	11,332	13,562
Group Type								
Single Specialty	99	21	9,900	3,857	6,756	9,007	12,278	15,771
Multispecialty	145	47	9,073	2,953	6,912	9,362	11,051	12,648
Geographic Section (All Pracs)								
Eastern	13	6	8,412	2,738	6,318	8,509	10,559	11,920
Midwest	70	18	9,841	3,654	7,467	9,378	11,749	14,750
Southern	91	24	10,062	3,451	7,211	9,788	11,979	14,741
Western	70	20	8,312	2,750	6,451	8,094	10,097	11,793

Cardiology: Invasive/Interventional

Table 79A: Compensation

	Phys	Med Pracs	Mean	Std. Dev.	25th %tile	Median	75th %tile	90th %tile
Overall	627	161	$537,858	$221,905	$392,590	$485,006	$630,000	$880,473
Group Type								
Single Specialty	394	83	$519,253	$205,820	$385,869	$469,778	$611,225	$795,881
Multispecialty	233	78	$569,319	$243,980	$409,735	$500,000	$651,987	$958,997
Geographic Section (All Pracs)								
Eastern	88	32	$469,892	$153,687	$381,172	$455,586	$548,835	$605,767
Midwest	171	44	$562,038	$253,060	$406,650	$511,141	$620,990	$992,162
Southern	206	48	$606,860	$243,119	$421,763	$543,228	$772,558	$946,591
Western	162	37	$461,511	$143,929	$371,177	$440,000	$523,927	$648,960

Table 79B: Collections for Professional Charges (TC/NPP Excluded)

	Phys	Med Pracs	Mean	Std. Dev.	25th %tile	Median	75th %tile	90th %tile
Overall	207	55	$835,374	$356,328	$583,393	$793,914	$972,989	$1,290,414
Group Type								
Single Specialty	109	21	$779,817	$334,833	$530,682	$730,364	$967,990	$1,226,889
Multispecialty	98	34	$897,167	$370,802	$703,501	$817,491	$1,001,253	$1,591,561
Geographic Section (All Pracs)								
Eastern	35	11	$887,232	$320,011	$677,214	$848,913	$1,032,118	$1,374,817
Midwest	72	20	$878,134	$425,853	$562,982	$801,162	$1,024,124	$1,672,535
Southern	56	13	$829,839	$341,846	$583,393	$814,555	$1,003,973	$1,259,043
Western	44	11	$731,196	$248,989	$567,941	$711,608	$876,630	$1,066,288

Table 79C: Compensation to Collections Ratio (TC/NPP Excluded)

	Phys	Med Pracs	Mean	Std. Dev.	25th %tile	Median	75th %tile	90th %tile
Overall	189	51	.657	.152	.536	.656	.771	.870
Group Type								
Single Specialty	100	20	.650	.166	.518	.628	.783	.893
Multispecialty	89	31	.666	.136	.564	.673	.756	.856
Geographic Section (All Pracs)								
Eastern	34	11	.594	.131	.494	.566	.678	.779
Midwest	69	18	.702	.152	.607	.716	.813	.921
Southern	47	12	.670	.157	.539	.683	.789	.872
Western	39	10	.619	.140	.522	.618	.716	.828

Table 79D: Physician Work RVUs (CMS RBRVS Method) (NPP Excluded)

	Phys	Med Pracs	Mean	Std. Dev.	25th %tile	Median	75th %tile	90th %tile
Overall	299	79	11,430	5,058	8,359	10,225	13,015	18,126
Group Type								
Single Specialty	149	27	11,215	5,096	8,575	9,784	12,265	17,419
Multispecialty	150	52	11,645	5,028	7,916	10,896	13,949	19,496
Geographic Section (All Pracs)								
Eastern	36	15	11,166	6,328	7,529	9,228	11,405	23,976
Midwest	88	20	12,766	5,638	9,062	11,118	15,012	20,958
Southern	94	23	11,778	4,332	9,196	11,058	14,386	17,430
Western	81	21	9,694	4,026	7,195	9,108	11,507	13,519

Cardiology: Noninvasive

Table 80A: Compensation

	Phys	Med Pracs	Mean	Std. Dev.	25th %tile	Median	75th %tile	90th %tile
Overall	516	138	$418,451	$138,842	$330,514	$410,784	$509,374	$598,576
Group Type								
Single Specialty	260	63	$427,172	$139,666	$346,140	$426,746	$531,406	$589,500
Multispecialty	256	75	$409,594	$137,708	$319,631	$393,375	$500,003	$603,466
Geographic Section (All Pracs)								
Eastern	187	36	$400,021	$129,376	$319,631	$400,000	$493,277	$590,694
Midwest	158	44	$455,916	$126,640	$375,963	$468,124	$548,908	$598,865
Southern	111	39	$420,658	$159,868	$299,126	$400,281	$529,463	$639,178
Western	60	19	$373,151	$135,057	$328,338	$375,707	$399,818	$492,218

Table 80B: Collections for Professional Charges (TC/NPP Excluded)

	Phys	Med Pracs	Mean	Std. Dev.	25th %tile	Median	75th %tile	90th %tile
Overall	151	44	$613,980	$268,094	$422,813	$568,695	$742,769	$986,782
Group Type								
Single Specialty	63	19	$628,914	$304,817	$383,798	$568,695	$768,086	$1,182,940
Multispecialty	88	25	$603,288	$239,646	$424,702	$562,071	$740,417	$968,891
Geographic Section (All Pracs)								
Eastern	69	11	$625,292	$268,332	$408,241	$592,342	$768,010	$1,015,843
Midwest	38	16	$596,827	$240,179	$455,256	$554,876	$671,985	$977,924
Southern	36	13	$600,925	$291,915	$365,620	$568,695	$690,907	$1,062,600
Western	8	4	*	*	*	*	*	*

Table 80C: Compensation to Collections Ratio (TC/NPP Excluded)

	Phys	Med Pracs	Mean	Std. Dev.	25th %tile	Median	75th %tile	90th %tile
Overall	132	42	.672	.179	.537	.675	.796	.937
Group Type								
Single Specialty	51	18	.644	.186	.493	.607	.772	.944
Multispecialty	81	24	.690	.173	.592	.688	.800	.937
Geographic Section (All Pracs)								
Eastern	63	10	.667	.186	.498	.676	.800	.941
Midwest	34	16	.664	.159	.583	.674	.758	.870
Southern	27	12	.729	.186	.587	.739	.906	.985
Western	8	4	*	*	*	*	*	*

Table 80D: Physician Work RVUs (CMS RBRVS Method) (NPP Excluded)

	Phys	Med Pracs	Mean	Std. Dev.	25th %tile	Median	75th %tile	90th %tile
Overall	241	70	8,005	3,767	5,352	7,274	9,849	12,847
Group Type								
Single Specialty	85	25	9,452	4,450	6,029	8,854	11,620	15,634
Multispecialty	156	45	7,216	3,076	5,170	6,721	8,747	11,027
Geographic Section (All Pracs)								
Eastern	96	20	8,143	4,277	5,177	6,897	10,010	13,789
Midwest	68	19	8,007	3,584	5,379	7,218	9,972	12,310
Southern	49	18	8,538	3,511	5,728	8,257	11,033	12,896
Western	28	13	6,590	2,304	5,124	6,743	8,458	9,844

Dermatology

Table 81A: Compensation

	Phys	Med Pracs	Mean	Std. Dev.	25th %tile	Median	75th %tile	90th %tile
Overall	361	128	$400,834	$195,891	$271,484	$357,945	$467,764	$680,096
Group Type								
Single Specialty	27	11	$450,154	$257,160	$284,630	$377,450	$572,174	$821,075
Multispecialty	334	117	$396,847	$190,021	$270,434	$356,462	$461,081	$666,318
Geographic Section (All Pracs)								
Eastern	63	23	$346,365	$178,595	$241,217	$290,570	$454,263	$594,831
Midwest	94	42	$442,126	$192,823	$293,119	$391,815	$572,035	$762,117
Southern	58	24	$442,711	$241,958	$258,955	$362,628	$571,799	$819,681
Western	146	39	$381,115	$176,877	$288,400	$361,122	$430,427	$540,790

Table 81B: Collections for Professional Charges (TC/NPP Excluded)

	Phys	Med Pracs	Mean	Std. Dev.	25th %tile	Median	75th %tile	90th %tile
Overall	151	64	$838,717	$386,282	$603,635	$738,110	$1,002,420	$1,414,670
Group Type								
Single Specialty	14	5	$755,246	$431,124	$451,762	$718,110	$1,007,214	$1,492,153
Multispecialty	137	59	$847,247	$382,121	$605,148	$745,386	$1,002,864	$1,426,239
Geographic Section (All Pracs)								
Eastern	23	10	$686,526	$243,440	$490,764	$637,366	$859,144	$1,031,257
Midwest	45	18	$890,182	$363,810	$613,416	$855,369	$1,127,740	$1,429,763
Southern	38	17	$856,229	$380,492	$602,334	$734,170	$1,007,469	$1,517,212
Western	45	19	$850,251	$457,967	$619,595	$716,247	$964,408	$1,639,130

Table 81C: Compensation to Collections Ratio (TC/NPP Excluded)

	Phys	Med Pracs	Mean	Std. Dev.	25th %tile	Median	75th %tile	90th %tile
Overall	148	62	.532	.135	.459	.513	.589	.715
Group Type								
Single Specialty	13	5	.669	.202	.536	.691	.823	.946
Multispecialty	135	57	.519	.120	.454	.508	.574	.699
Geographic Section (All Pracs)								
Eastern	23	10	.552	.150	.477	.518	.633	.820
Midwest	44	18	.530	.117	.464	.524	.608	.716
Southern	37	16	.564	.124	.471	.533	.663	.751
Western	44	18	.498	.148	.409	.474	.573	.669

Table 81D: Physician Work RVUs (CMS RBRVS Method) (NPP Excluded)

	Phys	Med Pracs	Mean	Std. Dev.	25th %tile	Median	75th %tile	90th %tile
Overall	213	78	8,224	5,120	5,306	7,113	9,458	12,755
Group Type								
Single Specialty	20	5	8,185	4,748	5,104	6,915	10,411	16,092
Multispecialty	193	73	8,228	5,168	5,306	7,113	9,403	12,577
Geographic Section (All Pracs)								
Eastern	47	12	7,147	2,780	4,752	6,708	9,163	11,195
Midwest	56	25	8,432	3,939	5,531	7,741	10,096	14,452
Southern	33	13	8,650	4,761	6,101	8,004	9,727	15,670
Western	77	28	8,547	6,837	5,133	6,840	9,181	14,348

Emergency Medicine

Table 82A: Compensation

	Phys	Med Pracs	Mean	Std. Dev.	25th %tile	Median	75th %tile	90th %tile
Overall	976	60	$260,790	$76,117	$217,827	$256,800	$302,397	$353,246
Group Type								
Single Specialty	379	17	$266,434	$87,362	$203,995	$264,116	$327,692	$370,983
Multispecialty	597	43	$257,207	$67,857	$222,500	$253,561	$290,542	$338,904
Geographic Section (All Pracs)								
Eastern	240	15	$242,112	$58,110	$210,340	$239,778	$262,961	$322,171
Midwest	220	21	$284,275	$71,315	$236,912	$276,827	$336,677	$376,441
Southern	146	9	$243,908	$90,919	$168,480	$256,800	$305,670	$352,498
Western	370	15	$265,603	$78,507	$222,900	$263,598	$298,828	$356,020

Table 82B: Collections for Professional Charges (TC/NPP Excluded)

	Phys	Med Pracs	Mean	Std. Dev.	25th %tile	Median	75th %tile	90th %tile
Overall	280	20	$307,788	$110,699	$235,266	$302,599	$391,470	$446,732
Group Type								
Single Specialty	165	8	$299,483	$99,095	$233,494	$297,642	$373,058	$427,800
Multispecialty	115	12	$319,704	$124,985	$236,161	$316,793	$399,021	$483,983
Geographic Section (All Pracs)								
Eastern	74	6	$296,687	$118,218	$230,431	$268,990	$322,153	$536,903
Midwest	55	6	$346,961	$102,150	$275,115	$338,032	$431,097	$472,903
Southern	25	1	$288,924	$91,308	$221,639	$316,793	$352,464	$398,483
Western	126	7	$300,952	$110,522	$227,224	$318,643	$398,380	$430,373

Table 82C: Compensation to Collections Ratio (TC/NPP Excluded)

	Phys	Med Pracs	Mean	Std. Dev.	25th %tile	Median	75th %tile	90th %tile
Overall	193	19	.702	.197	.536	.729	.867	.940
Group Type								
Single Specialty	117	8	.694	.209	.525	.733	.860	.940
Multispecialty	76	11	.715	.178	.561	.722	.872	.942
Geographic Section (All Pracs)								
Eastern	50	6	.643	.253	.378	.732	.883	.917
Midwest	39	6	.751	.166	.566	.760	.902	.971
Southern	20	1	*	*	*	*	*	*
Western	84	6	.703	.183	.536	.722	.846	.950

Table 82D: Physician Work RVUs (CMS RBRVS Method) (NPP Excluded)

	Phys	Med Pracs	Mean	Std. Dev.	25th %tile	Median	75th %tile	90th %tile
Overall	281	25	6,686	2,447	4,939	6,516	8,403	9,716
Group Type								
Single Specialty	46	2	*	*	*	*	*	*
Multispecialty	235	23	6,678	2,530	4,747	6,512	8,494	9,970
Geographic Section (All Pracs)								
Eastern	117	7	6,452	2,208	5,049	6,248	7,630	9,015
Midwest	93	12	6,745	2,603	4,526	7,011	8,604	9,874
Southern	25	1	*	*	*	*	*	*
Western	46	5	6,124	2,290	4,383	6,120	8,265	9,231

Endocrinology/Metabolism

Table 83A: Compensation

	Phys	Med Pracs	Mean	Std. Dev.	25th %tile	Median	75th %tile	90th %tile
Overall	291	137	$211,550	$67,221	$167,980	$199,006	$246,099	$302,168
Group Type								
Single Specialty	18	11	$217,238	$71,722	$162,082	$210,601	$276,442	$321,302
Multispecialty	273	126	$211,174	$67,036	$168,490	$197,186	$245,965	$298,968
Geographic Section (All Pracs)								
Eastern	69	35	$188,610	$58,007	$151,871	$177,815	$212,249	$261,265
Midwest	69	33	$216,749	$76,881	$160,905	$209,364	$248,936	$315,580
Southern	81	40	$222,387	$70,725	$174,964	$204,863	$260,757	$327,491
Western	72	29	$216,357	$56,935	$182,200	$210,746	$248,106	$296,554

Table 83B: Collections for Professional Charges (TC/NPP Excluded)

	Phys	Med Pracs	Mean	Std. Dev.	25th %tile	Median	75th %tile	90th %tile
Overall	121	66	$366,803	$122,064	$281,378	$357,810	$419,402	$514,071
Group Type								
Single Specialty	9	6	*	*	*	*	*	*
Multispecialty	112	60	$369,706	$123,274	$281,109	$366,168	$420,206	$513,838
Geographic Section (All Pracs)								
Eastern	27	15	$366,649	$119,877	$318,783	$359,276	$424,217	$452,839
Midwest	29	17	$345,327	$121,232	$260,528	$339,139	$400,197	$518,606
Southern	44	23	$388,675	$121,284	$302,516	$370,919	$442,794	$550,558
Western	21	11	$350,834	$128,551	$273,748	$338,776	$435,736	$539,316

Table 83C: Compensation to Collections Ratio (TC/NPP Excluded)

	Phys	Med Pracs	Mean	Std. Dev.	25th %tile	Median	75th %tile	90th %tile
Overall	118	64	.570	.145	.478	.581	.682	.740
Group Type								
Single Specialty	8	6	*	*	*	*	*	*
Multispecialty	110	58	.565	.146	.474	.566	.674	.742
Geographic Section (All Pracs)								
Eastern	26	15	.516	.147	.413	.498	.633	.707
Midwest	28	16	.591	.108	.536	.593	.647	.738
Southern	44	23	.583	.168	.477	.589	.708	.800
Western	20	10	.578	.123	.479	.579	.699	.745

Table 83D: Physician Work RVUs (CMS RBRVS Method) (NPP Excluded)

	Phys	Med Pracs	Mean	Std. Dev.	25th %tile	Median	75th %tile	90th %tile
Overall	191	88	4,712	1,473	3,748	4,519	5,696	6,710
Group Type								
Single Specialty	9	6	*	*	*	*	*	*
Multispecialty	182	82	4,714	1,476	3,747	4,556	5,698	6,690
Geographic Section (All Pracs)								
Eastern	44	20	4,600	1,609	3,819	4,481	5,756	6,867
Midwest	52	24	4,311	1,270	3,237	4,242	5,099	6,050
Southern	48	23	5,553	1,503	4,365	5,344	6,368	7,641
Western	47	21	4,400	1,188	3,456	4,324	5,220	5,815

Family Practice (with OB)

Table 84A: Compensation

	Phys	Med Pracs	Mean	Std. Dev.	25th %tile	Median	75th %tile	90th %tile
Overall	789	141	$199,650	$66,332	$150,725	$187,393	$233,616	$290,016
Group Type								
Single Specialty	95	27	$205,027	$74,861	$145,716	$187,396	$273,205	$310,039
Multispecialty	694	114	$198,914	$65,103	$152,814	$187,170	$230,933	$283,404
Geographic Section (All Pracs)								
Eastern	97	20	$168,452	$43,686	$134,783	$159,330	$197,908	$217,522
Midwest	386	67	$211,326	$71,784	$158,760	$195,268	$251,886	$314,824
Southern	149	20	$204,116	$58,260	$167,940	$190,012	$237,045	$283,593
Western	157	34	$185,981	$62,958	$140,564	$174,146	$222,774	$274,695

Table 84B: Collections for Professional Charges (TC/NPP Excluded)

	Phys	Med Pracs	Mean	Std. Dev.	25th %tile	Median	75th %tile	90th %tile
Overall	323	65	$401,049	$168,965	$300,675	$374,925	$464,810	$609,654
Group Type								
Single Specialty	37	10	$370,809	$122,810	$282,051	$356,141	$449,858	$507,313
Multispecialty	286	55	$404,961	$173,829	$303,567	$380,933	$469,380	$625,838
Geographic Section (All Pracs)								
Eastern	22	6	$323,820	$73,707	$314,099	$331,354	$372,753	$409,042
Midwest	145	26	$443,341	$200,274	$326,759	$400,009	$516,256	$736,419
Southern	65	11	$365,937	$101,645	$305,985	$360,228	$428,048	$514,488
Western	91	22	$377,409	$153,486	$256,778	$374,916	$464,810	$584,210

Table 84C: Compensation to Collections Ratio (TC/NPP Excluded)

	Phys	Med Pracs	Mean	Std. Dev.	25th %tile	Median	75th %tile	90th %tile
Overall	309	63	.523	.146	.429	.502	.623	.732
Group Type								
Single Specialty	37	10	.530	.155	.367	.530	.675	.737
Multispecialty	272	53	.522	.145	.429	.501	.615	.730
Geographic Section (All Pracs)								
Eastern	22	6	.508	.102	.440	.488	.585	.670
Midwest	139	26	.521	.146	.439	.517	.604	.726
Southern	63	11	.583	.164	.449	.609	.690	.810
Western	85	20	.486	.128	.398	.462	.545	.695

Table 84D: Physician Work RVUs (CMS RBRVS Method) (NPP Excluded)

	Phys	Med Pracs	Mean	Std. Dev.	25th %tile	Median	75th %tile	90th %tile
Overall	552	77	4,785	1,482	3,868	4,664	5,555	6,691
Group Type								
Single Specialty	32	9	4,744	1,239	4,307	4,650	5,299	6,261
Multispecialty	520	68	4,787	1,497	3,857	4,664	5,586	6,739
Geographic Section (All Pracs)								
Eastern	77	12	4,177	1,217	3,329	4,181	4,978	5,841
Midwest	264	36	4,903	1,513	3,877	4,732	5,638	6,774
Southern	125	10	5,011	1,393	4,118	4,949	5,947	6,774
Western	86	19	4,639	1,589	3,357	4,543	5,301	7,014

Family Practice (without OB)

Table 85A: Compensation

	Phys	Med Pracs	Mean	Std. Dev.	25th %tile	Median	75th %tile	90th %tile
Overall	5,959	630	$187,953	$72,042	$139,457	$173,812	$220,472	$283,010
Group Type								
Single Specialty	947	272	$180,771	$77,378	$130,487	$162,375	$213,403	$293,925
Multispecialty	5,012	358	$189,310	$70,915	$140,643	$176,233	$221,117	$281,701
Geographic Section (All Pracs)								
Eastern	1,087	154	$172,338	$69,158	$129,808	$156,782	$195,130	$257,586
Midwest	2,100	188	$187,750	$70,508	$140,000	$173,782	$220,750	$280,456
Southern	1,451	193	$199,122	$78,534	$144,118	$182,589	$235,859	$306,148
Western	1,321	95	$188,855	$66,872	$143,357	$182,322	$220,302	$276,143

Table 85B: Collections for Professional Charges (TC/NPP Excluded)

	Phys	Med Pracs	Mean	Std. Dev.	25th %tile	Median	75th %tile	90th %tile
Overall	2,463	294	$370,720	$145,562	$285,507	$363,214	$449,157	$547,754
Group Type								
Single Specialty	362	123	$368,857	$117,691	$292,669	$365,625	$441,355	$516,545
Multispecialty	2,101	171	$371,042	$149,863	$284,638	$362,402	$451,265	$551,399
Geographic Section (All Pracs)								
Eastern	447	64	$341,129	$115,395	$283,939	$343,568	$396,128	$479,499
Midwest	761	80	$384,019	$133,664	$302,580	$383,126	$463,187	$553,860
Southern	640	95	$366,547	$164,874	$260,849	$331,559	$431,259	$570,487
Western	615	55	$380,116	$154,660	$308,819	$389,872	$470,411	$555,159

Table 85C: Compensation to Collections Ratio (TC/NPP Excluded)

	Phys	Med Pracs	Mean	Std. Dev.	25th %tile	Median	75th %tile	90th %tile
Overall	2,330	290	.508	.146	.413	.487	.582	.707
Group Type								
Single Specialty	361	123	.497	.133	.400	.486	.577	.673
Multispecialty	1,969	167	.510	.148	.415	.487	.582	.717
Geographic Section (All Pracs)								
Eastern	429	64	.507	.130	.425	.480	.553	.687
Midwest	736	79	.512	.142	.415	.501	.590	.692
Southern	619	95	.564	.168	.457	.544	.669	.800
Western	546	52	.438	.100	.368	.434	.496	.554

Table 85D: Physician Work RVUs (CMS RBRVS Method) (NPP Excluded)

	Phys	Med Pracs	Mean	Std. Dev.	25th %tile	Median	75th %tile	90th %tile
Overall	3,629	300	4,800	1,926	3,701	4,600	5,606	6,796
Group Type								
Single Specialty	311	98	4,737	1,428	3,787	4,657	5,535	6,552
Multispecialty	3,318	202	4,805	1,966	3,684	4,591	5,625	6,815
Geographic Section (All Pracs)								
Eastern	651	80	4,530	1,501	3,596	4,488	5,362	6,191
Midwest	1,389	92	4,708	1,678	3,646	4,468	5,513	6,873
Southern	804	75	5,102	1,808	3,950	4,930	6,102	7,289
Western	785	53	4,876	2,605	3,674	4,620	5,500	6,659

Family Practice: Ambulatory Only (no inpatient work)

Table 86A: Compensation

	Phys	Med Pracs	Mean	Std. Dev.	25th %tile	Median	75th %tile	90th %tile
Overall	236	28	$170,721	$61,879	$134,784	$158,106	$190,067	$224,716
Group Type								
Single Specialty	20	7	$208,075	$84,033	$138,090	$178,500	$246,601	$350,706
Multispecialty	216	21	$167,262	$58,476	$132,040	$157,266	$187,828	$218,410
Geographic Section (All Pracs)								
Eastern	33	7	$137,643	$28,293	$121,459	$130,474	$155,385	$172,912
Midwest	34	4	$171,777	$70,006	$128,002	$153,509	$198,016	$238,063
Southern	91	9	$188,414	$74,065	$141,976	$167,360	$208,998	$282,802
Western	78	8	$163,614	$44,168	$138,597	$162,265	$186,382	$202,286

Table 86B: Collections for Professional Charges (TC/NPP Excluded)

	Phys	Med Pracs	Mean	Std. Dev.	25th %tile	Median	75th %tile	90th %tile
Overall	72	9	$365,991	$150,058	$266,756	$333,154	$429,047	$573,963
Group Type								
Single Specialty	7	3	*	*	*	*	*	*
Multispecialty	65	6	$346,096	$123,332	$263,886	$330,522	$405,880	$489,436
Geographic Section (All Pracs)								
Eastern	26	4	$320,240	$90,720	$258,022	$312,275	$383,615	$489,390
Midwest	1	1	*	*	*	*	*	*
Southern	42	3	$366,207	$144,911	$261,881	$333,154	$434,616	$631,871
Western	3	1	*	*	*	*	*	*

Table 86C: Compensation to Collections Ratio (TC/NPP Excluded)

	Phys	Med Pracs	Mean	Std. Dev.	25th %tile	Median	75th %tile	90th %tile
Overall	71	9	.523	.122	.423	.528	.618	.667
Group Type								
Single Specialty	6	3	*	*	*	*	*	*
Multispecialty	65	6	.534	.118	.433	.531	.622	.678
Geographic Section (All Pracs)								
Eastern	26	4	.456	.129	.390	.417	.486	.677
Midwest	1	1	*	*	*	*	*	*
Southern	41	3	.581	.079	.526	.596	.633	.685
Western	3	1	*	*	*	*	*	*

Table 86D: Physician Work RVUs (CMS RBRVS Method) (NPP Excluded)

	Phys	Med Pracs	Mean	Std. Dev.	25th %tile	Median	75th %tile	90th %tile
Overall	77	10	4,031	1,426	3,074	3,773	4,875	5,771
Group Type								
Single Specialty	1	1	*	*	*	*	*	*
Multispecialty	76	9	4,027	1,435	3,071	3,768	4,884	5,772
Geographic Section (All Pracs)								
Eastern	29	6	3,461	898	2,895	3,576	4,237	4,529
Midwest	22	1	*	*	*	*	*	*
Southern	8	2	*	*	*	*	*	*
Western	18	1	*	*	*	*	*	*

Gastroenterology

Table 87A: Compensation

	Phys	Med Pracs	Mean	Std. Dev.	25th %tile	Median	75th %tile	90th %tile
Overall	887	198	$457,053	$184,066	$331,697	$418,139	$541,784	$715,593
Group Type								
Single Specialty	320	39	$450,070	$193,074	$306,298	$431,228	$552,159	$717,565
Multispecialty	567	159	$460,994	$178,836	$343,710	$412,511	$532,568	$714,796
Geographic Section (All Pracs)								
Eastern	146	39	$437,336	$192,085	$294,731	$396,697	$526,225	$747,892
Midwest	263	59	$499,658	$196,397	$366,274	$466,130	$623,153	$814,807
Southern	195	52	$433,451	$173,425	$304,614	$407,539	$532,568	$679,080
Western	283	48	$443,895	$168,805	$347,120	$404,300	$467,312	$688,442

Table 87B: Collections for Professional Charges (TC/NPP Excluded)

	Phys	Med Pracs	Mean	Std. Dev.	25th %tile	Median	75th %tile	90th %tile
Overall	375	102	$762,298	$280,402	$587,000	$743,867	$905,751	$1,141,749
Group Type								
Single Specialty	129	18	$729,397	$285,682	$592,653	$709,954	$858,203	$1,125,785
Multispecialty	246	84	$779,551	$276,615	$573,350	$755,773	$937,356	$1,151,820
Geographic Section (All Pracs)								
Eastern	52	19	$703,830	$248,427	$554,863	$683,408	$872,482	$1,048,867
Midwest	140	28	$815,799	$336,601	$601,058	$790,006	$1,059,255	$1,253,809
Southern	108	32	$724,768	$209,326	$596,787	$727,054	$838,449	$971,749
Western	75	23	$757,010	$262,224	$588,440	$761,662	$909,908	$1,105,087

Table 87C: Compensation to Collections Ratio (TC/NPP Excluded)

	Phys	Med Pracs	Mean	Std. Dev.	25th %tile	Median	75th %tile	90th %tile
Overall	357	98	.580	.151	.471	.562	.682	.792
Group Type								
Single Specialty	122	17	.547	.178	.421	.512	.651	.851
Multispecialty	235	81	.597	.132	.496	.580	.689	.776
Geographic Section (All Pracs)								
Eastern	46	18	.556	.121	.454	.558	.640	.723
Midwest	139	28	.558	.142	.467	.547	.641	.751
Southern	105	31	.623	.160	.502	.600	.727	.860
Western	67	21	.575	.162	.448	.513	.712	.808

Table 87D: Physician Work RVUs (CMS RBRVS Method) (NPP Excluded)

	Phys	Med Pracs	Mean	Std. Dev.	25th %tile	Median	75th %tile	90th %tile
Overall	491	121	8,779	3,085	6,812	8,381	10,428	12,733
Group Type								
Single Specialty	136	12	8,667	3,682	6,499	8,260	10,778	13,860
Multispecialty	355	109	8,822	2,828	6,964	8,440	10,387	12,592
Geographic Section (All Pracs)								
Eastern	101	22	9,475	3,706	6,988	8,714	11,648	14,927
Midwest	171	35	8,219	2,738	6,693	8,118	9,718	11,576
Southern	87	29	9,437	2,843	7,566	9,663	11,320	13,297
Western	132	35	8,540	2,993	6,507	7,975	10,136	12,765

Hematology/Oncology

Table 88A: Compensation

	Phys	Med Pracs	Mean	Std. Dev.	25th %tile	Median	75th %tile	90th %tile
Overall	460	111	$449,520	$261,932	$291,899	$363,428	$515,784	$777,783
Group Type								
Single Specialty	77	16	$633,376	$385,812	$325,000	$571,359	$837,648	$1,265,348
Multispecialty	383	95	$412,556	$211,281	$285,425	$348,780	$485,096	$646,720
Geographic Section (All Pracs)								
Eastern	102	22	$422,256	$201,562	$250,798	$373,300	$539,370	$694,308
Midwest	108	39	$487,617	$267,238	$309,122	$413,974	$531,371	$946,838
Southern	113	26	$503,148	$308,607	$320,124	$429,790	$544,880	$964,628
Western	137	24	$395,551	$244,393	$297,070	$324,000	$387,745	$578,739

Table 88B: Collections for Professional Charges (TC/NPP Excluded)

	Phys	Med Pracs	Mean	Std. Dev.	25th %tile	Median	75th %tile	90th %tile
Overall	174	48	$688,240	$624,253	$322,184	$526,461	$798,385	$1,106,276
Group Type								
Single Specialty	39	4	$939,032	$888,832	$470,376	$609,180	$923,742	$2,974,552
Multispecialty	135	44	$615,788	$505,450	$296,355	$502,280	$773,490	$969,075
Geographic Section (All Pracs)								
Eastern	40	9	$525,953	$383,284	$225,709	$422,759	$789,776	$955,957
Midwest	48	19	$806,101	$542,610	$435,579	$750,641	$911,949	$1,290,725
Southern	59	12	$582,345	$484,016	$377,724	$495,098	$609,118	$894,489
Western	27	8	$950,534	$1,074,570	$293,847	$490,537	$878,033	$3,166,268

Table 88C: Compensation to Collections Ratio (TC/NPP Excluded)

	Phys	Med Pracs	Mean	Std. Dev.	25th %tile	Median	75th %tile	90th %tile
Overall	107	39	.615	.214	.451	.637	.784	.883
Group Type								
Single Specialty	25	5	.578	.249	.337	.627	.806	.857
Multispecialty	82	34	.626	.202	.507	.638	.780	.890
Geographic Section (All Pracs)								
Eastern	19	7	.608	.198	.436	.601	.790	.873
Midwest	26	14	.619	.283	.422	.646	.874	.986
Southern	39	11	.677	.160	.574	.686	.808	.890
Western	23	7	.512	.187	.319	.577	.659	.718

Table 88D: Physician Work RVUs (CMS RBRVS Method) (NPP Excluded)

	Phys	Med Pracs	Mean	Std. Dev.	25th %tile	Median	75th %tile	90th %tile
Overall	241	62	4,973	1,636	3,608	4,903	5,993	7,302
Group Type								
Single Specialty	38	5	5,144	1,571	3,871	5,096	6,042	7,446
Multispecialty	203	57	4,940	1,650	3,499	4,852	5,928	7,299
Geographic Section (All Pracs)								
Eastern	56	10	4,398	1,702	3,185	3,709	5,612	7,233
Midwest	60	21	5,460	1,618	4,261	5,327	7,116	7,574
Southern	65	13	5,235	1,649	4,138	5,200	6,391	7,467
Western	60	18	4,738	1,389	3,737	4,906	5,472	6,527

Hospitalist: Family Practice

Table 89A: Compensation

	Phys	Med Pracs	Mean	Std. Dev.	25th %tile	Median	75th %tile	90th %tile
Overall	53	16	$201,663	$57,148	$166,000	$194,259	$235,101	$283,988
Group Type								
Single Specialty	2	2	*	*	*	*	*	*
Multispecialty	51	14	$202,121	$58,094	$162,000	$194,259	$236,170	$284,120
Geographic Section (All Pracs)								
Eastern	6	3	*	*	*	*	*	*
Midwest	16	4	$217,814	$43,061	$190,953	$209,305	$249,232	$291,008
Southern	24	7	$198,995	$73,955	$118,602	$197,498	$250,112	$317,773
Western	7	2	*	*	*	*	*	*

Table 89B: Collections for Professional Charges (TC/NPP Excluded)

	Phys	Med Pracs	Mean	Std. Dev.	25th %tile	Median	75th %tile	90th %tile
Overall	15	5	$206,629	$68,486	$171,145	$190,000	$239,657	$327,567
Group Type								
Single Specialty	2	2	*	*	*	*	*	*
Multispecialty	13	3	$208,512	$73,756	$167,039	$187,045	$245,605	$355,956
Geographic Section (All Pracs)								
Midwest	12	*	*	*	*	*	*	*
Southern	3	3	*	*	*	*	*	*

Table 89C: Compensation to Collections Ratio (TC/NPP Excluded)

	Phys	Med Pracs	Mean	Std. Dev.	25th %tile	Median	75th %tile	90th %tile
Overall	6	4	*	*	*	*	*	*
Group Type								
Single Specialty	1	1	*	*	*	*	*	*
Multispecialty	5	3	*	*	*	*	*	*
Geographic Section (All Pracs)								
Midwest	4	2	*	*	*	*	*	*
Southern	2	2	*	*	*	*	*	*

Table 89D: Physician Work RVUs (CMS RBRVS Method) (NPP Excluded)

	Phys	Med Pracs	Mean	Std. Dev.	25th %tile	Median	75th %tile	90th %tile
Overall	28	8	4,430	1,424	3,072	4,342	5,481	6,449
Group Type								
Single Specialty	1	1	*	*	*	*	*	*
Multispecialty	27	7	4,502	1,399	3,311	4,418	5,492	6,458
Geographic Section (All Pracs)								
Eastern	1	1	*	*	*	*	*	*
Midwest	13	*	*	*	*	*	*	*
Southern	14	5	4,850	1,328	4,259	5,058	5,686	6,625

Hospitalist: Internal Medicine

Table 90A: Compensation

	Phys	Med Pracs	Mean	Std. Dev.	25th %tile	Median	75th %tile	90th %tile
Overall	1,185	148	$206,768	$56,086	$172,999	$197,872	$227,878	$275,067
Group Type								
Single Specialty	131	18	$233,838	$52,417	$197,147	$228,088	$273,482	$295,785
Multispecialty	1,054	130	$203,403	$55,635	$171,016	$194,300	$223,105	$266,678
Geographic Section (All Pracs)								
Eastern	266	35	$185,476	$40,374	$159,798	$181,443	$214,125	$238,767
Midwest	330	45	$204,275	$54,994	$173,000	$193,971	$225,333	$259,797
Southern	249	36	$234,116	$58,910	$196,920	$219,170	$264,324	$318,185
Western	340	32	$205,816	$57,673	$172,779	$191,819	$222,353	$294,378

Table 90B: Collections for Professional Charges (TC/NPP Excluded)

	Phys	Med Pracs	Mean	Std. Dev.	25th %tile	Median	75th %tile	90th %tile
Overall	603	84	$197,521	$82,847	$145,060	$186,528	$239,554	$311,406
Group Type								
Single Specialty	114	15	$234,722	$80,420	$179,557	$228,509	$275,296	$345,231
Multispecialty	489	69	$188,848	$81,061	$137,532	$179,720	$226,674	$304,355
Geographic Section (All Pracs)								
Eastern	111	18	$199,284	$72,750	$150,153	$193,082	$239,129	$288,690
Midwest	140	25	$212,088	$74,679	$163,599	$204,001	$247,853	$325,154
Southern	167	25	$217,996	$81,772	$167,632	$205,901	$261,848	$316,019
Western	185	16	$166,956	$86,968	$116,510	$156,660	$204,379	$267,631

Table 90C: Compensation to Collections Ratio (TC/NPP Excluded)

	Phys	Med Pracs	Mean	Std. Dev.	25th %tile	Median	75th %tile	90th %tile
Overall	248	67	.813	.139	.717	.843	.930	.974
Group Type								
Single Specialty	60	14	.822	.138	.736	.860	.940	.985
Multispecialty	188	53	.809	.140	.713	.838	.929	.972
Geographic Section (All Pracs)								
Eastern	51	14	.796	.160	.687	.791	.948	.992
Midwest	69	21	.810	.135	.718	.808	.937	.980
Southern	74	21	.794	.138	.667	.827	.917	.959
Western	54	11	.857	.116	.793	.890	.941	.972

Table 90D: Physician Work RVUs (CMS RBRVS Method) (NPP Excluded)

	Phys	Med Pracs	Mean	Std. Dev.	25th %tile	Median	75th %tile	90th %tile
Overall	784	98	4,091	1,550	3,000	3,943	5,017	6,293
Group Type								
Single Specialty	83	12	5,149	1,251	4,437	5,377	6,173	6,461
Multispecialty	701	86	3,966	1,535	2,927	3,804	4,722	6,142
Geographic Section (All Pracs)								
Eastern	164	24	3,964	1,586	2,686	3,952	4,988	6,259
Midwest	237	31	4,030	1,579	3,023	3,822	4,638	6,180
Southern	133	19	5,378	1,451	4,500	5,435	6,393	7,018
Western	250	24	3,548	1,111	2,772	3,454	4,189	5,083

Hospitalist: Internal Medicine (fewer than 250 Ambulatory Encounters)

Table 91A: Compensation

	Phys	Med Pracs	Mean	Std. Dev.	25th %tile	Median	75th %tile	90th %tile
Overall	50	7	$265,422	$85,316	$179,459	$251,626	$333,490	$377,337
Group Type								
Multispecialty	50	7	$265,422	$85,316	$179,459	$251,626	$333,490	$377,337
Geographic Section (All Pracs)								
Eastern	3	1	*	*	*	*	*	*
Midwest	3	1	*	*	*	*	*	*
Southern	27	3	$278,453	$94,491	$179,999	$299,565	$339,775	$422,920
Western	17	2	*	*	*	*	*	*

Table 91B: Collections for Professional Charges (TC/NPP Excluded)

	Phys	Med Pracs	Mean	Std. Dev.	25th %tile	Median	75th %tile	90th %tile
Overall	20	4	$118,522	$126,317	$34,086	$37,610	$234,866	$263,217
Group Type								
Multispecialty	20	4	$118,522	$126,317	$34,086	$37,610	$234,866	$263,217
Geographic Section (All Pracs)								
Midwest	3	1	*	*	*	*	*	*
Southern	4	1	*	*	*	*	*	*
Western	13	2	*	*	*	*	*	*

Table 91C: Compensation to Collections Ratio (TC/NPP Excluded)

	Phys	Med Pracs	Mean	Std. Dev.	25th %tile	Median	75th %tile	90th %tile
Overall	7	2	*	*	*	*	*	*
Group Type								
Multispecialty	7	2	*	*	*	*	*	*
Geographic Section (All Pracs)								
Midwest	3	1	*	*	*	*	*	*
Southern	4	1	*	*	*	*	*	*

Table 91D: Physician Work RVUs (CMS RBRVS Method) (NPP Excluded)

	Phys	Med Pracs	Mean	Std. Dev.	25th %tile	Median	75th %tile	90th %tile
Overall	45	5	4,970	1,368	3,967	4,932	5,777	6,907
Group Type								
Multispecialty	45	5	4,970	1,368	3,967	4,932	5,777	6,907
Geographic Section (All Pracs)								
Midwest	3	1	*	*	*	*	*	*
Southern	25	2	*	*	*	*	*	*
Western	17	2	*	*	*	*	*	*

Hospitalist: Pediatrics

Table 92A: Compensation

	Phys	Med Pracs	Mean	Std. Dev.	25th %tile	Median	75th %tile	90th %tile
Overall	97	19	$162,439	$47,341	$137,500	$161,000	$175,065	$202,491
Group Type								
Single Specialty	9	1	*	*	*	*	*	*
Multispecialty	88	18	$162,761	$47,935	$136,250	$162,000	$175,049	$200,186
Geographic Section (All Pracs)								
Eastern	6	2	*	*	*	*	*	*
Midwest	10	5	$170,759	$39,583	$147,659	$169,819	$201,315	$226,982
Southern	32	6	$176,902	$71,396	$144,713	$170,392	$180,447	$218,203
Western	49	6	$151,828	$24,687	$130,000	$154,145	$166,320	$186,177

Table 92B: Collections for Professional Charges (TC/NPP Excluded)

	Phys	Med Pracs	Mean	Std. Dev.	25th %tile	Median	75th %tile	90th %tile
Overall	29	9	$106,978	$52,151	$67,740	$116,741	$139,967	$165,168
Group Type								
Single Specialty	9	1	*	*	*	*	*	*
Multispecialty	20	8	$105,523	$60,935	$48,500	$110,426	$144,149	$202,721
Geographic Section (All Pracs)								
Eastern	4	1	*	*	*	*	*	*
Midwest	7	4	*	*	*	*	*	*
Southern	10	2	*	*	*	*	*	*
Western	8	2	*	*	*	*	*	*

Table 92C: Compensation to Collections Ratio (TC/NPP Excluded)

	Phys	Med Pracs	Mean	Std. Dev.	25th %tile	Median	75th %tile	90th %tile
Overall	4	3	*	*	*	*	*	*
Group Type								
Multispecialty	4	3	*	*	*	*	*	*
Geographic Section (All Pracs)								
Eastern	2	1	*	*	*	*	*	*
Southern	1	1	*	*	*	*	*	*
Western	1	1	*	*	*	*	*	*

Table 92D: Physician Work RVUs (CMS RBRVS Method) (NPP Excluded)

	Phys	Med Pracs	Mean	Std. Dev.	25th %tile	Median	75th %tile	90th %tile
Overall	67	15	2,144	983	1,368	2,280	2,882	3,508
Group Type								
Single Specialty	9	1	*	*	*	*	*	*
Multispecialty	58	14	2,106	1,031	1,338	1,826	2,921	3,565
Geographic Section (All Pracs)								
Eastern	6	2	*	*	*	*	*	*
Midwest	9	4	*	*	*	*	*	*
Southern	22	4	2,123	843	1,695	1,797	2,738	3,413
Western	30	5	2,069	1,140	976	1,676	3,144	3,555

Infectious Disease

Table 93A: Compensation

	Phys	Med Pracs	Mean	Std. Dev.	25th %tile	Median	75th %tile	90th %tile
Overall	213	68	$202,840	$58,949	$158,084	$192,454	$245,627	$268,837
Group Type								
Single Specialty	22	9	$237,133	$74,791	$180,774	$227,666	$281,037	$374,588
Multispecialty	191	59	$198,890	$55,743	$157,260	$189,687	$242,328	$265,529
Geographic Section (All Pracs)								
Eastern	53	21	$191,910	$48,861	$155,992	$189,010	$227,666	$264,463
Midwest	91	19	$185,713	$51,949	$148,816	$175,838	$212,535	$257,979
Southern	26	13	$233,135	$64,153	$182,979	$206,800	$265,649	$338,242
Western	43	15	$234,239	$63,151	$194,700	$242,000	$260,809	$290,166

Table 93B: Collections for Professional Charges (TC/NPP Excluded)

	Phys	Med Pracs	Mean	Std. Dev.	25th %tile	Median	75th %tile	90th %tile
Overall	53	28	$299,631	$143,301	$187,732	$274,396	$376,731	$487,330
Group Type								
Single Specialty	18	7	$306,988	$107,548	$204,698	$323,488	$389,272	$468,302
Multispecialty	35	21	$295,848	$159,937	$169,063	$263,487	$348,840	$518,545
Geographic Section (All Pracs)								
Eastern	21	10	$261,082	$129,788	$157,558	$208,084	$366,899	$487,758
Midwest	11	6	$358,345	$221,835	$164,655	$233,026	$519,023	$762,926
Southern	13	7	$302,458	$89,096	$266,791	$302,751	$356,308	$408,266
Western	8	5	*	*	*	*	*	*

Table 93C: Compensation to Collections Ratio (TC/NPP Excluded)

	Phys	Med Pracs	Mean	Std. Dev.	25th %tile	Median	75th %tile	90th %tile
Overall	43	23	.696	.163	.563	.698	.835	.892
Group Type								
Single Specialty	15	6	.708	.206	.557	.721	.881	.981
Multispecialty	28	17	.689	.138	.573	.681	.800	.864
Geographic Section (All Pracs)								
Eastern	13	6	.690	.200	.476	.784	.858	.879
Midwest	10	6	.748	.165	.618	.776	.875	.964
Southern	12	6	.695	.113	.612	.660	.767	.913
Western	8	5	*	*	*	*	*	*

Table 93D: Physician Work RVUs (CMS RBRVS Method) (NPP Excluded)

	Phys	Med Pracs	Mean	Std. Dev.	25th %tile	Median	75th %tile	90th %tile
Overall	134	39	4,348	1,602	3,290	3,988	4,910	6,890
Group Type								
Single Specialty	8	4	*	*	*	*	*	*
Multispecialty	126	35	4,273	1,465	3,309	3,973	4,808	6,782
Geographic Section (All Pracs)								
Eastern	29	13	4,358	1,776	3,158	3,968	4,943	6,075
Midwest	79	12	3,999	1,225	3,221	3,768	4,319	5,947
Southern	8	5	*	*	*	*	*	*
Western	18	9	4,826	1,941	3,175	4,460	6,268	8,082

Internal Medicine: General

Table 94A: Compensation

	Phys	Med Pracs	Mean	Std. Dev.	25th %tile	Median	75th %tile	90th %tile
Overall	4,745	461	$201,603	$76,495	$149,875	$190,547	$236,879	$295,394
Group Type								
Single Specialty	375	92	$206,903	$89,741	$143,269	$182,121	$254,737	$337,341
Multispecialty	4,370	369	$201,148	$75,244	$150,000	$191,204	$236,241	$292,482
Geographic Section (All Pracs)								
Eastern	981	112	$179,005	$71,086	$132,740	$163,365	$212,645	$264,394
Midwest	1,189	138	$203,482	$83,942	$147,877	$188,261	$242,299	$307,025
Southern	1,028	125	$212,704	$85,364	$153,680	$197,307	$253,886	$323,035
Western	1,547	86	$207,112	$63,702	$164,860	$203,791	$239,942	$279,552

Table 94B: Collections for Professional Charges (TC/NPP Excluded)

	Phys	Med Pracs	Mean	Std. Dev.	25th %tile	Median	75th %tile	90th %tile
Overall	1,837	218	$351,457	$137,430	$264,273	$345,265	$423,456	$511,995
Group Type								
Single Specialty	142	34	$325,635	$141,503	$245,853	$309,164	$388,964	$522,948
Multispecialty	1,695	184	$353,621	$136,906	$266,722	$350,359	$426,142	$510,489
Geographic Section (All Pracs)								
Eastern	369	42	$324,421	$126,964	$239,702	$324,828	$407,347	$472,156
Midwest	575	67	$377,177	$140,169	$286,409	$367,581	$448,904	$551,224
Southern	479	66	$348,310	$140,533	$252,222	$335,442	$413,413	$521,031
Western	414	43	$343,474	$133,364	$263,563	$357,288	$423,960	$492,697

Table 94C: Compensation to Collections Ratio (TC/NPP Excluded)

	Phys	Med Pracs	Mean	Std. Dev.	25th %tile	Median	75th %tile	90th %tile
Overall	1,709	212	.545	.148	.440	.527	.629	.746
Group Type								
Single Specialty	129	32	.581	.137	.487	.569	.648	.769
Multispecialty	1,580	180	.542	.148	.435	.524	.626	.744
Geographic Section (All Pracs)								
Eastern	342	41	.535	.162	.430	.492	.613	.785
Midwest	564	67	.539	.138	.445	.535	.615	.710
Southern	440	64	.599	.149	.493	.585	.696	.812
Western	363	40	.495	.124	.407	.478	.566	.668

Table 94D: Physician Work RVUs (CMS RBRVS Method) (NPP Excluded)

	Phys	Med Pracs	Mean	Std. Dev.	25th %tile	Median	75th %tile	90th %tile
Overall	2,613	229	4,711	1,797	3,546	4,554	5,632	6,779
Group Type								
Single Specialty	155	33	4,601	1,921	3,433	4,484	5,529	7,346
Multispecialty	2,458	196	4,718	1,789	3,554	4,563	5,635	6,748
Geographic Section (All Pracs)								
Eastern	648	51	4,396	1,903	2,994	4,308	5,520	6,571
Midwest	677	66	4,780	1,692	3,623	4,633	5,613	6,876
Southern	599	62	5,283	2,022	4,043	4,988	6,282	7,802
Western	689	50	4,443	1,426	3,542	4,391	5,243	6,065

Internal Medicine: Ambulatory Only (no inpatient work)

Table 95A: Compensation

	Phys	Med Pracs	Mean	Std. Dev.	25th %tile	Median	75th %tile	90th %tile
Overall	39	16	$174,735	$45,359	$132,038	$181,291	$205,800	$237,225
Group Type								
Single Specialty	1	1	*	*	*	*	*	*
Multispecialty	38	15	$175,551	$45,677	$131,832	$181,682	$205,800	$239,403
Geographic Section (All Pracs)								
Eastern	18	6	$180,703	$40,804	$148,238	$180,691	$199,694	$261,038
Midwest	4	3	*	*	*	*	*	*
Southern	12	4	$193,831	$44,004	$185,968	$205,800	$205,800	$252,467
Western	5	3	*	*	*	*	*	*

Table 95B: Collections for Professional Charges (TC/NPP Excluded)

	Phys	Med Pracs	Mean	Std. Dev.	25th %tile	Median	75th %tile	90th %tile
Overall	14	7	$378,351	$386,120	$233,428	$275,808	$392,237	$1,085,961
Group Type								
Multispecialty	14	7	$378,351	$386,120	$233,428	$275,808	$392,237	$1,085,961
Geographic Section (All Pracs)								
Eastern	6	3	*	*	*	*	*	*
Midwest	2	2	*	*	*	*	*	*
Southern	5	1	*	*	*	*	*	*
Western	1	1	*	*	*	*	*	*

Table 95C: Compensation to Collections Ratio (TC/NPP Excluded)

	Phys	Med Pracs	Mean	Std. Dev.	25th %tile	Median	75th %tile	90th %tile
Overall	12	5	.531	.219	.385	.513	.648	.900
Group Type								
Multispecialty	12	5	.531	.219	.385	.513	.648	.900
Geographic Section (All Pracs)								
Eastern	5	2	*	*	*	*	*	*
Midwest	1	1	*	*	*	*	*	*
Southern	5	1	*	*	*	*	*	*
Western	1	1	*	*	*	*	*	*

Table 95D: Physician Work RVUs (CMS RBRVS Method) (NPP Excluded)

	Phys	Med Pracs	Mean	Std. Dev.	25th %tile	Median	75th %tile	90th %tile
Overall	21	9	3,853	1,304	2,977	3,587	4,876	5,649
Group Type								
Multispecialty	21	9	3,853	1,304	2,977	3,587	4,876	5,649
Geographic Section (All Pracs)								
Eastern	17	5	4,155	1,204	3,214	4,214	5,060	5,831
Midwest	2	2	*	*	*	*	*	*
Western	2	2	*	*	*	*	*	*

Nephrology

Table 96A: Compensation

	Phys	Med Pracs	Mean	Std. Dev.	25th %tile	Median	75th %tile	90th %tile
Overall	277	80	$305,602	$109,873	$223,077	$299,121	$354,528	$446,793
Group Type								
Single Specialty	64	9	$301,147	$117,505	$200,310	$308,943	$380,635	$446,657
Multispecialty	213	71	$306,941	$107,729	$229,369	$297,513	$351,447	$446,952
Geographic Section (All Pracs)								
Eastern	70	18	$285,010	$116,100	$183,900	$245,364	$389,677	$452,551
Midwest	69	27	$318,350	$120,490	$231,254	$307,214	$353,431	$502,050
Southern	44	17	$354,694	$134,144	$281,051	$317,926	$420,710	$524,286
Western	94	18	$288,600	$70,842	$235,630	$298,923	$329,562	$369,894

Table 96B: Collections for Professional Charges (TC/NPP Excluded)

	Phys	Med Pracs	Mean	Std. Dev.	25th %tile	Median	75th %tile	90th %tile
Overall	96	34	$429,101	$208,293	$239,282	$432,795	$546,015	$714,108
Group Type								
Single Specialty	13	2	*	*	*	*	*	*
Multispecialty	83	32	$467,066	$198,381	$327,984	$459,158	$560,851	$731,219
Geographic Section (All Pracs)								
Eastern	17	7	$484,337	$233,224	$325,947	$415,472	$662,025	$885,781
Midwest	25	9	$461,781	$224,518	$335,982	$459,158	$545,495	$800,264
Southern	32	12	$467,629	$183,096	$326,529	$508,991	$582,573	$683,939
Western	22	6	$293,243	$149,635	$182,267	$220,411	$434,932	$543,852

Table 96C: Compensation to Collections Ratio (TC/NPP Excluded)

	Phys	Med Pracs	Mean	Std. Dev.	25th %tile	Median	75th %tile	90th %tile
Overall	69	32	.667	.189	.544	.662	.812	.948
Group Type								
Single Specialty	6	2	*	*	*	*	*	*
Multispecialty	63	30	.649	.186	.532	.638	.767	.947
Geographic Section (All Pracs)								
Eastern	15	7	.635	.164	.561	.593	.697	.963
Midwest	21	8	.674	.169	.562	.663	.785	.945
Southern	21	12	.710	.188	.559	.691	.892	.968
Western	12	5	.618	.251	.329	.674	.862	.924

Table 96D: Physician Work RVUs (CMS RBRVS Method) (NPP Excluded)

	Phys	Med Pracs	Mean	Std. Dev.	25th %tile	Median	75th %tile	90th %tile
Overall	117	51	7,268	3,000	5,320	6,471	9,499	11,347
Group Type								
Single Specialty	2	1	*	*	*	*	*	*
Multispecialty	115	50	7,328	2,991	5,440	6,488	9,513	11,415
Geographic Section (All Pracs)								
Eastern	21	9	5,901	2,636	3,713	5,770	6,856	10,559
Midwest	40	18	7,787	2,899	5,531	8,046	9,528	11,663
Southern	30	12	8,222	3,588	5,612	8,211	10,955	13,795
Western	26	12	6,472	2,099	5,378	6,226	7,931	9,734

Neurology

Table 97A: Compensation

	Phys	Med Pracs	Mean	Std. Dev.	25th %tile	Median	75th %tile	90th %tile
Overall	637	185	$260,536	$108,122	$191,154	$227,670	$294,586	$412,170
Group Type								
Single Specialty	126	34	$268,084	$117,641	$199,141	$237,411	$289,597	$465,000
Multispecialty	511	151	$258,676	$105,683	$189,994	$225,000	$297,223	$405,534
Geographic Section (All Pracs)								
Eastern	183	40	$238,885	$100,443	$178,250	$212,538	$256,151	$390,910
Midwest	147	53	$278,159	$120,163	$193,974	$242,985	$325,740	$440,958
Southern	135	49	$290,572	$131,492	$201,645	$248,300	$345,851	$504,695
Western	172	43	$244,937	$71,687	$199,630	$227,795	$280,720	$342,164

Table 97B: Collections for Professional Charges (TC/NPP Excluded)

	Phys	Med Pracs	Mean	Std. Dev.	25th %tile	Median	75th %tile	90th %tile
Overall	246	83	$428,845	$195,879	$287,463	$405,408	$540,487	$712,058
Group Type								
Single Specialty	44	13	$380,971	$201,407	$200,390	$347,809	$540,576	$650,000
Multispecialty	202	70	$439,273	$193,594	$298,711	$412,042	$540,688	$746,994
Geographic Section (All Pracs)								
Eastern	69	19	$358,138	$189,308	$210,797	$320,610	$456,554	$681,652
Midwest	79	26	$465,852	$202,491	$309,931	$461,710	$557,788	$765,691
Southern	49	20	$460,385	$175,994	$330,488	$430,734	$549,392	$697,375
Western	49	18	$437,208	$192,193	$302,553	$417,412	$551,952	$704,301

Table 97C: Compensation to Collections Ratio (TC/NPP Excluded)

	Phys	Med Pracs	Mean	Std. Dev.	25th %tile	Median	75th %tile	90th %tile
Overall	221	79	.602	.157	.485	.573	.697	.836
Group Type								
Single Specialty	30	10	.592	.162	.424	.597	.713	.831
Multispecialty	191	69	.603	.156	.486	.565	.694	.854
Geographic Section (All Pracs)								
Eastern	57	18	.632	.152	.515	.642	.731	.838
Midwest	73	25	.595	.125	.502	.581	.656	.777
Southern	45	20	.615	.171	.476	.561	.767	.885
Western	46	16	.562	.186	.409	.519	.699	.872

Table 97D: Physician Work RVUs (CMS RBRVS Method) (NPP Excluded)

	Phys	Med Pracs	Mean	Std. Dev.	25th %tile	Median	75th %tile	90th %tile
Overall	376	105	5,391	2,034	4,023	5,154	6,425	8,214
Group Type								
Single Specialty	56	15	5,896	2,288	4,190	5,737	7,299	9,460
Multispecialty	320	90	5,302	1,977	4,006	5,069	6,303	8,107
Geographic Section (All Pracs)								
Eastern	126	24	5,160	1,986	3,683	5,030	6,407	7,751
Midwest	98	30	5,268	1,856	3,853	5,246	6,469	7,649
Southern	67	24	6,396	2,529	4,483	5,849	8,721	10,459
Western	85	27	5,082	1,612	4,045	5,007	6,016	7,120

Obstetrics/Gynecology

Table 98A: Compensation

	Phys	Med Pracs	Mean	Std. Dev.	25th %tile	Median	75th %tile	90th %tile
Overall	2,012	307	$302,362	$115,661	$222,647	$280,629	$360,099	$450,289
Group Type								
Single Specialty	443	85	$312,142	$127,866	$216,698	$296,138	$389,727	$478,245
Multispecialty	1,569	222	$299,600	$111,863	$225,407	$277,631	$351,335	$445,052
Geographic Section (All Pracs)								
Eastern	375	68	$261,713	$103,443	$190,563	$237,053	$323,640	$401,731
Midwest	569	102	$323,449	$127,473	$235,558	$307,381	$398,522	$480,108
Southern	410	73	$318,905	$119,681	$224,563	$300,100	$391,399	$477,049
Western	658	64	$296,984	$101,797	$235,449	$278,674	$330,055	$410,520

Table 98B: Collections for Professional Charges (TC/NPP Excluded)

	Phys	Med Pracs	Mean	Std. Dev.	25th %tile	Median	75th %tile	90th %tile
Overall	624	127	$615,886	$258,464	$454,517	$588,871	$739,322	$942,272
Group Type								
Single Specialty	102	27	$598,952	$228,726	$452,650	$573,174	$718,897	$915,531
Multispecialty	522	100	$619,195	$263,958	$454,932	$589,365	$749,287	$944,103
Geographic Section (All Pracs)								
Eastern	113	25	$497,644	$169,719	$378,545	$474,802	$561,015	$726,857
Midwest	221	45	$653,640	$243,850	$499,000	$621,335	$810,774	$993,225
Southern	148	31	$663,618	$279,203	$496,683	$652,492	$744,200	$1,028,643
Western	142	26	$601,472	$286,703	$431,106	$601,255	$746,333	$942,884

Table 98C: Compensation to Collections Ratio (TC/NPP Excluded)

	Phys	Med Pracs	Mean	Std. Dev.	25th %tile	Median	75th %tile	90th %tile
Overall	603	125	.497	.135	.403	.483	.580	.671
Group Type								
Single Specialty	100	27	.531	.145	.436	.548	.610	.720
Multispecialty	503	98	.491	.132	.399	.476	.573	.662
Geographic Section (All Pracs)								
Eastern	113	25	.481	.138	.387	.450	.562	.702
Midwest	218	45	.511	.121	.419	.510	.584	.663
Southern	148	31	.516	.158	.396	.509	.617	.724
Western	124	24	.465	.118	.400	.458	.520	.605

Table 98D: Physician Work RVUs (CMS RBRVS Method) (NPP Excluded)

	Phys	Med Pracs	Mean	Std. Dev.	25th %tile	Median	75th %tile	90th %tile
Overall	885	153	7,117	2,566	5,404	6,850	8,392	10,282
Group Type								
Single Specialty	115	27	7,187	2,633	5,738	6,763	8,066	9,326
Multispecialty	770	126	7,107	2,558	5,329	6,864	8,457	10,398
Geographic Section (All Pracs)								
Eastern	176	30	6,422	2,595	4,634	5,870	7,785	9,298
Midwest	303	52	6,890	2,426	5,064	6,676	8,376	10,176
Southern	152	30	8,305	2,910	6,420	7,852	9,777	12,045
Western	254	41	7,158	2,241	5,797	6,853	8,209	9,574

Obstetrics/Gynecology: Gynecology (only)

Table 99A: Compensation

	Phys	Med Pracs	Mean	Std. Dev.	25th %tile	Median	75th %tile	90th %tile
Overall	211	94	$226,545	$98,195	$151,852	$209,867	$279,622	$376,261
Group Type								
Single Specialty	35	20	$231,351	$109,550	$161,315	$205,104	$293,425	$403,882
Multispecialty	176	74	$225,589	$96,092	$150,774	$213,451	$279,571	$374,378
Geographic Section (All Pracs)								
Eastern	56	24	$206,077	$81,055	$148,104	$200,000	$251,669	$307,171
Midwest	82	28	$266,196	$99,850	$189,688	$251,771	$341,608	$407,652
Southern	50	28	$199,822	$97,312	$139,091	$187,206	$237,294	$337,958
Western	23	14	$193,105	$89,989	$128,628	$183,000	$228,175	$330,224

Table 99B: Collections for Professional Charges (TC/NPP Excluded)

	Phys	Med Pracs	Mean	Std. Dev.	25th %tile	Median	75th %tile	90th %tile
Overall	67	36	$464,869	$211,869	$336,934	$421,995	$582,317	$808,323
Group Type								
Single Specialty	3	3	*	*	*	*	*	*
Multispecialty	64	33	$462,522	$209,549	$337,929	$411,246	$562,508	$811,295
Geographic Section (All Pracs)								
Eastern	8	5	*	*	*	*	*	*
Midwest	25	13	$598,882	$239,468	$445,457	$569,222	$811,295	$946,192
Southern	24	13	$356,625	$153,846	$245,634	$349,462	$416,621	$568,690
Western	10	5	$416,064	$115,545	$341,982	$368,719	$530,420	$577,920

Table 99C: Compensation to Collections Ratio (TC/NPP Excluded)

	Phys	Med Pracs	Mean	Std. Dev.	25th %tile	Median	75th %tile	90th %tile
Overall	66	35	.503	.155	.411	.466	.566	.721
Group Type								
Single Specialty	2	2	*	*	*	*	*	*
Multispecialty	64	33	.502	.155	.410	.466	.558	.725
Geographic Section (All Pracs)								
Eastern	8	5	*	*	*	*	*	*
Midwest	24	12	.497	.105	.427	.480	.551	.680
Southern	24	13	.584	.199	.438	.545	.690	.919
Western	10	5	.388	.057	.359	.371	.434	.482

Table 99D: Physician Work RVUs (CMS RBRVS Method) (NPP Excluded)

	Phys	Med Pracs	Mean	Std. Dev.	25th %tile	Median	75th %tile	90th %tile
Overall	126	47	5,779	2,275	4,188	5,421	6,765	8,497
Group Type								
Single Specialty	11	6	8,597	4,032	5,133	8,009	13,152	13,391
Multispecialty	115	41	5,510	1,847	4,180	5,358	6,463	7,890
Geographic Section (All Pracs)								
Eastern	32	13	5,324	1,981	3,960	5,431	6,252	7,580
Midwest	56	12	6,151	1,702	4,742	6,192	7,527	8,420
Southern	19	11	7,004	3,589	4,450	5,285	8,710	13,381
Western	19	11	4,227	1,595	3,152	3,766	5,312	6,620

Ophthalmology

Table 100A: Compensation

	Phys	Med Pracs	Mean	Std. Dev.	25th %tile	Median	75th %tile	90th %tile
Overall	589	146	$349,766	$164,380	$245,415	$315,982	$407,705	$586,957
Group Type								
Single Specialty	180	38	$368,213	$176,917	$242,116	$338,655	$456,290	$634,939
Multispecialty	409	108	$341,648	$158,095	$245,415	$307,192	$398,869	$524,943
Geographic Section (All Pracs)								
Eastern	87	25	$311,719	$166,522	$215,600	$275,000	$355,839	$527,934
Midwest	179	51	$393,803	$178,089	$262,636	$360,802	$462,179	$663,934
Southern	140	40	$360,080	$181,296	$211,275	$343,038	$436,262	$634,939
Western	183	30	$316,890	$119,608	$250,573	$301,035	$345,272	$424,507

Table 100B: Collections for Professional Charges (TC/NPP Excluded)

	Phys	Med Pracs	Mean	Std. Dev.	25th %tile	Median	75th %tile	90th %tile
Overall	168	59	$761,667	$344,151	$515,836	$669,795	$959,176	$1,247,812
Group Type								
Single Specialty	34	11	$881,789	$327,279	$602,067	$849,402	$1,192,042	$1,315,656
Multispecialty	134	48	$731,188	$342,808	$505,375	$637,084	$874,004	$1,209,395
Geographic Section (All Pracs)								
Eastern	29	10	$757,574	$381,345	$518,459	$643,923	$889,942	$1,344,219
Midwest	56	20	$778,389	$289,119	$555,826	$698,120	$989,815	$1,217,291
Southern	48	18	$775,353	$358,471	$529,033	$702,591	$970,187	$1,309,650
Western	35	11	$719,532	$382,843	$466,679	$574,183	$839,725	$1,298,227

Table 100C: Compensation to Collections Ratio (TC/NPP Excluded)

	Phys	Med Pracs	Mean	Std. Dev.	25th %tile	Median	75th %tile	90th %tile
Overall	170	59	.475	.137	.374	.456	.545	.650
Group Type								
Single Specialty	36	12	.431	.129	.349	.414	.506	.568
Multispecialty	134	47	.487	.137	.378	.469	.562	.670
Geographic Section (All Pracs)								
Eastern	31	10	.442	.167	.341	.395	.483	.713
Midwest	58	21	.527	.126	.442	.511	.586	.710
Southern	48	18	.460	.137	.372	.417	.521	.654
Western	33	10	.437	.098	.350	.436	.518	.570

Table 100D: Physician Work RVUs (CMS RBRVS Method) (NPP Excluded)

	Phys	Med Pracs	Mean	Std. Dev.	25th %tile	Median	75th %tile	90th %tile
Overall	211	70	8,288	4,143	5,871	7,655	9,627	12,220
Group Type								
Single Specialty	11	3	12,562	9,231	7,831	10,652	12,725	34,200
Multispecialty	200	67	8,053	3,573	5,822	7,524	9,520	12,118
Geographic Section (All Pracs)								
Eastern	41	11	8,808	6,348	5,849	7,260	9,084	13,622
Midwest	86	29	8,462	3,440	6,246	7,806	10,487	12,638
Southern	35	15	8,742	3,729	6,248	7,967	10,957	15,163
Western	49	15	7,221	3,019	4,915	7,203	8,859	11,527

Orthopedic Surgery: General

Table 101A: Compensation

	Phys	Med Pracs	Mean	Std. Dev.	25th %tile	Median	75th %tile	90th %tile
Overall	1,029	240	$497,136	$233,403	$359,654	$446,303	$595,643	$799,883
Group Type								
Single Specialty	329	84	$507,123	$229,824	$342,003	$472,606	$658,134	$782,207
Multispecialty	700	156	$492,442	$235,083	$368,450	$439,970	$561,922	$800,265
Geographic Section (All Pracs)								
Eastern	154	46	$460,223	$227,345	$308,351	$414,389	$562,276	$765,000
Midwest	312	77	$557,342	$247,732	$378,204	$525,513	$685,178	$851,125
Southern	200	61	$468,044	$239,656	$313,382	$405,394	$593,673	$763,994
Western	363	56	$477,077	$209,724	$371,900	$434,088	$514,728	$761,933

Table 101B: Collections for Professional Charges (TC/NPP Excluded)

	Phys	Med Pracs	Mean	Std. Dev.	25th %tile	Median	75th %tile	90th %tile
Overall	355	98	$815,387	$315,870	$620,382	$797,705	$1,023,055	$1,220,832
Group Type								
Single Specialty	99	27	$794,050	$262,101	$634,466	$787,742	$948,867	$1,123,545
Multispecialty	256	71	$823,638	$334,459	$611,556	$803,919	$1,043,854	$1,268,831
Geographic Section (All Pracs)								
Eastern	56	18	$779,198	$284,313	$585,575	$765,812	$1,003,874	$1,134,635
Midwest	109	28	$912,662	$319,439	$694,736	$900,502	$1,122,441	$1,395,587
Southern	100	30	$821,483	$295,485	$623,371	$794,987	$1,035,051	$1,203,582
Western	90	22	$713,319	$320,878	$449,976	$717,028	$924,135	$1,126,942

Table 101C: Compensation to Collections Ratio (TC/NPP Excluded)

	Phys	Med Pracs	Mean	Std. Dev.	25th %tile	Median	75th %tile	90th %tile
Overall	343	95	.593	.142	.494	.575	.675	.791
Group Type								
Single Specialty	92	26	.605	.182	.468	.545	.722	.909
Multispecialty	251	69	.588	.124	.499	.577	.663	.760
Geographic Section (All Pracs)								
Eastern	55	18	.556	.121	.494	.531	.636	.714
Midwest	107	28	.625	.165	.510	.614	.716	.893
Southern	98	29	.569	.129	.477	.569	.651	.742
Western	83	20	.603	.129	.509	.586	.672	.798

Table 101D: Physician Work RVUs (CMS RBRVS Method) (NPP Excluded)

	Phys	Med Pracs	Mean	Std. Dev.	25th %tile	Median	75th %tile	90th %tile
Overall	454	110	8,633	3,413	6,462	8,256	10,504	13,147
Group Type								
Single Specialty	88	21	8,632	2,622	7,111	8,652	10,173	12,064
Multispecialty	366	89	8,633	3,581	6,281	8,186	10,567	13,656
Geographic Section (All Pracs)								
Eastern	68	20	8,608	4,021	5,605	8,215	11,505	14,082
Midwest	143	35	8,360	2,994	6,662	7,987	9,851	12,322
Southern	66	18	9,474	3,421	7,194	9,523	11,685	13,953
Western	177	37	8,549	3,456	6,392	8,178	10,388	12,578

Orthopedic Surgery: Sports Medicine

Table 102A: Compensation

	Phys	Med Pracs	Mean	Std. Dev.	25th %tile	Median	75th %tile	90th %tile
Overall	195	82	$610,641	$299,155	$404,515	$553,344	$773,722	$1,000,396
Group Type								
Single Specialty	122	54	$618,478	$299,257	$403,714	$560,609	$805,736	$1,012,836
Multispecialty	73	28	$597,544	$300,591	$389,424	$537,388	$743,274	$954,956
Geographic Section (All Pracs)								
Eastern	50	24	$527,048	$214,077	$361,462	$464,259	$625,294	$811,486
Midwest	39	21	$687,460	$346,486	$435,862	$621,384	$936,020	$1,215,415
Southern	51	18	$604,397	$300,968	$441,579	$563,866	$736,310	$928,281
Western	55	19	$637,954	$316,300	$398,906	$551,171	$845,171	$1,075,761

Table 102B: Collections for Professional Charges (TC/NPP Excluded)

	Phys	Med Pracs	Mean	Std. Dev.	25th %tile	Median	75th %tile	90th %tile
Overall	53	29	$950,250	$395,245	$729,952	$946,000	$1,153,015	$1,336,863
Group Type								
Single Specialty	33	19	$936,318	$278,034	$759,604	$946,000	$1,124,818	$1,266,822
Multispecialty	20	10	$973,239	$544,478	$579,904	$957,990	$1,278,681	$1,583,326
Geographic Section (All Pracs)								
Eastern	24	11	$965,102	$310,475	$744,981	$975,951	$1,193,864	$1,416,582
Midwest	7	6	*	*	*	*	*	*
Southern	9	6	*	*	*	*	*	*
Western	13	6	$849,098	$345,759	$595,879	$934,999	$1,096,903	$1,247,096

Table 102C: Compensation to Collections Ratio (TC/NPP Excluded)

	Phys	Med Pracs	Mean	Std. Dev.	25th %tile	Median	75th %tile	90th %tile
Overall	52	29	.586	.132	.509	.582	.638	.800
Group Type								
Single Specialty	33	19	.582	.141	.495	.577	.642	.813
Multispecialty	19	10	.592	.119	.545	.591	.621	.801
Geographic Section (All Pracs)								
Eastern	24	11	.534	.124	.463	.548	.601	.685
Midwest	7	6	*	*	*	*	*	*
Southern	9	6	*	*	*	*	*	*
Western	12	6	.687	.124	.588	.631	.812	.892

Table 102D: Physician Work RVUs (CMS RBRVS Method) (NPP Excluded)

	Phys	Med Pracs	Mean	Std. Dev.	25th %tile	Median	75th %tile	90th %tile
Overall	100	35	10,843	4,947	7,784	10,284	13,075	17,442
Group Type								
Single Specialty	41	17	12,746	4,899	9,629	12,076	14,627	20,257
Multispecialty	59	18	9,520	4,570	6,739	8,908	11,334	16,467
Geographic Section (All Pracs)								
Eastern	26	9	12,210	4,610	9,377	11,275	15,074	19,323
Midwest	20	11	11,140	4,716	8,826	10,793	12,581	18,936
Southern	19	5	11,720	7,017	6,327	10,905	16,782	21,248
Western	35	10	9,181	3,519	7,077	9,003	12,886	14,552

Otorhinolaryngology

Table 103A: Compensation

	Phys	Med Pracs	Mean	Std. Dev.	25th %tile	Median	75th %tile	90th %tile
Overall	541	159	$394,506	$186,754	$277,943	$345,210	$467,524	$641,344
Group Type								
Single Specialty	110	18	$398,511	$189,389	$247,336	$342,583	$496,897	$679,872
Multispecialty	431	141	$393,484	$186,284	$285,450	$345,951	$454,317	$626,181
Geographic Section (All Pracs)								
Eastern	66	22	$391,790	$177,597	$268,895	$335,650	$480,996	$637,434
Midwest	137	52	$433,223	$225,131	$283,447	$384,123	$520,197	$796,507
Southern	136	40	$425,425	$218,101	$269,673	$357,000	$531,251	$715,939
Western	202	45	$348,320	$115,943	$281,315	$335,434	$384,480	$499,435

Table 103B: Collections for Professional Charges (TC/NPP Excluded)

	Phys	Med Pracs	Mean	Std. Dev.	25th %tile	Median	75th %tile	90th %tile
Overall	199	75	$785,946	$323,145	$554,662	$717,891	$981,162	$1,260,965
Group Type								
Single Specialty	40	9	$904,104	$359,125	$616,138	$743,476	$1,242,750	$1,389,191
Multispecialty	159	66	$756,221	$307,573	$541,227	$717,891	$946,305	$1,204,800
Geographic Section (All Pracs)								
Eastern	37	10	$658,853	$160,780	$533,001	$644,577	$773,020	$883,665
Midwest	55	24	$775,490	$318,958	$541,227	$754,507	$987,309	$1,194,899
Southern	58	19	$904,619	$367,014	$593,329	$830,813	$1,242,766	$1,399,263
Western	49	22	$753,182	$325,977	$503,739	$717,891	$948,512	$1,258,397

Table 103C: Compensation to Collections Ratio (TC/NPP Excluded)

	Phys	Med Pracs	Mean	Std. Dev.	25th %tile	Median	75th %tile	90th %tile
Overall	200	73	.528	.158	.428	.508	.614	.734
Group Type								
Single Specialty	40	9	.441	.111	.365	.441	.505	.596
Multispecialty	160	64	.549	.161	.445	.527	.638	.769
Geographic Section (All Pracs)								
Eastern	37	10	.587	.171	.457	.559	.706	.837
Midwest	55	24	.557	.150	.442	.534	.620	.760
Southern	60	19	.503	.136	.428	.474	.566	.714
Western	48	20	.480	.166	.400	.498	.578	.633

Table 103D: Physician Work RVUs (CMS RBRVS Method) (NPP Excluded)

	Phys	Med Pracs	Mean	Std. Dev.	25th %tile	Median	75th %tile	90th %tile
Overall	231	88	7,353	2,745	5,460	7,116	8,932	11,004
Group Type								
Single Specialty	15	3	7,696	1,914	6,194	7,636	9,511	10,444
Multispecialty	216	85	7,329	2,795	5,312	7,043	8,930	11,156
Geographic Section (All Pracs)								
Eastern	35	11	8,230	2,683	5,971	7,774	10,929	12,101
Midwest	68	31	6,795	2,651	4,778	6,952	8,103	10,242
Southern	53	17	8,067	2,932	6,146	7,328	9,475	12,348
Western	75	29	6,946	2,555	5,084	6,331	8,857	10,243

Pathology: Anatomic and Clinical

Table 104A: Compensation

	Phys	Med Pracs	Mean	Std. Dev.	25th %tile	Median	75th %tile	90th %tile
Overall	210	26	$360,757	$165,267	$276,912	$319,405	$385,145	$538,460
Group Type								
Single Specialty	63	5	$447,763	$238,248	$280,788	$414,128	$560,000	$804,129
Multispecialty	147	21	$323,468	$101,626	$275,747	$313,723	$359,386	$433,706
Geographic Section (All Pracs)								
Eastern	38	7	$267,088	$93,989	$226,662	$258,920	$306,301	$324,826
Midwest	59	10	$364,507	$118,085	$285,046	$382,512	$433,400	$460,700
Southern	32	4	$508,360	$289,219	$289,196	$416,359	$707,951	$960,758
Western	81	5	$343,656	$107,508	$302,631	$319,766	$349,678	$506,688

Table 104B: Collections for Professional Charges (TC/NPP Excluded)

	Phys	Med Pracs	Mean	Std. Dev.	25th %tile	Median	75th %tile	90th %tile
Overall	58	9	$856,054	$795,845	$402,022	$560,156	$1,042,671	$2,229,051
Group Type								
Single Specialty	31	2	*	*	*	*	*	*
Multispecialty	27	7	$678,072	$429,020	$411,351	$501,770	$871,819	$1,228,825
Geographic Section (All Pracs)								
Eastern	17	2	*	*	*	*	*	*
Midwest	4	2	*	*	*	*	*	*
Southern	32	3	$1,049,232	$997,534	$284,468	$617,083	$1,764,678	$2,886,651
Western	5	2	*	*	*	*	*	*

Table 104C: Compensation to Collections Ratio (TC/NPP Excluded)

	Phys	Med Pracs	Mean	Std. Dev.	25th %tile	Median	75th %tile	90th %tile
Overall	42	9	.509	.247	.277	.495	.730	.847
Group Type								
Single Specialty	18	2	*	*	*	*	*	*
Multispecialty	24	7	.577	.218	.429	.530	.737	.887
Geographic Section (All Pracs)								
Eastern	15	2	*	*	*	*	*	*
Midwest	4	2	*	*	*	*	*	*
Southern	18	3	.395	.266	.174	.328	.585	.858
Western	5	2	*	*	*	*	*	*

Table 104D: Physician Work RVUs (CMS RBRVS Method) (NPP Excluded)

	Phys	Med Pracs	Mean	Std. Dev.	25th %tile	Median	75th %tile	90th %tile
Overall	73	13	5,658	2,400	3,736	5,518	7,075	8,550
Group Type								
Single Specialty	19	1	*	*	*	*	*	*
Multispecialty	54	12	5,856	2,685	3,233	6,043	7,740	8,849
Geographic Section (All Pracs)								
Eastern	24	4	6,479	2,507	4,607	6,797	7,767	10,133
Midwest	33	5	4,663	1,869	3,170	4,548	6,228	7,356
Southern	3	2	*	*	*	*	*	*
Western	13	2	*	*	*	*	*	*

Pediatrics: General

Table 105A: Compensation

	Phys	Med Pracs	Mean	Std. Dev.	25th %tile	Median	75th %tile	90th %tile
Overall	2,862	354	$196,936	$78,868	$143,512	$183,265	$233,520	$301,010
Group Type								
Single Specialty	622	81	$220,878	$99,361	$141,349	$208,451	$281,114	$355,801
Multispecialty	2,240	273	$190,288	$70,756	$144,015	$179,766	$222,420	$278,199
Geographic Section (All Pracs)								
Eastern	493	87	$173,107	$66,675	$129,205	$160,000	$204,330	$257,930
Midwest	848	109	$192,332	$70,958	$141,914	$181,997	$228,320	$286,867
Southern	746	89	$219,975	$98,598	$145,617	$203,247	$277,808	$353,866
Western	775	69	$194,957	$66,321	$154,372	$191,481	$220,457	$272,409

Table 105B: Collections for Professional Charges (TC/NPP Excluded)

	Phys	Med Pracs	Mean	Std. Dev.	25th %tile	Median	75th %tile	90th %tile
Overall	1,372	166	$428,278	$172,117	$309,036	$406,865	$523,377	$652,219
Group Type								
Single Specialty	398	39	$465,737	$187,691	$337,070	$444,191	$582,287	$715,076
Multispecialty	974	127	$412,972	$162,972	$302,237	$399,584	$493,467	$610,479
Geographic Section (All Pracs)								
Eastern	210	34	$388,627	$128,514	$289,727	$384,995	$460,481	$572,962
Midwest	417	48	$434,526	$165,476	$320,553	$410,465	$522,942	$631,086
Southern	447	48	$451,448	$176,950	$324,156	$427,543	$560,922	$687,192
Western	298	36	$412,721	$193,746	$297,511	$400,023	$516,210	$652,272

Table 105C: Compensation to Collections Ratio (TC/NPP Excluded)

	Phys	Med Pracs	Mean	Std. Dev.	25th %tile	Median	75th %tile	90th %tile
Overall	1,338	163	.474	.147	.369	.458	.566	.657
Group Type								
Single Specialty	393	39	.505	.158	.389	.503	.599	.691
Multispecialty	945	124	.462	.140	.360	.445	.543	.643
Geographic Section (All Pracs)								
Eastern	207	34	.453	.124	.353	.455	.533	.605
Midwest	412	48	.464	.149	.361	.435	.549	.647
Southern	449	48	.521	.144	.437	.521	.613	.693
Western	270	33	.429	.144	.337	.413	.470	.590

Table 105D: Physician Work RVUs (CMS RBRVS Method) (NPP Excluded)

	Phys	Med Pracs	Mean	Std. Dev.	25th %tile	Median	75th %tile	90th %tile
Overall	1,598	185	5,053	1,748	3,825	4,835	6,018	7,401
Group Type								
Single Specialty	252	25	5,344	2,055	3,929	5,263	6,675	8,120
Multispecialty	1,346	160	4,998	1,680	3,811	4,804	5,884	7,203
Geographic Section (All Pracs)								
Eastern	241	39	4,545	1,411	3,615	4,445	5,433	6,501
Midwest	513	65	4,893	1,731	3,716	4,642	5,733	7,120
Southern	494	42	5,748	1,910	4,355	5,670	7,026	8,240
Western	350	39	4,655	1,416	3,683	4,654	5,365	6,327

Physiatry (Physical Medicine and Rehabilitation)

Table 106A: Compensation

	Phys	Med Pracs	Mean	Std. Dev.	25th %tile	Median	75th %tile	90th %tile
Overall	248	98	$261,555	$123,901	$199,538	$234,338	$290,044	$379,687
Group Type								
Single Specialty	58	24	$302,500	$168,946	$187,805	$252,051	$351,466	$548,903
Multispecialty	190	74	$249,056	$103,841	$200,348	$226,775	$274,200	$350,563
Geographic Section (All Pracs)								
Eastern	41	23	$248,418	$145,604	$180,069	$216,803	$278,492	$359,895
Midwest	63	29	$261,908	$144,470	$175,313	$226,825	$302,698	$390,072
Southern	54	25	$280,770	$145,686	$180,722	$236,157	$345,965	$530,297
Western	90	21	$255,765	$74,565	$212,210	$239,833	$272,477	$327,215

Table 106B: Collections for Professional Charges (TC/NPP Excluded)

	Phys	Med Pracs	Mean	Std. Dev.	25th %tile	Median	75th %tile	90th %tile
Overall	95	42	$443,809	$219,562	$312,473	$396,000	$518,278	$744,671
Group Type								
Single Specialty	34	12	$452,355	$252,574	$303,719	$400,457	$456,128	$803,492
Multispecialty	61	30	$439,045	$200,933	$312,736	$380,092	$527,898	$765,468
Geographic Section (All Pracs)								
Eastern	15	10	$609,703	$351,153	$340,513	$427,905	$917,889	$1,196,842
Midwest	25	11	$386,953	$153,247	$265,886	$394,446	$444,096	$539,874
Southern	34	13	$392,752	$194,315	$281,535	$323,770	$419,532	$717,562
Western	21	8	$475,662	$139,993	$379,967	$472,598	$543,231	$689,584

Table 106C: Compensation to Collections Ratio (TC/NPP Excluded)

	Phys	Med Pracs	Mean	Std. Dev.	25th %tile	Median	75th %tile	90th %tile
Overall	89	40	.553	.134	.456	.545	.639	.731
Group Type								
Single Specialty	34	12	.572	.130	.479	.556	.635	.772
Multispecialty	55	28	.542	.136	.445	.539	.643	.732
Geographic Section (All Pracs)								
Eastern	16	10	.455	.114	.368	.464	.498	.651
Midwest	22	10	.625	.110	.543	.605	.730	.793
Southern	31	13	.576	.139	.509	.564	.643	.796
Western	20	7	.518	.113	.419	.504	.640	.685

Table 106D: Physician Work RVUs (CMS RBRVS Method) (NPP Excluded)

	Phys	Med Pracs	Mean	Std. Dev.	25th %tile	Median	75th %tile	90th %tile
Overall	114	48	5,408	2,429	3,460	4,963	6,986	9,095
Group Type								
Single Specialty	24	8	5,935	3,019	3,265	5,326	7,564	10,723
Multispecialty	90	40	5,267	2,245	3,546	4,829	6,313	8,781
Geographic Section (All Pracs)								
Eastern	17	8	6,751	3,484	4,045	5,713	8,200	13,209
Midwest	45	18	4,470	1,980	3,165	3,883	5,348	7,442
Southern	29	9	6,113	2,149	4,601	5,826	7,602	9,175
Western	23	13	5,360	1,975	4,108	5,155	6,159	7,955

Podiatry: General

Table 107A: Compensation

	Phys	Med Pracs	Mean	Std. Dev.	25th %tile	Median	75th %tile	90th %tile
Overall	145	88	$207,587	$86,037	$146,708	$185,819	$256,182	$335,014
Group Type								
Single Specialty	5	5	*	*	*	*	*	*
Multispecialty	140	83	$209,182	$86,788	$148,117	$186,065	$258,805	$339,794
Geographic Section (All Pracs)								
Eastern	12	10	$176,486	$67,794	$120,377	$160,080	$227,915	$297,968
Midwest	63	37	$202,095	$78,672	$141,430	$180,003	$237,021	$345,220
Southern	32	21	$219,258	$112,604	$146,444	$186,000	$276,656	$418,408
Western	38	20	$216,683	$76,684	$157,892	$199,493	$261,694	$342,745

Table 107B: Collections for Professional Charges (TC/NPP Excluded)

	Phys	Med Pracs	Mean	Std. Dev.	25th %tile	Median	75th %tile	90th %tile
Overall	78	46	$439,722	$187,949	$322,229	$415,156	$510,720	$686,949
Group Type								
Single Specialty	3	3	*	*	*	*	*	*
Multispecialty	75	43	$443,318	$190,795	$313,434	$427,482	$526,075	$692,373
Geographic Section (All Pracs)								
Eastern	2	2	*	*	*	*	*	*
Midwest	38	23	$418,439	$136,957	$326,566	$424,121	$491,879	$652,557
Southern	20	13	$492,905	$232,203	$299,442	$434,918	$589,200	$856,483
Western	18	8	$433,691	$231,742	$256,809	$418,780	$564,394	$783,464

Table 107C: Compensation to Collections Ratio (TC/NPP Excluded)

	Phys	Med Pracs	Mean	Std. Dev.	25th %tile	Median	75th %tile	90th %tile
Overall	74	45	.493	.111	.402	.488	.564	.636
Group Type								
Single Specialty	3	3	*	*	*	*	*	*
Multispecialty	71	42	.496	.110	.402	.494	.562	.637
Geographic Section (All Pracs)								
Eastern	2	2	*	*	*	*	*	*
Midwest	37	23	.508	.124	.395	.529	.590	.648
Southern	20	13	.525	.087	.437	.532	.589	.656
Western	15	7	.440	.062	.400	.444	.477	.553

Table 107D: Physician Work RVUs (CMS RBRVS Method) (NPP Excluded)

	Phys	Med Pracs	Mean	Std. Dev.	25th %tile	Median	75th %tile	90th %tile
Overall	96	51	4,889	1,983	3,492	4,756	5,976	6,910
Group Type								
Single Specialty	1	1	*	*	*	*	*	*
Multispecialty	95	50	4,901	1,989	3,492	4,758	6,003	6,916
Geographic Section (All Pracs)								
Eastern	4	3	*	*	*	*	*	*
Midwest	37	21	4,274	1,738	2,831	3,999	5,622	6,611
Southern	27	15	5,716	2,614	3,965	5,226	6,331	10,425
Western	28	12	4,904	1,370	3,895	4,770	6,149	6,837

Psychiatry: General

Table 108A: Compensation

	Phys	Med Pracs	Mean	Std. Dev.	25th %tile	Median	75th %tile	90th %tile
Overall	494	93	$200,518	$61,609	$159,364	$194,038	$230,486	$268,040
Group Type								
Single Specialty	44	5	$150,964	$32,794	$127,400	$149,722	$173,373	$198,141
Multispecialty	450	88	$205,363	$61,648	$165,120	$199,173	$234,990	$272,893
Geographic Section (All Pracs)								
Eastern	113	19	$188,884	$80,229	$149,950	$171,912	$198,900	$284,160
Midwest	153	40	$194,728	$66,588	$148,561	$180,001	$232,191	$280,452
Southern	54	19	$196,158	$51,576	$169,000	$183,349	$227,283	$259,117
Western	174	15	$214,517	$40,220	$188,649	$218,038	$239,267	$268,450

Table 108B: Collections for Professional Charges (TC/NPP Excluded)

	Phys	Med Pracs	Mean	Std. Dev.	25th %tile	Median	75th %tile	90th %tile
Overall	123	36	$196,689	$99,788	$126,364	$196,684	$250,248	$342,857
Group Type								
Single Specialty	16	2	*	*	*	*	*	*
Multispecialty	107	34	$189,843	$102,764	$111,820	$192,498	$245,034	$346,841
Geographic Section (All Pracs)								
Eastern	39	6	$138,577	$89,479	$43,431	$139,617	$197,307	$260,524
Midwest	29	12	$225,251	$89,203	$169,786	$214,895	$265,381	$359,689
Southern	34	13	$226,668	$109,054	$130,106	$224,861	$312,187	$379,375
Western	21	5	$216,632	$71,080	$174,678	$196,764	$251,381	$365,887

Table 108C: Compensation to Collections Ratio (TC/NPP Excluded)

	Phys	Med Pracs	Mean	Std. Dev.	25th %tile	Median	75th %tile	90th %tile
Overall	73	26	.714	.152	.617	.734	.830	.914
Group Type								
Single Specialty	15	2	*	*	*	*	*	*
Multispecialty	58	24	.718	.161	.604	.750	.844	.925
Geographic Section (All Pracs)								
Eastern	16	5	.719	.170	.624	.773	.840	.920
Midwest	18	8	.729	.141	.615	.760	.829	.930
Southern	19	8	.615	.121	.552	.619	.688	.792
Western	20	5	.790	.130	.714	.793	.878	.957

Table 108D: Physician Work RVUs (CMS RBRVS Method) (NPP Excluded)

	Phys	Med Pracs	Mean	Std. Dev.	25th %tile	Median	75th %tile	90th %tile
Overall	228	57	3,528	1,418	2,553	3,398	4,300	5,464
Group Type								
Single Specialty	15	2	*	*	*	*	*	*
Multispecialty	213	55	3,451	1,403	2,511	3,314	4,220	5,420
Geographic Section (All Pracs)								
Eastern	73	11	3,096	1,453	2,008	2,903	4,132	5,113
Midwest	99	27	3,697	1,352	2,854	3,446	4,257	5,606
Southern	25	9	4,678	1,189	3,649	4,451	5,805	6,426
Western	31	10	3,080	1,088	2,273	3,029	4,077	4,671

Pulmonary Medicine: General

Table 109A: Compensation

	Phys	Med Pracs	Mean	Std. Dev.	25th %tile	Median	75th %tile	90th %tile
Overall	253	100	$297,555	$115,250	$207,497	$274,358	$367,649	$452,453
Group Type								
Single Specialty	27	7	$312,521	$90,928	$236,442	$329,263	$391,297	$415,568
Multispecialty	226	93	$295,767	$117,860	$206,277	$273,180	$359,150	$465,379
Geographic Section (All Pracs)								
Eastern	49	22	$280,641	$98,231	$205,524	$270,133	$367,649	$411,797
Midwest	70	32	$335,418	$131,326	$248,872	$299,929	$415,705	$525,268
Southern	73	25	$290,965	$113,013	$195,205	$269,043	$359,199	$441,148
Western	61	21	$275,579	$102,264	$197,872	$266,511	$326,192	$413,419

Table 109B: Collections for Professional Charges (TC/NPP Excluded)

	Phys	Med Pracs	Mean	Std. Dev.	25th %tile	Median	75th %tile	90th %tile
Overall	123	51	$475,986	$215,680	$320,204	$446,582	$587,184	$808,427
Group Type								
Single Specialty	5	2	*	*	*	*	*	*
Multispecialty	118	49	$483,755	$214,856	$329,002	$450,459	$593,524	$811,633
Geographic Section (All Pracs)								
Eastern	20	7	$480,809	$276,830	$283,347	$370,732	$790,940	$901,957
Midwest	40	19	$524,440	$232,095	$383,363	$513,684	$648,193	$835,308
Southern	38	15	$447,512	$172,516	$345,565	$435,266	$545,542	$653,584
Western	25	10	$437,885	$188,811	$254,023	$448,979	$612,762	$699,351

Table 109C: Compensation to Collections Ratio (TC/NPP Excluded)

	Phys	Med Pracs	Mean	Std. Dev.	25th %tile	Median	75th %tile	90th %tile
Overall	113	48	.616	.164	.490	.587	.753	.870
Group Type								
Single Specialty	5	2	*	*	*	*	*	*
Multispecialty	108	46	.606	.160	.489	.576	.726	.857
Geographic Section (All Pracs)								
Eastern	19	7	.588	.209	.403	.565	.706	.913
Midwest	38	18	.638	.145	.523	.612	.752	.873
Southern	33	13	.603	.162	.486	.533	.764	.831
Western	23	10	.622	.162	.480	.639	.714	.878

Table 109D: Physician Work RVUs (CMS RBRVS Method) (NPP Excluded)

	Phys	Med Pracs	Mean	Std. Dev.	25th %tile	Median	75th %tile	90th %tile
Overall	170	66	7,355	3,149	5,076	6,773	9,369	11,483
Group Type								
Single Specialty	11	3	6,237	3,759	3,742	5,644	9,299	13,324
Multispecialty	159	63	7,432	3,102	5,212	7,038	9,493	11,485
Geographic Section (All Pracs)								
Eastern	26	13	7,123	4,436	3,991	6,089	8,123	13,436
Midwest	50	20	7,576	3,097	5,155	7,297	10,627	12,321
Southern	47	16	8,013	2,713	6,171	7,868	9,858	11,118
Western	47	17	6,590	2,652	4,730	5,939	7,736	9,604

Pulmonary Medicine: Critical Care

Table 110A: Compensation

	Phys	Med Pracs	Mean	Std. Dev.	25th %tile	Median	75th %tile	90th %tile
Overall	91	21	$316,023	$97,063	$256,250	$315,779	$366,085	$464,440
Group Type								
Single Specialty	7	4	*	*	*	*	*	*
Multispecialty	84	17	$313,064	$92,465	$261,893	$314,252	$365,145	$453,454
Geographic Section (All Pracs)								
Eastern	1	1	*	*	*	*	*	*
Midwest	39	7	$296,232	$70,914	$250,224	$290,763	$347,287	$390,180
Southern	18	6	$302,408	$41,896	$277,490	$312,603	$336,126	$349,447
Western	33	7	$346,414	$134,361	$212,154	$349,937	$467,114	$529,429

Table 110B: Collections for Professional Charges (TC/NPP Excluded)

	Phys	Med Pracs	Mean	Std. Dev.	25th %tile	Median	75th %tile	90th %tile
Overall	40	10	$402,019	$114,833	$314,278	$426,919	$475,050	$552,364
Group Type								
Single Specialty	4	2	*	*	*	*	*	*
Multispecialty	36	8	$403,371	$119,678	$283,542	$444,513	$476,230	$556,138
Geographic Section (All Pracs)								
Midwest	20	4	$458,994	$82,133	$378,576	$461,457	$499,286	$586,737
Southern	13	4	$338,634	$130,968	$250,726	$275,221	$466,486	$547,284
Western	7	2	*	*	*	*	*	*

Table 110C: Compensation to Collections Ratio (TC/NPP Excluded)

	Phys	Med Pracs	Mean	Std. Dev.	25th %tile	Median	75th %tile	90th %tile
Overall	28	8	.682	.156	.593	.680	.782	.888
Group Type								
Single Specialty	4	2	*	*	*	*	*	*
Multispecialty	24	6	.685	.160	.593	.691	.782	.907
Geographic Section (All Pracs)								
Midwest	20	4	.691	.172	.601	.700	.814	.925
Southern	6	3	*	*	*	*	*	*
Western	2	1	*	*	*	*	*	*

Table 110D: Physician Work RVUs (CMS RBRVS Method) (NPP Excluded)

	Phys	Med Pracs	Mean	Std. Dev.	25th %tile	Median	75th %tile	90th %tile
Overall	46	11	8,521	2,625	6,796	8,470	10,076	11,877
Group Type								
Single Specialty	1	1	*	*	*	*	*	*
Multispecialty	45	10	8,509	2,653	6,789	8,433	10,168	11,928
Geographic Section (All Pracs)								
Midwest	30	5	9,604	2,357	8,252	9,613	11,286	12,369
Southern	3	2	*	*	*	*	*	*
Western	13	4	6,517	1,729	4,768	6,803	8,085	8,381

Radiation Oncology

Table 111A: Compensation

	Phys	Med Pracs	Mean	Std. Dev.	25th %tile	Median	75th %tile	90th %tile
Overall	140	37	$528,225	$197,178	$366,911	$463,293	$668,188	$866,655
Group Type								
Single Specialty	20	5	$705,327	$225,773	$471,500	$866,555	$871,173	$871,173
Multispecialty	120	32	$498,709	$176,423	$363,232	$452,946	$583,426	$821,693
Geographic Section (All Pracs)								
Eastern	12	5	$401,558	$141,373	$307,750	$348,000	$477,145	$701,779
Midwest	27	12	$488,146	$174,528	$352,508	$427,000	$605,000	$806,016
Southern	35	9	$636,903	$198,094	$516,882	$631,669	$871,173	$871,173
Western	66	11	$510,020	$191,634	$369,000	$434,803	$597,587	$844,581

Table 111B: Collections for Professional Charges (TC/NPP Excluded)

	Phys	Med Pracs	Mean	Std. Dev.	25th %tile	Median	75th %tile	90th %tile
Overall	44	14	$588,754	$224,514	$420,530	$537,285	$807,452	$876,654
Group Type								
Single Specialty	14	4	$662,872	$151,133	$526,311	$652,572	$820,000	$839,209
Multispecialty	30	10	$554,166	$246,195	$329,309	$495,194	$777,231	$962,618
Geographic Section (All Pracs)								
Eastern	5	2	*	*	*	*	*	*
Midwest	9	4	*	*	*	*	*	*
Southern	12	4	$664,120	$230,719	$494,677	$625,743	$844,493	$1,011,273
Western	18	4	$449,525	$187,665	$320,531	$403,336	$559,281	$812,129

Table 111C: Compensation to Collections Ratio (TC/NPP Excluded)

	Phys	Med Pracs	Mean	Std. Dev.	25th %tile	Median	75th %tile	90th %tile
Overall	25	12	.739	.173	.636	.738	.908	.951
Group Type								
Single Specialty	6	3	*	*	*	*	*	*
Multispecialty	19	9	.768	.160	.641	.741	.934	.957
Geographic Section (All Pracs)								
Eastern	5	2	*	*	*	*	*	*
Midwest	8	4	*	*	*	*	*	*
Southern	5	3	*	*	*	*	*	*
Western	7	3	*	*	*	*	*	*

Table 111D: Physician Work RVUs (CMS RBRVS Method) (NPP Excluded)

	Phys	Med Pracs	Mean	Std. Dev.	25th %tile	Median	75th %tile	90th %tile
Overall	78	24	9,969	4,889	6,814	8,625	12,186	15,547
Group Type								
Single Specialty	14	2	*	*	*	*	*	*
Multispecialty	64	22	9,538	5,041	6,430	8,191	10,961	15,367
Geographic Section (All Pracs)								
Eastern	9	3	*	*	*	*	*	*
Midwest	13	7	9,338	4,009	6,650	8,269	11,183	16,928
Southern	22	6	13,671	6,095	9,967	13,783	15,703	22,964
Western	34	8	7,714	2,774	5,918	7,271	9,787	11,427

Radiology: Diagnostic-Inv

Table 112A: Compensation

	Phys	Med Pracs	Mean	Std. Dev.	25th %tile	Median	75th %tile	90th %tile
Overall	341	52	$507,508	$179,652	$404,177	$494,801	$611,064	$715,534
Group Type								
Single Specialty	189	19	$493,995	$174,235	$395,447	$512,000	$589,351	$699,601
Multispecialty	152	33	$524,310	$185,370	$407,310	$476,762	$640,877	$773,520
Geographic Section (All Pracs)								
Eastern	35	11	$458,381	$134,524	$366,345	$483,760	$526,115	$610,338
Midwest	58	15	$574,931	$183,982	$440,514	$565,304	$713,603	$859,887
Southern	137	13	$520,322	$212,687	$375,937	$517,000	$682,412	$730,363
Western	111	13	$471,954	$126,695	$411,595	$468,739	$533,335	$564,821

Table 112B: Collections for Professional Charges (TC/NPP Excluded)

	Phys	Med Pracs	Mean	Std. Dev.	25th %tile	Median	75th %tile	90th %tile
Overall	108	23	$746,360	$309,722	$569,315	$685,647	$863,972	$1,109,611
Group Type								
Single Specialty	74	11	$704,428	$252,350	$566,600	$671,207	$793,880	$1,043,044
Multispecialty	34	12	$837,625	$397,046	$580,717	$749,694	$984,397	$1,515,060
Geographic Section (All Pracs)								
Eastern	16	5	$685,434	$260,163	$566,421	$673,459	$801,637	$1,126,458
Midwest	13	5	$790,242	$404,903	$541,250	$793,860	$928,459	$1,537,119
Southern	38	7	$793,160	$381,603	$553,350	$661,182	$939,938	$1,508,978
Western	41	6	$712,847	$204,938	$576,334	$683,041	$767,586	$1,071,552

Table 112C: Compensation to Collections Ratio (TC/NPP Excluded)

	Phys	Med Pracs	Mean	Std. Dev.	25th %tile	Median	75th %tile	90th %tile
Overall	96	21	.675	.179	.528	.701	.801	.926
Group Type								
Single Specialty	66	9	.666	.188	.466	.708	.807	.919
Multispecialty	30	12	.694	.158	.572	.666	.799	.955
Geographic Section (All Pracs)								
Eastern	13	3	.682	.171	.551	.663	.826	.928
Midwest	11	5	.640	.190	.459	.639	.777	.947
Southern	33	7	.706	.146	.571	.727	.825	.916
Western	39	6	.656	.205	.450	.710	.793	.969

Table 112D: Physician Work RVUs (CMS RBRVS Method) (NPP Excluded)

	Phys	Med Pracs	Mean	Std. Dev.	25th %tile	Median	75th %tile	90th %tile
Overall	154	32	11,042	4,068	8,412	10,475	13,701	16,473
Group Type								
Single Specialty	82	11	11,412	3,912	9,141	10,454	13,198	17,204
Multispecialty	72	21	10,621	4,227	7,176	10,641	14,628	16,352
Geographic Section (All Pracs)								
Eastern	21	5	9,413	3,138	7,442	9,454	11,240	14,847
Midwest	33	11	9,851	3,978	7,197	9,022	12,206	15,518
Southern	47	10	11,659	3,724	9,596	11,066	14,579	16,612
Western	53	6	11,882	4,457	9,038	10,671	14,782	18,548

Radiology: Diagnostic-Non

Table 113A: Compensation

	Phys	Med Pracs	Mean	Std. Dev.	25th %tile	Median	75th %tile	90th %tile
Overall	874	85	$470,939	$160,903	$376,974	$450,658	$522,789	$687,357
Group Type								
Single Specialty	273	21	$467,065	$160,408	$374,446	$475,249	$543,270	$650,591
Multispecialty	601	64	$472,699	$161,230	$376,887	$436,535	$508,956	$690,186
Geographic Section (All Pracs)								
Eastern	164	17	$432,347	$167,474	$335,257	$398,708	$514,163	$721,360
Midwest	192	23	$510,791	$151,651	$429,485	$498,862	$566,902	$686,425
Southern	132	19	$458,921	$120,790	$399,410	$462,542	$521,613	$648,211
Western	386	26	$471,624	$170,238	$372,036	$428,722	$496,469	$792,117

Table 113B: Collections for Professional Charges (TC/NPP Excluded)

	Phys	Med Pracs	Mean	Std. Dev.	25th %tile	Median	75th %tile	90th %tile
Overall	228	33	$724,536	$396,022	$509,478	$664,825	$808,334	$1,074,993
Group Type								
Single Specialty	118	11	$670,958	$234,126	$518,209	$660,508	$794,015	$1,006,406
Multispecialty	110	22	$782,010	$511,211	$496,177	$686,430	$818,843	$1,410,964
Geographic Section (All Pracs)								
Eastern	58	5	$552,754	$212,679	$367,702	$543,873	$712,205	$845,968
Midwest	33	7	$695,805	$230,330	$513,075	$627,345	$774,325	$1,120,632
Southern	96	11	$801,428	$446,102	$575,246	$698,064	$881,636	$1,192,142
Western	41	10	$810,629	$495,211	$532,663	$707,037	$754,509	$1,470,378

Table 113C: Compensation to Collections Ratio (TC/NPP Excluded)

	Phys	Med Pracs	Mean	Std. Dev.	25th %tile	Median	75th %tile	90th %tile
Overall	207	32	.640	.200	.498	.665	.789	.896
Group Type								
Single Specialty	113	11	.638	.172	.469	.638	.766	.893
Multispecialty	94	21	.642	.229	.557	.675	.820	.897
Geographic Section (All Pracs)								
Eastern	46	5	.652	.197	.481	.606	.833	.934
Midwest	28	7	.780	.129	.746	.803	.879	.907
Southern	89	10	.624	.188	.519	.643	.745	.852
Western	44	10	.572	.223	.450	.668	.716	.865

Table 113D: Physician Work RVUs (CMS RBRVS Method) (NPP Excluded)

	Phys	Med Pracs	Mean	Std. Dev.	25th %tile	Median	75th %tile	90th %tile
Overall	421	50	9,801	4,107	6,824	9,377	12,193	14,894
Group Type								
Single Specialty	125	11	11,693	4,213	8,717	11,852	14,136	16,355
Multispecialty	296	39	9,002	3,794	6,363	8,313	11,066	13,939
Geographic Section (All Pracs)								
Eastern	111	10	8,664	3,393	6,067	8,311	10,910	12,938
Midwest	84	13	7,545	2,717	5,490	7,081	9,298	10,925
Southern	116	13	11,206	3,689	8,709	11,825	14,093	15,933
Western	110	14	11,189	4,911	7,582	10,600	13,314	18,802

Rheumatology

Table 114A: Compensation

	Phys	Med Pracs	Mean	Std. Dev.	25th %tile	Median	75th %tile	90th %tile
Overall	287	134	$238,574	$96,241	$176,497	$218,704	$273,966	$364,911
Group Type								
Single Specialty	22	11	$224,050	$116,150	$147,266	$183,478	$292,882	$388,006
Multispecialty	265	123	$239,780	$94,562	$179,160	$222,274	$273,150	$363,829
Geographic Section (All Pracs)								
Eastern	49	29	$217,403	$81,285	$164,096	$206,422	$257,663	$323,327
Midwest	80	42	$247,933	$107,484	$177,117	$222,056	$297,095	$413,012
Southern	68	34	$269,872	$117,515	$183,142	$246,821	$334,664	$400,837
Western	90	29	$218,134	$63,666	$175,757	$212,455	$248,037	$308,867

Table 114B: Collections for Professional Charges (TC/NPP Excluded)

	Phys	Med Pracs	Mean	Std. Dev.	25th %tile	Median	75th %tile	90th %tile
Overall	131	66	$429,864	$253,615	$273,757	$351,849	$501,442	$779,010
Group Type								
Single Specialty	13	6	$250,767	$83,305	$176,054	$238,517	$322,499	$392,051
Multispecialty	118	60	$449,595	$258,455	$284,695	$365,550	$511,804	$841,404
Geographic Section (All Pracs)								
Eastern	26	13	$405,252	$221,928	$274,658	$342,725	$518,719	$641,592
Midwest	45	22	$401,920	$186,326	$298,237	$363,347	$480,304	$610,809
Southern	35	21	$469,324	$319,702	$255,303	$338,495	$579,740	$1,021,416
Western	25	10	$450,516	$289,517	$261,418	$345,892	$551,016	$909,040

Table 114C: Compensation to Collections Ratio (TC/NPP Excluded)

	Phys	Med Pracs	Mean	Std. Dev.	25th %tile	Median	75th %tile	90th %tile
Overall	122	61	.569	.156	.474	.571	.655	.752
Group Type								
Single Specialty	13	6	.620	.180	.466	.552	.774	.920
Multispecialty	109	55	.563	.153	.477	.574	.653	.736
Geographic Section (All Pracs)								
Eastern	25	13	.567	.153	.504	.560	.608	.795
Midwest	42	20	.574	.136	.479	.568	.654	.758
Southern	33	19	.597	.191	.513	.641	.694	.819
Western	22	9	.521	.134	.419	.495	.630	.731

Table 114D: Physician Work RVUs (CMS RBRVS Method) (NPP Excluded)

	Phys	Med Pracs	Mean	Std. Dev.	25th %tile	Median	75th %tile	90th %tile
Overall	184	84	4,565	1,400	3,684	4,488	5,349	6,586
Group Type								
Single Specialty	12	5	3,146	845	2,421	2,994	3,970	4,439
Multispecialty	172	79	4,664	1,378	3,791	4,543	5,428	6,609
Geographic Section (All Pracs)								
Eastern	32	15	4,378	1,272	3,804	4,506	5,338	5,805
Midwest	61	29	4,301	1,410	3,411	4,246	4,928	5,994
Southern	36	19	5,325	1,418	4,123	5,373	6,263	7,152
Western	55	21	4,470	1,306	3,574	4,151	5,151	6,449

Surgery: General

Table 115A: Compensation

	Phys	Med Pracs	Mean	Std. Dev.	25th %tile	Median	75th %tile	90th %tile
Overall	1,024	257	$339,362	$129,732	$251,361	$316,909	$396,004	$499,180
Group Type								
Single Specialty	129	34	$300,385	$121,656	$222,409	$275,000	$352,713	$452,563
Multispecialty	895	223	$344,980	$129,958	$258,950	$322,707	$400,759	$503,118
Geographic Section (All Pracs)								
Eastern	150	49	$286,566	$114,201	$212,276	$264,415	$339,926	$410,157
Midwest	317	96	$379,200	$148,469	$274,095	$361,218	$457,550	$590,321
Southern	216	60	$314,941	$117,685	$235,578	$298,517	$380,198	$473,693
Western	341	52	$341,020	$112,196	$276,100	$325,427	$381,896	$446,873

Table 115B: Collections for Professional Charges (TC/NPP Excluded)

	Phys	Med Pracs	Mean	Std. Dev.	25th %tile	Median	75th %tile	90th %tile
Overall	460	131	$563,673	$207,356	$423,946	$535,803	$681,082	$853,538
Group Type								
Single Specialty	72	20	$524,623	$170,781	$431,873	$507,099	$611,250	$712,736
Multispecialty	388	111	$570,919	$212,859	$423,056	$542,356	$685,969	$867,141
Geographic Section (All Pracs)								
Eastern	84	24	$485,420	$135,973	$392,159	$480,788	$560,143	$618,403
Midwest	130	46	$651,371	$220,072	$491,843	$662,561	$792,676	$936,238
Southern	119	32	$574,045	$206,685	$424,641	$548,461	$698,232	$854,025
Western	127	29	$515,941	$201,109	$390,361	$479,707	$628,277	$801,077

Table 115C: Compensation to Collections Ratio (TC/NPP Excluded)

	Phys	Med Pracs	Mean	Std. Dev.	25th %tile	Median	75th %tile	90th %tile
Overall	425	124	.566	.140	.466	.543	.646	.770
Group Type								
Single Specialty	71	21	.540	.138	.430	.519	.646	.732
Multispecialty	354	103	.572	.140	.473	.550	.647	.774
Geographic Section (All Pracs)								
Eastern	78	24	.530	.125	.438	.505	.633	.698
Midwest	129	44	.553	.133	.455	.539	.633	.747
Southern	112	31	.552	.126	.466	.534	.630	.719
Western	106	25	.624	.157	.500	.594	.754	.865

Table 115D: Physician Work RVUs (CMS RBRVS Method) (NPP Excluded)

	Phys	Med Pracs	Mean	Std. Dev.	25th %tile	Median	75th %tile	90th %tile
Overall	568	148	7,424	2,705	5,792	7,170	8,843	10,964
Group Type								
Single Specialty	57	14	7,726	2,385	6,192	7,318	9,096	11,361
Multispecialty	511	134	7,390	2,739	5,754	7,136	8,839	10,945
Geographic Section (All Pracs)								
Eastern	90	29	6,573	3,014	5,342	6,541	8,010	10,378
Midwest	200	54	7,382	2,589	5,749	7,153	8,872	10,493
Southern	117	29	8,237	2,873	6,182	7,923	9,924	12,109
Western	161	36	7,361	2,379	5,859	7,097	8,343	10,157

Surgery: Cardiovascular

Table 116A: Compensation

	Phys	Med Pracs	Mean	Std. Dev.	25th %tile	Median	75th %tile	90th %tile
Overall	245	69	$479,624	$159,400	$382,950	$461,860	$560,180	$673,722
Group Type								
Single Specialty	94	23	$465,734	$171,926	$363,561	$447,841	$565,594	$684,769
Multispecialty	151	46	$488,271	$151,025	$401,005	$468,382	$556,730	$667,943
Geographic Section (All Pracs)								
Eastern	51	12	$444,280	$160,697	$320,000	$446,588	$522,567	$696,407
Midwest	60	22	$458,875	$119,428	$400,000	$460,633	$542,615	$592,214
Southern	81	24	$482,337	$159,082	$372,685	$452,277	$572,721	$692,532
Western	53	11	$532,979	$186,123	$405,200	$488,099	$608,505	$896,920

Table 116B: Collections for Professional Charges (TC/NPP Excluded)

	Phys	Med Pracs	Mean	Std. Dev.	25th %tile	Median	75th %tile	90th %tile
Overall	123	35	$598,666	$234,053	$414,483	$598,768	$789,601	$894,696
Group Type								
Single Specialty	62	14	$636,876	$239,318	$451,978	$668,534	$836,171	$957,893
Multispecialty	61	21	$559,830	$223,871	$381,490	$551,788	$739,268	$890,834
Geographic Section (All Pracs)								
Eastern	29	6	$500,921	$203,607	$355,240	$537,433	$643,675	$789,866
Midwest	26	10	$644,264	$180,254	$545,942	$673,657	$752,408	$910,793
Southern	43	12	$672,244	$259,239	$441,894	$757,543	$883,110	$970,991
Western	25	7	$538,074	$226,559	$355,969	$488,580	$735,500	$856,011

Table 116C: Compensation to Collections Ratio (TC/NPP Excluded)

	Phys	Med Pracs	Mean	Std. Dev.	25th %tile	Median	75th %tile	90th %tile
Overall	89	27	.664	.170	.533	.641	.809	.896
Group Type								
Single Specialty	49	12	.640	.171	.523	.589	.787	.896
Multispecialty	40	15	.694	.165	.560	.695	.821	.926
Geographic Section (All Pracs)								
Eastern	19	5	.770	.143	.624	.840	.876	.938
Midwest	24	9	.671	.171	.522	.712	.807	.869
Southern	35	8	.610	.113	.530	.569	.653	.787
Western	11	5	.634	.270	.320	.679	.932	.984

Table 116D: Physician Work RVUs (CMS RBRVS Method) (NPP Excluded)

	Phys	Med Pracs	Mean	Std. Dev.	25th %tile	Median	75th %tile	90th %tile
Overall	138	43	10,096	4,371	6,586	9,608	13,537	15,491
Group Type								
Single Specialty	39	11	10,512	4,135	8,152	11,388	13,939	14,837
Multispecialty	99	32	9,931	4,471	6,372	9,572	12,962	15,602
Geographic Section (All Pracs)								
Eastern	26	7	9,003	3,682	6,374	9,553	11,751	13,910
Midwest	35	14	10,813	4,635	6,692	10,801	13,921	17,566
Southern	36	14	9,897	4,078	6,479	8,545	14,200	15,583
Western	41	8	10,351	4,778	6,798	9,676	14,230	16,512

Surgery: Neurological

Table 117A: Compensation

	Phys	Med Pracs	Mean	Std. Dev.	25th %tile	Median	75th %tile	90th %tile
Overall	237	77	$721,458	$394,276	$483,067	$637,895	$841,047	$1,200,051
Group Type								
Single Specialty	46	13	$855,841	$441,659	$478,750	$712,497	$1,211,664	$1,385,962
Multispecialty	191	64	$689,094	$376,119	$483,133	$626,712	$802,000	$974,244
Geographic Section (All Pracs)								
Eastern	48	13	$603,208	$174,061	$480,783	$565,186	$728,715	$856,453
Midwest	43	22	$961,430	$616,847	$600,000	$807,650	$1,140,145	$1,596,700
Southern	66	22	$692,998	$397,949	$473,348	$605,981	$812,898	$1,300,000
Western	80	20	$686,903	$268,424	$483,000	$634,548	$815,034	$1,086,235

Table 117B: Collections for Professional Charges (TC/NPP Excluded)

	Phys	Med Pracs	Mean	Std. Dev.	25th %tile	Median	75th %tile	90th %tile
Overall	124	40	$1,010,801	$575,196	$557,710	$882,341	$1,351,656	$1,836,169
Group Type								
Single Specialty	39	9	$1,210,923	$667,924	$640,494	$1,162,287	$1,847,788	$1,955,994
Multispecialty	85	31	$918,980	$505,486	$523,066	$859,623	$1,184,888	$1,620,049
Geographic Section (All Pracs)								
Eastern	26	5	$930,124	$436,887	$542,327	$869,553	$1,227,029	$1,618,575
Midwest	23	13	$1,148,535	$671,375	$524,454	$1,053,756	$1,615,000	$2,099,267
Southern	39	14	$980,333	$623,799	$541,874	$865,730	$1,223,041	$1,884,356
Western	36	8	$1,014,077	$549,741	$645,007	$906,792	$1,335,130	$1,917,645

Table 117C: Compensation to Collections Ratio (TC/NPP Excluded)

	Phys	Med Pracs	Mean	Std. Dev.	25th %tile	Median	75th %tile	90th %tile
Overall	98	32	.660	.151	.552	.657	.756	.881
Group Type								
Single Specialty	33	7	.649	.160	.542	.656	.718	.887
Multispecialty	65	25	.665	.147	.559	.658	.771	.887
Geographic Section (All Pracs)								
Eastern	21	4	.657	.135	.533	.639	.744	.885
Midwest	19	11	.644	.177	.469	.658	.759	.898
Southern	29	11	.706	.127	.595	.687	.794	.920
Western	29	6	.626	.162	.518	.625	.720	.859

Table 117D: Physician Work RVUs (CMS RBRVS Method) (NPP Excluded)

	Phys	Med Pracs	Mean	Std. Dev.	25th %tile	Median	75th %tile	90th %tile
Overall	129	43	10,511	5,093	7,208	9,783	12,885	16,103
Group Type								
Single Specialty	19	3	12,077	7,231	7,400	11,027	15,688	18,492
Multispecialty	110	40	10,241	4,618	7,049	9,744	12,276	15,759
Geographic Section (All Pracs)								
Eastern	38	8	10,412	3,369	8,021	10,585	13,286	14,742
Midwest	25	13	10,238	4,339	5,924	9,048	13,594	16,888
Southern	18	8	11,980	7,930	7,272	9,394	12,767	23,353
Western	48	14	10,180	5,326	6,639	9,468	11,737	16,110

Surgery: Vascular

Table 118A: Compensation

	Phys	Med Pracs	Mean	Std. Dev.	25th %tile	Median	75th %tile	90th %tile
Overall	197	71	$390,563	$133,437	$306,680	$378,894	$468,333	$590,409
Group Type								
Single Specialty	25	10	$393,028	$141,115	$257,350	$374,776	$512,960	$608,849
Multispecialty	172	61	$390,204	$132,713	$309,865	$379,225	$466,592	$588,493
Geographic Section (All Pracs)								
Eastern	39	21	$371,380	$121,458	$290,775	$362,921	$443,291	$519,559
Midwest	47	17	$382,495	$120,432	$275,704	$362,500	$458,693	$580,244
Southern	53	18	$431,631	$171,497	$294,332	$430,316	$590,838	$642,744
Western	58	15	$372,472	$103,191	$328,863	$384,758	$413,704	$491,564

Table 118B: Collections for Professional Charges (TC/NPP Excluded)

	Phys	Med Pracs	Mean	Std. Dev.	25th %tile	Median	75th %tile	90th %tile
Overall	65	31	$601,325	$249,859	$415,531	$560,707	$787,583	$946,275
Group Type								
Single Specialty	5	4	*	*	*	*	*	*
Multispecialty	60	27	$610,558	$256,092	$414,180	$570,934	$798,700	$965,438
Geographic Section (All Pracs)								
Eastern	15	9	$636,965	$212,040	$495,995	$661,257	$808,711	$883,083
Midwest	21	7	$642,319	$228,492	$502,402	$578,826	$805,917	$992,616
Southern	21	9	$580,209	$285,792	$397,028	$445,341	$787,583	$1,077,411
Western	8	6	*	*	*	*	*	*

Table 118C: Compensation to Collections Ratio (TC/NPP Excluded)

	Phys	Med Pracs	Mean	Std. Dev.	25th %tile	Median	75th %tile	90th %tile
Overall	56	27	.564	.132	.481	.532	.666	.743
Group Type								
Single Specialty	4	3	*	*	*	*	*	*
Multispecialty	52	24	.567	.136	.473	.541	.681	.754
Geographic Section (All Pracs)								
Eastern	13	8	.544	.083	.482	.513	.600	.706
Midwest	20	6	.567	.154	.426	.600	.693	.767
Southern	16	8	.570	.104	.487	.540	.682	.729
Western	7	5	*	*	*	*	*	*

Urgent Care

Table 119A: Compensation

	Phys	Med Pracs	Mean	Std. Dev.	25th %tile	Median	75th %tile	90th %tile
Overall	407	78	$213,458	$75,869	$160,102	$204,528	$256,685	$306,563
Group Type								
Single Specialty	17	5	$191,406	$39,049	$161,318	$199,292	$215,545	$240,952
Multispecialty	390	73	$214,420	$76,959	$159,983	$204,704	$257,583	$309,962
Geographic Section (All Pracs)								
Eastern	26	11	$206,500	$79,825	$155,561	$183,632	$222,752	$329,593
Midwest	111	28	$231,006	$85,864	$165,018	$207,976	$286,108	$360,364
Southern	69	15	$193,313	$75,526	$152,110	$180,346	$219,925	$259,105
Western	201	24	$211,583	$67,625	$160,966	$212,125	$257,068	$289,960

Table 119B: Collections for Professional Charges (TC/NPP Excluded)

	Phys	Med Pracs	Mean	Std. Dev.	25th %tile	Median	75th %tile	90th %tile
Overall	215	35	$487,258	$167,831	$347,184	$475,370	$603,191	$709,673
Group Type								
Single Specialty	16	4	$392,651	$190,135	$264,603	$306,344	$540,240	$701,445
Multispecialty	199	31	$494,864	$164,082	$368,522	$479,585	$605,692	$730,071
Geographic Section (All Pracs)								
Eastern	9	4	*	*	*	*	*	*
Midwest	60	12	$490,669	$203,264	$304,962	$477,388	$641,948	$767,519
Southern	23	7	$447,491	$130,206	$383,230	$446,808	$541,369	$633,158
Western	123	12	$504,937	$152,255	$373,848	$503,114	$613,509	$714,859

Table 119C: Compensation to Collections Ratio (TC/NPP Excluded)

	Phys	Med Pracs	Mean	Std. Dev.	25th %tile	Median	75th %tile	90th %tile
Overall	215	35	.460	.130	.382	.439	.529	.612
Group Type								
Single Specialty	16	4	.468	.133	.347	.463	.592	.640
Multispecialty	199	31	.459	.130	.384	.439	.518	.611
Geographic Section (All Pracs)								
Eastern	9	4	*	*	*	*	*	*
Midwest	60	12	.505	.138	.425	.499	.594	.684
Southern	23	7	.496	.152	.432	.450	.489	.793
Western	123	12	.424	.108	.351	.415	.465	.562

Table 119D: Physician Work RVUs (CMS RBRVS Method) (NPP Excluded)

	Phys	Med Pracs	Mean	Std. Dev.	25th %tile	Median	75th %tile	90th %tile
Overall	332	52	5,397	2,150	3,798	5,015	6,657	8,476
Group Type								
Single Specialty	4	1	*	*	*	*	*	*
Multispecialty	328	51	5,417	2,155	3,808	5,053	6,685	8,491
Geographic Section (All Pracs)								
Eastern	15	5	5,965	1,938	3,952	6,445	7,382	9,020
Midwest	77	18	5,907	2,962	3,506	5,202	8,320	10,444
Southern	52	10	5,268	1,501	4,457	5,376	6,288	6,862
Western	188	19	5,178	1,881	3,715	4,819	6,470	7,901

Urology

Table 120A: Compensation

	Phys	Med Pracs	Mean	Std. Dev.	25th %tile	Median	75th %tile	90th %tile
Overall	557	150	$427,471	$192,729	$309,984	$388,125	$480,855	$644,304
Group Type								
Single Specialty	186	23	$453,127	$217,727	$339,945	$414,537	$505,761	$708,011
Multispecialty	371	127	$414,609	$177,815	$305,232	$378,606	$469,372	$633,078
Geographic Section (All Pracs)								
Eastern	86	31	$411,651	$171,633	$278,557	$384,584	$521,081	$683,472
Midwest	117	49	$429,017	$178,694	$295,788	$388,125	$501,924	$679,934
Southern	189	32	$468,575	$248,409	$329,817	$414,043	$488,955	$924,953
Western	165	38	$387,538	$116,851	$313,600	$380,000	$438,994	$539,371

Table 120B: Collections for Professional Charges (TC/NPP Excluded)

	Phys	Med Pracs	Mean	Std. Dev.	25th %tile	Median	75th %tile	90th %tile
Overall	236	68	$710,171	$285,037	$503,720	$662,204	$882,787	$1,102,827
Group Type								
Single Specialty	99	12	$676,179	$249,773	$493,738	$642,660	$845,090	$978,132
Multispecialty	137	56	$734,734	$306,568	$515,815	$670,101	$943,401	$1,157,981
Geographic Section (All Pracs)								
Eastern	30	11	$753,464	$337,136	$495,822	$703,225	$879,441	$1,361,063
Midwest	50	22	$764,710	$303,989	$602,952	$713,698	$956,101	$1,146,356
Southern	110	18	$666,300	$257,986	$476,336	$648,801	$845,384	$984,190
Western	46	17	$727,563	$282,186	$551,765	$655,900	$984,755	$1,108,878

Table 120C: Compensation to Collections Ratio (TC/NPP Excluded)

	Phys	Med Pracs	Mean	Std. Dev.	25th %tile	Median	75th %tile	90th %tile
Overall	230	65	.565	.138	.479	.556	.653	.736
Group Type								
Single Specialty	98	12	.571	.147	.474	.569	.685	.741
Multispecialty	132	53	.562	.131	.481	.550	.621	.728
Geographic Section (All Pracs)								
Eastern	30	11	.554	.112	.511	.544	.625	.664
Midwest	49	21	.563	.146	.468	.538	.612	.763
Southern	108	18	.586	.134	.491	.589	.684	.748
Western	43	15	.526	.151	.439	.516	.613	.734

Table 120D: Physician Work RVUs (CMS RBRVS Method) (NPP Excluded)

	Phys	Med Pracs	Mean	Std. Dev.	25th %tile	Median	75th %tile	90th %tile
Overall	256	84	8,604	3,126	6,437	8,222	10,417	12,848
Group Type								
Single Specialty	64	9	10,103	3,302	7,987	9,716	12,400	15,658
Multispecialty	192	75	8,105	2,906	6,089	7,761	9,965	12,220
Geographic Section (All Pracs)								
Eastern	61	17	9,174	3,664	6,386	9,492	11,598	15,045
Midwest	60	26	7,484	2,532	5,717	7,450	9,232	10,763
Southern	61	15	9,894	3,089	7,599	9,395	11,666	15,574
Western	74	26	7,979	2,642	6,293	7,921	9,627	12,107

Nonphysician Providers

Table 121: Nonphysician Provider Compensation

	NPPs	Med Pracs	Mean	Std. Dev.	25th %tile	Median	75th %tile	90th %tile
Audiologist	71	42	$77,575	$29,860	$57,276	$68,931	$94,000	$129,287
Cert Reg Nurse Anesthetist	1,669	60	$140,141	$24,151	$125,069	$140,000	$156,000	$171,000
Chiropractor	17	11	$113,774	$37,254	$90,723	$101,356	$135,457	$167,667
Dietician/Nutritionist	29	17	$47,531	$12,200	$36,327	$46,556	$56,590	$63,561
Midwife: Out-/In-patient	120	40	$85,998	$27,677	$69,880	$85,005	$94,650	$118,524
Midwife: Outpatient (only)	11	9	$72,418	$17,268	$58,385	$74,507	$85,633	$93,845
Midwife: Inpatient (only)	15	8	$81,515	$18,749	$67,583	$75,774	$95,235	$116,396
Nurse Practitioner	1,326	347	$78,595	$21,215	$66,483	$76,970	$90,000	$104,179
NP: Cardiology	26	13	$79,779	$15,570	$66,981	$79,583	$86,405	$101,495
NP: Family Practice (w/o OB)	38	13	$78,723	$31,274	$56,973	$76,461	$88,003	$114,314
NP: Gastroenterology	12	6	$74,784	$11,946	$65,732	$77,962	$82,146	$91,104
NP: Gerontology/Elder Health	16	5	$79,519	$7,145	$75,777	$80,435	$83,584	$90,172
NP: Hematology/Oncology	10	9	$93,209	$36,951	$73,143	$78,579	$99,791	$180,366
NP: Internal Medicine	55	24	$78,695	$21,357	$67,337	$78,945	$90,850	$98,415
NP: Pediatric/Child Health	51	21	$81,074	$28,934	$63,686	$80,258	$92,537	$129,257
NP: OB/GYN/Women's Health	60	26	$85,820	$32,166	$64,594	$79,138	$96,410	$128,431
Occupational Therapist	42	15	$59,163	$16,200	$47,644	$56,368	$71,131	$83,581
Optometrist	259	69	$140,558	$52,296	$107,970	$127,875	$161,285	$214,709
Perfusionist	12	4	$159,087	$44,279	$104,134	$183,787	$193,600	$196,664
Pharmacist	224	9	$105,276	$16,844	$100,552	$107,570	$115,669	$120,536
Physical Therapist	360	52	$67,543	$22,269	$55,155	$62,802	$74,437	$92,472
Physician Asst (surgical)	447	101	$97,207	$25,826	$81,089	$96,452	$109,600	$129,457
PA: Orthopedic	55	16	$93,550	$23,019	$78,555	$84,857	$104,443	$133,432
PA: Surg: General	11	7	$80,255	$13,576	$75,644	$81,778	$91,093	$94,208
Physician Asst (primary care)	707	185	$84,326	$26,379	$67,000	$81,052	$98,005	$116,253
PA: Family Practice (w/ OB)	50	17	$90,989	$34,188	$69,499	$86,226	$104,816	$145,166
PA: Family Practice (w/o OB)	42	8	$85,890	$17,155	$72,776	$85,357	$99,466	$105,948
PA: Internal Medicine	24	12	$73,365	$11,774	$61,500	$72,048	$82,036	$90,311
PA: Urgent Care	12	7	$99,642	$36,239	$79,083	$93,511	$100,408	$178,265
Phys Asst (nonsurg/nonprim care)	276	102	$84,173	$21,163	$72,635	$82,144	$93,883	$113,460
PA: Cardiology	11	6	$73,076	$20,840	$48,197	$77,907	$84,752	$108,018
Psychologist	228	45	$85,227	$34,514	$60,000	$83,423	$102,000	$130,594
Social Worker	154	27	$57,513	$22,129	$40,406	$53,023	$67,905	$81,248
Speech Therapist	7	3	*	*	*	*	*	*
Surgeon Assistant	12	8	$63,698	$19,110	$45,475	$61,744	$83,288	$89,130

Table 122: Nonphysician Provider Compensation by Group Type

	Single Specialty			Multispecialty		
	NPPs	Med Pracs	Median	NPPs	Med Pracs	Median
Audiologist	9	4	*	62	38	$71,086
Cert Reg Nurse Anesthetist	1,284	44	$140,000	385	16	$134,888
Chiropractor	1	1	*	16	10	$103,343
Dietician/Nutritionist	3	2	*	26	15	$42,672
Midwife: Out-/In-patient	20	6	$79,680	100	34	$85,051
Midwife: Outpatient (only)	3	3	*	8	6	*
Midwife: Inpatient (only)	7	3	*	8	5	*
Nurse Practitioner	273	141	$72,238	1,053	206	$77,987
NP: Cardiology	3	2	*	23	11	$79,829
NP: Family Practice (w/o OB)	1	1	*	37	12	$77,133
NP: Gastroenterology	*	*	*	12	6	$77,962
NP: Gerontology/Elder Health	*	*	*	16	5	$80,435
NP: Hematology/Oncology	*	*	*	10	9	$78,579
NP: Internal Medicine	*	*	*	55	24	$78,945
NP: Pediatric/Child Health	*	*	*	51	21	$80,258
NP: OB/GYN/Women's Health	5	3	*	55	23	$79,021
Occupational Therapist	5	3	*	37	12	$56,506
Optometrist	70	17	$137,831	189	52	$126,742
Perfusionist	*	*	*	12	4	$183,787
Pharmacist	2	1	*	222	8	$107,654
Physical Therapist	74	12	$71,420	286	40	$61,340
Physician Asst (surgical)	152	42	$92,457	295	59	$96,715
PA: Orthopedic	16	3	$79,828	39	13	$95,436
PA: Surg: General	*	*	*	11	7	$81,778
Physician Asst (primary care)	125	54	$78,090	582	131	$82,251
PA: Family Practice (w/ OB)	5	3	*	45	14	$88,873
PA: Family Practice (w/o OB)	*	*	*	42	8	$85,357
PA: Internal Medicine	*	*	*	24	12	$72,048
PA: Urgent Care	*	*	*	12	7	$93,511
Phys Asst (nonsurg/nonprim care)	112	45	$84,051	164	57	$80,815
PA: Cardiology	2	1	*	9	5	*
Psychologist	43	4	$47,008	185	41	$87,608
Social Worker	48	4	$40,100	106	23	$60,008
Speech Therapist	0	*	*	7	3	*
Surgeon Assistant	10	6	$66,599	2	2	*

Table 123: Nonphysician Provider Compensation by Hospital Ownership

	Hospital Owned			Not Hospital Owned		
	NPPs	Med Pracs	Median	NPPs	Med Pracs	Median
Audiologist	12	8	$73,077	59	34	$66,758
Cert Reg Nurse Anesthetist	154	5	$140,608	1,515	55	$140,000
Chiropractor	7	4	*	10	7	$114,833
Dietician/Nutritionist	4	2	*	25	15	$46,903
Midwife: Out-/In-patient	58	16	$84,138	62	24	$86,491
Midwife: Outpatient (only)	4	3	*	7	6	*
Midwife: Inpatient (only)	3	2	*	12	6	$74,093
Nurse Practitioner	498	140	$77,014	828	207	$76,937
NP: Cardiology	7	3	*	19	10	$81,000
NP: Family Practice (w/o OB)	10	5	$73,894	28	8	$77,324
NP: Gastroenterology	3	2	*	9	4	*
NP: Gerontology/Elder Health	*	*	*	16	5	$80,435
NP: Hematology/Oncology	1	1	*	9	8	*
NP: Internal Medicine	29	9	$80,749	26	15	$76,336
NP: Pediatric/Child Health	30	7	$74,642	21	14	$82,621
NP: OB/GYN/Women's Health	14	8	$78,382	46	18	$80,364
Occupational Therapist	14	4	$50,527	28	11	$64,250
Optometrist	60	16	$122,400	199	53	$128,696
Perfusionist	12	4	$183,787	*	*	*
Pharmacist	194	1	*	30	8	$109,025
Physical Therapist	157	8	$56,841	203	44	$70,741
Physician Asst (surgical)	87	25	$103,360	360	76	$94,025
PA: Orthopedic	13	3	$79,935	42	13	$88,794
PA: Surg: General	3	2	*	8	5	*
Physician Asst (primary care)	362	100	$84,296	345	85	$78,704
PA: Family Practice (w/ OB)	27	9	$77,301	23	8	$96,788
PA: Family Practice (w/o OB)	5	1	*	37	7	$82,926
PA: Internal Medicine	1	1	*	23	11	$71,998
PA: Urgent Care	4	3	*	8	4	*
Phys Asst (nonsurg/nonprim care)	53	31	$77,398	223	71	$82,763
PA: Cardiology	2	1	*	9	5	*
Psychologist	71	15	$86,937	157	30	$77,682
Social Worker	33	7	$57,026	121	20	$51,518
Speech Therapist	6	2	*	1	1	*
Surgeon Assistant	1	1	*	11	7	$64,814

Table 124: Nonphysician Provider Compensation by Geographic Section

	Eastern		Midwest		Southern		Western	
	NPPs	Median	NPPs	Median	NPPs	Median	NPPs	Median
Audiologist	18	$64,496	25	$69,554	14	$69,580	14	$71,980
Cert Reg Nurse Anesthetist	500	$137,800	412	$140,608	662	$140,000	95	$141,005
Chiropractor	1	*	12	$99,563	2	*	2	*
Dietician/Nutritionist	8	*	13	$38,556	4	*	4	*
Midwife: Out-/In-patient	15	$81,042	38	$92,333	38	$76,987	29	$79,048
Midwife: Outpatient (only)	4	*	1	*	3	*	3	*
Midwife: Inpatient (only)	6	*	6	*	*	*	3	*
Nurse Practitioner	366	$74,373	436	$77,033	250	$78,937	274	$80,160
NP: Cardiology	7	*	7	*	5	*	7	*
NP: Family Practice (w/o OB)	1	*	23	$72,000	8	*	6	*
NP: Gastroenterology	7	*	5	*	*	*	*	*
NP: Gerontology/Elder Health	2	*	11	*	1	*	2	*
NP: Hematology/Oncology	2	*	5	*	2	*	1	*
NP: Internal Medicine	21	$79,953	21	$77,929	9	*	4	*
NP: Pediatric/Child Health	9	*	27	$85,126	13	$65,106	2	*
NP: OB/GYN/Women's Health	8	*	26	$88,051	12	$73,697	14	$87,502
Occupational Therapist	6	*	7	*	13	$50,369	16	$71,687
Optometrist	40	$109,772	103	$144,234	49	$131,960	67	$126,731
Perfusionist	4	*	*	*	3	*	5	*
Pharmacist	1	*	200	*	6	*	17	$106,149
Physical Therapist	35	$64,700	209	$60,299	65	$60,063	51	$70,907
Physician Asst (surgical)	164	$98,679	117	$89,491	46	$95,898	120	$96,864
PA: Orthopedic	16	$82,310	14	$83,672	8	*	17	$102,310
PA: Surg: General	5	*	1	*	4	*	1	*
Physician Asst (primary care)	201	$76,700	239	$80,145	94	$84,475	173	$85,804
PA: Family Practice (w/ OB)	12	$65,687	28	$95,028	8	*	2	*
PA: Family Practice (w/o OB)	7	*	14	$96,915	12	*	9	*
PA: Internal Medicine	12	$63,000	5	*	3	*	4	*
PA: Urgent Care	*	*	7	*	*	*	5	*
Phys Asst (nonsurg/nonprim care)	78	$76,327	105	$81,262	42	$80,469	51	$89,979
PA: Cardiology	6	*	1	*	3	*	1	*
Psychologist	43	$85,500	161	$80,072	10	$108,873	14	$102,692
Social Worker	20	$58,424	108	$51,746	13	$51,124	13	$53,292
Speech Therapist	*	*	3	*	4	*	*	*
Surgeon Assistant	*	*	4	*	2	*	6	*

Table 125A: Nonphysician Provider Compensation by Size of Practice (50 or fewer FTE Physicians)

	4 or fewer		5 to 10		11 to 25		26 to 50	
	NPPs	Median	NPPs	Median	NPPs	Median	NPPs	Median
Audiologist	4	*	14	$59,358	1	*	12	$60,626
Cert Reg Nurse Anesthetist	6	*	144	$132,463	405	$137,800	162	$171,000
Chiropractor	3	*	*	*	0	*	2	*
Dietician/Nutritionist	1	*	*	*	4	*	9	*
Midwife: Out-/In-patient	7	*	15	$89,505	11	$72,415	16	$88,514
Midwife: Outpatient (only)	*	*	2	*	2	*	2	*
Midwife: Inpatient (only)	*	*	7	*	6	*	1	*
Nurse Practitioner	103	$72,549	132	$70,100	166	$79,149	192	$77,587
NP: Cardiology	2	*	*	*	1	*	*	*
NP: Family Practice (w/o OB)	*	*	6	*	*	*	7	*
NP: Gerontology/Elder Health	*	*	*	*	1	*	1	*
NP: Hematology/Oncology	*	*	*	*	1	*	*	*
NP: Internal Medicine	*	*	*	*	6	*	5	*
NP: Pediatric/Child Health	*	*	*	*	4	*	16	$86,020
NP: OB/GYN/Women's Health	1	*	1	*	5	*	13	$79,927
Occupational Therapist	1	*	2	*	3	*	1	*
Optometrist	18	$128,948	30	$139,582	29	$149,749	8	*
Pharmacist	*	*	*	*	5	*	*	*
Physical Therapist	3	*	20	$72,688	46	$71,119	18	$74,550
Physician Asst (surgical)	8	*	83	$90,985	81	$103,134	58	$104,426
PA: Orthopedic	4	*	*	*	12	*	3	*
Physician Asst (primary care)	53	$79,869	73	$82,800	90	$75,992	126	$74,608
PA: Family Practice (w/ OB)	7	*	*	*	1	*	10	$103,686
PA: Family Practice (w/o OB)	*	*	*	*	*	*	6	*
PA: Internal Medicine	*	*	*	*	1	*	8	*
PA: Urgent Care	*	*	*	*	2	*	1	*
Phys Asst (nonsurg/nonprim care)	16	$76,609	36	$88,369	42	$79,964	39	$84,926
PA: Cardiology	2	*	*	*	*	*	*	*
Psychologist	2	*	9	*	7	*	52	$49,289
Social Worker	1	*	1	*	15	$49,065	44	$40,100
Speech Therapist	0	*	*	*	*	*	*	*
Surgeon Assistant	*	*	7	*	4	*	*	*

Table 125B: Nonphysician Provider Compensation by Size of Practice (51 or more FTE Physicians)

	51 to 75		76 to 100		101 to 150		151 or more	
	NPPs	Median	NPPs	Median	NPPs	Median	NPPs	Median
Audiologist	12	$66,742	3	*	9	*	16	$95,863
Cert Reg Nurse Anesthetist	528	$140,000	2	*	173	*	249	$140,608
Chiropractor	1	*	0	*	*	*	11	$101,356
Dietician/Nutritionist	4	*	4	*	1	*	6	*
Midwife: Out-/In-patient	14	$73,475	7	*	8	*	42	$84,781
Midwife: Outpatient (only)	1	*	1	*	*	*	3	*
Midwife: Inpatient (only)	*	*	1	*	*	*	*	*
Nurse Practitioner	158	$77,416	82	$76,418	124	$74,053	369	$80,181
NP: Cardiology	2	*	8	*	9	*	4	*
NP: Family Practice (w/o OB)	2	*	1	*	12	$77,324	10	*
NP: Gastroenterology	*	*	3	*	3	*	6	*
NP: Gerontology/Elder Health	*	*	*	*	2	*	12	*
NP: Hematology/Oncology	2	*	2	*	1	*	4	*
NP: Internal Medicine	4	*	19	$80,749	12	$70,613	9	*
NP: Pediatric/Child Health	3	*	8	*	10	$65,687	10	$91,012
NP: OB/GYN/Women's Health	1	*	1	*	12	$72,908	26	$94,856
Occupational Therapist	6	*	2	*	23	$63,565	4	*
Optometrist	11	$149,986	7	*	17	$122,427	139	$125,992
Perfusionist	*	*	5	*	3	*	4	*
Pharmacist	18	$105,665	6	*	1	*	194	*
Physical Therapist	39	$66,607	16	$76,175	96	$65,414	122	$56,110
Physician Asst (surgical)	26	$80,523	26	$97,458	43	$90,000	122	$97,363
PA: Orthopedic	5	*	1	*	11	$100,599	19	$102,310
PA: Surg: General	*	*	2	*	6	*	3	*
Physician Asst (primary care)	58	$70,964	66	$91,227	34	$79,294	207	$86,550
PA: Family Practice (w/ OB)	5	*	10	*	*	*	17	$88,873
PA: Family Practice (w/o OB)	4	*	*	*	28	$77,917	4	*
PA: Internal Medicine	3	*	2	*	10	$72,185	*	*
PA: Urgent Care	3	*	1	*	1	*	4	*
Phys Asst (nonsurg/nonprim care)	47	$82,282	18	$74,804	30	$82,317	48	$79,943
PA: Cardiology	2	*	4	*	2	*	1	*
Psychologist	19	$97,152	13	$95,978	6	*	120	$86,938
Social Worker	14	$70,573	29	$58,011	11	*	39	$60,339
Speech Therapist	*	*	1	*	4	*	2	*
Surgeon Assistant	*	*	1	*	*	*	*	*

Table 126: Nonphysician Provider Compensation by Years in Specialty

	1 to 2 years		3 to 7 years		8 to 17 years		18 years or more	
	NPPs	Median	NPPs	Median	NPPs	Median	NPPs	Median
Audiologist	4	*	15	$71,105	14	$62,882	18	$68,422
Cert Reg Nurse Anesthetist	100	$150,311	272	$139,000	551	$141,418	349	$140,000
Chiropractor	1	*	0	*	7	*	2	*
Dietician/Nutritionist	3	*	4	*	6	*	3	*
Midwife: Out-/In-patient	3	*	13	$84,640	19	$88,192	6	*
Midwife: Outpatient (only)	1	*	3	*	*	*	1	*
Midwife: Inpatient (only)	1	*	1	*	8	*	3	*
Nurse Practitioner	96	$70,719	265	$75,266	336	$78,204	87	$81,664
NP: Cardiology	3	*	12	$82,823	3	*	1	*
NP: Family Practice (w/o OB)	3	*	8	*	8	*	3	*
NP: Gastroenterology	4	*	2	*	2	*	*	*
NP: Gerontology/Elder Health	1	*	*	*	3	*	2	*
NP: Hematology/Oncology	1	*	3	*	2	*	*	*
NP: Internal Medicine	3	*	11	$80,749	20	$79,449	6	*
NP: Pediatric/Child Health	1	*	4	*	13	$73,792	7	*
NP: OB/GYN/Women's Health	2	*	9	*	16	$74,597	11	$83,694
Occupational Therapist	1	*	8	*	7	*	2	*
Optometrist	7	*	35	$117,471	69	$126,005	77	$130,460
Perfusionist	*	*	1	*	*	*	*	*
Pharmacist	*	*	1	*	4	*	7	*
Physical Therapist	11	$65,909	40	$68,632	41	$73,029	40	$80,426
Physician Asst (surgical)	42	$79,163	88	$94,028	68	$101,151	31	$102,400
PA: Orthopedic	3	*	12	$80,772	11	$100,599	11	$82,305
PA: Surg: General	*	*	2	*	3	*	3	*
Physician Asst (primary care)	48	$74,195	129	$75,397	176	$84,227	61	$85,000
PA: Family Practice (w/ OB)	6	*	5	*	7	*	5	*
PA: Family Practice (w/o OB)	3	*	8	*	11	$86,115	4	*
PA: Internal Medicine	4	*	6	*	5	*	4	*
PA: Urgent Care	2	*	1	*	2	*	3	*
Phys Asst (nonsurg/nonprim care)	30	$78,270	71	$80,081	39	$79,990	28	$81,252
PA: Cardiology	1	*	*	*	5	*	1	*
Psychologist	5	*	37	$82,999	41	$92,478	40	$100,151
Social Worker	2	*	4	*	19	$72,802	22	$62,485
Speech Therapist	*	*	*	*	1	*	*	*
Surgeon Assistant	*	*	2	*	4	*	4	*

Table 127: Nonphysician Provider Compensation by Gender

	Male			Female		
	NPPs	Med Pracs	Median	NPPs	Med Pracs	Median
Audiologist	19	16	$91,996	51	30	$63,894
Cert Reg Nurse Anesthetist	178	25	$144,155	312	28	$132,463
Chiropractor	9	7	*	4	4	*
Dietician/Nutritionist	*	*	*	29	17	$46,556
Midwife: Out-/In-patient	*	*	*	82	35	$87,240
Midwife: Outpatient (only)	*	*	*	11	9	$74,507
Midwife: Inpatient (only)	1	1	*	13	7	$76,579
Nurse Practitioner	87	49	$85,430	1,110	322	$76,340
NP: Cardiology	2	2	*	23	12	$79,829
NP: Family Practice (w/o OB)	1	1	*	37	13	$75,788
NP: Gastroenterology	2	2	*	9	4	*
NP: Gerontology/Elder Health	1	1	*	15	4	$81,469
NP: Hematology/Oncology	*	*	*	10	9	$78,579
NP: Internal Medicine	1	1	*	54	23	$78,437
NP: Pediatric/Child Health	*	*	*	37	20	$73,792
NP: OB/GYN/Women's Health	*	*	*	59	25	$79,021
Occupational Therapist	7	3	*	23	12	$56,229
Optometrist	140	59	$147,217	61	38	$109,894
Perfusionist	7	3	*	2	2	*
Pharmacist	104	8	$111,808	120	7	$103,646
Physical Therapist	131	42	$72,923	149	34	$57,135
Physician Asst (surgical)	229	75	$102,400	196	71	$88,955
PA: Orthopedic	41	15	$89,231	14	9	$82,594
PA: Surg: General	3	2	*	8	6	*
Physician Asst (primary care)	238	115	$91,261	400	140	$75,034
PA: Family Practice (w/ OB)	16	11	$89,231	24	13	$86,841
PA: Family Practice (w/o OB)	10	5	$100,222	32	7	$80,360
PA: Internal Medicine	4	3	*	20	10	$68,448
PA: Urgent Care	5	5	*	7	5	*
Phys Asst (nonsurg/nonprim care)	78	45	$89,219	150	73	$78,359
PA: Cardiology	3	3	*	8	5	*
Psychologist	112	33	$93,906	90	29	$70,955
Social Worker	41	16	$61,192	94	21	$50,629
Speech Therapist	*	*	*	1	1	*
Surgeon Assistant	4	3	*	7	6	*

Table 128: Nonphysician Provider Retirement Benefits

	NPPs	Med Pracs	Mean	Std. Dev.	25th %tile	Median	75th %tile	90th %tile
Audiologist	56	33	$5,327	$2,571	$3,369	$4,800	$7,051	$9,134
Cert Reg Nurse Anesthetist	1,372	51	$16,846	$7,237	$11,300	$17,135	$20,435	$23,824
Chiropractor	11	7	$7,503	$4,778	$3,075	$7,195	$10,423	$16,402
Dietician/Nutritionist	16	11	$3,064	$1,722	$1,701	$3,197	$4,118	$5,793
Midwife: Out-/In-patient	72	32	$5,980	$3,212	$3,161	$4,948	$7,726	$10,673
Midwife: Outpatient (only)	8	8	*	*	*	*	*	*
Midwife: Inpatient (only)	13	6	$5,558	$3,370	$3,216	$3,832	$9,311	$10,811
Nurse Practitioner	891	278	$5,852	$3,762	$3,230	$4,744	$7,688	$10,905
NP: Cardiology	22	11	$5,179	$2,121	$3,540	$5,528	$6,928	$7,880
NP: Family Practice (w/o OB)	28	8	$3,964	$1,857	$2,853	$3,930	$4,850	$6,207
NP: Gastroenterology	8	4	*	*	*	*	*	*
NP: Gerontology/Elder Health	14	4	$5,242	$797	$4,512	$5,037	$5,975	$6,340
NP: Hematology/Oncology	7	7	*	*	*	*	*	*
NP: Internal Medicine	51	23	$6,802	$4,434	$3,312	$5,845	$8,350	$14,427
NP: Pediatric/Child Health	50	20	$5,163	$2,699	$3,155	$4,854	$6,540	$9,330
NP: OB/GYN/Women's Health	49	22	$6,551	$3,300	$4,036	$6,185	$8,580	$12,137
Occupational Therapist	15	10	$3,452	$1,758	$2,143	$2,769	$5,139	$6,557
Optometrist	188	54	$14,387	$9,423	$7,211	$11,388	$19,725	$32,064
Perfusionist	5	2	*	*	*	*	*	*
Pharmacist	28	7	$5,962	$2,733	$4,733	$4,990	$8,693	$9,947
Physical Therapist	167	37	$5,801	$3,252	$3,488	$5,050	$7,090	$10,515
Physician Asst (surgical)	266	80	$7,502	$3,432	$4,844	$7,075	$9,627	$11,840
PA: Orthopedic	55	15	$7,639	$3,908	$4,273	$7,337	$9,251	$14,179
PA: Surg: General	11	7	$4,600	$2,409	$3,496	$4,555	$4,736	$9,765
Physician Asst (primary care)	499	147	$6,253	$3,966	$3,093	$5,391	$8,521	$11,768
PA: Family Practice (w/ OB)	37	15	$6,571	$3,671	$3,642	$5,931	$8,660	$12,166
PA: Family Practice (w/o OB)	30	5	$4,762	$1,466	$3,726	$4,361	$5,462	$7,261
PA: Internal Medicine	19	10	$4,270	$1,835	$3,000	$3,488	$5,998	$7,272
PA: Urgent Care	9	6	*	*	*	*	*	*
Phys Asst (nonsurg/nonprim care)	198	83	$6,670	$4,522	$3,476	$5,419	$8,926	$13,252
PA: Cardiology	11	6	$5,573	$4,594	$1,870	$4,850	$7,607	$14,748
Psychologist	137	31	$7,840	$3,763	$5,231	$6,886	$9,990	$13,034
Social Worker	65	16	$5,177	$4,791	$3,061	$4,079	$5,897	$9,080
Speech Therapist	3	2	*	*	*	*	*	*
Surgeon Assistant	10	7	$5,581	$2,369	$3,394	$6,373	$7,550	$8,202

Table 129: Nonphysician Provider Retirement Benefits by Group Type

	Single Specialty			Multispecialty		
	NPPs	Med Pracs	Median	NPPs	Med Pracs	Median
Audiologist	9	4	*	47	29	$5,560
Cert Reg Nurse Anesthetist	1,200	41	$15,230	172	10	$18,338
Chiropractor	1	1	*	10	6	$7,258
Dietician/Nutritionist	3	2	*	13	9	$3,274
Midwife: Out-/In-patient	19	6	$4,670	53	26	$5,292
Midwife: Outpatient (only)	3	3	*	5	5	*
Midwife: Inpatient (only)	7	3	*	6	3	*
Nurse Practitioner	216	122	$4,406	675	156	$4,850
NP: Cardiology	3	2	*	19	9	$5,609
NP: Family Practice (w/o OB)	0	*	*	28	8	$3,930
NP: Gastroenterology	*	*	*	8	4	*
NP: Gerontology/Elder Health	*	*	*	14	4	$5,037
NP: Hematology/Oncology	*	*	*	7	7	*
NP: Internal Medicine	*	*	*	51	23	$5,845
NP: Pediatric/Child Health	*	*	*	50	20	$4,854
NP: OB/GYN/Women's Health	4	2	*	45	20	$6,185
Occupational Therapist	4	3	*	11	7	$2,739
Optometrist	43	12	$9,039	145	42	$12,185
Perfusionist	*	*	*	5	2	*
Pharmacist	2	1	*	26	6	$5,060
Physical Therapist	45	9	$5,435	122	28	$4,960
Physician Asst (surgical)	126	36	$6,937	140	44	$7,128
PA: Orthopedic	16	3	$7,831	39	12	$7,126
PA: Surg: General	*	*	*	11	7	$4,555
Physician Asst (primary care)	102	49	$3,508	397	98	$5,876
PA: Family Practice (w/ OB)	4	3	*	33	12	$6,555
PA: Family Practice (w/o OB)	*	*	*	30	5	$4,361
PA: Internal Medicine	*	*	*	19	10	$3,488
PA: Urgent Care	*	*	*	9	6	*
Phys Asst (nonsurg/nonprim care)	87	39	$6,535	111	44	$4,932
PA: Cardiology	2	1	*	9	5	*
Psychologist	4	3	*	133	28	$6,947
Social Worker	8	3	*	57	13	$4,371
Speech Therapist	0	*	*	3	2	*
Surgeon Assistant	8	5	*	2	2	*

page 267

Table 130: Nonphysician Provider Collections for Professional Charges (TC Excluded)

	NPPs	Med Pracs	Mean	Std. Dev.	25th %tile	Median	75th %tile	90th %tile
Audiologist	27	19	$143,347	$104,654	$53,718	$133,534	$213,575	$320,893
Cert Reg Nurse Anesthetist	199	15	$190,915	$66,842	$128,053	$219,103	$240,932	$253,551
Chiropractor	5	4	*	*	*	*	*	*
Dietician/Nutritionist	14	10	$61,458	$30,536	$39,376	$62,681	$81,502	$106,584
Midwife: Out-/In-patient	39	21	$223,982	$105,293	$161,630	$219,783	$285,999	$334,864
Midwife: Outpatient (only)	8	6	*	*	*	*	*	*
Midwife: Inpatient (only)	4	3	*	*	*	*	*	*
Nurse Practitioner	612	188	$185,876	$103,623	$107,968	$180,218	$254,773	$324,630
NP: Cardiology	14	8	$109,929	$66,589	$51,463	$90,256	$151,210	$225,702
NP: Family Practice (w/o OB)	25	8	$192,298	$82,185	$133,001	$178,654	$245,705	$330,483
NP: Gastroenterology	6	3	*	*	*	*	*	*
NP: Gerontology/Elder Health	5	3	*	*	*	*	*	*
NP: Hematology/Oncology	7	7	*	*	*	*	*	*
NP: Internal Medicine	47	18	$176,408	$71,657	$124,520	$163,846	$235,969	$294,057
NP: Pediatric/Child Health	28	15	$221,374	$86,494	$147,061	$201,865	$273,668	$354,116
NP: OB/GYN/Women's Health	33	18	$178,601	$89,783	$122,048	$168,698	$238,850	$281,086
Occupational Therapist	25	10	$146,515	$115,744	$80,255	$107,873	$155,648	$319,135
Optometrist	93	34	$327,649	$136,361	$237,087	$316,906	$402,056	$481,958
Perfusionist	1	1	*	*	*	*	*	*
Pharmacist	2	2	*	*	*	*	*	*
Physical Therapist	135	30	$213,739	$103,024	$142,344	$190,002	$271,456	$367,422
Physician Asst (surgical)	178	59	$181,844	$138,086	$85,715	$143,723	$238,592	$348,299
PA: Orthopedic	39	14	$205,949	$128,595	$99,945	$189,577	$287,825	$420,837
PA: Surg: General	10	6	$91,475	$41,527	$69,627	$88,135	$131,980	$145,608
Physician Asst (primary care)	291	100	$230,742	$127,583	$136,513	$217,584	$315,685	$411,805
PA: Family Practice (w/ OB)	23	13	$210,081	$110,003	$128,485	$210,822	$280,670	$377,562
PA: Family Practice (w/o OB)	30	4	$292,987	$87,731	$242,287	$297,401	$357,277	$398,917
PA: Internal Medicine	16	7	$229,567	$80,617	$167,062	$213,213	$251,170	$396,615
PA: Urgent Care	7	4	*	*	*	*	*	*
Phys Asst (nonsurg/nonprim care)	106	49	$215,631	$137,356	$106,982	$207,099	$316,156	$380,846
PA: Cardiology	7	5	*	*	*	*	*	*
Psychologist	70	22	$124,175	$66,590	$76,477	$121,049	$175,039	$214,756
Social Worker	35	11	$126,201	$53,880	$92,222	$126,270	$153,985	$177,066
Speech Therapist	1	1	*	*	*	*	*	*
Surgeon Assistant	11	7	$46,407	$18,855	$36,367	$44,698	$52,604	$82,530

Table 131: Nonphysician Provider Collections for Professional Charges (TC Excluded) by Group Type

	Single Specialty			Multispecialty		
	NPPs	Med Pracs	Median	NPPs	Med Pracs	Median
Audiologist	3	1	*	24	18	$108,080
Cert Reg Nurse Anesthetist	187	9	$219,103	12	6	$102,580
Chiropractor	1	1	*	4	3	*
Dietician/Nutritionist	1	1	*	13	9	$62,473
Midwife: Out-/In-patient	6	2	*	33	19	$205,099
Midwife: Outpatient (only)	2	2	*	6	4	*
Midwife: Inpatient (only)	0	*	*	4	3	*
Nurse Practitioner	118	79	$171,633	494	109	$181,755
NP: Cardiology	3	2	*	11	6	$90,913
NP: Family Practice (w/o OB)	0	*	*	25	8	$178,654
NP: Gastroenterology	*	*	*	6	3	*
NP: Gerontology/Elder Health	*	*	*	5	3	*
NP: Hematology/Oncology	*	*	*	7	7	*
NP: Internal Medicine	*	*	*	47	18	$163,846
NP: Pediatric/Child Health	*	*	*	28	15	$201,865
NP: OB/GYN/Women's Health	2	2	*	31	16	$168,698
Occupational Therapist	5	3	*	20	7	$100,189
Optometrist	8	4	*	85	30	$316,962
Perfusionist	*	*	*	1	1	*
Pharmacist	0	*	*	2	2	*
Physical Therapist	30	8	$329,676	105	22	$183,303
Physician Asst (surgical)	84	28	$125,876	94	31	$147,693
PA: Orthopedic	5	3	*	34	11	$192,164
PA: Surg: General	*	*	*	10	6	$88,135
Physician Asst (primary care)	67	30	$251,282	224	70	$209,233
PA: Family Practice (w/ OB)	5	3	*	18	10	$227,368
PA: Family Practice (w/o OB)	*	*	*	30	4	$297,401
PA: Internal Medicine	*	*	*	16	7	$213,213
PA: Urgent Care	*	*	*	7	4	*
Phys Asst (nonsurg/nonprim care)	29	17	$70,575	77	32	$217,874
PA: Cardiology	2	1	*	5	4	*
Psychologist	1	1	*	69	21	$121,641
Social Worker	2	2	*	33	9	$128,316
Speech Therapist	0	*	*	1	1	*
Surgeon Assistant	9	5	*	2	2	*

Table 132: Nonphysician Provider Compensation to Collections Ratio (TC Excluded)

	NPPs	Med Pracs	Mean	Std. Dev.	25th %tile	Median	75th %tile	90th %tile
Audiologist	17	12	.450	.246	.224	.358	.659	.842
Cert Reg Nurse Anesthetist	143	12	.686	.151	.552	.745	.780	.780
Chiropractor	5	4	*	*	*	*	*	*
Dietician/Nutritionist	12	9	.618	.204	.458	.593	.786	.950
Midwife: Out-/In-patient	34	21	.419	.131	.323	.373	.472	.642
Midwife: Outpatient (only)	6	5	*	*	*	*	*	*
Midwife: Inpatient (only)	4	3	*	*	*	*	*	*
Nurse Practitioner	513	170	.422	.177	.296	.369	.512	.690
NP: Cardiology	9	6	*	*	*	*	*	*
NP: Family Practice (w/o OB)	25	8	.423	.128	.316	.405	.517	.622
NP: Gastroenterology	6	3	*	*	*	*	*	*
NP: Gerontology/Elder Health	1	1	*	*	*	*	*	*
NP: Hematology/Oncology	6	6	*	*	*	*	*	*
NP: Internal Medicine	47	18	.474	.176	.360	.433	.489	.831
NP: Pediatric/Child Health	30	16	.330	.104	.267	.308	.376	.459
NP: OB/GYN/Women's Health	29	17	.403	.131	.317	.375	.457	.613
Occupational Therapist	25	11	.562	.251	.359	.498	.818	.961
Optometrist	91	34	.490	.166	.377	.480	.619	.713
Perfusionist	1	1	*	*	*	*	*	*
Pharmacist	2	2	*	*	*	*	*	*
Physical Therapist	133	30	.370	.151	.267	.336	.439	.590
Physician Asst (surgical)	137	51	.549	.245	.363	.477	.783	.899
PA: Orthopedic	35	11	.477	.192	.324	.439	.568	.798
PA: Surg: General	5	4	*	*	*	*	*	*
Physician Asst (primary care)	251	96	.364	.150	.261	.317	.432	.562
PA: Family Practice (w/ OB)	20	13	.386	.127	.283	.356	.452	.630
PA: Family Practice (w/o OB)	30	4	.305	.097	.248	.278	.321	.459
PA: Internal Medicine	16	7	.332	.077	.290	.342	.385	.425
PA: Urgent Care	7	4	*	*	*	*	*	*
Phys Asst (nonsurg/nonprim care)	86	43	.384	.153	.285	.344	.451	.627
PA: Cardiology	3	3	*	*	*	*	*	*
Psychologist	52	20	.650	.147	.519	.621	.793	.875
Social Worker	32	8	.559	.147	.437	.554	.656	.773
Speech Therapist	1	1	*	*	*	*	*	*
Surgeon Assistant	2	2	*	*	*	*	*	*

Table 133: Nonphysician Provider Gross Charges (TC Excluded)

	NPPs	Med Pracs	Mean	Std. Dev.	25th %tile	Median	75th %tile	90th %tile
Audiologist	33	22	$231,081	$145,326	$112,972	$199,930	$304,959	$484,024
Cert Reg Nurse Anesthetist	453	19	$263,822	$199,859	$60,069	$247,260	$472,135	$524,048
Chiropractor	10	6	$470,384	$203,435	$364,610	$410,454	$480,512	$969,897
Dietician/Nutritionist	20	11	$76,796	$54,227	$29,660	$73,222	$107,076	$163,547
Midwife: Out-/In-patient	56	27	$403,103	$172,221	$279,361	$372,088	$486,926	$613,608
Midwife: Outpatient (only)	8	6	*	*	*	*	*	*
Midwife: Inpatient (only)	4	3	*	*	*	*	*	*
Nurse Practitioner	797	209	$303,393	$164,166	$187,850	$288,063	$398,597	$531,377
NP: Cardiology	16	10	$193,199	$112,065	$100,582	$130,303	$271,501	$386,781
NP: Family Practice (w/o OB)	33	10	$304,266	$159,065	$188,090	$284,650	$376,545	$581,293
NP: Gastroenterology	10	5	$327,129	$118,857	$229,200	$341,116	$409,544	$519,315
NP: Gerontology/Elder Health	15	4	$170,743	$36,179	$140,902	$176,900	$200,884	$216,072
NP: Hematology/Oncology	9	8	*	*	*	*	*	*
NP: Internal Medicine	45	19	$284,121	$106,607	$206,836	$250,610	$355,221	$467,825
NP: Pediatric/Child Health	34	18	$394,228	$183,377	$236,487	$361,031	$534,979	$717,956
NP: OB/GYN/Women's Health	49	20	$310,569	$116,365	$225,769	$294,700	$381,140	$482,219
Occupational Therapist	27	12	$300,664	$170,662	$187,519	$253,043	$323,950	$549,464
Optometrist	138	44	$509,266	$192,144	$361,828	$502,197	$610,810	$787,794
Perfusionist	1	1	*	*	*	*	*	*
Pharmacist	2	2	*	*	*	*	*	*
Physical Therapist	156	35	$394,106	$186,603	$265,780	$361,200	$489,893	$662,490
Physician Asst (surgical)	235	68	$436,671	$301,550	$206,830	$355,391	$605,761	$876,626
PA: Orthopedic	42	13	$609,770	$366,945	$323,943	$501,788	$834,718	$1,249,305
PA: Surg: General	10	6	$403,836	$261,860	$225,374	$370,209	$568,315	$843,020
Physician Asst (primary care)	387	115	$373,386	$188,988	$232,425	$354,742	$480,346	$651,660
PA: Family Practice (w/ OB)	42	15	$397,946	$177,284	$242,868	$424,719	$512,135	$635,685
PA: Family Practice (w/o OB)	35	5	$461,178	$145,257	$332,524	$476,909	$558,173	$649,601
PA: Internal Medicine	14	7	$369,105	$132,871	$291,834	$354,562	$397,949	$613,667
PA: Urgent Care	7	4	*	*	*	*	*	*
Phys Asst (nonsurg/nonprim care)	139	58	$329,325	$227,127	$131,963	$312,816	$448,320	$697,757
PA: Cardiology	7	5	*	*	*	*	*	*
Psychologist	156	28	$227,221	$100,018	$165,612	$224,638	$286,669	$367,604
Social Worker	77	17	$203,535	$70,954	$147,997	$206,075	$252,125	$293,798
Speech Therapist	3	2	*	*	*	*	*	*
Surgeon Assistant	11	7	$103,535	$89,983	$41,591	$80,981	$164,878	$288,410

Table 134: Nonphysician Provider Gross Charges (TC Excluded) by Group Type

	Single Specialty			Multispecialty		
	NPPs	Med Pracs	Median	NPPs	Med Pracs	Median
Audiologist	3	1	*	30	21	$193,379
Cert Reg Nurse Anesthetist	330	9	$322,447	123	10	$126,098
Chiropractor	1	1	*	9	5	*
Dietician/Nutritionist	1	1	*	19	10	$72,935
Midwife: Out-/In-patient	6	2	*	50	25	$371,386
Midwife: Outpatient (only)	2	2	*	6	4	*
Midwife: Inpatient (only)	0	*	*	4	3	*
Nurse Practitioner	119	79	$266,258	678	130	$291,911
NP: Cardiology	2	2	*	14	8	$130,303
NP: Family Practice (w/o OB)	0	*	*	33	10	$284,650
NP: Gastroenterology	*	*	*	10	5	$341,116
NP: Gerontology/Elder Health	*	*	*	15	4	$176,900
NP: Hematology/Oncology	*	*	*	9	8	*
NP: Internal Medicine	*	*	*	45	19	$250,610
NP: Pediatric/Child Health	*	*	*	34	18	$361,031
NP: OB/GYN/Women's Health	2	2	*	47	18	$294,700
Occupational Therapist	5	3	*	22	9	$244,749
Optometrist	8	4	*	130	40	$506,982
Perfusionist	*	*	*	1	1	*
Pharmacist	0	*	*	2	2	*
Physical Therapist	30	8	$525,555	126	27	$335,308
Physician Asst (surgical)	82	28	$487,479	153	40	$300,885
PA: Orthopedic	5	1	*	37	12	$536,602
PA: Surg: General	*	*	*	10	6	$370,209
Physician Asst (primary care)	69	30	$380,953	318	85	$348,048
PA: Family Practice (w/ OB)	5	3	*	37	12	$436,660
PA: Family Practice (w/o OB)	*	*	*	35	5	$476,909
PA: Internal Medicine	*	*	*	14	7	$354,562
PA: Urgent Care	*	*	*	7	4	*
Phys Asst (nonsurg/nonprim care)	33	18	$155,445	106	40	$336,768
PA: Cardiology	2	1	*	5	4	*
Psychologist	2	2	*	154	26	$225,668
Social Worker	2	2	*	75	15	$207,617
Speech Therapist	0	*	*	3	2	*
Surgeon Assistant	9	5	*	2	2	*

Table 135: Nonphysician Provider Gross Charges (TC Excluded) by Geographic Section

	Eastern		Midwest		Southern		Western	
	NPPs	Median	NPPs	Median	NPPs	Median	NPPs	Median
Audiologist	10	$222,881	12	$186,802	5	*	6	*
Cert Reg Nurse Anesthetist	176	$60,069	162	$466,648	108	$429,072	7	*
Chiropractor	1	*	8	*	1	*	0	*
Dietician/Nutritionist	4	*	12	$58,285	3	*	1	*
Midwife: Out-/In-patient	8	*	36	$390,289	4	*	8	*
Midwife: Outpatient (only)	4	*	0	*	3	*	1	*
Midwife: Inpatient (only)	1	*	3	*	*	*	0	*
Nurse Practitioner	201	$241,405	298	$278,672	135	$290,491	163	$328,192
NP: Cardiology	3	*	7	*	5	*	1	*
NP: Family Practice (w/o OB)	1	*	20	$228,998	7	*	5	*
NP: Gastroenterology	5	*	5	*	*	*	*	*
NP: Gerontology/Elder Health	2	*	11	*	0	*	2	*
NP: Hematology/Oncology	1	*	5	*	2	*	1	*
NP: Internal Medicine	17	$261,113	18	$244,938	7	*	3	*
NP: Pediatric/Child Health	8	*	13	$534,196	12	$245,813	1	*
NP: OB/GYN/Women's Health	8	*	22	$296,585	10	$260,924	9	*
Occupational Therapist	5	*	7	*	0	*	15	$267,152
Optometrist	20	$466,558	68	$496,597	25	$531,822	25	$530,920
Perfusionist	0	*	*	*	0	*	1	*
Pharmacist	1	*	0	*	1	*	0	*
Physical Therapist	23	$461,036	91	$308,095	12	$452,172	30	$408,176
Physician Asst (surgical)	70	$384,800	73	$266,646	24	$556,957	68	$526,827
PA: Orthopedic	17	$345,719	8	*	7	*	10	*
PA: Surg: General	5	*	1	*	4	*	0	*
Physician Asst (primary care)	99	$360,927	131	$346,891	40	$267,085	117	$385,144
PA: Family Practice (w/ OB)	12	$352,871	25	$449,370	3	*	2	*
PA: Family Practice (w/o OB)	6	*	9	*	12	*	8	*
PA: Internal Medicine	9	*	1	*	3	*	1	*
PA: Urgent Care	*	*	3	*	*	*	4	*
Phys Asst (nonsurg/nonprim care)	35	$155,445	56	$341,363	20	$244,788	28	$434,253
PA: Cardiology	2	*	1	*	3	*	1	*
Psychologist	30	$77,802	105	$229,423	8	*	13	$217,395
Social Worker	9	*	57	$203,499	8	*	3	*
Speech Therapist	*	*	3	*	0	*	*	*
Surgeon Assistant	*	*	4	*	2	*	5	*

Table 136: Nonphysician Provider Compensation to Gross Charges Ratio (TC Excluded)

	NPPs	Med Pracs	Mean	Std. Dev.	25th %tile	Median	75th %tile	90th %tile
Audiologist	27	17	.378	.198	.190	.345	.546	.680
Cert Reg Nurse Anesthetist	244	19	.367	.121	.308	.355	.396	.484
Chiropractor	10	6	.238	.072	.223	.239	.273	.335
Dietician/Nutritionist	14	11	.485	.163	.358	.437	.646	.706
Midwife: Out-/In-patient	56	27	.258	.101	.200	.241	.310	.382
Midwife: Outpatient (only)	7	6	*	*	*	*	*	*
Midwife: Inpatient (only)	4	3	*	*	*	*	*	*
Nurse Practitioner	734	201	.294	.146	.192	.252	.348	.505
NP: Cardiology	18	10	.490	.225	.263	.533	.687	.748
NP: Family Practice (w/o OB)	33	10	.296	.105	.215	.287	.368	.436
NP: Gastroenterology	10	5	.257	.094	.189	.205	.346	.415
NP: Gerontology/Elder Health	15	4	.485	.126	.426	.449	.493	.706
NP: Hematology/Oncology	8	7	*	*	*	*	*	*
NP: Internal Medicine	49	19	.289	.100	.214	.264	.341	.375
NP: Pediatric/Child Health	36	18	.208	.074	.169	.199	.218	.299
NP: OB/GYN/Women's Health	49	20	.281	.084	.228	.258	.321	.393
Occupational Therapist	29	12	.249	.103	.176	.241	.281	.371
Optometrist	133	44	.303	.122	.210	.272	.356	.478
Perfusionist	1	1	*	*	*	*	*	*
Pharmacist	2	2	*	*	*	*	*	*
Physical Therapist	149	33	.198	.071	.142	.182	.235	.284
Physician Asst (surgical)	214	66	.282	.180	.156	.226	.359	.537
PA: Orthopedic	41	12	.206	.105	.118	.179	.291	.398
PA: Surg: General	9	6	*	*	*	*	*	*
Physician Asst (primary care)	370	111	.253	.111	.173	.230	.292	.404
PA: Family Practice (w/ OB)	37	14	.232	.070	.187	.205	.287	.331
PA: Family Practice (w/o OB)	33	5	.203	.074	.140	.185	.278	.313
PA: Internal Medicine	16	7	.207	.062	.173	.211	.262	.285
PA: Urgent Care	7	4	*	*	*	*	*	*
Phys Asst (nonsurg/nonprim care)	120	55	.307	.196	.170	.231	.353	.662
PA: Cardiology	5	4	*	*	*	*	*	*
Psychologist	140	27	.406	.142	.312	.400	.443	.573
Social Worker	75	15	.327	.103	.254	.303	.389	.470
Speech Therapist	3	2	*	*	*	*	*	*
Surgeon Assistant	7	6	*	*	*	*	*	*

Table 137: Nonphysician Provider Compensation to Gross Charges Ratio (TC Excluded) by Group Type

	Single Specialty			Multispecialty		
	NPPs	Med Pracs	Median	NPPs	Med Pracs	Median
Audiologist	3	1	*	24	16	.350
Cert Reg Nurse Anesthetist	188	9	.355	56	10	.390
Chiropractor	1	1	*	9	5	*
Dietician/Nutritionist	1	1	*	13	10	.419
Midwife: Out-/In-patient	6	2	*	50	25	.243
Midwife: Outpatient (only)	2	2	*	5	4	*
Midwife: Inpatient (only)	0	*	*	4	3	*
Nurse Practitioner	102	71	.227	632	130	.258
NP: Cardiology	3	2	*	15	8	.527
NP: Family Practice (w/o OB)	0	*	*	33	10	.287
NP: Gastroenterology	*	*	*	10	5	.205
NP: Gerontology/Elder Health	*	*	*	15	4	.449
NP: Hematology/Oncology	*	*	*	8	7	*
NP: Internal Medicine	*	*	*	49	19	.264
NP: Pediatric/Child Health	*	*	*	36	18	.199
NP: OB/GYN/Women's Health	2	2	*	47	18	.258
Occupational Therapist	5	3	*	24	9	.248
Optometrist	8	4	*	125	40	.269
Perfusionist	*	*	*	1	1	*
Pharmacist	0	*	*	2	2	*
Physical Therapist	29	8	.145	120	25	.203
Physician Asst (surgical)	81	28	.218	133	38	.247
PA: Orthopedic	5	1	*	36	11	.175
PA: Surg: General	*	*	*	9	6	*
Physician Asst (primary care)	60	28	.186	310	83	.240
PA: Family Practice (w/ OB)	4	3	*	33	11	.205
PA: Family Practice (w/o OB)	*	*	*	33	5	.185
PA: Internal Medicine	*	*	*	16	7	.211
PA: Urgent Care	*	*	*	7	4	*
Phys Asst (nonsurg/nonprim care)	25	17	.245	95	38	.231
PA: Cardiology	0	*	*	5	4	*
Psychologist	2	2	*	138	25	.399
Social Worker	1	1	*	74	14	.301
Speech Therapist	0	*	*	3	2	*
Surgeon Assistant	5	4	*	2	2	*

Table 138: Nonphysician Provider Ambulatory Encounters

	NPPs	Med Pracs	Mean	Std. Dev.	25th %tile	Median	75th %tile	90th %tile
Audiologist	38	22	1,393	754	710	1,322	2,046	2,570
Cert Reg Nurse Anesthetist	156	7	281	260	139	216	318	522
Chiropractor	11	7	5,840	4,207	1,946	5,397	9,371	12,686
Dietician/Nutritionist	14	7	632	301	434	634	861	1,073
Midwife: Out-/In-patient	63	29	1,383	814	925	1,233	1,875	2,417
Midwife: Outpatient (only)	8	7	*	*	*	*	*	*
Midwife: Inpatient (only)	7	5	*	*	*	*	*	*
Nurse Practitioner	914	264	2,314	1,238	1,457	2,339	3,179	3,918
NP: Cardiology	19	11	1,203	756	747	928	1,567	2,458
NP: Family Practice (w/o OB)	35	12	2,493	1,304	1,368	2,514	3,322	4,299
NP: Gastroenterology	7	4	*	*	*	*	*	*
NP: Gerontology/Elder Health	12	3	1,199	295	986	1,125	1,287	1,824
NP: Hematology/Oncology	9	8	*	*	*	*	*	*
NP: Internal Medicine	52	22	2,283	871	1,713	2,241	2,879	3,435
NP: Pediatric/Child Health	34	17	2,824	1,343	1,975	2,653	3,608	4,204
NP: OB/GYN/Women's Health	49	21	2,300	728	1,856	2,415	2,776	3,303
Occupational Therapist	26	9	2,029	1,104	1,395	1,660	2,221	4,244
Optometrist	155	51	4,101	1,747	2,919	3,934	5,071	6,226
Perfusionist	1	1	*	*	*	*	*	*
Pharmacist	1	1	*	*	*	*	*	*
Physical Therapist	154	32	2,664	1,342	1,873	2,456	3,331	4,672
Physician Asst (surgical)	213	64	1,218	979	319	1,010	1,988	2,681
PA: Orthopedic	45	14	1,426	1,196	195	1,169	2,591	3,020
PA: Surg: General	8	4	*	*	*	*	*	*
Physician Asst (primary care)	518	141	2,891	1,487	1,962	2,906	3,767	4,623
PA: Family Practice (w/ OB)	50	17	3,322	1,188	2,325	3,282	4,200	4,794
PA: Family Practice (w/o OB)	41	7	3,254	745	2,648	3,371	3,705	4,072
PA: Internal Medicine	14	8	2,501	974	1,649	2,314	3,336	4,044
PA: Urgent Care	10	5	4,048	1,134	2,999	3,985	4,620	6,313
Phys Asst (nonsurg/nonprim care)	150	69	2,113	1,532	702	1,893	3,309	4,239
PA: Cardiology	7	5	*	*	*	*	*	*
Psychologist	157	29	1,147	466	903	1,171	1,386	1,722
Social Worker	82	19	1,117	377	911	1,112	1,343	1,576
Speech Therapist	3	2	*	*	*	*	*	*
Surgeon Assistant	2	2	*	*	*	*	*	*

Table 139: Nonphysician Provider Ambulatory Encounters by Group Type

	Single Specialty			Multispecialty		
	NPPs	Med Pracs	Median	NPPs	Med Pracs	Median
Audiologist	3	1	*	35	21	1,230
Cert Reg Nurse Anesthetist	109	5	216	47	2	*
Chiropractor	1	1	*	10	6	5,576
Dietician/Nutritionist	1	1	*	13	6	726
Midwife: Out-/In-patient	14	5	1,469	49	24	1,223
Midwife: Outpatient (only)	3	3	*	5	4	*
Midwife: Inpatient (only)	2	1	*	5	4	*
Nurse Practitioner	194	113	1,890	720	151	2,410
NP: Cardiology	2	2	*	17	9	928
NP: Family Practice (w/o OB)	1	1	*	34	11	2,585
NP: Gastroenterology	*	*	*	7	4	*
NP: Gerontology/Elder Health	*	*	*	12	3	1,125
NP: Hematology/Oncology	*	*	*	9	8	*
NP: Internal Medicine	*	*	*	52	22	2,241
NP: Pediatric/Child Health	*	*	*	34	17	2,653
NP: OB/GYN/Women's Health	2	2	*	47	19	2,415
Occupational Therapist	3	1	*	23	8	1,869
Optometrist	36	10	3,881	119	41	3,934
Perfusionist	*	*	*	1	1	*
Pharmacist	0	*	*	1	1	*
Physical Therapist	28	6	2,747	126	26	2,395
Physician Asst (surgical)	73	28	1,372	140	36	940
PA: Orthopedic	10	2	*	35	12	2,071
PA: Surg: General	*	*	*	8	4	*
Physician Asst (primary care)	92	40	2,972	426	101	2,860
PA: Family Practice (w/ OB)	5	3	*	45	14	3,203
PA: Family Practice (w/o OB)	*	*	*	41	7	3,371
PA: Internal Medicine	*	*	*	14	8	2,314
PA: Urgent Care	*	*	*	10	5	3,985
Phys Asst (nonsurg/nonprim care)	38	27	1,899	112	42	1,892
PA: Cardiology	2	1	*	5	4	*
Psychologist	2	2	*	155	27	1,169
Social Worker	5	3	*	77	16	1,143
Speech Therapist	0	*	*	3	2	*
Surgeon Assistant	2	2	*	0	*	*

Table 140: Nonphysician Provider Hospital Encounters

	NPPs	Med Pracs	Mean	Std. Dev.	25th %tile	Median	75th %tile	90th %tile
Audiologist	4	2	*	*	*	*	*	*
Cert Reg Nurse Anesthetist	106	5	229	80	209	242	275	314
Chiropractor	1	1	*	*	*	*	*	*
Dietician/Nutritionist	0	*	*	*	*	*	*	*
Midwife: Out-/In-patient	36	17	86	95	12	53	140	251
Midwife: Outpatient (only)	4	3	*	*	*	*	*	*
Midwife: Inpatient (only)	6	5	*	*	*	*	*	*
Nurse Practitioner	128	53	326	416	62	156	371	955
NP: Cardiology	15	8	180	180	7	122	396	438
NP: Family Practice (w/o OB)	4	4	*	*	*	*	*	*
NP: Gastroenterology	3	2	*	*	*	*	*	*
NP: Gerontology/Elder Health	1	1	*	*	*	*	*	*
NP: Hematology/Oncology	6	5	*	*	*	*	*	*
NP: Internal Medicine	7	6	*	*	*	*	*	*
NP: Pediatric/Child Health	5	4	*	*	*	*	*	*
NP: OB/GYN/Women's Health	4	3	*	*	*	*	*	*
Occupational Therapist	1	1	*	*	*	*	*	*
Optometrist	8	5	*	*	*	*	*	*
Perfusionist	1	1	*	*	*	*	*	*
Pharmacist	0	*	*	*	*	*	*	*
Physical Therapist	4	3	*	*	*	*	*	*
Physician Asst (surgical)	90	24	216	175	91	194	285	379
PA: Orthopedic	27	8	30	44	1	6	44	117
PA: Surg: General	7	3	*	*	*	*	*	*
Physician Asst (primary care)	36	19	248	260	58	130	379	728
PA: Family Practice (w/ OB)	15	8	63	96	2	7	118	241
PA: Family Practice (w/o OB)	2	2	*	*	*	*	*	*
PA: Internal Medicine	2	2	*	*	*	*	*	*
PA: Urgent Care	0	*	*	*	*	*	*	*
Phys Asst (nonsurg/nonprim care)	46	22	257	309	55	127	362	656
PA: Cardiology	6	4	*	*	*	*	*	*
Psychologist	21	9	71	88	22	37	87	187
Social Worker	9	3	*	*	*	*	*	*
Speech Therapist	0	*	*	*	*	*	*	*
Surgeon Assistant	1	1	*	*	*	*	*	*

Table 141: Nonphysician Provider Hospital Encounters by Group Type

	Single Specialty			Multispecialty		
	NPPs	Med Pracs	Median	NPPs	Med Pracs	Median
Audiologist	0	*	*	4	2	*
Cert Reg Nurse Anesthetist	58	2	*	48	3	272
Chiropractor	0	*	*	1	1	*
Dietician/Nutritionist	0	*	*	0	*	*
Midwife: Out-/In-patient	14	5	107	22	12	33
Midwife: Outpatient (only)	1	1	*	3	2	*
Midwife: Inpatient (only)	2	1	*	4	4	*
Nurse Practitioner	37	19	324	91	34	145
NP: Cardiology	2	1	*	13	7	52
NP: Family Practice (w/o OB)	1	1	*	3	3	*
NP: Gastroenterology	*	*	*	3	2	*
NP: Gerontology/Elder Health	*	*	*	1	1	*
NP: Hematology/Oncology	*	*	*	6	5	*
NP: Internal Medicine	*	*	*	7	6	*
NP: Pediatric/Child Health	*	*	*	5	4	*
NP: OB/GYN/Women's Health	0	*	*	4	3	*
Occupational Therapist	0	*	*	1	1	*
Optometrist	2	2	*	6	3	*
Perfusionist	*	*	*	1	1	*
Pharmacist	0	*	*	0	*	*
Physical Therapist	0	*	*	4	3	*
Physician Asst (surgical)	16	8	155	74	16	201
PA: Orthopedic	10	2	*	17	6	3
PA: Surg: General	*	*	*	7	3	*
Physician Asst (primary care)	8	5	*	28	14	121
PA: Family Practice (w/ OB)	4	3	*	11	5	11
PA: Family Practice (w/o OB)	*	*	*	2	2	*
PA: Internal Medicine	*	*	*	2	2	*
PA: Urgent Care	*	*	*	0	*	*
Phys Asst (nonsurg/nonprim care)	16	9	112	30	13	168
PA: Cardiology	2	1	*	4	3	*
Psychologist	0	*	*	21	9	37
Social Worker	0	*	*	9	3	*
Speech Therapist	0	*	*	0	*	*
Surgeon Assistant	0	*	*	1	1	*

page 279

Table 142: Nonphysician Provider Surgery/Anesthesia Cases

	NPPs	Med Pracs	Mean	Std. Dev.	25th %tile	Median	75th %tile	90th %tile
Audiologist	3	3	*	*	*	*	*	*
Cert Reg Nurse Anesthetist	401	15	312	359	14	45	598	675
Chiropractor	1	1	*	*	*	*	*	*
Dietician/Nutritionist	0	*	*	*	*	*	*	*
Midwife: Out-/In-patient	26	11	186	97	115	164	270	340
Midwife: Outpatient (only)	5	4	*	*	*	*	*	*
Midwife: Inpatient (only)	6	4	*	*	*	*	*	*
Nurse Practitioner	281	91	297	403	56	123	384	806
NP: Cardiology	6	4	*	*	*	*	*	*
NP: Family Practice (w/o OB)	19	5	278	373	11	18	509	957
NP: Gastroenterology	1	1	*	*	*	*	*	*
NP: Gerontology/Elder Health	2	2	*	*	*	*	*	*
NP: Hematology/Oncology	3	3	*	*	*	*	*	*
NP: Internal Medicine	23	12	70	128	6	26	46	340
NP: Pediatric/Child Health	22	10	80	80	23	51	106	226
NP: OB/GYN/Women's Health	30	13	183	171	69	145	231	364
Occupational Therapist	5	4	*	*	*	*	*	*
Optometrist	57	22	68	76	19	41	86	177
Perfusionist	1	1	*	*	*	*	*	*
Pharmacist	0	*	*	*	*	*	*	*
Physical Therapist	27	9	14	14	3	9	22	37
Physician Asst (surgical)	111	37	379	284	165	333	495	743
PA: Orthopedic	31	10	468	282	280	412	637	911
PA: Surg: General	8	5	*	*	*	*	*	*
Physician Asst (primary care)	199	53	243	273	71	124	272	716
PA: Family Practice (w/ OB)	25	10	111	92	47	97	143	224
PA: Family Practice (w/o OB)	28	5	324	405	65	88	685	1,132
PA: Internal Medicine	9	5	*	*	*	*	*	*
PA: Urgent Care	1	1	*	*	*	*	*	*
Phys Asst (nonsurg/nonprim care)	54	23	540	538	105	316	923	1,427
PA: Cardiology	3	3	*	*	*	*	*	*
Psychologist	3	2	*	*	*	*	*	*
Social Worker	0	*	*	*	*	*	*	*
Speech Therapist	1	1	*	*	*	*	*	*
Surgeon Assistant	4	4	*	*	*	*	*	*

Table 143: Nonphysician Provider Surgery/Anesthesia Cases by Group Type

	Single Specialty			Multispecialty		
	NPPs	Med Pracs	Median	NPPs	Med Pracs	Median
Audiologist	0	*	*	3	3	*
Cert Reg Nurse Anesthetist	397	13	45	4	2	*
Chiropractor	0	*	*	1	1	*
Dietician/Nutritionist	0	*	*	0	*	*
Midwife: Out-/In-patient	5	3	*	21	8	182
Midwife: Outpatient (only)	2	2	*	3	2	*
Midwife: Inpatient (only)	2	1	*	4	3	*
Nurse Practitioner	43	30	92	238	61	134
NP: Cardiology	0	*	*	6	4	*
NP: Family Practice (w/o OB)	0	*	*	19	5	18
NP: Gastroenterology	*	*	*	1	1	*
NP: Gerontology/Elder Health	*	*	*	2	2	*
NP: Hematology/Oncology	*	*	*	3	3	*
NP: Internal Medicine	*	*	*	23	12	26
NP: Pediatric/Child Health	*	*	*	22	10	51
NP: OB/GYN/Women's Health	1	1	*	29	12	146
Occupational Therapist	0	*	*	5	4	*
Optometrist	16	4	44	41	18	41
Perfusionist	*	*	*	1	1	*
Pharmacist	0	*	*	0	*	*
Physical Therapist	0	*	*	27	9	9
Physician Asst (surgical)	41	20	351	70	17	303
PA: Orthopedic	13	3	298	18	7	588
PA: Surg: General	*	*	*	8	5	*
Physician Asst (primary care)	37	17	105	162	36	141
PA: Family Practice (w/ OB)	5	3	*	20	7	107
PA: Family Practice (w/o OB)	*	*	*	28	5	88
PA: Internal Medicine	*	*	*	9	5	*
PA: Urgent Care	*	*	*	1	1	*
Phys Asst (nonsurg/nonprim care)	5	5	*	49	18	372
PA: Cardiology	0	*	*	3	3	*
Psychologist	0	*	*	3	2	*
Social Worker	0	*	*	0	*	*
Speech Therapist	0	*	*	1	1	*
Surgeon Assistant	2	2	*	2	2	*

Table 144: Nonphysician Provider Total RVUs (TC Excluded)

	NPPs	Med Pracs	Mean	Std. Dev.	25th %tile	Median	75th %tile	90th %tile
Audiologist	14	10	1,578	769	1,061	1,382	2,017	3,098
Cert Reg Nurse Anesthetist	465	11	2,112	2,076	175	2,387	2,718	4,314
Chiropractor	3	1	*	*	*	*	*	*
Dietician/Nutritionist	7	5	*	*	*	*	*	*
Midwife: Out-/In-patient	24	10	5,027	1,639	3,819	4,927	5,605	8,137
Midwife: Outpatient (only)	1	1	*	*	*	*	*	*
Midwife: Inpatient (only)	1	1	*	*	*	*	*	*
Nurse Practitioner	385	96	4,816	2,643	2,701	4,759	6,639	8,246
NP: Cardiology	5	3	*	*	*	*	*	*
NP: Family Practice (w/o OB)	13	5	5,363	2,141	4,044	5,185	5,922	9,690
NP: Gastroenterology	3	2	*	*	*	*	*	*
NP: Gerontology/Elder Health	10	1	*	*	*	*	*	*
NP: Hematology/Oncology	4	4	*	*	*	*	*	*
NP: Internal Medicine	27	9	3,902	1,478	2,890	3,777	4,614	6,287
NP: Pediatric/Child Health	23	9	7,265	3,185	5,439	6,695	8,863	10,521
NP: OB/GYN/Women's Health	23	7	5,301	2,268	3,708	5,042	6,352	8,360
Occupational Therapist	16	5	4,132	1,940	2,841	3,515	4,439	7,633
Optometrist	58	19	11,257	3,702	8,453	11,796	14,004	15,779
Perfusionist	1	1	*	*	*	*	*	*
Pharmacist	1	1	*	*	*	*	*	*
Physical Therapist	56	15	5,321	2,524	3,765	5,143	6,225	7,666
Physician Asst (surgical)	146	36	4,509	3,001	2,498	3,650	6,426	8,837
PA: Orthopedic	27	8	5,343	2,541	2,880	5,147	6,968	8,594
PA: Surg: General	7	3	*	*	*	*	*	*
Physician Asst (primary care)	218	63	6,102	2,859	4,129	6,151	8,009	9,964
PA: Family Practice (w/ OB)	28	6	6,769	2,370	5,151	7,009	8,522	10,022
PA: Family Practice (w/o OB)	26	3	7,183	1,690	6,370	7,500	8,603	9,207
PA: Internal Medicine	8	4	*	*	*	*	*	*
PA: Urgent Care	1	1	*	*	*	*	*	*
Phys Asst (nonsurg/nonprim care)	71	28	4,464	2,768	2,039	4,250	6,586	8,385
PA: Cardiology	8	4	*	*	*	*	*	*
Psychologist	62	11	3,824	1,368	3,053	3,744	4,340	5,619
Social Worker	40	8	3,136	764	2,500	3,194	3,603	4,271
Speech Therapist	0	*	*	*	*	*	*	*
Surgeon Assistant	8	4	*	*	*	*	*	*

Table 145: Nonphysician Provider Compensation to Total RVUs Ratio (CMS RBRVS Method) (TC Excluded)

	NPPs	Med Pracs	Mean	Std. Dev.	25th %tile	Median	75th %tile	90th %tile
Audiologist	16	11	$53.83	$22.21	$36.04	$52.70	$69.84	$85.64
Cert Reg Nurse Anesthetist	465	11	$342.54	$359.57	$49.93	$49.93	$793.39	$794.29
Chiropractor	3	1	*	*	*	*	*	*
Dietician/Nutritionist	7	5	*	*	*	*	*	*
Midwife: Out-/In-patient	24	10	$18.98	$5.14	$14.91	$18.64	$24.38	$25.68
Midwife: Outpatient (only)	1	1	*	*	*	*	*	*
Midwife: Inpatient (only)	1	1	*	*	*	*	*	*
Nurse Practitioner	381	96	$36.35	$202.27	$12.21	$16.16	$26.68	$49.54
NP: Cardiology	5	3	*	*	*	*	*	*
NP: Family Practice (w/o OB)	13	5	$15.73	$4.97	$12.03	$15.83	$20.07	$23.52
NP: Gastroenterology	3	2	*	*	*	*	*	*
NP: Gerontology/Elder Health	10	1	*	*	*	*	*	*
NP: Hematology/Oncology	4	4	*	*	*	*	*	*
NP: Internal Medicine	27	9	$20.68	$6.45	$16.12	$20.48	$24.44	$32.24
NP: Pediatric/Child Health	23	9	$11.31	$3.95	$7.97	$11.81	$14.38	$16.10
NP: OB/GYN/Women's Health	23	7	$19.97	$7.18	$11.12	$23.40	$25.63	$27.70
Occupational Therapist	18	6	$17.70	$5.73	$15.17	$17.60	$19.99	$23.85
Optometrist	56	19	$13.84	$5.66	$9.84	$11.66	$16.66	$21.78
Perfusionist	1	1	*	*	*	*	*	*
Pharmacist	1	1	*	*	*	*	*	*
Physical Therapist	54	14	$16.25	$9.32	$10.88	$13.19	$19.16	$25.03
Physician Asst (surgical)	130	36	$29.67	$16.71	$15.68	$25.21	$38.95	$57.96
PA: Orthopedic	27	8	$22.12	$11.47	$12.26	$18.64	$31.16	$39.66
PA: Surg: General	7	3	*	*	*	*	*	*
Physician Asst (primary care)	212	62	$18.36	$14.06	$11.15	$13.42	$19.07	$32.96
PA: Family Practice (w/ OB)	26	6	$14.87	$4.78	$12.29	$13.67	$15.35	$24.18
PA: Family Practice (w/o OB)	26	3	$11.80	$3.22	$9.37	$11.67	$13.78	$16.73
PA: Internal Medicine	8	4	*	*	*	*	*	*
PA: Urgent Care	1	1	*	*	*	*	*	*
Phys Asst (nonsurg/nonprim care)	71	28	$1,452.03	$7,017.62	$14.17	$17.68	$37.70	$93.81
PA: Cardiology	8	4	*	*	*	*	*	*
Psychologist	60	11	$27.02	$10.32	$19.96	$25.96	$28.85	$37.51
Social Worker	40	8	$20.13	$4.45	$17.02	$18.37	$21.28	$29.05
Speech Therapist	0	*	*	*	*	*	*	*
Surgeon Assistant	8	4	*	*	*	*	*	*

Table 146: Nonphysician Provider Work RVUs (CMS RBRVS Method)

	NPPs	Med Pracs	Mean	Std. Dev.	25th %tile	Median	75th %tile	90th %tile
Audiologist	21	14	145	148	32	115	228	385
Cert Reg Nurse Anesthetist	44	3	56	34	20	66	82	95
Chiropractor	12	7	3,108	626	2,749	2,938	3,704	4,206
Dietician/Nutritionist	8	5	*	*	*	*	*	*
Midwife: Out-/In-patient	53	24	3,204	1,188	2,253	2,919	3,958	4,659
Midwife: Outpatient (only)	6	5	*	*	*	*	*	*
Midwife: Inpatient (only)	5	4	*	*	*	*	*	*
Nurse Practitioner	802	184	2,435	1,283	1,508	2,421	3,284	4,099
NP: Cardiology	15	7	1,615	1,094	796	1,147	1,977	3,750
NP: Family Practice (w/o OB)	21	9	2,786	1,254	1,797	2,695	3,470	4,643
NP: Gastroenterology	8	4	*	*	*	*	*	*
NP: Gerontology/Elder Health	15	4	1,724	324	1,606	1,712	1,923	2,189
NP: Hematology/Oncology	6	5	*	*	*	*	*	*
NP: Internal Medicine	36	16	2,444	949	1,615	2,422	3,109	3,678
NP: Pediatric/Child Health	26	13	3,723	1,537	2,822	3,519	4,327	6,325
NP: OB/GYN/Women's Health	53	21	2,393	779	1,906	2,321	2,959	3,359
Occupational Therapist	18	6	2,262	1,069	1,523	2,011	2,503	4,109
Optometrist	135	42	4,676	1,666	3,613	4,535	5,609	6,403
Perfusionist	1	1	*	*	*	*	*	*
Pharmacist	1	1	*	*	*	*	*	*
Physical Therapist	112	21	2,583	1,140	1,709	2,596	3,348	3,965
Physician Asst (surgical)	234	56	2,594	1,909	1,266	2,141	3,359	5,161
PA: Orthopedic	44	12	2,585	1,366	1,179	2,598	3,747	4,398
PA: Surg: General	8	4	*	*	*	*	*	*
Physician Asst (primary care)	411	109	3,169	1,449	2,170	3,056	4,032	5,036
PA: Family Practice (w/ OB)	46	14	3,525	1,227	2,485	3,673	4,298	5,190
PA: Family Practice (w/o OB)	37	6	3,583	959	2,680	3,795	4,346	4,830
PA: Internal Medicine	13	7	2,663	1,084	1,897	2,727	3,587	4,231
PA: Urgent Care	9	4	*	*	*	*	*	*
Phys Asst (nonsurg/nonprim care)	145	49	2,451	1,504	1,163	2,311	3,556	4,453
PA: Cardiology	10	5	1,341	1,111	416	1,079	1,934	3,471
Psychologist	162	29	2,449	838	2,003	2,478	2,854	3,511
Social Worker	97	21	2,205	659	1,813	2,192	2,593	3,014
Speech Therapist	3	2	*	*	*	*	*	*
Surgeon Assistant	10	6	1,326	778	676	1,214	1,797	2,824

Table 147: Nonphysician Provider Work RVUs (CMS RBRVS Method) by Group Type

	Single Specialty			Multispecialty		
	NPPs	Med Pracs	Median	NPPs	Med Pracs	Median
Audiologist	0	*	*	21	14	115
Cert Reg Nurse Anesthetist	43	2	*	1	1	*
Chiropractor	1	1	*	11	6	2,873
Dietician/Nutritionist	0	*	*	8	5	*
Midwife: Out-/In-patient	10	3	3,007	43	21	2,919
Midwife: Outpatient (only)	1	1	*	5	4	*
Midwife: Inpatient (only)	2	1	*	3	3	*
Nurse Practitioner	100	61	2,072	702	123	2,446
NP: Cardiology	2	1	*	13	6	1,457
NP: Family Practice (w/o OB)	0	*	*	21	9	2,695
NP: Gastroenterology	*	*	*	8	4	*
NP: Gerontology/Elder Health	*	*	*	15	4	1,712
NP: Hematology/Oncology	*	*	*	6	5	*
NP: Internal Medicine	*	*	*	36	16	2,422
NP: Pediatric/Child Health	*	*	*	26	13	3,519
NP: OB/GYN/Women's Health	5	3	*	48	18	2,205
Occupational Therapist	0	*	*	18	6	2,011
Optometrist	5	2	*	130	40	4,524
Perfusionist	*	*	*	1	1	*
Pharmacist	0	*	*	1	1	*
Physical Therapist	1	1	*	111	20	2,618
Physician Asst (surgical)	42	16	2,184	192	40	2,141
PA: Orthopedic	9	2	*	35	10	2,964
PA: Surg: General	*	*	*	8	4	*
Physician Asst (primary care)	58	28	3,503	353	81	3,017
PA: Family Practice (w/ OB)	5	3	*	41	11	3,741
PA: Family Practice (w/o OB)	*	*	*	37	6	3,795
PA: Internal Medicine	*	*	*	13	7	2,727
PA: Urgent Care	*	*	*	9	4	*
Phys Asst (nonsurg/nonprim care)	22	10	810	123	39	2,636
PA: Cardiology	2	1	*	8	4	*
Psychologist	1	1	*	161	28	2,480
Social Worker	2	2	*	95	19	2,192
Speech Therapist	0	*	*	3	2	*
Surgeon Assistant	8	4	*	2	2	*

Table 148: Nonphysician Provider Compensation to Work RVUs Ratio (CMS RBRVS Method)

	NPPs	Med Pracs	Mean	Std. Dev.	25th %tile	Median	75th %tile	90th %tile
Audiologist	21	14	$1,872.71	$2,562.87	$409.03	$716.04	$1,584.16	$7,375.18
Cert Reg Nurse Anesthetist	66	6	$4,000.77	$7,034.17	$187.46	$1,744.19	$3,653.94	$10,323.87
Chiropractor	12	7	$32.49	$2.77	$32.09	$33.14	$33.77	$35.90
Dietician/Nutritionist	8	5	*	*	*	*	*	*
Midwife: Out-/In-patient	53	24	$32.11	$9.84	$24.36	$31.39	$39.14	$44.13
Midwife: Outpatient (only)	6	5	*	*	*	*	*	*
Midwife: Inpatient (only)	5	4	*	*	*	*	*	*
Nurse Practitioner	802	182	$102.95	$392.88	$24.06	$31.28	$48.43	$110.13
NP: Cardiology	15	7	$67.11	$42.03	$34.91	$52.61	$83.86	$138.98
NP: Family Practice (w/o OB)	21	9	$34.81	$14.54	$23.82	$32.46	$40.64	$60.23
NP: Gastroenterology	8	4	*	*	*	*	*	*
NP: Gerontology/Elder Health	15	4	$47.16	$6.61	$43.88	$47.15	$49.93	$57.01
NP: Hematology/Oncology	6	5	*	*	*	*	*	*
NP: Internal Medicine	36	16	$35.26	$13.20	$27.95	$33.51	$37.42	$49.89
NP: Pediatric/Child Health	26	13	$22.22	$8.27	$16.07	$20.39	$27.18	$32.17
NP: OB/GYN/Women's Health	53	21	$37.65	$13.58	$27.98	$34.66	$43.93	$50.37
Occupational Therapist	20	7	$32.79	$12.31	$27.74	$30.57	$36.65	$56.80
Optometrist	135	42	$31.83	$12.85	$24.44	$27.00	$36.36	$49.77
Perfusionist	1	1	*	*	*	*	*	*
Pharmacist	1	1	*	*	*	*	*	*
Physical Therapist	112	22	$33.73	$35.76	$21.13	$26.46	$37.13	$46.54
Physician Asst (surgical)	234	56	$77.93	$171.29	$29.21	$45.50	$77.52	$139.71
PA: Orthopedic	44	12	$47.17	$22.21	$30.45	$39.21	$66.79	$81.88
PA: Surg: General	8	4	*	*	*	*	*	*
Physician Asst (primary care)	404	108	$33.71	$25.55	$22.01	$26.84	$34.07	$53.89
PA: Family Practice (w/ OB)	46	14	$27.93	$11.44	$18.78	$25.80	$30.36	$48.75
PA: Family Practice (w/o OB)	37	6	$25.66	$9.66	$17.95	$23.55	$28.23	$43.11
PA: Internal Medicine	13	7	$37.85	$25.50	$22.16	$29.08	$46.85	$91.10
PA: Urgent Care	9	4	*	*	*	*	*	*
Phys Asst (nonsurg/nonprim care)	145	49	$763.99	$4,940.33	$24.77	$32.60	$63.14	$157.42
PA: Cardiology	10	5	$83.08	$44.71	$47.22	$69.75	$125.73	$149.55
Psychologist	158	28	$39.97	$14.63	$32.68	$36.37	$41.63	$60.64
Social Worker	93	20	$30.79	$11.28	$23.60	$28.18	$34.36	$42.19
Speech Therapist	3	2	*	*	*	*	*	*
Surgeon Assistant	10	6	$60.36	$32.66	$28.88	$59.08	$80.40	$123.61

Appendices

Appendix A: Abbreviations, Acronyms and Geographic Sections

Abbreviations and Acronyms

%tile	percentile	NP	nurse practitioner
anes	anesthesiology/anesthesia	NPP	nonphysician provider
asst	assistant	OB	obstetrics
cert	certified	OB/GYN	obstetrics/gynecology
CMS	Centers for Medicare & Medicaid Services	ortho	orthopedic
comp	compensation	PA	physician assistant
crit	critical	ped	pediatrics
DO	Doctor of Osteopathy	PhD	Doctor of Philosophy
FP	family practice	phys	physician/physical
FTE	full-time equivalent	PPMC	Physician Practice Management Company
Gyn	gynecology	pracs	practice(s)
Hem/Onc	hematology/oncology	RBRVS	Resource Based Relative Value Scale
IM	internal medicine	recon	reconstruction
intvl	interventional	reg	registered
inv	invasive	rehab	rehabilitation
MD	Doctor of Medicine	repro	reproductive
med	medical/medicine	RVU	relative value unit(s)
MGMA	Medical Group Management Association	std dev	standard deviation
MSO	Management Services Organization	surg	surgery
NAPR	National Association of Physician Recruiters	TC	technical component
noninv	noninvasive	w/	with
nonprim	nonprimary	w/o	without
nonsurg	nonsurgical		

Geographic Sections

Eastern Section:	Western Section:	Midwest Section:	Southern Section:
Connecticut	Alaska	Illinois	Alabama
Delaware	Arizona	Indiana	Arkansas
District of Columbia	California	Iowa	Florida
Maine	Colorado	Michigan	Georgia
Maryland	Hawaii	Minnesota	Kansas
Massachusetts	Idaho	Nebraska	Kentucky
New Hampshire	Montana	North Dakota	Louisiana
New Jersey	Nevada	Ohio	Mississippi
New York	New Mexico	South Dakota	Missouri
North Carolina	Oregon	Wisconsin	Oklahoma
Pennsylvania	Utah		South Carolina
Rhode Island	Washington		Tennessee
Vermont	Wyoming		Texas
Virginia			
West Virginia			

Appendix B: Terms Used in the Report

Adjusted charges
The total amounts expected to be paid by patients or third-party payers. Calculate this measure by taking gross charges and subtracting the adjustments from third-party payers and charge restrictions from Medicare/Medicaid.

Administrative or governance
Administrative or governance responsibility that encompasses nonclinical administrative, strategic, leadership or oversight for the practice. Typically, this term describes the nonclinical activities of physicians.

Ambulatory encounters (see also encounters)
Documented face-to-face contact between a patient and a provider who exercises independent judgment in the provision of services to the individual. If a patient with the same diagnosis sees two different providers on the same day, it is one encounter. If a patient sees two different providers on the same day for two different diagnoses, then it is considered two encounters. Ambulatory encounters are those performed in the following Centers for Medicare and Medicaid Services (CMS) place of service codes:

      11 – Office
      12 – Home
      22 – Outpatient hospital
      23 – Emergency room
      24 – Ambulatory surgical center
      31 – Skilled nursing facility
      32 – Nursing facility
      33 – Custodial care facility
      34 – Hospice
      50 – Federally qualified health center
      52 – Psychiatric facility partial hospitalization
      53 – Community mental health facility
      54 – Intermediate care facility for mentally retarded
      55 – Residential substance abuse treatment facility
      56 – Psychiatric residential treatment center
      62 – Comprehensive outpatient rehabilitation facility
      65 – End stage renal disease treatment facility
      71 – State or local public health clinic
      72 – Rural health clinic
      81 – Independent laboratory

ASA units
The American Society of Anesthesiologists (ASA) units that consist of three components for each procedure – base unit, time in 15-minute increments and risk factors.

Base salary plus incentive
Payment of a guaranteed base salary along with an incentive component that must be earned. The incentive is awarded based on one or more criteria such as individual production, performance or patient satisfaction.

Business corporation
A for-profit organization recognized by law as a business entity separate and distinct from its shareholders. Shareholders need not be licensed in the profession practiced by the corporation.

Capitation contract
A contract in which the practice agrees to provide medical services to a defined population for a fixed price per beneficiary per month, regardless of actual services provided. Capitation contracts, which always contain an element of risk, include HMO, Medicare and Medicaid.

Clinical activities

Those activities performed by the physician in which patients are seen in the office, outpatient clinic, emergency room, nursing home, operating room or labor and delivery; any time spent on hospital rounds, telephone conversations with patients, consultations with providers, interpretation of diagnostic tests and chart review. Should also include "on-call" hours if the physician is required to be present in the medical facility such as a medical clinic or hospital.

Clinical full-time equivalent (FTE)

A measure based upon the number of hours worked on clinical activities for each provider. A provider cannot be more than 1.0 FTE, but may be less. For example, a physician administrator who is 80 percent clinical and 20 percent administrative would be 0.8 clinical FTE; a physician with a normal workweek of 32 hours (4 days) working in a clinic or hospital for 32 hours would be 1.0 clinical FTE; a physician with a normal workweek of 50 hours (5 days) working 32 clinical or hospital hours would be a 0.64 clinical FTE (32 divided by 50 hours).

Clinical science department

A unit of organization in a medical school with an independent chair and single budget. The department's mission is to conduct teaching, research and/or clinical activities related to the entire spectrum of health care delivery to humans, from prevention through treatment. Residents in training or fellows may be present.

Clinical service hours

Weekly hours during which a clinician is involved in direct patient care and a patient bill is generated and a fee-for-service equivalent charge is created for the practice.

Collections for professional charges

The actual dollars collected that can be attributed to a physician for all professional services. Includes fee-for-service collections, allocated capitation payments, administration of chemotherapy drugs and administration of immunizations. However, this measure should not include collections on drug charges, including vaccinations, allergy injections and immunizations, as well as chemotherapy and antinauseant drugs, the technical component associated with any laboratory, radiology, medical diagnostic or surgical procedure collections, collections attributed to nonphysician providers, infusion-related collections, facility fees, supplies, revenue associated with the sale of hearing aids, eyeglasses or contact lenses.

Community outreach

Direct involvement in community service activities to promote better public health and build rapport between health providers and members of their communities.

Compensation pool

An allocation of a compensation plan that is equal to the total practice revenues net of practice overhead expenses. To calculate: practice revenues – practice expense = compensation pool.

Encounters (see also ambulatory and hospital encounters)

A documented, face-to-face contact between a patient and a provider who exercises independent judgment in the provision of services to the individual in an ambulatory or hospital setting. If a patient with the same diagnosis sees two different providers on the same day, it is one encounter. If a patient sees two different providers on the same day for two different diagnoses, then it is considered two encounters. Encounters should include only procedures from the evaluation and management chapter (CPT codes 99201–99499) or the medicine chapter (CPT codes 90800–99199) of the *Physicians' Current Procedural Terminology, Fourth Edition,* copyrighted by the American Medical Association (AMA).

Equal share of practice compensation pool (see also compensation pool)

Each physician allocated an equal share of the money available in the compensation pool.

Established primary care physician

A physician with more than two years in a primary care specialty. Primary care is comprised of family practice, geriatrics, internal medicine and pediatrics. The count of the number of years should begin at the time the physician completes the latter of residency or fellowship.

Established specialist

A physician with more than two years in a specialty other than primary care. The count of the number of years should begin at the time the physician completes the latter of residency or fellowship.

Fiscal year

The corporate year established by the practice for business purposes. For many practices, this is January through December of the same year.

Freestanding ambulatory surgery center

A freestanding entity that is specifically licensed to provide surgery services that are performed on a same-day outpatient basis. A freestanding ambulatory surgery center does not employ physicians.

Full-time equivalent (FTE) physician (see also part-time physician)

A full-time equivalent physician who works the number of hours the practice considers to be the minimum for a normal workweek, which could be 37.5, 40, 50 hours or some other standard.

Government

A government organization at the federal, state or local level. Government funding is not a sufficient criterion. Government ownership is the key factor. An example would be a medical clinic at a federal, state or county correctional facility.

Health Maintenance Organization (HMO)

An insurance company that accepts responsibility for providing and delivering a predetermined set of comprehensive health maintenance and treatment services to a voluntarily enrolled population for a negotiated and fixed periodic premium.

Hospital

An inpatient facility that admits patients for overnight stays, incurs nursing care costs and generates bed per day revenues.

Hospital encounters (see also encounters)

A documented face-to-face contact between a patient and a provider who exercises independent judgment in the provision of services to the individual. If a patient with the same diagnosis sees two different providers on the same day, it is one encounter. If a patient sees two different providers on the same day for two different diagnoses, then it is considered two encounters. Hospital encounters should be reported only if performed in the following Centers for Medicare & Medicaid Services (CMS) place of service codes:

      21 – Inpatient hospital
      25 – Birthing center
      26 – Military treatment facility
      51 – Inpatient psychiatric facility
      61 – Comprehensive inpatient rehabilitation facility

Hours worked per week

The number of hours an individual, such as a physician, works during a normal (typical) workweek.

Independent Practice Association (IPA)

An association or network of licensed providers and/or medical practices. An IPA is usually a unique legal entity, most often operating on a for-profit basis. Typically, the primary purpose of the IPA is to secure and maintain contractual relationships between providers and health plans.

Insurance company

An organization that indemnifies an insured party against a specified loss in return for premiums paid as stipulated by a contract.

Integrated Delivery System (IDS)

A network of organizations that provide or coordinate and arrange for the provision of a continuum of health care services to consumers and are willing to be held clinically and fiscally responsible for the outcomes and the health status of the populations served. Generally consisting of hospitals, physician groups, health plans, home health agencies, hospices, skilled nursing facilities or other provider entities, these networks may be built through virtual integration processes encompassing contractual arrangements and strategic alliances as well as through direct ownership. An emerging description of this same type of entity is Integrated Delivery Network (IDN).

Limited liability company
A legal entity that is a hybrid between a corporation and a partnership, because it provides limited liability to owners, like a corporation, while passing profits and losses through to owners, like a partnership.

Management Services Organization (MSO)
An entity organized to provide various forms of practice management and administrative support services to health care providers. These services may include centralized billing and collections services, management information services and other components of the managed care infrastructure. MSOs do not actually deliver health care services. MSOs may be jointly or solely owned and sponsored by physicians, hospitals or other parties. Some MSOs also purchase assets of affiliated physicians and enter into long-term management service arrangements with a provider network. Some expand their ownership base by involving outside investors to help capitalize the development of such practice infrastructure.

Medical school
A medical school is an institution that trains physicians and awards medical and osteopathic degrees.

Metropolitan area (50,000 to 250,000)
The community in which the practice is located is a metropolitan statistical area (MSA) or Census Bureau defined urbanized area with a population of 50,000 to 250,000.

Metropolitan area (250,001 to 1,000,000)
The community in which the practice is located is a metropolitan statistical area (MSA) or Census Bureau defined urbanized area with a population of 250,001 to 1,000,000.

Metropolitan area (more than 1,000,000)
The community in which the practice is located is a primary metropolitan statistical area (PMSA) having a population of more than 1,000,000.

Modifier
A factor that causes an increase or decrease to RVU values such as modifiers 21, 22, 51 and 80 for additional complexity or multiple procedures.

Multispecialty practice with primary and specialty care
A medical practice that consists of physicians practicing in different specialties, including at least one primary care specialty listed below. Family practice: general, family practice: sports medicine, family practice: urgent care, family practice: with obstetrics, family practice: without obstetrics, geriatrics, internal medicine: general, pediatrics: adolescent medicine, pediatrics: general and pediatrics: sports medicine.

Multispecialty practice with primary care only
A medical practice that consists of physicians practicing in more than one of the primary care specialties listed in multispecialty with primary and specialty care or the surgical specialties of obstetrics/gynecology, gynecology (only) and obstetrics (only).

Multispecialty with specialty care only
A medical practice that consists of physicians practicing in different specialties, none of which are the primary care specialties listed under multispecialty practice with primary and specialty care and multispecialty practice with primary care only.

New physician
A physician with less than two years in a specialty. The count of the number of years should begin at the time the physician completes the latter of residency or fellowship.

Nonmetropolitan area (fewer than 50,000)
The community in which the practice is located is generally referred to as "rural." It is located outside of a metropolitan statistical area (MSA), as defined by the United States Office of Management and Budget, and has a population of less than 50,000.

Nonphysician provider (NPP)
Specially trained and licensed providers who can provide medical care and billable services. Examples of nonphysician providers include audiologists, Certified Registered Nurse Anesthetists (CRNAs), dieticians/nutritionists, midwives, nurse practitioners, occupational therapists, optometrists, physical therapists, physician assistants, psychologists, social workers, speech therapists and surgeon's assistants.

Not-for-profit corporation/foundation
An organization that has obtained special exemption under Section 501(c) of the Internal Revenue Code that qualifies the organization to be exempt from federal income taxes. To qualify as a tax-exempt organization, a practice or faculty practice plan would have to provide evidence of a charitable, educational or research purpose.

Part-time physician (see also full-time equivalent physician)
A part-time physician works less than the number of hours considered to be a normal workweek. To compute the FTE of a part-time physician, divide the total hours worked by the physician by the number of hours that your medical practice considers to be a normal workweek. For example, a physician working in a clinic or hospital on behalf of the practice for 30 hours compared to a normal workweek of 40 hours would be 0.75 FTE (30 divided by 40 hours). A physician working fulltime for three months during a year would be 0.25 FTE (3 divided by 12 months). A medical director devoting 50 percent effort to clinical activity would be 0.5 FTE.

Partnership
An organization where two or more individuals have agreed that they will share profits, losses, assets and liabilities, although not necessarily on an equal basis. The partnership agreement may or may not be formalized in writing.

Patient satisfaction
Patient evaluation of clinical services.

Peer review
A review process of physician clinical performance provided by a panel of physicians.

Physician
Any doctor of medicine (MD) or doctor of osteopathy (DO) who is duly licensed and qualified under the law of jurisdiction in which treatment is received.

Physician patient panel
The number of patients, regardless of payer, assigned to a physician.

Physician Practice Management Company (PPMC)
Publicly held or entrepreneurial-directed enterprises that acquire total or partial ownership interests in physician organizations. PPMCs are a type of MSO, however the motivations, goals, strategies and structures arising from their unequivocal ownership character — development of growth and profits for their investors, not for participating providers — differentiate them from other MSO models.

Physician work RVUs (see also Relative Value Units (RVUs))
The physician work component of the total RVU that includes physician work RVUs for all professional medical and surgical services; for the professional component of laboratory, radiology, medical diagnostic and surgical procedures; and all procedures performed by the medical practice, for both fee-for-service and capitation patients and for all payers.

Productivity-based option
Provider compensation based wholly or partially upon individual physician output measurements.

Professional activities
Those services performed by the physician including both clinical and nonclinical time.

Professional corporation/association
A for-profit organization recognized by law as a business entity separate and distinct from its shareholders. Shareholders must be licensed in the profession practiced by the organization.

Professional gross charges

Gross patient charges are the full dollar value, at the practice's established undiscounted rates, of services provided to all patients before reduction by charitable adjustments, professional courtesy adjustments, contractual adjustments, employee discounts and bad debts. For both Medicare participating and nonparticipating providers, gross charges should include the practice's full, undiscounted charge and not the Medicare limiting charge.

Relative Value Units (RVUs)

Relative value units are nonmonetary, relative units of measure that indicate the value of health care services and relative difference in resources consumed when providing different procedures and services. RVUs assign relative values or weights to medical procedures primarily for the purpose of the reimbursement of services performed. They are used as a standardized method of analyzing resources involved in the provision of services or procedures.

Retirement benefit contributions

All employer contributions to retirement plans including defined benefit and contribution plans, 401(k), 403(b) and Keogh Plans, and any nonqualified funded retirement plan. For defined benefit plans, estimate the employer's contribution made on behalf of each plan participant by multiplying the employer's total contribution by each plan participant's compensation divided by the total compensation of all plan participants. This measure does not include employer contributions to social security mandated by the Federal Insurance Contributions Act (FICA); voluntary employee contributions that are an allocation of salary to a 401(k), 403(b) or Keogh Plan; the dollar value of any other fringe benefits paid by the practice, such as life and health insurance and automobile allowances.

Technical component (TC) (see also RVUs)

Modifier-TC, when attached to an appropriate CPT code, represents the technical component of the procedure and includes the cost of equipment and supplies to perform that procedure. This modifier corresponds to the equipment/facility part of a given procedure.

Total compensation

The amount reported as direct compensation on a W2, 1099 or K1 (for partnerships) plus all voluntary salary reductions, such as 401(k), 403(b), Section 125 Tax Savings Plan and Medical Savings Plan. The amount should include salary, bonus and/or incentive payments, research stipends, honoraria and distribution of profits. However, it does not include the dollar value of expense reimbursements, fringe benefits paid by the medical practice such as retirement plan contributions, life and health insurance, automobile allowances or any employer contributions to a 401(k), 403(b) or Keogh Plan.

Total medical revenue (collections)

The sum of fee-for-service collections, capitation payments and other medical activity revenues.

Undiscounted rates

The full retail prices before Medicare/Medicaid charge restrictions, third-party payer such as commercial insurance and/or managed care organization contractual adjustments, and other charitable, professional courtesy or employee adjustments.

University

An institution of higher learning with teaching and research facilities comprising undergraduate, graduate and professional schools.

Weeks worked per year

The number of weeks the physician works during the year.

Years in specialty

The number of years each physician and nonphysician provider has practiced in a specialty. The count of the number of years should begin at the time the physician completes the latter of residency or fellowship.

Appendix C: Formulas and Methodology

Formulas

Full-Time Provider: 0.8 – 1.0 clinical FTE

Part-Time Provider: 0.4 – 0.6 clinical FTE

Compensation to Collections Ratio:

$$\frac{\text{Compensation}}{\text{Collections}}$$

Compensation per Total RVU:

$$\frac{\text{Compensation}}{\text{Total RVU}}$$

Compensation per Physician Work RVU:

$$\frac{\text{Compensation}}{\text{Physician Work RVU}}$$

Collections per Total RVU:

$$\frac{\text{Collections}}{\text{Total RVU}}$$

Collections per Physician Work RVU:

$$\frac{\text{Collections}}{\text{Physician Work RVU}}$$

Work RVUs per Total Encounters Ratio:

$$\frac{\text{Work RVUs}}{(\text{Ambulatory Encounters} + \text{Hospital Encounters} + \text{Surgery/Anesthesia Cases})}$$

Total RVUs per Total Encounters Ratio:

$$\frac{\text{Total RVUs}}{(\text{Ambulatory Encounters} + \text{Hospital Encounters} + \text{Surgery/Anesthesia Cases})}$$

Methodology

Data Editing

A critical aspect of the survey process is the editing phase. Editing identifies reporting errors, mathematical miscalculations, inconsistencies and extreme values for follow-up and resolution. Practices that identified themselves as freestanding ambulatory surgery centers, academics or a nonphysician organization were reclassified as ineligible for inclusion in the survey report.

Guidelines were developed to structure the editing process. MGMA Survey Operations examined all questionnaires. Data representing outliers were investigated by telephone, e-mail or fax for follow-up and either corrected or suppressed from the database.

In 2007, MGMA Survey Operations changed methodology for trimming extreme values. In doing so, outlier identification is more repeatable from year to year as well as adjusted as the data moves over time. This will provide greater reliability in future trending data. The other key to this method is to avoid a shift in the median due to unbalanced trimming. By trimming equally from either side of the array, the median is static while the mean trends toward the median. The trim also evaluates each value with respect to the specialty it represents: in this manner, trims are made within the context of other data in a specialty, as opposed to looking at the entire data set to determine minimum and maximum values.

As a first step we eliminated any data that was a clear outlier for certain variables. This included any compensation less than $30,000. The next step in the trimming process is to identify what specialties should be trimmed for each variable. This is done by evaluating each specialty for several indicators of possible outliers. These criteria include standard deviation as a percent of the median, standard deviation as a percent of the mean, difference between mean and median as a percent of the median and range as a percent of the median. If any of these ratios exceed predetermined values for a given specialty, extreme values will be identified and removed by the trim program.

The trim program creates two scores by which the data will be evaluated within each specialty. The first score is the normal score, which is computed by subtracting the mean from the value and dividing by the standard deviation of the original data set. The second computation is the proportional score. This is similar to a percentile ranking, but is evaluated on a continuous scale as opposed to using only 99 discrete values. Within each specialty the proportion score is computed on the following formula:

$$\frac{(r - 3/8)}{(w + 1/4)}$$

where r is the rank of the value within the specialty, and w is the number of cases within the specialty.

These scores are then evaluated based on the following criteria:

Number of physicians responding within specialty	Normal scores used	Proportion scores used	Estimated data points trimmed
16 thru 50	-2.25 thru 2.25	.0400 thru .9600	1–4
51 thru 100	-2.25 thru 2.25	.0250 thru .9750	2–4
101 thru 300	-2.50 thru 2.50	.0150 thru .9850	2–8
301 thru 1000	-2.75 thru 2.75	.0100 thru .9900	6–20
1001 thru 2000	-3.00 thru 3.00	.0050 thru .9950	10–20
2001 or more	-3.00 thru 3.00	.0025 thru .9975	10–24

Additionally, specialties with fewer than 15 responding physicians required manual editing. Expert MGMA staff evaluates these specialties individually and suppresses extreme values, as deemed necessary.

For example, in 2007, nephrology had 292 respondents. If identified as having potential outliers in total compensation, compensation would be trimmed for any value with a proportion score under .0150 or above .9850, as well as any value with a normal score below -2.50 or above 2.50. In nephrology this would include the four values that are on each end of the array. These would be represented by ranks 1, 2, 3, 4, 289, 290, 291 and 292.

Limitations of the Data

It is recommended to use caution in interpreting the data in this report. The report is based on a voluntary response by primarily MGMA member practices and data may not be representative of all providers in medical practices. Providers in the responding organizations may have different compensation and productivity than providers in practices that did not respond to the survey or were not MGMA members. Additionally, note that the respondent sample varies from year to year. Therefore, conclusions about longitudinal trends or year-to-year fluctuations in summary statistics may not be appropriate.

Appendix D: MGMA Survey Products

Survey Reports

Academic Practice Compensation and Production Survey for Faculty and Management

Provides compensation and productivity levels for medical school physician faculty. The report also contains clinical science department and practice plan managerial compensation and benefit information.

Ambulatory Surgery Center Performance Survey

Provides ambulatory surgery center (ASC) administrators, consultants and others with data that can be used to evaluate ASC performance and help make policy decisions about ASC operations.

Cost Survey

Summarizes the financial performance and productivity of responding medical practices. Significant measures contained in the report are: staffing ratios, medical revenue, staff salary costs, total operating costs, revenue after operating costs, provider costs and net practice income/loss. Accounts receivable, payer mix, collection percentages, financial ratios and balance sheet information are also included.

The Cost Survey is also the basis for additional reports. An in-depth analysis of "better performing" medical group practices is presented in a companion publication, the *Performance and Practices of Successful Medical Groups*. Also, studies have been conducted of various clinical specialties and special interest groups within MGMA:
  • Cost Survey for Anesthesia Practices;
  • Cost Survey for Cardiovascular/Thoracic Surgery and Cardiology Practices;
  • Cost Survey for Integrated Delivery Systems;
  • Cost Survey for Obstetrics and Gynecology Practices;
  • Cost Survey for Orthopedic Practices;
  • Cost Survey for Pediatric Practices; and
  • Cost Survey for Urology Practices.

Freestanding Diagnostic Imaging Center Performance Survey

Provides information to evaluate different aspects of freestanding diagnostic imaging center (FDIC) performance and to help make policy decisions about FDIC operations.

Management Compensation Survey

Includes compensation, bonus and retirement benefit amounts for physician executives and for middle and upper-level manager positions.

Payer Performance Survey

Helps practices assess the reimbursement for office-based evaluation and management (E&M) services. Contains comparative information on physician service reimbursement, data categorized by specialty, revenue and key payer satisfaction indicators and satisfaction measures by region, experience, payer guidelines and revenue.

Performance and Practices of Successful Medical Groups

Provides benchmarking data on better performing medical groups and identifies the business practices and behaviors these groups employ to achieve success.

Physician Compensation and Production Survey

Reports individual physician and nonphysician provider compensation data. This survey report also has productivity data including professional gross charges, ambulatory encounters, hospital encounters, surgical/anesthesia cases, total Resource-Based Relative Value Scale (RBRVS) units and physician work Relative Value Units (RVUs). Ratios of compensation to gross charges and compensation per physician work RVU are also calculated.

Interactive Reports

Physician Compensation and Production Interactive Report
The CD features more data than its printed counterpart and offers custom reports that are simple to generate. It is easy to analyze and benchmark with the built-in comparison tools and the customizable compensation and productivity tracking tool. The user has the option to export tabular information to spreadsheet formats and generate graphs for reports and presentations. Management compensation data are now available on a special version of the Physician Compensation and Production Interactive Report.

Cost Survey Interactive Report
The CD features a larger range of data points per table than the printed version and the built-in comparison tools make analysis and benchmarking easy. Data for geographic regions and states are available by selected indicators. The user has the option to export tabular information to spreadsheet formats and generate graphs for reports and presentations.

Academic Practice Compensation and Production for Faculty and Management Interactive Report
The CD features more data points than the printed report. It has built-in tools for estimating compensation and department benchmarks. The user has the option to export tabular information to spreadsheet formats and generate graphs for reports and presentations.

Custom Analysis and Market Research
Our survey instruments collect vast amounts of data — more than what appears in our printed reports and interactive CDs. Therefore, we can generate more detailed reports that we can tailor to your needs. If you want a specific report — perhaps data by region, group size, revenue size or other variable — call us for a price quote toll-free at 877.ASK.MGMA (275.6462), ext. 895.

To order MGMA products, visit the *Store* on mgma.com or call toll-free 877.ASK.MGMA (275.6462), ext. 888.

Appendix E: Compensation and Production Survey: 2008 Questionnaire Based on 2007 Data

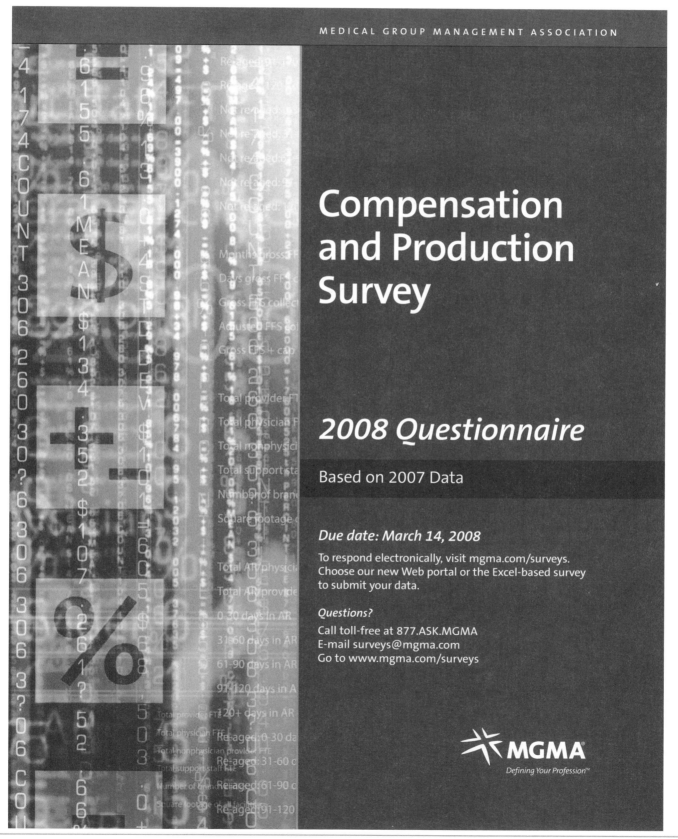

MEDICAL GROUP MANAGEMENT ASSOCIATION

Compensation and Production Survey

2008 Questionnaire

Based on 2007 Data

Due date: March 14, 2008

To respond electronically, visit mgma.com/surveys. Choose our new Web portal or the Excel-based survey to submit your data.

Questions?

Call toll-free at 877.ASK.MGMA
E-mail surveys@mgma.com
Go to www.mgma.com/surveys

MGMA
Defining Your Profession™

Medical Group Management Association®
Compensation and Production Survey: 2008 Questionnaire Based on 2007 Data

Instructions

Refer to the *Compensation and Production Survey: 2008 Guide to the Questionnaire Based on 2007 Data* (Guide) for definitions and instructions for completing the questionnaire.

If your organization is a Management Services Organization (MSO), Physician Practice Management Company (PPMC), hospital, integrated health care system and/or a medical practice consisting of more than one legal entity, please read the instructions in the Guide.

R Designates questions required for inclusion in the report. Failure to answer any of the required questions will deem the submitted data ineligible.

2007 Fiscal Year Definition

All the questions on this questionnaire refer to the 2007 fiscal year. This is typically January 2007 through December 2007. If your practice uses an alternative fiscal year, you are encouraged to use it in your responses.

R 1. For the purposes of reporting the information in this questionnaire, what fiscal year was used?

Beginning month$_a$ ☐   Beginning year$_b$ ☐   *through* Ending month$_c$ ☐   Ending year$_d$ ☐

Medical Practice Information

Answer the following questions in the way that best describes your practice at the end of the 2007 fiscal year.

R 2. What was your practice type? (select only one)
- ☐ Single specialty $_1$
- ☐ Multispecialty with primary and specialty care $_2$
- ☐ Multispecialty with primary care only $_3$
- ☐ Multispecialty with specialty care only $_4$

R 3. If you answered "Single specialty" for question 2, what specialty was your practice?
[ ]

R 4. Was your organization a freestanding ambulatory surgery center only? Answer "No" if the ambulatory surgery center was a unit of the medical practice.
- ☐ Yes $_1$
- ☐ No $_2$

R 5. Was your practice a medical school faculty practice plan and/or clinical science department?
- ☐ Yes $_1$
- ☐ No $_2$

6. Was your practice affiliated with a medical school?
- ☐ Yes $_1$
- ☐ No $_2$

*Please indicate the name and location of your parent organization (owner) on questions 44-47.

7. Did an MSO, PPMC, Independent Practice Association or other type of management organization provide services to your practice?
- ☐ Yes $_1$
- ☐ No $_2$

8. What was the legal organization of your practice? (select only one)
- ☐ Business corporation $_1$
- ☐ Limited liability company $_2$
- ☐ Not-for-profit corporation/foundation $_3$
- ☐ Partnership $_4$
- ☐ Professional corporation/association $_5$
- ☐ Sole proprietorship $_6$
- ☐ Other $_7$ [ ]

R 9. Who was the majority owner of your practice? (select only one)
- ☐ Government $_1$
- ☐ *Hospital/integrated delivery system (IDS) $_2$
- ☐ Insurance company or health maintenance organization (HMO) $_3$
- ☐ *MSO or PPMC $_4$
- ☐ Physicians $_5$
- ☐ *University or medical school $_6$
- ☐ *Other $_7$ [ ]

Medical Group Management Association®
Compensation and Production Survey: 2008 Questionnaire Based on 2007 Data

Medical Practice Information (continued)

10. **If you are a hospital/IDS, MSO or PPMC, and/ or a medical practice with more than one legal entity, do you have a centralized administrative department?**

    ☐ Yes₁

    ☐ No₂

11. **Which population designation best describes the area surrounding the primary location of your practice? If your practice had multiple sites, choose the option that represents the location with the largest number of full-time-equivalent (FTE) physicians. (select only one)**

    ☐ Nonmetropolitan (fewer than 50,000)₁

    ☐ Metropolitan (50,000 to 250,000)₂

    ☐ Metropolitan (250,001 to 1,000,000)₃

    ☐ Metropolitan (more than 1,000,000)₄

12. **Did your practice derive revenue from capitation contracts?**

    ☐ Yes₁

    ☐ No₂

13. **If you answered "Yes" to question 12, what percentage of your practice's total medical revenue was derived from capitation contracts?**

    ☐☐☐ % capitation

R 14. **What was the total medical revenue (collections) for your practice?**

    $ _____ total medical revenue

R 15. **How many FTE physicians were in your practice?**

    _____ physicians

R 16. **How many FTE nonphysician providers were in your practice?**

    _____ nonphysician providers

17. **Does your practice intend to change its physician compensation method within the next fiscal year?**

    ☐ Yes₁

    ☐ No₂

18. **If compensation is productivity-based, how was production measured? (select all that apply)**

    ☐ Gross charges ₐ

    ☐ Adjusted charges ᵦ

    ☐ Collections for professional charges ᵪ

    ☐ Number of patient encounters ᵨ

    ☐ Size of physician's patient panel ₑ

    ☐ Number of RVUs ᶠ

    ☐ Other ₉ _____

19. **If compensation is based on a structured incentive/bonus, what was the basis for the incentive/bonus? (select all that apply)**

    ☐ Patient satisfaction ₐ

    ☐ Peer review ᵦ

    ☐ Administrative/governance responsibility ᵪ

    ☐ Service quality ᵨ

    ☐ Seniority in the medical practice ₑ

    ☐ Community outreach ᶠ

    ☐ Other ₉ _____

Electronic Health Records (EHR)

20. **How did the health/medical records system store information for the majority of patients served by the practice? If the practice used multiple technologies, choose the system used for the majority of your patients' medical records. (select only one)**

    ☐ Paper medical records/charts filed in record cabinet.₁

    ☐ Computer-based system in which paper records/charts are scanned and scanned documents are filed electronically. This system can be described as a document imaging management system (DIMS).₂

    ☐ An EHR system that stores patient medical and demographic information in a computer database that is accessed by computer terminals or other electronic means. An EHR may also incorporate features of a DIMS.₃

    ☐ Hybrid (inception and cross between paper and electronic). This would include any increments or transactions between electronic and paper.₄

    ☐ Other ₅ _____

21. **If you indicated that you used an EHR, how many years has the EHR been in place?**

    _____ years

Medical Group Management Association®
Compensation and Production Survey: 2008 Questionnaire Based on 2007 Data

Physician Compensation and Production Matrix

The Guide contains additional instructions. The matrix should be completed only for providers who have worked the entire 12-month period reported in question 1. If your practice has more than 12 providers, you are encouraged to submit responses using the Excel- or Web-based version. Visit mgma.com/surveys to download the survey. You must fill in data for at least one provider or one management position in the management compensation matrix.

	1 Provider Tracking Number	2 R Specialty Code (use codes below)	3 R Total Compensation	4 Retirement Benefits (exclude FICA)	5 Partner/ Shareholder in Practice	6 Compensation Method (use codes on next page)	7 Years in Specialty	8 Gender	9 R % Billable Clinical	10 Clinical Svc. Hrs. Worked per Week	11 Physician had on-call duties	12 Weeks Worked per Year
1			$	$	Y N			M F			Y N	
2			$	$	Y N			M F			Y N	
3			$	$	Y N			M F			Y N	
4			$	$	Y N			M F			Y N	
5			$	$	Y N			M F			Y N	
6			$	$	Y N			M F			Y N	
7			$	$	Y N			M F			Y N	
8			$	$	Y N			M F			Y N	
9			$	$	Y N			M F			Y N	
10			$	$	Y N			M F			Y N	
11			$	$	Y N			M F			Y N	
12			$	$	Y N			M F			Y N	

For each provider, select one specialty code where they spent 50% or more time.

Physician Specialty List

Allergy/Immunology 1
Anesthesiology 2*
Anesthesiology: Pain Management 3*
Anesthesiology: Pediatric 4*
Cardiology: Electrophysiology 5
Cardiology: Invasive 6
Cardiology: Inv-Intervntnl 7
Cardiology: Noninvasive 8
Critical Care: Intensivist 9
Dentistry 10
Dermatology 11
Dermatology: Mohs Surgery 12
Emergency Medicine 13
Endocrinology/Metabolism 14
Family Practice (with OB) 15
Family Practice (without OB) 16
Family Practice: Ambulatory Only
   (no inpatient work) 16.1
Family Practice: Sports Medicine 17
Family Practice: Urgent Care 18
Gastroenterology 19
Gastroenterology: Hepatology 20
Genetics 21
Geriatrics 22
Hematology/Oncology 23
Hematology/Oncology: Oncology (only) 24
Hospice/Palliative Care 24.1
Hospitalist: Family Practice 24.2
Hospitalist: Internal Medicine 24.3
Hospitalist: Internal Medicine-Pediatrics 24.4
Hospitalist: Pediatrics 24.5

Hyperbaric Medicine/Wound Care 24.9
Infectious Disease 25
Internal Medicine: General 26
Internal Medicine: Ambulatory Only
   (no inpatient work) 26.1
Internal Medicine: Pediatrics 28
Nephrology 29
Neurology 30
Obstetrics/Gynecology: General 31
OB/GYN: Gynecology (only) 32
OB/GYN: Gynecological Oncology 33
OB/GYN: Maternal & Fetal Medicine 34
OB/GYN: Reproductive Endocrinology 35
Occupational Medicine 36
Ophthalmology 37
Ophthalmology: Pediatric 38
Ophthalmology: Retina 39
Orthopedic (nonsurgical) 40
Orthopedic Surgery: General 41
Orthopedic Surgery: Foot & Ankle 42
Orthopedic Surgery: Hand 43
Orthopedic Surgery: Hip & Joint 44
Orthopedic Surgery: Oncology 45
Orthopedic Surgery: Pediatric 46
Orthopedic Surgery: Spine 47
Orthopedic Surgery: Trauma 48
Orthopedic Surgery: Sports Medicine 49
Otorhinolaryngology 50
Otorhinolaryngology: Pediatric 51
Pathology: Anatomic and Clinical 52
Pathology: Anatomic 53

Pathology: Clinical 54
Pediatrics: General 55
Pediatrics: Adolescent Medicine 56
Pediatrics: Allergy/Immunology 57
Pediatrics: Cardiology 58
Pediatrics: Child Development 59
Pediatrics: Clinical & Lab Immunology 60
Pediatrics: Critical Care/Intensivist 61
Pediatrics: Emergency Medicine 62
Pediatrics: Endocrinology 63
Pediatrics: Gastroenterology 64
Pediatrics: Genetics 65
Pediatrics: Hematology/Oncology 66
Pediatrics: Infectious Disease 68
Pediatrics: Neonatal Medicine 69
Pediatrics: Nephrology 70
Pediatrics: Neurology 71
Pediatrics: Pulmonology 72
Pediatrics: Rheumatology 73
Pediatrics: Sports Medicine 74
Physiatry (Physical Med & Rehab) 75
Podiatry: General 76
Podiatry: Surgery-Foot & Ankle 77
Podiatry: Surgery-Forefoot Only 78
Psychiatry: General 79
Psychiatry: Child & Adolescent 80
Psychiatry: Forensic 81
Psychiatry: Geriatric 82
Pulmonary Medicine: General 83
Pulmonary Medicine: Critical Care 84
Pulmonary Med: General & Critical Care . 110

Please refer to the Guide for more information.

Medical Group Management Association®
Compensation and Production Survey: 2008 Questionnaire Based on 2007 Data

Physician Compensation and Production Matrix (continued)

For questions 13 and 14, TC = Technical Component for laboratory, radiology, medical diagnostic and surgical procedures. Question 21 refers to questions 13 through 20.

13 Collections for Professional Charges	14 Professional Gross Charges	15 **R** Level of TC included in 13 and 14 (circle one)	16 Ambulatory Encounters	17 Hospital Encounters	18 Surgery/ Anesthesia Cases	19 Total RVUs*	20 Physician Work RVUs	21 **R** Nonphysician Provider Productivity (included in 13-20)	22 Half-day Clinical Sessions (direct patient coverage)	
$	$	0% 1-10% >10%						Y N		1
$	$	0% 1-10% >10%						Y N		2
$	$	0% 1-10% >10%						Y N		3
$	$	0% 1-10% >10%						Y N		4
$	$	0% 1-10% >10%						Y N		5
$	$	0% 1-10% >10%						Y N		6
$	$	0% 1-10% >10%						Y N		7
$	$	0% 1-10% >10%						Y N		8
$	$	0% 1-10% >10%						Y N		9
$	$	0% 1-10% >10%						Y N		10
$	$	0% 1-10% >10%						Y N		11
$	$	0% 1-10% >10%						Y N		12

Physician Specialty List (continued)

Radiation Oncology 85
Radiology: Diagnostic-Invasive 86
Radiology: Diagnostic-Noninvasive 87
Radiology: Nuclear Medicine 88
Rheumatology 89
Sleep Medicine 90
Surgery: General 91
Surgery: Bariatric 91.5
Surgery: Cardiovascular 92
Surgery: Cardiovascular-Pediatric 93
Surgery: Colon and Rectal 94
Surgery: Neurological 95
Surgery: Oncology 96
Surgery: Oral 97
Surgery: Pediatric 98
Surgery: Plastic & Reconstruction 99
Surgery: Plastic & Reconstr-Hand 100
Surgery: Plastic & Reconstr-Pediatric 101

Surgery: Thoracic (primary) 102
Surgery: Transplant 103
Surgery: Trauma 104
Surgery: Trauma-Burn 105
Surgery: Endovascular 111
Surgery: Vascular (primary) 106
Urgent Care 107
Urology 108
Urology: Pediatric 109
Other Physician Specialty
 (write in column 2) 112

Nonphysician Provider List
Audiologist 115
Certified Reg. Nurse Anesthetist 116
Dietician/Nutritionist 117
Nurse Midwife: Outpatient/inpatient
 deliveries 118

Nurse Midwife: Outpatient (only) 119
Nurse Midwife: Inpatient (only) 120
Nurse Practitioner 121*
Occupational Therapist 122
Optometrist 123
Orthotist/Prosthetist 124
Perfusionist 125
Pharmacist 126
Physical Therapist 127
Physician Assistant (surgical) 128*
Physician Assistant (primary care) 129*
Physician Assistant (non-surg,
 non-primary care) 130*
Psychologist 131
Social Worker 132
Speech Therapist 133
Surgeon Assistant 134
Other nonphysician provider 135
 (write in column 2)

Compensation Method: Select the choice that best describes the compensation method for each provider listed in the matrix, and place the corresponding number in question 6. The Guide contains additional information for answering questions in this section.

1 100% production less allocated overhead
2 50-99% production less allocated overhead
3 1-49% production less allocated overhead
4 100% production-based share of practice compensation pool
5 50-99% production-based share of practice compensation pool
6 1-49% production-based share of practice compensation pool

7 100% equal share of practice compensation pool
8 50-99% base salary plus incentive
9 1-49% base salary plus incentive
10 100% straight/guaranteed salary
11 Other (describe compensation method in Comments section on pg. 8)

Please refer to the Guide for more information.

Medical Group Management Association®
Compensation and Production Survey: 2008 Questionnaire Based on 2007 Data

Management Compensation Matrix

The Guide contains additional instructions. The matrix requests information for executives, managerial staff, specialists and supervisors who held the same position for the entire 12-month reporting period and were employed on a

1 Employee Tracking Code	2 [R] Position Title (use codes below)	3 Centralized Staff Position	4 [R] Total Compensation (include bonus/incentive)	5 Bonus/Incentive Amount	6 Retirement Benefits (exclude FICA)	7 Compensation Method (use codes on next page)
1		Y N	$	$	$	
2		Y N	$	$	$	
3		Y N	$	$	$	
4		Y N	$	$	$	
5		Y N	$	$	$	
6		Y N	$	$	$	
7		Y N	$	$	$	
8		Y N	$	$	$	
9		Y N	$	$	$	
10		Y N	$	$	$	

Select one position that best describes each individual's responsibilities from the list below, and place the corresponding number in question 2. The Guide contains position descriptions.

Physician Executive Positions
Associate/Assistant Medical Director 3
Medical Director 2
Physician Chief Executive Officer (CEO)/President 1

Executive Management Position
Administrator 5
Assistant Administrator 9
Chief Executive Officer (CEO)/Executive Director 4
Chief Financial Officer (CFO) 8
Chief Information Officer (CIO) 47
Chief Operating Officer (COO) 7
MSO Administrator/Executive Director 6

Senior Management Positions
Ambulatory/Clinical Services Director 10
Branch/Satellite Clinic Director 48
Building and Grounds Director 11
Business Services Director 12
Clinical Research Director 13
Compliance Director 14
Education and Training Director 15
Finance Director 16
Human Resources Director 17
Information Systems Director 18
Laboratory Services Director 19
Managed Care Director 20
Marketing and Sales Director 21
Medical Records Director 22
Nursing Services Director 23
Physician Recruitment Director 49
Quality Improvement/Quality Assurance Director 24
Radiology Services Director 25
Reimbursement Director 26

General Management Positions
Benefits Manager 27
Branch/Satellite Clinic Manager 28
Business Office Manager 29
Clinical Department Manager 30
Clinic Research Manager 31
General Accounting Manager 32
Laboratory Services Manager 33
Materials Management Manager 34
Medical Records Manager 35
Nursing Manager 36
Office Manager 37
Operations Manager 38
Patient Accounting Manager 39
Radiology Services Manager 40
Training/Education Manager 41

Specialists
Benefits/Payroll Specialist 42
Marketing/Communication Specialist 43

Supervisors
Business Office Supervisor 44
Clinic Supervisor 45
Front Office Supervisor 50
Nursing Supervisor 46

Other: (please list the title and describe the position in Comments on pg. 8) 51

Medical Group Management Association®
Compensation and Production Survey: 2008 Questionnaire Based on 2007 Data

Management Compensation Matrix (continued)

full-time basis. If your practice has more than 10 management staff, you are encouraged to submit responses using the Excel- or Web-based version. Visit mgma.com/surveys to download the survey.

8 Formal Education (use codes below)	9 Years of Management Experience	10 Gender	11 ACMPE Status (use codes below)	12 MGMA National Member	Phys. Exec., Exec. Mgmt., Sr. Mgmt. Positions ONLY 13 Professional Organization Fees	Physician Executives ONLY 14 Percentage of Time Admin Clinical	
_____	_____	M F	_____	Y N	$ _____	____ % ____ %	1
_____	_____	M F	_____	Y N	$ _____	____ % ____ %	2
_____	_____	M F	_____	Y N	$ _____	____ % ____ %	3
_____	_____	M F	_____	Y N	$ _____	____ % ____ %	4
_____	_____	M F	_____	Y N	$ _____	____ % ____ %	5
_____	_____	M F	_____	Y N	$ _____	____ % ____ %	6
_____	_____	M F	_____	Y N	$ _____	____ % ____ %	7
_____	_____	M F	_____	Y N	$ _____	____ % ____ %	8
_____	_____	M F	_____	Y N	$ _____	____ % ____ %	9
_____	_____	M F	_____	Y N	$ _____	____ % ____ %	10

Compensation Method: Select the choice that best describes the compensation method for each individual listed in question 2, and place the corresponding number in question 7.

1   Hourly
2   Straight salary only (no bonus)
3   Base salary + discretionary bonus (e.g., end-of-year bonus)
4   Base salary + percentage of practice productivity and/or physician income (formula bonus)
5   Base salary + percentage of practice's net profit (formula bonus)
6   Base salary + other formula bonus (e.g., number of patient visits, patient satisfaction, etc.)
7   Base salary + deferred compensation (e.g., trusts, stock options, etc.)
8   Base salary + combination of discretionary and formula bonuses + deferred compensation
9   Other (describe the compensation method in Comments on pg. 8)

Formal Education: Select the highest level of formal education attained by each individual, and place the corresponding number in question 8.
1   High school diploma or the equivalent
2   Associate degree or other two-year degree
3   Bachelor's degree or other four-year degree
4   Master's degree
5   PhD, JD, EdD
6   MD, DO
7   MD or DO (with Master's degree)
8   Other (describe the education level in Comments on pg. 8)

ACMPE Status: Select each individual's status in the American College of Medical Practice Executives (ACMPE), the professional credentialing arm of MGMA, and place the corresponding number in question 11.
1   Not affiliated
2   Nominee
3   Certified (CMPE)
4   Fellow (FACMPE)

Medical Group Management Association®
Compensation and Production Survey: 2008 Questionnaire Based on 2007 Data

Report Recipient

Organizations will be mailed a Respondent Ranking Report and a complimentary copy of the survey report as a benefit of participation. To ensure this confidential information reaches the appropriate individual, indicate below the recipient's name, organization, and mailing address in the spaces provided, if different from the information appearing on the mailing label. Provide complete information.

34. Name _____
35. Title _____
36. Organization _____
37. Address _____
38. City _____
39. State _____ 40. ZIP _____
41. Telephone number (_____) _____
42. E-mail address _____
43. MGMA member # _____

Questionnaire Contact

Provide contact information for the individual who completed this questionnaire, as well as the name of the observed practice for which data are reported.

22. Name _____
23. Title _____
24. Telephone number (_____) _____
25. Fax number (_____) _____
26. E-mail address _____
R 27. Observed Practice Name _____
28. Address _____
29. City _____
30. State _____ 31. ZIP _____
32. Provide the Federal Tax ID # for the observed practice.
_____
33. Number of hours required to complete this questionnaire _____

Parent Organization Information

The observed medical practice is the medical practice for which data are reported on this questionnaire. If you indicated in question 9, ownership of the observed practice by a 'hospital/integrated delivery system,' 'MSO,' 'PPMC,' 'university' or 'other' type of organization, provide the name of the parent organization (owner) and its location in the spaces provided below.

44. Parent Name _____
45. Address _____
46. City _____
47. State _____

Comments

_____
_____
_____
_____
_____
_____
_____
_____
_____

MGMA use only

GSN:
Database ID:
P=
M=

Appendix F: Compensation and Production Survey: 2008 Guide to the Questionnaire Based on 2007 Data

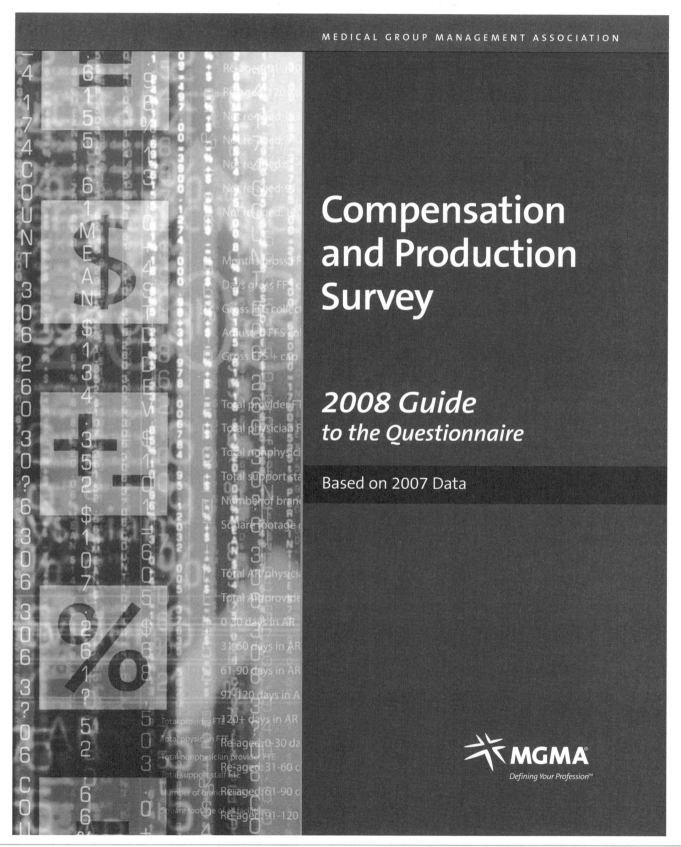

MEDICAL GROUP MANAGEMENT ASSOCIATION

Compensation and Production Survey

2008 Guide
to the Questionnaire

Based on 2007 Data

MGMA
Defining Your Profession™

Medical Group Management Association®
Compensation and Production Survey: 2008 Guide to the Questionnaire Based on 2007 Data

Frequently Asked Questions

What is the purpose of this survey questionnaire?
This survey questionnaire collects data for the *Physician Compensation and Production Survey: 2008 Report Based on 2007 Data* and the *Management Compensation Survey: 2008 Report Based on 2007 Data*. These reports provide comparison data on physician and nonphysician provider compensation and production, as well as managerial compensation to help evaluate decisions in a medical practice.

Who is conducting this survey?
Medical Group Management Association (MGMA) Survey Operations.

Who should complete this survey?
One questionnaire should be completed by the medical practice.

If your organization is an Integrated Delivery System (IDS), hospital, Management Services Organization (MSO), Physician Practice Management Company (PPMC), Independent Practice Association (IPA) or other entity that owns, manages or provides services to medical practices, **one questionnaire should be completed for each medical practice that you own, manage or service.**

Academic practices, faculty practice plans and clinical science departments associated with medical schools should **not** participate in this survey. Freestanding ambulatory surgery centers (ASC) also should **not** participate in this survey. Instead, they should participate respectively in the *Academic Practice Compensation and Production Survey: 2008 Questionnaire Based on 2008 Data* or the *Ambulatory Surgery Center Performance Survey: 2008 Questionnaire Based on 2007 Data*.

Questionnaires should not be submitted for departments within multispecialty practices. A questionnaire must represent a complete medical practice.

Do I need to answer all of the questions on the survey?
We would appreciate receiving the requested information on your organization, to the extent you can provide it. The quality of our reported results depends upon the completeness and accuracy of every response.

Questions with an **R** next to the number are required. Therefore, if any of the following questions are omitted the respondent's questionnaire will be considered

incomplete and ineligible for data inclusion:
    Fiscal year
    Practice type
    Single-specialty (if applicable)
    Freestanding ambulatory surgery center
    Medical school faculty practice plan/clinical science department
    Majority owner
    Total medical revenue
    Full-time equivalent physicians
    Full-time equivalent nonphysician providers
    Specialty code (physician matrix)
    Total compensation (physician matrix)
    Percent billable clinical (physician matrix)
    Level of TC included in 13 and 14
    Nonphysician provider productivity (physician matrix)
    Position title (management matrix)
    Total compensation (management matrix)
    Observed practice name (questionnaire contact)

What if I am unsure about how to answer a question properly?
Refer to the Guide. For any questions about the survey questionnaire, call MGMA Survey Operations toll-free, 877.275.6462, ext. 895, or e-mail surveys@mgma.com.

Are all survey data confidential?
Yes. The MGMA and the MGMA Center for Research Policy on Data Confidentiality states: All data submitted to MGMA or to the MGMA Center for Research will be kept confidential. All submitted data and related materials that identify a specific organization or individual will be safeguarded and will not be published or voluntarily released within the public domain without written permission.

Only summary statistics will be published. A summary statistic will be reported only if there are sufficient responses and if the anonymity of those submitting data is protected.

When is my response due?
The due date is March 14, 2008. The survey results will be much more useful to you if we can report the results on a timely basis. We have a very tight schedule for obtaining responses, processing the data and publishing the *2008 Physician Compensation and Production*

Medical Group Management Association®
Compensation and Production Survey: 2008 Guide to the Questionnaire Based on 2007 Data

Survey Report and the 2008 Management Compensation Survey Report. Therefore, we would sincerely appreciate you giving this survey a high priority and returning your completed questionnaire as soon as you can.

Can the data be submitted electronically?
Yes. Visit mgma.com/surveys and follow the directions to access the Web-based or Excel-based versions on the screen.

Where do I send a completed questionnaire?
Use the enclosed reply envelope and mail the completed questionnaire to the MGMA Survey Operations Department, 104 Inverness Terrace East, Englewood, CO 80112-5306. Or you may fax your response to 303.784.6100, Attention: Survey Operations. If you used the Excel-based version, you may e-mail your response to surveys@mgma.com. Be sure to keep a photocopy of the completed questionnaire for your reference. If you complete the Web-based version, follow the instructions on the screen to submit it.

Medical Group Management Association®
Compensation and Production Survey: 2008 Guide to the Questionnaire Based on 2007 Data

Definitions

2007 Fiscal Year Definition

1. **For the purposes of reporting the information in this questionnaire, what fiscal year was used?**
For many practices, this is January 2007 through December 2007. If your practice uses an alternative fiscal year, you are encouraged to use it in your responses. Do not report data for periods less than 12 months.

   If your medical practice was involved in a merger or acquisition during 2007 and you cannot assemble 12 months of practice data, you may not be able to participate this year. Please call MGMA Survey Operations if you are uncertain about your eligibility to participate.

Medical Practice Information

2. **What was your practice type? (select only one)**
Single specialty: A medical practice that focuses its clinical work in one specialty. The determining factor for classifying the type of specialty is the focus of clinical work and not necessarily the specialties of the physicians in the practice. For example, a single specialty neurosurgery practice may include a neurologist and a radiologist.

   Practices that include only the subspecialties of internal medicine should be classified as a single specialty internal medicine practice. Internal medicine subspecialties include:
   Allergy and immunology
   Cardiology
   Endocrinology/metabolism
   Gastroenterology
   Hematology/oncology
   Infectious disease
   Nephrology
   Pulmonary disease
   Rheumatology
   Multispecialty with primary and specialty care: A medical practice which consists of physicians practicing in different specialties, including at least one primary care specialty listed below.
   Family practice: general
   Family practice: sports medicine
   Family practice: urgent care
   Family practice: with obstetrics
   Family practice: without obstetrics

   Geriatrics
   Internal medicine: general
   Internal medicine: urgent care
   Pediatrics: adolescent medicine
   Pediatrics: general
   Pediatrics: sports medicine
   Multispecialty with primary care only: A medical practice that consists of physicians practicing in more than one of the primary care specialties listed above or the surgical specialties of
   Obstetrics/gynecology
   Gynecology (only)
   Obstetrics (only)
   Multispecialty with specialty care only: A medical practice, which consists of physicians practicing in different specialties, none of which are the primary care specialties listed above.

3. **If you answered "Single specialty" for question 2, what specialty was your practice?**
State the name of the single specialty that most closely describes your practice.

4. **Was your organization a freestanding ambulatory surgery center only? Answer "No" if the ambulatory surgery center was a unit of the medical practice.**
An ambulatory surgery center (ASC) is a freestanding entity that is specifically licensed to provide surgery services that are performed on a same-day outpatient basis. An ASC does not employ physicians.

5. **Was your practice a medical school faculty practice plan and/or clinical science department?**
Answer "Yes" if your practice was a medical school faculty practice plan and/or clinical science department.

   A faculty practice plan is the organization that manages the business functions of a medical school faculty's clinical practices. The plan performs a range of services including billing, collections, contract negotiations and the distribution of income. Practice plans may form a separate legal organization or may be affiliated with the medical school through a clinical science department or teaching hospital. Faculty associated with the

Medical Group Management Association®
Compensation and Production Survey: 2008 Guide to the Questionnaire Based on 2007 Data

practice plan must provide patient care as part of the clinical department teaching or research programs that result in the granting of a doctor of medicine (MD) degree.

A clinical science department is a unit of organization in a medical school with an independent chair and a single budget. The department's missions are to educate medical students and residents and to conduct research and/or clinical activities related to the entire spectrum of health care delivery to humans, from prevention through treatment.

6. **Was your practice affiliated with a medical school?**
Answer "Yes" if your practice had a relationship in which:
- Clinicians from the medical group practice hold nontenure appointments on a medical school faculty and/or are part of a health system that is associated with a medical school that grants an MD degree; and
- A legal standing with a medical school, faculty practice plan, or clinical science department existed.
Answer "No" if you are a:
- Medical practice that provided residency rotations, but did not meet the above criteria.

7. **Did an MSO, PPMC or an Independent Practice Association (IPA) provide services to your practice?**
Answer "Yes" if your practice had a contract with an MSO, PPMC or IPA to provide services to your practice.

Management Services Organizations (MSO), Physician Practice Management Companies (PPMC), etc.
An MSO is an entity organized to provide various forms of practice management and administrative support services to health care providers. These services may include centralized billing and collections services, management information services and other components of the managed care infrastructure. MSOs do not actually deliver health care services. MSOs may be jointly or solely owned and sponsored by physicians, hospitals or other parties. Some MSOs also purchase assets of affiliated physicians and enter into long-term

management service arrangements with a provider network. Some expand their ownership base by involving outside investors to help capitalize the development of such practice infrastructure.

PPMCs are usually publicly held or entrepreneurial directed enterprises that acquire total or partial ownership interests in physician organizations. PPMCs are a type of MSO, however the motivations, goals, strategies, and structures arising from their unequivocal ownership character - development of growth and profits for their investors, not for participating providers — differentiate them from other MSO models.

An IPA is an association or network of licensed providers and/or medical practices. An IPA is usually a unique legal entity, most often operating on a for-profit basis. Typically, the primary purpose of the IPA is to secure and maintain contractual relationships between providers and health plans.

If your organization is an MSO, PPMC, IPA or other type of management organization, you should complete one questionnaire for each medical practice that you manage or service. You may make as many photocopies of this questionnaire as necessary or call MGMA Survey Operations to receive additional copies.

When completing a questionnaire on behalf of a managed practice, identify the parent organization (owner) by completing the Parent Organization Information section of the questionnaire.

8. **What was the legal organization of your practice? (select only one)**
Business corporation: A for-profit organization recognized by law as a business entity separate and distinct from its shareholders. Shareholders need not be licensed in the profession practiced by the corporation.
Limited liability company: A legal entity that is a hybrid between a corporation and a partnership, because it provides limited liability to owners like a corporation while passing profits and losses through to owners like a partnership.
Not-for-profit corporation/foundation: An organization that has obtained special exemption under Section 501(c) of the Internal Revenue Service

Medical Group Management Association®
Compensation and Production Survey: 2008 Guide to the Questionnaire Based on 2007 Data

code that qualifies the organization to be exempt from federal income taxes. To qualify as a tax-exempt organization, a practice or faculty practice plan would have to provide evidence of a charitable, educational or research purpose.

Partnership: An unincorporated organization where two or more individuals have agreed that they will share profits, losses, assets and liabilities, although not necessarily on an equal basis. The partnership agreement may or may not be formalized in writing.

Professional corporation/association: A for-profit organization recognized by law as a business entity separate and distinct from its shareholders. Shareholders must be licensed in the profession practiced by the organization.

Sole proprietorship: An organization with a single owner who is responsible for all profit, losses, assets and liabilities.

Other: Describe the legal organization in the "other" box.

9. **Who was the majority owner of your practice? (select only one)**
Government: A governmental organization at the federal, state or local level. Government funding is not a sufficient criterion. Government ownership is the key factor. An example would be a medical clinic at a federal, state or county correctional facility.

Hospital/integrated delivery system (IDS): An IDS is a network of organizations that provide or coordinate and arrange for the provision of a continuum of health care services to consumers and are willing to be held clinically and fiscally responsible for the outcomes and the health status of the populations served. Generally consisting of hospitals, physician groups, health plans, home health agencies, hospices, skilled nursing facilities, or other provider entities, these networks may be built through "virtual" integration processes encompassing contractual arrangements and strategic alliances as well as through direct ownership.

A hospital is an inpatient facility that admits patients for overnight stays, incurs nursing care costs and generates bed-day revenues.

If your organization is an IDS or hospital that owns and/or manages medical practices, you should complete one questionnaire for each practice that you own or manage. Also, you may want to complete the *Cost Survey for Integrated Delivery System Practices: 2008 Questionnaire Based on 2007 Data.*

When completing a questionnaire on behalf of an owned practice, identify the parent organization (owner) by completing the Parent Organization Information section of the questionnaire.

Insurance company or health maintenance organization (HMO): An insurance company is an organization that indemnifies an insured party against a specified loss in return for premiums paid, as stipulated by a contract. An HMO is an insurance company that accepts responsibility for providing and delivering a predetermined set of comprehensive health maintenance and treatment services to a voluntarily enrolled population for a negotiated and fixed periodic premium.

MSO or PPMC: If your practice is owned by an MSO or PPMC, indicate the name and location of your parent organization (owner) on questions 44-47.

Physicians: Any MD or doctor of osteopathy (DO) who is duly licensed and qualified under the law of jurisdiction in which treatment is received.

University or medical school: A university is an institution of higher learning with teaching and research facilities comprising undergraduate, graduate and professional schools. A medical school is an institution that trains physicians and awards medical and osteopathic degrees. If your practice is owned by a university or medical school, indicate the name and location of your parent organization (owner) on questions 44-47.

Other: Describe the type of entity in the "Other" box.

10. **If you are a hospital/IDS, MSO or PPMC, and/or a medical practice with more than one legal entity, do you have a centralized administrative department?**
Answer "Yes" if you have a centralized administrative department that provides leadership and has the authority/responsibility for the operations of the various physician practices within the entity. This department would provide oversight and encompass many or all of the following types of activities: establishing policies, negotiating managed care agreements, strategic planning, physician contracting, approving expenditures, as well as affording any other resources required to manage the physician practices.

Medical Group Management Association®
Compensation and Production Survey: 2008 Guide to the Questionnaire Based on 2007 Data

11. **Which population designation best describes the area surrounding the primary location of your practice? If your practice had multiple sites, choose the option that represents the location with the largest number of full-time-equivalent (FTE) physicians. (select only one)**
Nonmetropolitan (fewer than 50,000): The community in which the practice is located is generally referred to as "rural". It is located outside of a "metropolitan statistical area" (MSA), as defined by the United States Office of Management and Budget, and has a population less than 50,000.
Metropolitan (50,000 to 250,000): The community in which the practice is located is an MSA or Census Bureau defined urbanized area with a population of 50,000 to 250,000.
Metropolitan (250,001 to 1,000,000): The community in which the practice is located is an MSA or Census Bureau defined urbanized area with a population of 250,001 to 1,000,000.
Metropolitan (more than 1,000,000): The community in which the practice is located is a "primary metropolitan statistical area" (PMSA) with a population of more than 1,000,000.

12. **Did your practice derive revenue from capitation contracts?** Answer "Yes" if your practice derives revenue from capitation contracts. A capitation contract is a contract in which the practice agrees to provide medical services to a defined population for a fixed price per beneficiary per month, regardless of actual services provided. Capitation contracts, which always contain an element of risk, include HMO, Medicare and Medicaid capitation contracts.

13. **If you answered "Yes" to question 12, what percentage of your practice's total medical revenue was derived from capitation contracts?** Report the percentage of your total medical revenue that was derived from capitation contracts.

14. **What was the total medical revenue (collections) for your practice?** Report the net of gross practice revenue, refunds, returned checks, contractual discounts and allowances, bad debts and write-offs. Total medical revenue is the sum of fee-for-service collections, capitation payments, and other medical activity revenues.

15. **How many FTE physicians were in your practice?** Report the number of FTE physicians in your practice. An FTE physician works whatever number of hours the practice considers to be the minimum for a normal workweek, which could be 37.5, 40, 50 hours or some other standard. To compute the FTE of a part-time physician divide the total hours worked by the physician by the number of hours that your medical practice considers to be a normal workweek. For example, a physician working in a clinic or hospital on behalf of the practice for 30 hours compared to a normal workweek of 40 hours would be 0.75 FTE (30 divided by 40 hours). A physician working full-time for three months during a year would be 0.25 FTE (3 divided by 12 months). A medical director devoting 50% effort to clinical activity would be 0.5 FTE. **Do not report a physician as more than 1.0 FTE regardless of the number of hours worked.**
Include:
1. Practice physicians such as shareholders/partners, salaried associates, employed and contracted physicians and locum tenens; and
2. Only physicians involved in clinical care.
Do not include:
1. Full-time physician administrators.

16. **How many FTE nonphysician providers were in your practice?** Report the number of FTE nonphysician providers in your practice. Nonphysician providers are specially trained and licensed providers who can provide medical care and billable services. Examples of nonphysician providers include audiologists, Certified Registered Nurse Anesthetists (CRNAs), dieticians/nutritionists, midwives, nurse practitioners, occupational therapists, optometrists, physical therapists, physician assistants, psychologists, social workers, speech therapists and surgeon assistants. To compute the number of nonphysician providers see the definition for FTE physicians given in question 15.

17. **Does your practice intend to change its physician compensation method within the next fiscal year?** Answer "Yes" if the current method of determining your physicians' compensation will change in the next fiscal year.

Medical Group Management Association®
Compensation and Production Survey: 2008 Guide to the Questionnaire Based on 2007 Data

18. If compensation is productivity-based, how was production measured? (select all that apply)

Gross charges: Gross charges are the full value, at the practice's undiscounted rates, of all services provided. Undiscounted rates are the full retail prices before Medicare/Medicaid charge restrictions, third-party payer (such as commercial insurance and/or managed care organization) contractual adjustments, and other charitable, professional courtesy or employee adjustments.

Adjusted charges: (gross charges *minus* contractual discounts/allowances) Adjusted charges are the total amounts expected to be paid by patients or third-party payers. This figure can be calculated by taking gross charges and subtracting the adjustments from third-party payer's and charge restrictions from Medicare/Medicaid.

Collections for professional charges: Amount of revenue attributed to a physician for their professional services to patients.

Number of patient encounters: A documented, face-to-face contact between a patient and a provider who exercises independent judgment in the provision of services to the individual. If the patient with the same diagnosis sees two different providers on the same day, it is one encounter. If patient sees two different providers on the same day for two different diagnoses, then it is considered two encounters.

Size of physician's patient panel: The number of patients, regardless of payer, assigned to a primary care physician.

Number of RVUs: The number of relative value units (RVU), as measured by the Resource Based Relative Value Scale (RBRVS). The RBRVS units may be measured either as physician work units or total units.

Other: If your practice's production is measured other than the options provided, describe the measurement used in the "Other" box.

19. If compensation is based on a structured incentive/bonus, what was the basis for the incentive/bonus? (select all that apply)

Patient satisfaction: Evaluation of clinical services by patients who assess their degree of satisfaction.

Peer review: An internal review process of practice providers by a panel of group physicians.

Administrative/governance responsibility: If a physician holds administrative or governance responsibility, and receives a bonus or incentive payment for their nonclinical administrative and governance work.

Service quality: Some measurement decided by the practice on the quality of a physician's service to patients.

Seniority in the medical practice: The length of time a physician has been with the practice.

Community outreach: Direct involvement in community service activities.

Other: If your practice's incentive/bonus is other than the options provided, describe the measurement used in the "Other" box.

Electronic Health Records (EHR)

20. How did the health/medical records system store information for the majority of patients served by the practice? If the practice used multiple technologies, choose the system used for the majority of your patients' medical records. (select only one)

Choose the method in which the practice stored the health/medical records for the majority of patients served by the practice.

A fully operational EHR would include the following four functions:

- Collect patient data;
- Display test results;
- Allow providers to enter medical orders and prescriptions; and
- Aid physicians in making treatment decisions.

21. If you indicated that you used an EHR, how many years has the EHR been in place?

Indicate, in whole numbers, the number of years the EHR was in place.

Physician Compensation and Production Matrix

The matrix requests information for questions 1 through 22. Complete the matrix for all providers who worked for your medical practice the entire 12 months indicated in question 1. Make sure that all physician administrators are also reported in the Management Matrix, if 50% or more of their time is spent administratively.

ATTENTION: Equal-share anesthesiology practices should follow instructions provided in this packet.

Medical Group Management Association®
Compensation and Production Survey: 2008 Guide to the Questionnaire Based on 2007 Data

The following question numbers apply to the matrices.

Question 1 - Provider tracking number

Indicate your medical practice's internal tracking number such as the last four numbers of a SSN or initials for each individual. This number may be numeric, alpha or a combination of both and may be up to six digits long. This number will make it easier to interpret the Respondent Ranking Report. If you do not have a unique identifier, create a series of letters and numbers such as 12345x.

Question 2 - Specialty code

Select only one specialty for each physician and nonphysician provider using the specialty codes listed below the matrix. A provider should be classified in the specialty or subspecialty where the provider spends 50% or more time. If you select "Other", please indicate the specialty.

For nurse practitioners and physician assistants, select the appropriate code number and provide the specialty area where at least 50% of their time is being spent such as acute care, adult, emergency, family practice, gerontologic/elder health, neonatal/perinatal, occupational health, oncology, pediatric/child health, psychiatric/mental health, school/college health or women's health.

Question 3 - Total compensation

State the amount reported as direct compensation on a W2, 1099, or K1 (for partnerships) plus all voluntary salary reductions such as 401(k), 403(b), Section 125 Tax Savings Plan, or Medical Savings Plan. The amount reported should include salary, bonus and/or incentive payments, research stipends, honoraria and distribution of profits.

Do not include:
1. The dollar value of expense reimbursements, fringe benefits paid by the medical practice such as retirement plan contributions, life and health insurance, or automobile allowances, or any employer contributions to a 401(k), 403(b) or Keogh Plan.

Question 4 - Retirement benefits (exclude FICA)

Report all employer contributions to retirement plans including defined benefit and contribution plans, 401(k), 403(b) and Keogh Plans, and any non-qualified funded retirement plan. For defined benefit plans, estimate the employer's contribution made on behalf of each plan participant by multiplying the employer's total contribution by each plan participant's compensation divided by the total compensation of all plan participants.

Do not include:
1. Employer contributions to social security mandated by the Federal Insurance Contributions Act (FICA);
2. Voluntary employee contributions that are an allocation of salary to a 401(k), 403(b), or Keogh Plan; or
3. The dollar value of any other fringe benefits paid by the practice, such as life and health insurance or automobile allowances.

Question 5 - Partner/shareholder in practice

Answer "Yes" if the physician has a partner, shareholder, or other ownership status in the practice, regardless of the particular form of legal entity used for the practice. Partner and shareholder status represents ownership in which the physician agrees to share profits, losses, assets and liabilities, although not necessarily on an equal basis. Shareholder status also includes formal possession of shares in the practice.

Question 6 - Compensation method

From the options listed select the choice that best describes the compensation method for the provider. For each provider, select the compensation plan/financial funds flow model that best represents the compensation plan from the following broad types of plans:

Production less allocated overhead: This compensation plan allocates a portion of practice revenues to each individual physician, and subtracts an allocated portion of practice expenses to determine each individual physician's compensation. Such plans tend to treat each physician as a separate economic unit for compensation plan purposes; commonly use cost accounting and similar methods; and may be referred to as "individualistic" compensation plans. The basic calculation is Physician Revenues - Physician Expenses = Physician Compensation.

Medical Group Management Association®
Compensation and Production Survey: 2008 Guide to the Questionnaire Based on 2007 Data

Production-based share of practice compensation pool: This compensation plan uses a methodology to allocate a "compensation pool" which is equal to the total practice revenues net of practice overhead expenses to determine physician compensation. Such plans generally treat practice overhead as a cost of doing business that is borne by the group as a whole and not allocated to individual physicians (with the potential exception of physician-specific direct expenses). Such plans may be referred to as "team" or "group-oriented" compensation plans. The basic calculation is Practice Revenues - Practice Expense = Compensation Pool.

100% Equal share of practice compensation pool: This compensation plan allocates to each physician an equal share of the money available in the compensation pool. Refer to the definition of "compensation pool" above.

Base plus incentive: This compensation plan involves the payment of a guaranteed base salary, coupled with an incentive component in which the incentive is "at risk" or must be earned, and may be awarded based on one or more criteria including individual production, unit/department and/or organization performance, patient satisfaction, citizenship, and other factors.

Straight/guaranteed salary: This compensation plan pays 100% of the provider's compensation via a fixed salary.

Other: If your compensation method is other than the options provided, describe the compensation method in the Comments section of the questionnaire.

Question 7 - Years in specialty
Report the number of years each physician and nonphysician provider has practiced in the specialty. The count of the number of years should begin at the time the physician completes the latter of the residency or fellowship.

Question 8 - Gender
Select the gender for this individual.

Question 9 - Percent billable clinical
Report in whole numbers the billable clinical percent for each provider listed in question 1. Billable clinical percent can be calculated a variety of ways. In general, the calculations are all the same - the clinical effort divided by the total effort. Often, the

difference between formulas equals the units of measurement such as hours per day or sessions per week. Clinical effort and activities include direct patient care and consultation, individually or in a team-care setting, where a patient bill is generated or a fee-for-service equivalent charge is recorded.

Question 10 - Clinical service hours worked per week
Clinical service hours refer to weekly hours during which a clinician is involved in direct patient care where a patient bill is generated and a fee-for-service equivalent charge is created for the practice. Clinical service hours include seeing patients in the office, outpatient clinic, emergency room, nursing home, operating room, labor and delivery, and time spent on hospital rounds.
Include:
1. Capitated (HMO) contracts;
2. Indigent and professional courtesy care;
3. Clinical or ancillary services;
4. Dictation and chart documentation; and
5. Clinical services delivered at VA facilities where a patient bill is generated.

Do not include:
1. On-call time regardless of whether physician is on- or off-site;
2. Nonbillable clinical activities where a patient bill is not generated nor a fee-for-service equivalent charge recorded such as pro bono clinical activities performed at VA facilities;
3. Telephone conversations with patients, consultations with providers, interpretation of diagnostic tests and chart reviews;
4. Research activities including specific research, training, and other projects that are separately budgeted and accounted for by the medical practice;
5. Performing administrative activities or support activities in a medical practice; or
6. Case conferences.

Indicate the number of clinical service hours the physician works during a normal (typical) work week.

Question 11 - Physician had on-call duties
If the physician has on-call responsibilities, select "Yes." If the physician does not participate in on-call, select "No."

Medical Group Management Association®
Compensation and Production Survey: 2008 Guide to the Questionnaire Based on 2007 Data

Question 12 - Weeks worked per year
Estimate to the nearest week the number of weeks the provider was engaged in professional activities in the practice.
Include:
1. Clinical and nonclinical time.

Do not include:
1. Vacation, sick leave, medical or continuing education.

Question 13 - Collections for professional charges
Report amount of collections attributed to a physician for all professional services.
Include:
1. Fee-for-service collections;
2. Allocated capitation payments;
3. Administration of chemotherapy drugs; and
4. Administration of immunizations.

Do not include:
1. Collections on drug charges, including vaccinations, allergy injections, and immunizations, as well as chemotherapy and antinauseant drugs;
2. The technical component (TC) associated with any laboratory, radiology, medical diagnostic or surgical procedure collections. If your practice cannot break this out, report collections and answer the appropriate response in question 15;
3. Collections attributed to nonphysician providers. If your practice cannot break this out, report collections and answer "Yes" in question 21;
4. Infusion-related collections;
5. Facility fees;
6. Supplies; or
7. Revenue associated with the sale of hearing aids, eyeglasses, contact lenses, etc.

Important: If collections are reported in question 13, respondents must complete questions 15 and 21.

Question 14 - Professional gross charges
Report the total gross patient charges attributed to a physician for all professional services. Gross patient charges are the full dollar value, at the practice's established undiscounted rates, of services provided to all patients, before reduction by charitable adjustments, professional courtesy adjustments, contractual adjustments, employee discounts, bad debts, etc. For both Medicare participating and nonparticipating providers, gross charges should include the practice's full, undiscounted charge and not the Medicare limiting charge.
Include:
1. Fee-for-service charges;
2. In-house equivalent gross fee-for-service charges for capitated patients;
3. Administration of chemotherapy drugs; and
4. Administration of immunizations.

Do not include:
1. Charges for drugs, including vaccinations, allergy, injections, and immunizations as well as chemotherapy and antinauseant drugs;
2. The technical component associated with any laboratory, radiology, medical diagnostic or surgical procedure. If your practice cannot break this out, report gross charges and answer the appropriate response in question 15;
3. Charges attributed to nonphysician providers. If your practice cannot break this out, report gross charges and answer Y for "Yes" in question 21;
4. Infusion-related charges;
5. Facility fees;
6. Supplies; or
7. Charges associated with the sale of hearing aids, eyeglasses, contact lenses, etc.

Important: If gross charges are reported in question 14 respondents must complete questions 15 and 21.

Question 15 - Level of TC included in collections for professional charges and professional gross charges
Collections for professional charges and gross charges for laboratory, radiology, medical diagnostic and surgical procedures may have two components: the physician's professional charge such as interpretation and the technical charge for the operation and use of the equipment. If collections for professional charges and gross charges in questions 13 and 14 do not include the TC, referred to as professional services only billing, select "0%." If collections for professional charges and gross charges does include the TC, referred to as global fee billing, indicate the approximate percentage of charges represented by the TC by selecting either "1-10%" or ">10%."

Questions 16 and 17 - Encounters
A documented, face-to-face contact between a patient and a provider who exercises independent

Medical Group Management Association®
Compensation and Production Survey: 2008 Guide to the Questionnaire Based on 2007 Data

judgment in the provision of services to the individual. If a patient sees multiple providers on the same day for the same set of problems/diagnoses, it is considered one encounter. If a patient with multiple problems/diagnoses sees multiple providers on the same day and each provider manages a different set of problems/diagnoses, then it can be considered as multiple encounters.

Include:
1. Pre- and post-operative visits and other visits associated with a global charge;
2. For diagnostic radiologists, report the total number of procedures or reads, regardless of place of service; and
3. For obstetrics care, where a single CPT-4 code is used for a global service, count each ambulatory contact as a separate ambulatory encounter (e.g., each prenatal visit and postnatal visit is an ambulatory encounter). Count the delivery as a single surgical case.

Do not include:
1. Ambulatory encounters attributed to nonphysician providers. If your practice cannot break this out, report encounters and answer "Yes" in question 21;
2. Encounters for the physician specialties of pathology or diagnostic radiology. (see #2 under "Include" above);
3. Encounters that include procedures from the surgery chapter (CPT codes 10021-69979) or anesthesia chapter (CPT codes 00100-01999). Report these as surgery/anesthesia cases in question 18;
4. Number of procedures, since a single encounter can generate multiple procedures;
5. Visits where there is not an identifiable contact between a patient and a physician or nonphysician provider such as when the patient comes into the practice solely for an injection, vein puncture, EKG, or EEG administered by an RN or technician;
6. Administration of chemotherapy drugs; or
7. Administration of immunizations.

Question 16 - Ambulatory encounters
Report total number of encounters, using the previous definition, with the following Centers for Medicare and Medicaid Services (CMS) place of service codes:
11 Office

12 Home
20 Urgent Care Facility
22 Outpatient Hospital
23 Emergency Room
24 Ambulatory Surgical Center
31 Skilled Nursing Facility
32 Nursing Facility
33 Custodial Care Facility
34 Hospice
50 Federally Qualified Health Center
52 Psychiatric Facility Partial Hospitalization
53 Community Mental Health Facility
54 Intermediate Care Facility for Mentally Retarded
55 Residential Substance Abuse Treatment Facility
56 Psychiatric Residential Treatment Center
62 Comprehensive Outpatient Rehabilitation Facility
65 End Stage Renal Disease Treatment Facility
71 State or Local Public Health Clinic
72 Rural Health Clinic
81 Independent Laboratory

Important: If ambulatory encounters are reported in question 16, respondents must complete question 21.

Question 17 - Hospital encounters
Report the total number of encounters, using the previous definition, with the following CMS place of service codes:
21 Inpatient Hospital
25 Birthing Center
26 Military Treatment Facility
51 Inpatient Psychiatric Facility
61 Comprehensive Inpatient Rehabilitation Facility

Question 18 - Surgery/anesthesia cases
Report the total surgery/anesthesia cases performed annually by each provider. A surgery/anesthesia case is a case between a provider and a patient where at least one procedure performed is a procedure from the surgery chapter (CPT codes 10021-69979) or anesthesia chapter (CPT codes 00100-01999) of the Current Procedural Terminology, Fourth Edition, copyrighted by the American Medical Association (AMA).

Note that the number of cases, not procedures, should be counted since a case may consist of multiple procedures. Surgery/anesthesia cases include cases performed on an inpatient or outpatient basis, regardless of facility or site. For anesthesia

Medical Group Management Association®
Compensation and Production Survey: 2008 Guide to the Questionnaire Based on 2007 Data

care teams, an anesthesiologist who supervises one or more CRNAs, include total care team cases.

Questions 19 and 20 - RVUs

Report the RVUs, as measured by the RBRVS, not weighted by a conversion factor, attributed to all professional services. An RVU is a nonmonetary standard unit of measure that indicates the value of services provided by physicians, nonphysician providers, and other health care professionals. The RVU system is explained in detail in the December 1, 2006 *Federal Register*, pages 69624 to 70251. Addendum B: Relative Value Units (RVUs) and Related Information presents a table of RVUs by CPT code. Your billing system vendor should be able to load these RVUs into your system if you are not yet using RVUs for management analysis. When answering this question, note the following:

- The RVUs published in the December 1, 2006, *Federal Register*, effective for calendar year 2007, should be used; and
- The total RVUs for a given procedure consist of three components:
  - Physician work RVUs;
  - Practice expense (PE) RVUs; and
  - Malpractice RVUs.

Thus, total RVUs = physician work RVUs + practice expense RVUs + malpractice RVUs.

For 2006, there were two different types of practice expense RVUs:
1. Fully implemented nonfacility practice expense RVUs; and
2. Fully implemented facility practice expense RVUs.

"Nonfacility" refers to RVUs associated with a medical practice that is not affiliated with a hospital and does not utilize a split billing system that itemizes facility (hospital) charges and professional charges. "Nonfacility" also applies to services performed in settings other than a hospital, skilled nursing facility or ambulatory surgery center. You should report total RVUs in question 19 that are a function of "nonfacility" practice expense RVUs.

"Facility" refers to RVUs associated with a hospital affiliated medical practice that utilizes a split billing fee schedule where facility (hospital) charges and professional charges are billed separately. "Facility" also refers to services performed in a hospital, skilled nursing facility or ambulatory surgery center. Do not report total RVUs in question 19 that are a function of "facility" practice expense RVUs. If you are a hospital affiliated medical practice that utilizes a split billing fee schedule, you should report your total RVUs in question 19 as if you were a medical practice not affiliated with a hospital.

To summarize, there are two different types of total RVUs that you could potentially report in question 19:
1. Fully implemented nonfacility total RVUs; and
2. Fully implemented facility total RVUs.

The Federal Register Addendum B presents six columns of RVU data. The column labeled "Physician work RVUs" is what you should report when answering question 20, "Physician work RVUs."

Any adjustments to RVU values through periodic adjustments and updates made by CMS should be included.

Question 19 - Total RVUs
Include:
1. RVUs for the "physician work RVUs", " practice expense", and "malpractice RVUs" including any adjustments made as a result of modifier usage;
2. RVUs for all professional medical and surgical services performed by physicians, nonphysician providers and other physician extenders such as nurses and medical assistants;
3. RVUs for the professional component of laboratory, radiology, medical diagnostic and surgical procedures;
4. For anesthesiology groups, provide the American Society of Anesthesiologists (ASA) units for surgical anesthesia units.
   - The ASA units for a given procedure consist of three components:
     - Base unit;
     - Time in 15-minute increments; and
     - Risk factors.
5. For procedures with either no listed CPT code or with an RVU value of zero, RVUs can be estimated by dividing the total gross charges for the unlisted or unvalued procedures by the

Medical Group Management Association®
Compensation and Production Survey: 2008 Guide to the Questionnaire Based on 2007 Data

practice's known average charge per RVU for all procedures that are listed and valued;

6. RVUs for procedures for both fee-for-service and capitation patients; and
7. RVUs for all payers, not just Medicare.

Do not include:
1. RVUs for other scales such as McGraw-Hill or California;
2. The TC associated with any medical diagnostic, laboratory, radiology, or surgical procedure;
3. RVUs attributed to nonphysician providers. If your practice cannot break this out, report RVUs and answer "Yes" in question 21; or
4. RVUs where the Geographic Practice Cost Index (GPCI) equals any value other than one. The GPCI must be set to 1.000 (neutral).

Question 20 - Physician work RVUs
Include:
1. RVUs for the "physician work RVUs" only including any adjustments made as a result of modifier usage;
2. Physician work RVUs for all professional medical and surgical services performed by providers;
3. Physician work RVUs for the professional component of laboratory, radiology, medical diagnostic and surgical procedures;
4. Physician work RVUs for all procedures performed by the medical practice. For procedures with either no listed CPT code or with an RVU value of zero, RVUs can be estimated by dividing the total gross charges for the unlisted or unvalued procedures by the practice's known average charge per RVU for all procedures that are listed and valued;
5. Physician work RVUs for procedures for both fee-for-service and capitation patients;
6. Physician work RVUs for all payers, not just Medicare;
7. Physician work RVUs for purchased procedures from external providers on behalf of the practice's fee-for-service patients; and
8. Anesthesia practices should provide the physician work component of the RVU for flat fee procedures only such as lines, blocks, critical care visits, intubations and post-operative management care.

Do not include:
1. RVUs for "malpractice RVUs";
2. RVUs for other scales such as McGraw-Hill or California;

3. RVUs for purchased procedures from external providers on behalf of the practice's capitation patients;
4. RVUs that have been weighted by a conversion factor. Do not weigh the RVUs by a conversion factor; or
5. RVUs where the Geographic Practice Cost Index (GPCI) equals any value other than one. The GPCI must be set to 1.000 (neutral).

Important: If physician work RVUs in question 20 are reported, respondents must complete question 21.

Question 21 - Nonphysician provider productivity
For physicians, state if the productivity measures (questions 13 though 20) include productivity attributed to a nonphysician provider working under a physician's supervision by selecting "Yes" or "No." For nonphysician providers, state whether the productivity measures include productivity attributed to another nonphysician provider by selecting "Yes" or "No."

Question 22 - Half-day clinical sessions (direct patient coverage)
Half-day clinical sessions are blocks of time during which a physician can be scheduled for or is involved in direct patient care (contact) where a patient bill is generated and a fee-for-service equivalent charge is created for the practice. Clinical sessions include seeing patients in the office, outpatient clinic, emergency room, nursing home, operating room, labor and delivery, and time spent on hospital rounds. Indicate the number of half-day sessions per week to consider your physician an FTE.

Do not include:
1. On-call time

Management Compensation Matrix
The matrix requests information for executives, managerial staff, specialists and supervisors who held the same position for the entire 12-month reporting period and were employed on a full-time basis.

Administrative personnel working directly for the observed practice should continue to be reported in the questionnaire representing their specific medical practice.

Medical Group Management Association®
Compensation and Production Survey: 2008 Guide to the Questionnaire Based on 2007 Data

Question 1 - Employee tracking code

Indicate your medical practice's internal tracking number such as the last four numbers of a SSN or initials for each individual. This number may be numeric, alpha or a combination of both and may be up to six digits long. This number will make it easier to interpret the Respondent Ranking Report. If you do not have a unique identifier, create a series of letters and numbers such as 12345x.

Question 2 - Position title

Select one position that best describes each individual's responsibilities. The numbers by the positions described below correspond to the positions listed on the questionnaire. **Positions are listed in alphabetical order within each management level.** If the position is other than the options provided, write his/her position in question 2 and describe the position in the Comments section of the questionnaire.

Physician Executive Positions

Associate/Assistant Medical Director: (3)
- Position requires candidate to be a licensed physician;
- Time is devoted to both administrative duties and the delivery of health care services;
- Typically assists the Medical Director in all respects, from the administration of medical care and clinical services to utilization review and medical protocol development. If there are multiple Associate/Assistant Medical Directors, the functional areas of medical administration are usually divided up among physicians with this position title; and
- Usually reports to the Medical Director and/or Physician Chief Executive Officer (CEO)/President.

Medical Director: (2)
- Position requires candidate to be a licensed physician;
- The senior medical administrative position within a medical group practice;
- Physician's time is devoted to both administrative duties and the delivery of health care services;
- In larger organizations there may be more than one Medical Director;
- Responsible for all activities related to the delivery of medical care and clinical services such as cost management, utilization review, quality assurance and medical protocol development;
- Typically oversees the activities of group physicians, including the recruiting and credentialing processes; and
- Usually reports to the Physician CEO/President and/or to the governing body of the organization.

Physician CEO/President: (1)
- Position requires candidate to be a licensed physician;
- Usually found in larger practices or in some form of an integrated system or network such as Physician Hospital Organization (PHO) and MSO;
- Since administrative duties are substantial, the delivery of health care services is minimal;
- Develops and monitors organizational policy with other management personnel and board of directors;
- Responsible for the overall operation of the organization, including patient care and contract relations;
- Oversees activities related to the growth and expansion of the organization;
- Plays a major role in the organization's strategic process;
- Typically serves as the liaison between the organization, the community and the board of directors;
- Oversees a team of senior management personnel; and
- Usually reports to the governing body of the organization.

Executive Management Positions

Administrator: (5)
- The top nonphysician professional administrative position with less authority than a CEO;
- Maintains broad responsibilities for all administrative functions of the medical group, including operations, marketing, finance, managed care/third party contracting, physician compensation and reimbursement, human resources, medical and business information systems and planning and development;
- Typically oversees management personnel with direct responsibilities for the specific functional areas of the organization; and
- Reports to the governing body of the organization.

Medical Group Management Association®
Compensation and Production Survey: 2008 Guide to the Questionnaire Based on 2007 Data

Assistant Administrator: (9)

- Provides assistance to the CEO and/or Practice Administrator with the management of one or more functional areas of the medical practice such as administration, managed care, human resources, marketing, patient accounting or operations;
- Has a more limited scope of responsibility than a chief operating officer (COO);
- A medical group may have multiple assistant administrators;
- Responsible for assisting the CEO and/or Practice Administrator in accomplishing organizational objectives; and
- Usually reports to the senior administrative officer.

Chief Executive Officer (CEO)/Executive Director: (4)

- Highest nonphysician executive position in the organization;
- Typically found in larger practices, or in some form of an integrated system such as PHO and MSO;
- Develops and monitors organizational policy in conjunction with other management personnel and board of directors;
- Responsible for the overall operation of the organization, including patient care, contract relations and activities that relate to the future growth of the organization such as strategic planning and marketing;
- Oversees a team of senior management personnel who have direct responsibility for specific functional areas of the organization;
- Typically serves as a liaison between the organization and staff members, businesses, individuals in the community and board of directors; and
- Reports to the governing body of the organization.

Chief Financial Officer (CFO): (8)

- Usually the organization's senior financial position;
- Develops financial policies and oversees their implementation;
- Typically monitors a variety of financial activities, including budgeting, analysis, accounting, billing, payer contracting, collections and the preparation of tax returns;
- Usually prepares or oversees the preparation of annual reports and long-term projections to ensure that the organization's financial obligations are met;

- May obtain funds for capital development;
- May hold a designation as a Certified Public Accountant (CPA); and
- Usually reports to the senior administrative officer, or to the governing body of the organization.

Chief Information Officer (CIO): (47)

- Usually found in large organizations;
- The top level contact in information systems development and solutions;
- Contributes to general business planning regarding technology;
- Accountable for directing data integrity and confidentiality of the medical practice's patient care information;
- Identifies new developments in information systems technology, and strategizes organizational modifications;
- Requires a masters or bachelors degree in MIS or CIS or a related field; and
- Usually reports to the CEO.

Chief Operating Officer (COO): (7)

- Consults, advises and assists the CEO and/or Practice Administrator in providing leadership and direction in planning, directing and coordinating both patient and non-patient care activities;
- May be the second senior administrative position, and assume the duties of the top administrator when necessary;
- Oversees the daily operations of the medical practice and/or other affiliated health care organizations;
- Responsibilities may include facilities management, business services, human resources management; and
- Usually reports to the senior administrative officer, or in some cases, to the governing body of the organization.

MSO Administrator/Executive Director: (6)

- Oversees all activities of a hospital or investor-owned MSO, that provides practice management services to physician practices and clinics;
- Responsibilities range from the daily operations of multiple sites to developing strategic plans;
- Monitors the marketing of MSO services to physician clients;
- Typically serves as a liaison between various organization levels, from the physicians to the governing entities of the organization such as a

Medical Group Management Association®
Compensation and Production Survey: 2008 Guide to the Questionnaire Based on 2007 Data

hospital or health system, investors in the MSO and board of directors;
- Oversees the provision of management services to newly integrated practices; and
- Usually reports to the governing body of the MSO.

Senior Management Positions

Ambulatory/Clinical Services Director: (10)
- A clinical operations position;
- Monitors the daily operations of the organization's clinical function;
- Develops, implements and monitors policies and procedures;
- Monitors the activities of the nonphysician technical staff such as radiology and laboratory technicians;
- May oversee the medical records staff; and
- Usually reports to CFO or senior administrative officer.

Branch/Satellite Clinic Director: (48)
- Oversees the administrative and operations activities of multiple clinical practice sites;
- Develops financial policy for the clinical operation in concert with the organization's top financial officer;
- Oversees the implementation of the organization's policies and procedures, including budget management, human resources management, and compliance with state and federal regulations;
- Supervises clinic managers and indirectly supervises clinic staff; and
- Usually reports to COO or senior administrative position.

Building and Grounds Director: (11)
- Usually found in an organization with a facilities or building services department;
- Develops and implements policies and procedures related to the organization's physical facilities such as buildings;
- Oversees related activities such as building maintenance, housekeeping, grounds preservation; and
- Usually reports to COO.

Business Services Director: (12)
- Usually found in large organizations;
- Directs and coordinates business office activities in an organization that has a top administrator;

- Monitors the medical billing system;
- Oversees areas of responsibility such as third-party reimbursement, physician billing, collections, contract administration and management reporting; and
- Usually reports to the senior administrative officer or to the organization's top financial position.

Clinical Research Director: (13)
- Analyzes and summarizes clinical data and outcomes, with responsibility for research design, methodology and data collection protocols;
- Prepares grant proposals;
- Participates in investigator meetings, seminars and regional or national research conferences;
- Coordinates the activities of associates and investigators to ensure compliance with protocols and overall research objectives; and
- Usually reports to Medical Director or senior administrative officer.

Compliance Director: (14)
- Develops, plans, organizes and administers programs to comply with applicable state and federal statues, regulations, policies and procedures within the organization to ensure administrative and operational objectives are met;
- Identifies operational business risk issues;
- Develops a Corporate Compliance Plan, the Code of Conduct Handbook; and
- Usually reports to the CFO or COO.

Education and Training Director: (15)
- Only found in very large organizations with multiple locations;
- Supervises Training Managers;
- Develops and delivers education and training programs for the training needs of the organization's staff and patients;
- Evaluates programs to determine whether the training goals and objectives have been met;
- Monitors the delivery of on-going programs; and
- Usually reports to Human Resources Director or COO.

Finance Director: (16)
- Responsible for preparing financial statements and all general accounting functions;
- Develops, implements and monitors tax compliance, for example, income, sales, use, etc.,

Medical Group Management Association®
Compensation and Production Survey: 2008 Guide to the Questionnaire Based on 2007 Data

and has payroll oversight;
- Responsible for internal accounting policies and procedures;
- Supervises financial department;
- Directs all statistical analysis and reporting including monthly operating and medical management statistics; and
- Reports to CFO.

Human Resources Director: (17)
- Usually found in larger practices;
- Oversees all functions of an established human resources department within an organization;
- Using the organization's objectives and philosophies as a guide, develops, implements and coordinates policies relating to all aspects of personnel administration. This includes recruitment, salary and benefits administration, EEO/AA and labor law compliance and employee relations; and
- Usually reports to the senior administrative officer.

Information Systems Director: (18)
- Implements and monitors all activities that relate to the organization's information system, including functions such as physician practice billing, scheduling, data processing, networking and system security;
- Oversees or resolves systems implementation and integration issues;
- Performs programming tasks when necessary; and
- Usually reports to the CFO, CIO, or to the senior administrative officer.

Laboratory Services Director: (19)
- Responsible for all activities related to the operations of a laboratory or several laboratories, from the initiation and implementation of test procedures to the oversight of laboratory personnel;
- May perform and monitor testing procedures in addition to administrative duties:
- Monitors budget activities that relate to the laboratory function; and
- Usually reports to the COO or to the senior administrative officer.

Managed Care Director: (20)
- Initiates and maintains relationships with managed care organizations as well as physician and ancillary providers;
- Develops and directs all managed care activities of the organization, including contract negotiations, product development and capitation payment procedures;
- May oversee risk and utilization management activities or claims administration for professional/ medical purchased services; and
- Usually reports to the organization's Medical Director or the senior administrative officer.

Marketing and Sales Director: (21)
- The top marketing position in an organization with a distinct marketing and sales function;
- Typically found in larger organizations;
- May oversee the communications function;
- Develops marketing policies and programs that reflect the organization's goals and objectives;
- Oversees or conducts research designed to evaluate the organization's market position;
- Directs the implementation of policies and procedures that relate to the promotion of the organization;
- Performs administrative tasks such as department budgeting and supervises the Marketing/ Communication specialist; and
- Usually reports to the senior administrative officer.

Medical Records Director: (22)
- The individual in this position usually holds professional licensure in the area of medical records management;
- Usually found in large organizations and is considered part of the senior management team;
- Responsible for medical records library such as patient records;
- Oversees all medical records personnel;
- Monitors budget activities that relate to the medical records function; and
- Usually reports to the COO.

Nursing Services Director: (23)
- Oversees all aspects of the organization's nursing practices;
- Typically found in large organizations;
- Is part of the senior management team;
- In most cases, requires certification as a Registered Nurse (RN);
- Oversees the nursing staff; and
- Usually reports to the COO.

Medical Group Management Association®
Compensation and Production Survey: 2008 Guide to the Questionnaire Based on 2007 Data

Physician Recruitment Director: (49)

- Researchers for, and recruitment of, physicians and other allied health personnel;
- Completes the entire recruitment cycle from initial contact to contract by organizing schedules, problem resolution, spouse and children considerations, travel, hotel arrangements, meals, references, license, housing, banking and all other general hosting of candidates; and
- Reports to the Sr. Vice President , Vice President of Human Resources.

Quality Improvement/Quality Assurance Director: (24)

- Develops and monitors programs designed to improve the quality of health care delivery e.g., outcome measurement;
- Develops policies and procedures designed to measure the quantitative and qualitative aspects of health care delivery;
- More likely to be found in larger organizations with some degree of integration with other health care organizations; and
- Usually reports to the CFO or to the senior administrative officer.

Radiology Services Director: (25)

- Usually found in large organizations with several radiology departments;
- Responsible for all activities relating to the delivery of radiological services, including the development of policies and procedures;
- Oversees radiology personnel activities;
- Monitors the quality of all film products used;
- Monitors budget activities related to the radiology departments; and
- Usually reports to the COO or to the senior administrative officer.

Reimbursement Director: (26)

- Oversees payment services for the practice, including establishing and maintaining the practice's fee schedules and fees that relate to managed care activities;
- Conducts regular analyses of reimbursement rates;
- Oversees coding activities; and
- Usually reports to the Managed Care Director, the CFO, or the senior administrative officer.

General Management Positions

Benefits Manager: (27)

- Oversees all aspects of the organization's salary/ wage administration program as well as the benefits program;
- Determines eligibility for the benefits program;
- May provide assistance and information to employees with the selection of benefits and filing claims; and
- Usually assists and reports to the Human Resources Director.

Branch/Satellite Clinic Manager: (28)

- Oversees the daily administrative and operations activities of an assigned clinic in an organization with multiple clinics;
- Prepares the clinic's annual budget and supervises clinic staff;
- Oversees financial transactions such as purchasing supplies; and
- Usually reports to the COO or senior administrative position.

Business Office Manager: (29)

- Responsible for directing and coordinating the overall functions of the Business Office;
- The top Business Office position in a mid-size or small organization without a Director of Business Services;
- Exercises general supervision over business office staff;
- Plans and directs registration, patient insurance, billing and collections and data processing to ensure accurate patient billing and efficient account collection; and
- Reports to the Finance Director or Business Services Director.

Clinical Department Manager: (30)

- Manages operation of one or more medical/ surgical departments, ancillary service departments or an ambulatory surgery facility;
- Usually found in larger practices;
- Assists with budget planning and approves department expenditures;
- May supervise department nonmedical staff; and
- Usually reports to the COO or the Nursing Services Director.

Medical Group Management Association®
Compensation and Production Survey: 2008 Guide to the Questionnaire Based on 2007 Data

Clinic Research Manager: (31)
- Collects and analyzes clinical data and outcomes;
- The top Clinic Research position in a mid-size or small organization without a Clinical Research Director; and
- Usually reports to the Medical Director, the senior administrative officer or the Clinical Research Director.

General Accounting Manager: (32)
- The second or third financial position in the organization;
- Assists the CFO or Finance Director with the financial responsibilities of the organization;
- Develops and oversees activities related to implementing and maintaining the integrity of the organization's financial reporting system;
- Assists with or oversees the budgeting process; and
- Usually reports to the CFO, Finance Director or in smaller organizations, to the senior administrative officer.

Laboratory Services Manager: (33)
- The top laboratory position in a mid-size or small organization without a Laboratory Services Director;
- Responsible for the activities related to the delivery of laboratory services;
- Monitors the quality of services, products, supplies used;
- May monitor budget activities related to the laboratory department; and
- Reports to the COO, senior administrative officer or Laboratory Services Director.

Materials Management Manager: (34)
- Usually found in organizations with a separate purchasing department or function;
- Oversees all activities that involve the acquisition of equipment and supplies;
- May monitor budget activities, including the capital equipment budget; and
- Usually reports to the CFO.

Medical Records Manager: (35)
- The top Medical Records position in a mid-size or small organization without a Medical Records Director;
- Oversees and coordinates all activities of the medical library, from maintenance tasks to the movement of patient records;
- Oversees all medical records personnel;
- May monitor budget activities that relate to the medical records function; and
- Usually reports to the COO, Medical Records Director or Practice Administrator.

Nursing Manager: (36)
- Responsible for managing, supervising and administering the patient/nursing services in the practice;
- In most cases, requires certification as a Registered Nurse (RN);
- Supervises nursing staff; and
- Reports to the Practice Administrator in smaller organization and the Nursing Services Director in larger organizations.

Office Manager: (37)
- Manages the nonmedical activities of a larger medical practice;
- Typically found in a practice that does not have a Practice Administrator;
- The focus of this position usually rests on the daily operations of the organization;
- May oversee some financial activities such as billing and collections; and
- Usually reports to the Practice Administrator, or the Business Services Director.

Operations Manager: (38)
- Assists the top operations administrator;
- Coordinates and directs the overall operation of specific departments;
- Coordinates between departments to ensure that the organization meets internal and external regulatory requirements; and
- Usually reports to the COO or the senior administrative officer.

Patient Accounting Manager: (39)
- Manages the billing process and billing staff for the practice;
- Manages insurance and other reimbursement functions; and
- Usually reports to the Reimbursement Director or the CFO.

Medical Group Management Association®
Compensation and Production Survey: 2008 Guide to the Questionnaire Based on 2007 Data

Radiology Services Manager: (40)

- Not a Director or Senior Management level position;
- The top Radiology position in a mid-size or small organization without a Radiology Director;
- Responsible for activities related to the delivery of radiological services;
- Monitors the quality of all film products used;
- May monitor budget activities related to the radiology departments; and
- Reports to the COO, the senior administrative officer or the Radiology Services Director.

Training/Education Manager: (41)

- Assists in delivering education and training programs for staff members and patients;
- Helps to identify the training needs;
- Evaluates programs to determine whether the goals and objectives have been met;
- Monitors the delivery of on-going programs; and
- Usually reports to the Training/Education Director or the COO.

Specialists

Benefits/Payroll Specialist: (42)

- Oversees the entire payroll system, which includes implementing and converting the payroll system for newly acquired sites;
- Recommends policies and standards that pertain to payroll activities;
- Responsible for the accuracy of the payroll system; and
- Usually reports to the Benefits Manager or Human Resources Manager.

Marketing/Communication Specialist: (43)

- Usually found in organizations in which there is a separate publications/communications function;
- In some organizations, this person may be known as the "Public Relations Manager" and may report to the top marketing and sales position;
- Represents the organization at all media and other public relations events;
- May oversee the activities of public relations/ communications staff; and
- Usually reports to the Marketing and Sales Director, the COO, or the senior administrative officer.

Supervisors

Business Office Supervisor: (44)

- Responsible for supervising and coordinating activities of the business office;
- This position may be implemented in a multiple clinic setting;
- Supervises assigned business office staff; and
- Reports to the Business Office Manager or the Practice Administrator.

Clinic Supervisor: (45)

- Exercises supervision over assigned staff;
- Responsible for supervising and coordinating day to day activities of the clinic; and
- Reports to the Branch/Satellite Manager or the Practice Administrator.

Front Office Supervisor: (50)

- Responsible for supervising the front office
- Maintains and coordinates the policies and procedures;
- Training and daily activities of front office staff; and
- Reports to the Office Manager, Operations Manager or the Administrator

Nursing Supervisor: (46)

- Supervises a staff of nurses;
- In larger organization, may be one of several supervisors;
- Splits time between patient care and supervision of staff;
- Responsibilities are more limited than the Nursing Manager; and
- Reports to the Nursing Manager, the Nursing Services Director or the Practice Administrator.

Other: (51)

If your practice's position is other than the options provided, write his/her position in column 2 and describe the position in the Comments section of the questionnaire.

Question 3 - Centralized staff position

If you answered "Yes" to question 10 in the Medical Practice Information section, select "Yes" if the employee was part of the centralized administrative department. Select "No" if the employee worked

Medical Group Management Association®
Compensation and Production Survey: 2008 Guide to the Questionnaire Based on 2007 Data

directly for the observed practice. Refer to question 10 for the definition of "centralized administrative department."

Administrative personnel working directly for the observed practice should continue to be reported in the questionnaire representing their specific medical practice.

Question 4 - Total compensation
State the amount reported as direct compensation on a W2, 1099, or K1 (for partnerships) plus all voluntary salary reductions such as 401(k), 403(b), Section 125 Tax Savings Plan, or Medical Savings Plan. The amount reported should include salary, bonus and/or incentive payments, research stipends, honoraria and distribution of profits.
Do not include:
1. The dollar value of expense reimbursements, fringe benefits paid by the medical practice such as retirement plan contributions, life and health insurance, or automobile allowances, or any employer contributions to a 401(k), 403(b) or Keogh Plan.

Question 5 - Bonus/incentive amount
Report the total dollar amount of any bonus or incentive payments received by each individual. The amount listed as a bonus/incentive should be included in total compensation, question 4.

Question 6 - Retirement benefits
Report all employer contributions to retirement plans including defined benefit and contribution plans, 401(k), 403(b) and Keogh Plans, and any nonqualified funded retirement plan. For defined benefit plans, estimate the employer's contribution made on behalf of each plan participant by multiplying the employer's total contribution by each plan participant's compensation divided by the total compensation of all plan participants.
Do not include:
1. Employer contributions to social security mandated by the Federal Insurance Contributions Act (FICA);
2. Voluntary employee contributions that are an allocation of salary to a 401(k), 403(b), or Keogh Plan; or
3. The dollar value of any other fringe benefits paid

by the practice, such as life and health insurance or automobile allowances.

Question 7 - Compensation method
From the options listed select the choice that best describes the compensation method for each individual. If the compensation method falls under "Other," write his/her compensation method in the Comments section of the questionnaire.

Question 8 - Formal education
From the options listed select the highest level of formal education attained by each individual. If the education level falls under "Other," write his/her education level in the Comments section of the questionnaire.

Question 9 - Years of management experience
Report the total years of management experience in health care delivery, health care administration and/or business administration for each individual.

Question 10 - Gender
Report the gender for this individual.

Question 11 - ACMPE status
From the options listed select the appropriate status designation in the American College of Medical Practice Executives (ACMPE), the professional credentialing arm of MGMA, for this individual.

Question 12 - MGMA national member
Report whether the individual listed is a national MGMA member.

Complete question 13 for Physician Executives, Executive Management and Senior Management positions ONLY.

Question 13 - Professional organization fees
Report the dollar amount paid for professional organization dues and memberships, and educational conference fees and travel expenses related to those conferences over the fiscal year for each physician executive, executive management and senior management position listed. If your organization uses the MGMA *Chart of Accounts for Health Care Organizations*, report the amounts by employee aggregated from: general ledger accounts 5845,

Medical Group Management Association®
Compensation and Production Survey: 2008 Guide to the Questionnaire Based on 2007 Data

5855, and 5860, for Executive Management positions and Senior Management positions; and general ledger accounts 8245, 8255, and 8260 for Physician Executive positions.

Complete question 14 for Physician Executive positions ONLY.

Question 14 - Percentage of time administrative and clinical

List the percentage of time spent performing administrative duties and clinical care responsibilities. For example, a physician executive spending approximately 70% of their time in an administrative capacity and 30% of their time performing clinical functions should report 70% on the "Admin" line and 30% on the "Clinical" line.

Questionnaire Contact

22-31. If we need to clarify any responses, it would be helpful to have the name of the person who is most familiar with the completed questionnaire. Provide complete information.

32. Provide the Federal Tax ID # for the observed practice.

Provide the Federal Tax ID # for the observed practice reported in the questionnaire. This

information will be used for internal tracking purposes only, and will not be released under any circumstances.

33. Hours to complete

Add together the total number of hours for each individual who worked on this questionnaire.

Report Recipient

Respondent Ranking Reports contain customized comparisons of an organization's self-reported data to median values compiled from the survey results. The individual identified on the questionnaire label will receive the Respondent Ranking Report and complimentary survey report for your organization. If this information is incorrect, provide complete information on lines 34 through 43 for the appropriate recipient.

Parent Organization Information

The observed medical practice is the medical practice for which data are reported. If you indicated in question 9, ownership of the observed practice by a 'hospital/integrated delivery system', 'MSO', 'PPMC', 'University' or 'Other' type of organization, provide the name and location of the parent organization (owner) in the spaces provided. Complete information on questions 44 to 47.

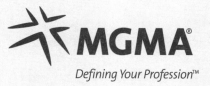